TAYLOR'S 10-MINUTE DIAGNOSIS MANUAL

SYMPTOMS AND SIGNS IN THE
TIME-LIMITED ENCOUNTER

Second Edition

TAYLOR'S 10-MINUTE DIAGNOSIS MANUAL
SYMPTOMS AND SIGNS IN THE TIME-LIMITED ENCOUNTER
Second Edition

Editors

Paul M. Paulman, MD
Professor/Predoctoral Director
Department of Family Medicine
University of Nebraska Medical Center
Omaha, Nebraska

Audrey A. Paulman, MD
Clinical Associate Professor
Department of Family Medicine
University of Nebraska Medical Center
Omaha, Nebraska

Jeffrey D. Harrison, MD
Program Director, Rural Residency Program
Department of Family Medicine
University of Nebraska Medical Center
Omaha, Nebraska

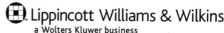
. Lippincott Williams & Wilkins
a Wolters Kluwer business
Philadelphia · Baltimore · New York · London
Buenos Aires · Hong Kong · Sydney · Tokyo

Acquisitions Editor: Sonya Seigafuse
Managing Editor: Nancy Winter
Developmental Editor: Martha Cushman
Project Manager: Alicia Jackson
Manufacturing Manager: Kathleen Brown
Marketing Manager: Kimberly Schonberger
Cover Designer: Larry Didona
Design Coordinator: Terry Mallon
Production Services: Laserwords Private Limited, Chennai, India
Printer: R.R. Donnelley Crawfordsville

© 2007 by LIPPINCOTT WILLIAMS & WILKINS, a Wolters Kluwer business

530 Walnut Street
Philadelphia, PA 19106, USA
LWW.com

1st edition, © 1999 Williams & Wilkins

Printed in the USA

Library of Congress Cataloging-in-Publication Data

Taylor's 10-minute diagnosis manual : symptoms and signs in the time-
   limited encounter / editors, Paul M. Paulman, Audrey A. Paulman,
   Jeffrey D. Harrison.—2nd ed.
     p. ; cm.
   Rev. ed. of: The 10-minute diagnosis manual / editor, Robert B. Taylor. c2000.
   Includes bibliographical references and index.
   ISBN-13: 978-0-7817-6944-0
   ISBN-10: 0-7817-6944-2
   1. Symptoms—Handbooks, manuals, etc. 2. Diagnosis—Handbooks,
manuals, etc. I. Paulman, Paul M., 1953–. II. Paulman, Audrey A.
III. Harrison, Jeffrey D. IV. Taylor, Robert B. V. 10-minute
diagnosis manual. VI. Title: 10-minute diagnosis manual. VII. Title: Ten-minute diagnosis manual.
   [DNLM: 1. Diagnosis—Handbooks.   WB 39 T247 2007]
RC69.A18 2007
616.07′5—dc22
                                                           2006022133

                                             10 9 8 7 6 5 4 3 2 1

This book is dedicated to our children, Roger, Kate, Craig, and Adam, who inspire us

CONTENTS

1: PRINCIPLES OF THE 10-MINUTE DIAGNOSIS
Robert B. Taylor

2: UNDIFFERENTIATED PROBLEMS
Richard H. Hurd

3: MENTAL HEALTH PROBLEMS
Jim Medder

4: PROBLEMS RELATED TO THE NERVOUS SYSTEM
Michael A. Myers

5: EYE PROBLEMS
Shou Ling Leong

6: EAR, NOSE, AND THROAT PROBLEMS
Frank S. Celestino

7: CARDIOVASCULAR PROBLEMS
Joann E. Schaefer

8: RESPIRATORY PROBLEMS
Joseph E. Scherger

9: GASTROINTESTINAL PROBLEMS
Michael R. Spieker

10: RENAL AND UROLOGIC PROBLEMS
R. Whitney Curry, Jr.

11: PROBLEMS RELATED TO THE FEMALE REPRODUCTIVE SYSTEM
Kathryn M. Andolsek

12: MUSCULOSKELETAL PROBLEMS
Laeth Nasir

13: DERMATOLOGIC PROBLEMS
Michael L. O'Dell

14: ENDOCRINE AND METABOLIC PROBLEMS
Richard D. Blondell

15: VASCULAR AND LYMPHATIC SYSTEM PROBLEMS
Gregory J. Babbe

16: LABORATORY ABNORMALITIES: HEMATOLOGY AND URINE DETERMINATIONS
Carol A. LaCroix

17: LABORATORY ABNORMALITIES: BLOOD CHEMISTRY AND IMMUNOLOGY
Judith A. Fisher

18: DIAGNOSTIC IMAGING ABNORMALITIES
Enrique S. Fernandez

Samuel B. Adkins III, MD
Associate Clinical Professor
Department of Family Medicine
University of Texas Medical Branch
Galveston, Texas
Director, Family Medicine Residency
Austin Medical Education Program
Austin, Texas
12.3 Hip Pain

Paul V. Aitken, Jr., MD, MPH
Associate Professor
Department of Family
and Community Medicine
Penn State University College of Medicine
Hershey, Philadelphia;
Program Director
Residency in Family
and Community Medicine
Penn State University
Good Samaritan Hospital
Lebanon, Philadelphia
11.3 Chronic Pelvic Pain
11.4 Dysmenorrhea

Iman S. Al-Jabi, MD
Faculty Member and Lecturer
Department of Community
and Family Medicine
University of Jordan
Amman, Jordan
12.1 Arthralgia

Karthryn M. Andolsek, MD, MPH
Clinical Professor
Department of Community
and Family Medicine
Duke University School of Medicine;
Associate Director
Department of Graduate
Medical Education
Duke University Hospital
Durham, North Carolina
11.5 Menorrhagia

Mark D. Andrews, MD
Associate Professor
Department of Family Medicine
Wake Forest University School of Medicine
Winston-Salem, North Carolina
6.1 Halitosis

Kamlesh G. Ansingkar, MD, MSHI
Final Year Resident
Department of Family Medicine
Creighton University Medical Center
Omaha, Nebraska
7.10 Pericardial Friction Rub

Elisabeth L. Backer, MD
Clinical Associate Professor
Department of Family Medicine
University of Nebraska Medical Center
Omaha, Nebraska
*16.3 Erythrocyte Sedimentation Rate And
C-Reactive Protein*

James R. Barrett, MD
Professor
Department of Family
and Preventive Medicine
University of Oklahoma
Health Sciences Center
Oklahoma city, Oklahoma
12.7 Neck Pain

Sandra B. Baumberger, MD
Chief Resident
Department of Family Medicine
Creighton University Medical School
Creighton University Medical Center
Omaha, Nebraska
7.11 Raynaud's Disease

Thomas C. Bent, MD
Associate Clinical Professor
Department of Family Medicine
University of California, Irvine
Orange, California;
Medical Director, Chief Operating Officer
Laguna Beach Community Clinic
Laguna Beach, California
8.9 Wheezing

Charles S. Blackadar, MD
Clinical Assistant Professor
Department of Family Medicine
University of Washington
Seattle, Washington;
Staff Faculty Physician
Puget Sound Family Medicine Residency
Bremerton Naval Hospital
Bremerton, Washington
9.7 Upper Gastrointestinal Bleeding

Douglas G. Browning, MD
Assistant Professor
Department of Family
and Community Medicine
Wake Forest University
School of Medicine;
Assistant Professor
Department of Family
and Community Medicine
North Carolina Baptist Hospital
Winston-Salem, North Carolina
6.4 Nosebleed

Charles L. Bryner, Jr., MD, PhD
Department of Family Medicine
Orange Park Medical Center
Orange Park, Florida
9.12 Steatorrhea

Jennifer J. Buescher, MD, MSPH
Faculty
Department of Clarkson Family Medicine;
Physician
Department of Family Medicine
The Nebraska Medical Center
Omaha, Nebraska
2.8 Hypersomnia
2.9 Insomnia
2.10 Nausea and Vomiting

Kendall M. Campbell, MD
Assistant Professor
Department of Community Health
and Family Medicine
University of Florida College of Medicine
Gainesville, Florida
10.8 Scrotal Mass

Sandra M. Carr-Johnson, MD
Chief
Clinical Education and Services
Program Director
Family Medicine Resident
Southern Regional Area Health Center
Fayetteville, North Carolina
11.9 Vaginal Discharge

Katrina Carter, MD
Department of Family Medicine
Nebraska Medical Center
Omaha, Nebraska
16.1 Anemia
16.5 Polycythemia

Frank S. Celestino, MD
Associate Professor
Department of Family
and Community Medicine
Wake Forest University
School of Medicine;
Attending Physician
Department of Family
and Community Medicine
North Carolina Baptist Hospital
Winston-Salem, North Carolina
6.9 Vertigo

Ku-Lang Chang, MB, BCH
Clinical Assistant Professor
Department of Family Medicine
University of Florida College of Medicine
Gainesville, Florida
10.2 Hematuria

Brian Coleman, MD
Assistant Professor
Department of Family
and Preventive Medicine
University of Oklahoma
Health Sciences Center,
Oklahoma City, Oklahoma
12.7 Neck Pain

David R. Congdon, MD
Assistant Program Director
Puget Sound Family Medicine Residency
Bremerton Naval Hospital
Bremerton, Washington
9.1 Abdominal Pain

Joyce A. Copeland, MD
Clinical Associate Professor
Department of Family Medicine
Duke University School of Medicine
Durham, North Carolina
11.2 Breast Mass
*11.6 Nipple Discharge In The
Nonpregnant Female*

Ronnie Coutinho, MD
Assistant Professor
Department of Advanced Introduction to
Clinical Medicine
Ross University School of Medicine
Edison, New Jersey
18.2 Mediastinal Mass

Ronald D. Craig, MD, FAAFP, Diplomate ABFP
Faculty Physician
Lincoln Medical Education Partnership
Buffalo, New York
4.8 Stroke
4.9 Tremors

J. Steven Cramer, MD, MS
Associate Clinical Professor
Department of Family Medicine
State University of New York at Buffalo
Buffalo, New York
14.1 Diabetes Mellitus

Peter F. Cronholm, MD, MSCE
Physician
Department of Family Medicine and
Community Health
Penn Presbyterian Medical Center;
Assistant Professor
Department of Family Medicine and
Community Health
University of Pennsylvania Health System
Philadelphia
17.1 Alkaline Phosphatase, Elevated
17.2 Aminotransferase Levels, Elevated
17.3 Antinuclear Antibody Titer, Elevated
17.6 Hypercalcemia

L. Gail Curtis, MD
Assistant Professor
Department of Family
and Community Medicine
Wake Forest University Medical Center
Winston-Salem, North Carolina
6.3 Hoarseness

Tanika L. Day, MD
Clinical Associate
Department of Community
and Family Medicine
Duke University Medical Center
Durham, North Carolina
11.1 Amenorrhea

Ronald F. Dommermuth MD
Associate Clinical Professor
Department of Family Medicine
University of Washington;
Program Director
Puget Sound Family Medicine Residency
Naval Hospital Bremerton;
Staff Physician
Department of Family Medicine
Naval Hospital Bremerton
Bremerton, Washington
9.10 Jaundice

Alexandra Duke, DO
Assistant Clinical Professor
Department of Family Medicine
University of California, Irvine College of
Medicine
Irvine, California
8.8 Stridor

Mike Dukelow, MD
Creighton Family Healthcare Omaha,
Nebraska
7.12 Tachycardia

Kristy D. Edwards, MD, CWS
Assistant Professor
Department of Family Medicine
University of Nebraska
Nebraska Medical Center;
Omaha, Nebraska
15.1 Lymphadenopathy, Generalized
15.2 Lymphadenopathy, Localized

Chad Ezzell, MD
Sports Medicine Fellow
Department of Family
and Community Medicine
Wake Forest University
School of Medicine;
Sports Medicine Fellow
Department of Family
and Community Medicine
North Carolina Baptist Hospital
Winston-Salem, North Carolina
6.4 Nosebleed

David B. Feller, MD
Assistant Professor
Department of Family Medicine
University of Florida College
of Medicine
Gainesville, Florida
10.7 Priapism

Tina M. Flores, MD
Assistant Professor
Department of Family Medicine
University of Nebraska
Medical Center
Omaha, Nebraska
16.2 Eosinophilia

Norman Benjamin Fredrick, MD
Assistant Professor
Department of Family
and Community Medicine
Pennsylvania State University
College of Medicine;
Faculty
Milton S. Hershey Medical Center
Hershey, Pennsylvania
5.1 Blurred Vision
5.3 Diplopia

Marcia W. Funderburk, MD
Associate Professor
Department of Community Health
and Family Medicine
University of Florida Health Science
Center/Jacksonville;
Associate Professor
Department of Community Health and
Family Medicine
Shands at Jacksonville
Jacksonville, Florida
10.6 Oliguria and Anuria

Mark F. Giglio, MD
Associate Clinical Professor
Department of Family Medicine
University of California, Irvine College of
Medicine
Irvine, California
8.4 Pleural Effusion

Mark D. Goodman, MD
Assistant Professor
Department of Family Medicine
Creighton University;
Creighton University Medical Center
Omaha, Nebraska

Heath A. Grames, PhD
Assistant Professor
Department of Child and Family Studies
University of Southern Mississippi
Hattiesburg, Mississippi
3.3 Suicide Risk

Sara Graybill, MD
Department of Family Medicine
University of Nebraska Medical Center
Omaha, Nebraska
16.4 Neutropenia

Christian Kyle Haefele, MD, FAAFP
Faculty Physician
Lincoln Family Medicine Program
Lincoln Medical Education Partnership
Lincoln, Nebraska
4.4 Dementia
4.5 Memory Impairment

Thomas J. Hansen, MD
Program Director, Assistant Professor
Department of Family Medicine
Creighton University
Medical Center
Omaha, Nebraska
7.1 Atypical Chest Pain

Stephen J. Hartsock, MD
Advanced Occupational Medicine
Specialists
Chicago, Illinois
12.2 Calf Pain

Robert L. Hatch, MD, MPH
Associate Professor
Department of Community Health
and Family Medicine
University of Florida College
of Medicine
Gainesville, Florida
10.8 Scrotal Mass

Raymond D. Heller, MD
Assistant Professor
Department of Family Medicine
Creighton University
Omaha, Nebraska
7.8 Hypertension

David C. Holub, MD
Clinical Assistant Professor
Department of Family
and Community Medicine
Pennsylvania State University
College of Medicine
Hershey, Pennsylvania;
Associate Program Director
Family and Community Medicine
Residency Program
Good Samaritan Hospital
Lebanon, Pennsylvania
5.6 Pupillary Inequality
5.7 The Red Eye
5.8 Scotoma

Karen Hughes, MD
Attending Faculty
Department of Family Medicine
North Mississippi Medical Center Family
Medicine Residency;
Attending Physician
Department of Family Medicine
North Mississippi Medical Center
Tupelo, Mississippi
13.1 Alopecia
13.4 Pigmentation Disorders

Richard H. Hurd, MD
Director
Department of Clarkson Family Medicine;
Physician
Department of Family Medicine
Nebraska Medical Center
Omaha, Nebraska
2.2 Dizziness
2.11 Night Sweats

Scott Ippolito, MD
Associate Dean of Clinical Sciences
Ross University School of Medicine
Dominica, West Indies
18.3 Osteopenia

Kimberly J. Jarzynka, MD
Assistant Professor
Department of Family Medicine
University of Nebraska Medical Center
Omaha, Nebraska
15.4 Splenomegaly

Amy K. Jespersen, MD
Director
Department of Clarkson Family Medicine;
Physician
Department of Family Medicine
Nebraska Medical Center
Omaha, Nebraska
2.5 Fatigue
2.13 Weight Loss

Andrew D. Jones, MD
Faculty Physician
Department of Family Medicine
Exempla Saint Joseph Hospital Family
Medicine Residency Program;
Exempla Saint Joseph Hospital
Denver, Colorado
12.9 Shoulder Pain

Victoria S. Kaprielian, MD
Clinical Professor
Department of Community
and Family Medicine
Duke University School of Medicine;
Attending Staff
Duke University Hospital
Durham, North Carolina
11.8 Postmenopausal Bleeding

Martina Kelly, MD, MRCGP, MICGP
Lecturer
Department of General Practice
University College Cork
Cork, Ireland
12.8 Polymyalgia

Mary D. Knudtson, DNSC, NP
Professor, Director of FNP Program
Department of Family Medicine
University of California, Irvine
College of Medicine
Irvine, California
8.3 Hemoptysis

Charles M. Kodner, MD
Associate Professor
Department of Family
and Geriatric Medicine
University of Louisville School
of Medicine
Louisville, Kentucky
14.2 Gynecomastia

David C. Krulak, MD, MPH

9.4 Diarrhea

Louis Kuritzky, MD
Clinical Assistant Professor
Department of Community Health
and Family Medicine
University of Florida
Gainesville, Florida
10.3 Impotence

Carol A. Lacroix, MD
Clinical Assistant Professor
Department of Family Medicine
University of Nebraska Medical Center
Omaha, Nebraska
16.6 Proteinuria

Kathryn M. Larsen, MD
Clinical Professor
Department of Family Medicine
University of California, Irvine
College of Medicine
Irvine, California;
Chair
University of California, Irvine
Medical Center
Orange, California
8.3 Hemoptysis

Joseph T. LaVan, MD
Faculty
Department of Family Medicine
Puget Sound Family Medicine Residency
Bremerton, Washington;
Faculty
Department of Family Medicine
Madigan Army Medical Center
Tacoma, Washington
9.3 Constipation

Peter R. Lewis, MD
Associate Professor
Department of Family
and Community Medicine
Penn State University College of Medicine;
Physician
Department of Family
and Community Medicine
Milton S. Hershey Medical Center
Hershey, Pennsylvania
5.2 Corneal Foreign Body
5.4 Nystagmus
5.5 Papilledema

Désirée A. Lie, MD, MSEd
Clinical Professor
Department of Family Medicine
University of California, Irvine
Orange, California
8.1 Cough

Richard W. Lord, MD
Assistant Professor
Department of Family
and Community Medicine
Wake Forest University
School of Medicine;
Assistant Professor
Department of Family
and Community Medicine
North Carolina Baptist Hospital
Winston-Salem, North Carolina
6.5 Pharyngitis

Jelyn W. Lu, MD
Resident
Creighton Medical School
Omaha, Nebraska
7.6 Diastolic Heart Murmurs

William M. Lucas, MD
Attending Staff
Department of Family Medicine
Puget Sound Family Medicine
Residency
Bremertor Naval Hospital
Bremertor, Washington
9.2 Ascites

James R. Lundy, MD
Clinical Assistant Professor
Department of Family Medicine
University of Mississippi Medical Center
Jackson, Mississippi;
Faculty of Family Medicine Residency
Program
North Mississippi Medical Center
Tupelo, Mississippi
13.3 Maculopapular Rash
13.5 Pruritis

Chris Madden, MD
Longs Peak Sports and Family Medicine;
Assistant Clinical Faculty
Department of Family Medicine
University of Colorado Health Sciences
Longmont, Colorado
12.4 Knee Pain

Barbara A. Majeroni, MD
Associate Clinical Professor
Department of Family Medicine
State University of New York
at Buffalo;
Attending Physician
Erie County Medical Center
Buffalo, New York
14.8 Hyperthyroidism/Thyrotoxicosis

Andrea Manyon, MD
Clinical Associate Professor
Department of Family Medicine
University of Buffalo
Buffalo, NewYork
14.1 Diabetes Mellitus

Gail S. Marion, PA-C, PhD
Assistant Professor
Department of Family
and Community Medicine
Wake Forest University
School of Medicine;
Assistant Professor
Department of Family
and Community Medicine
North Carolina Baptist Hospital
Winston-Salem, North Carolina
6.6 Rhinitis

Roger Massie, MD
Faculty
Department of Clarkson Family Medicine;
Physician
Department of Family Medicine
The Nebraska Medical Center
Omaha, Nebraska
2.3 Edema
2.12 Syncope

Tahany Maurice-Habashy, MD
Private practice
Orange County, California
8.8 Stridor

Ronald McCoy, MBBS
General Practitioner and Medical Educator
Royal Australian College of General
Practitioners
South Melbourne, Victoria, Australia
12.5 Low Back Pain

Lou Ann McStay, MD
Assistant Professor
Department of Family Medicine
Creighton University Medical School;
Active Staff
Department of Family Medicine
Creighton University Medical Center
Omaha, Nebraska
7.4 Cardiomegaly

Albert A. Meyer, MD
Associate Professor
Department of Family Medicine
University of North Carolina
School of Medicine
Chapel Hill, North Carolina;
Family Medicine Faculty
Residency in Family Medicine
New Hanover Regional Medical Center
Wilmington, North Carolina
11.3 Chronic Pelvic Pain
11.4 Dysmenorrhea

Joseph A. Moran, MB, BCh, BAO, MCLSC, MRCGP, MICGP
Lecturer
Department of General Practice
University College Cork
Cork, Ireland
12.8 Polymyalgia

Soraya P. Nasraty, MD
Medical Director
Department of Family
and Geriatric Medicine
University of Louisville
Active Staff
Department of Family Medicine
Jewish Hospital, Norton Hospital,
and University of Louville Hospital
Louisville, Kentucky
14.5 Polydipsia

Sara Neal, MD
Assistant Director of Residency Training
Department of Family
and Community Medicine
Wake Forest University School of Medicine
Winston-Salem, North Carolina
6.8 Tinnitus

Mark R. Needham, MD
Saint Johns Hospital
Santa Monica, California
18.1 Bone Cyst
18.4 Solitary Pulmonary Nodule

Janis F. Neuman, MD
Kaiser Permanente Medical Group
Riverside, California
8.2 Cyanosis

Vincent H. Ober, Jr., BS, MD
Assistant Clinical Professor
Department of Community Health
and Family Medicine
University of Florida College of Medicine
Jacksonville, Florida
10.5 Nocturia

Michael L. O'Dell, MD, MSHA
Chair and Program Director
Department of Family Medicine
NMMC Family Medicine Residency;
Chair, Family Medicine
Department of Family Medicine
North Mississippi Medical Center
Tupelo, Mississippi
13.6 Rash Accompanied by Fever
13.8 Vesicular and Bullous Eruptions

Nicole J. Otto, MD
Staff Physician
Student Health Services
University of Pennsylvania
Clinical Associate Professor
Department of Family Medicine
Hospital of the University of Pennsylvania
Pennsylvania, Philadelphia
17.4 Brain Natriuretic Peptide
07.5 D-Dimer

Trish Palmer, MD
Assistant Professor, Sports Medicine
Department of Family Medicine at Rush
Midwest Orthopedics
at Rush
Chicago, Illinois
12.6 Monoarticular Joint Pain

Pamela L. Pentin, MD
Assistant Clinical Professor
Department of Family Medicine
University of Washington
School of Medicine
Seattle, Washington;
Faculty Physician
Department of Family Medicine
Naval Hospital Bremerton
Bremerton, Washington
9.6 Epigastric Distress

T. Ray Perrine, MS, MD FAAFP
Faculty Attending
Family Medicine Residency Center
North Mississippi Medical Center;
Active Staff
Department of Family Medicine
North Mississippi Medical Center
Tupelo, Mississippi
13.2 Erythema Multiforme
13.7 Urticaria

Kenneth D. Peters, MD
Faculty
Department of Clarkson Family Medicine;
Physician
Department of Family Medicine
The Nebraska Medical Center
Omaha, Nebraska
2.4 Falls
2.7 Headaches

Carlos A. Prendes, Jr., MD
Assistant Professor
Department of Family Medicine
Creighton University;
Staff
Creighton University Medical Center
Omaha, Nebraska
7.7 Systemic Heart Murmurs

Layne A. Prest, BA, MA, PhD
Associate Professor
Department of Family Medicine
University of Nebraska Medical Center;
UNMC Physicians
Department of Family Medicine
Nebraska Health System
Omaha, Nebraska
3.1 Anxiety

David M. Quillen, MD
Assistant Professor
Department of Community Health
and Family Medicine
University of Florida
Gainesville, Florida
10.1 Dysuria

Kalyanakrishnan Ramakrishnan, MD
Associate Professor
Department of Family
and Preventive Medicine
University of Oklahoma
Health Sciences Center
Oklahoma City, Oklahoma
12.9 Shoulder Pain

Richard Rathe, MD
Associate Professor
Department of Family Medicine
University of Florida College of Medicine
Gainesville, Florida
10.4 Urinary Incontinence in Adults

Robert R. Rauner, MD, FAAFP
Faculty Physician
Lincoln Family Medicine Program
Lincoln Medical Education Partnership
Lincoln, Nebraska
4.1 Ataxia
4.2 Coma
4.3 Paresthesia and Dyesthesia

Jeri R. Reid, MD
Assistant Professor
Department of Family
and Geriatric Medicine
University of Louisville
Louisville, Kentucky
14.6 Thyroid Enlargement/Goiter
14.7 Thyroid Nodule

W. David Robinson, PhD
Assistant Professor
Department of Family Medicine
University of Nebraska Medical Center
Omaha, Nebraska
3.2 Depression

Christine Romascan, DO
Assistant Clinical Professor
Department of Family Medicine
University of Washington
Seattle, Washington;
Staff Physician
Department of Family Medicine
Naval Hospital Bremerton
Bremerton, Washington
9.11 Rectal Bleeding

George PN Samraj, MD, MRCOG
Associate Professor
Department of Family Medicine
University of Florida
Gainesville, Florida
10.10 Urethral Discharge

Hemant K. Satpathy, MD
Assistant Professor
Department of Family Practice
Creighton University Medical School
Omaha, Nebraska
7.5 Congestive Heart Failure

Chhabi Satpathy, MD
Lecturer
Department of Cardiology
SCB Medical College
Cuttack, Orissa, India
7.5 Congestive Heart Failure

Siegfried O. F. Schmidt, MD, PhD, FAAFP
Associate Professor and Medical Director
Department of Community Health
and Family Medicine
University of Florida
Hampton Oaks Medical
Plaza Family Medicine
Staff Physician
Department of Medicine
Shands at AGH and Shands at UF
Gainesville, Florida
10.2 Hematuria

Michael D. Schooff, MD
Associate Director
Clarkson Family Medicine
Residency Program
Omaha, Nebraska
2.1 Anorexia
2.6 Fever

Perry W. Sexton, MD
Staff Physician
Student Health Services
University of Pennsylvania
Staff Physician
Department of Family Medicine
Penn, Presbyterian Hospital
Pennsylvania, Philadelphia
17.4 Brain Natriuretic Peptide
17.5 D-Dimer

Sanjeev Sharma, MD
Assistant Professor
Department of Family Medicine
Creighton University Medical Center
Omaha, Nebraska
7.2 Chest Pain

Hal S. Shimazu, MD
Clinical Professor
Department of Family Medicine
University of California, Irvine
Tustin, California

John L. Smith, MD
Assistant Professor
Department of Family Medicine
University of Nebraska
College of Medicine
Omaha, Nebraska
15.3 Petechiae and Purpura

Brian A. Smoley, MD
Faculty Development Fellow
Department of Family Medicine
Madigan Army Medical Center
Tacoma, Washington
9.8 Hepatitis

John G. Spangler, MD
Assistant Professor
Department of Family
and Community Medicine
Wake Forest University School of Medicine
Winston-Salem, North Carolina
6.7 Stomatitis

Rebecca L. Spaulding, MD
Clinical Instructor
Department of Family Medicine University
of North Carolina
School of Medicine, Chapel Hill;
Faculty
Department of Family Medicine and Sports
Medicine
Moses Cone Health System
Greensboro, North Carolina
12.2 Calf Pain

Michael R. Spieker, MD
Associate Clinical Professor
Department of Family Medicine
University of Washington
Seattle, Washington;
Staff Physician
Department of Family Medicine
Naval Hospital Bremerton
Bremerton, Washington
9.5 Dysphagia

Joseph B. Straton, MD, MSCE
Assistant Professor
Department of Family Medicine and
Community Health
University of Pennsylvania
Pennsylvania, Philadelphia
17.1 Alkaline Phosphatase, Elevated
17.2 Aminotransferase Levels, Elevated
17.3 Antinuclear Antibody Titer, Elevated
17.6 Hypercalcemia

Teresa Stump, DO

16.7 Thrombocytopenia

Robert M. Theal, MD
Assistant Chief of Service
Department of Family Medicine
Kaiser Foundation Hospital
Fontana, California
8.7 Shortness of Breath

Fidel A. Valea, MD
Associate Professor
Residency Program Director
Department of Obstetrics and Gynecology
Duke University Medical Center;
Duke University Medical Center
Durham, North Carolina
11.7 PAP Smear Abnormality

Charles Vega, MD
Associate Clinical Professor
Department of Family Medicine
University of California, Irvine
Orange, California
8.6 Pneumothorax

Les Veskrna, MD
Faculty Physician
Lincoln Family Medicine Program
Lincoln Medical Education Partnership
Lincoln, Nebraska
4.3 Delirium
4.7 Seizures

David Webner, MD
Assistant Professor
Department of Family Medicine
University of Pennsylvania
Assistant Professor
Department of Family Medicine
University of Pennsylvania Health System
Pennsylvania, Philadelphia
17.7 Hyperkalemia
17.8 Hypokalemia

Stephen F. Wheeler, MChE, MD
Associate Professor
Department of Family
and Geriatric Medicine
University of Louisville School of Medicine
Louisville, Kentucky
14.4 Hypothyroidism
14.6 Thyroid Enlargement/Goiter
14.7 Thyroid Nodule
14.8 Hyperthyroidism/Thyrotoxicosis

Darryl G. White, MD
Assistant Clinical Professor
Department of Family Medicine
UT Health Science Center San Antonio;
Staff Physician, Chief
Department of Family Medicine
Valley Baptist Medical Center
Harlingen, Texas
9.9 Hepatomegaly

George R. Wilson, MD
Associate Professor and Associate Chair
Community Health and Family Medicine
University of Florida College of Medicine;
Chief
Department of Family Medicine
and Occupational Medicine
Shands at Jacksonville Medical Center
Jacksonville, Florida
10.9 Scrotal Pain

John Winters, MD
Resident
Creighton Medical School
Omaha, Nebraska
7.9 Palpitations

Kathryn M. Andolsek, MD, MPH
Clinical Professor
Department of Community
and Family Medicine
Duke University School of Medicine;
Associate Director
Graduate Medical Education
Duke University Hospital
Durham, North Carolina
11. *Problems Related to the Female
Reproductive System*

Gregory J. Babbe, MD
Assistant Professor
Department of Family Medicine
University of Nebraska Medical Center
Omaha, Nebraska
15. *Vascular and Lymphatic System
Problems*

Richard D. Blondell, MD
Associate Professor
Department of Family Medicine
StateUniversity of New York at Buffalo;
Attending Physician
Department of Chemical Dependency
Erie County Medical Center
Buffalo, New York
14. *Endocrine and Metabolic Problems*

Frank S. Celestino, MD
Associate Professor
Department of Family
and Community Medicine
Wake Forest University
School of Medicine;
Attending Physician
Department of Family
and Community Medicine
North Carolina Baptist Hospital
Winston-Salem, North Carolina
6.9 *Ear, Nose, and Throat Problems*

R. Whitney Curry, Jr., MD
Professor and Chairman
Department of Community Health
and Family Medicine
University of Florida
Gainesville, Florida
10. *Renal and Urologic Problems*

Enrique S. Fernandez, MD, MSEd
Associate Professor
Department of Clinical Family Medicine
and Community Health
Uiversity of Miami School of Medicine
Miami, Florida
Diagnostic Imaging Abnormalities
18. *Diagnostic Imaging Abnormalities*

Judith A. Fisher, MD
Assistant Professor
Department of Family Practice
and Community Medicine
University of Pennsylvania School of
Medicine
Philadelphia, Pennsylvania
17. *Labarotory Abnormalities: Blood
Chemistry and Immunology*

Richard H. Hurd, MD
Director
Department of Clarkson Family Medicine;
Physician
Department of Family Medicine
Nebraska Medical Center
Omaha, Nebraska
2. *Undifferentiated Problems*

Carol A. LaCroix, MD
Clinical Assistant Professor
Department of Family Medicine
University of Nebraska Medical Center
Omaha, Nebraska
16. *Laboratory Abnormalities:
Hematology and Urine Determinations*

Shou Ling Leong, MD
Professor
Department of Family
and Community Medicine
Penn State College of Medicine;
Professor
Family and Community Medicine
Milton S. Hershey Medical Center
Hershey, Philadelphia
5. Eye Problems

Jim Medder, MD, MPH
Associate Professor
Department of Family Medicine
University of Nebraska Medical Center
Omaha, Nebraska
3. Mental Health Problems

Michael A. Myers, MD
Program Director
Lincoln Family Medicine Program
Lincoln Medical Education Partnership
Lincoln, Nebraska
4. Problems Related to the Nervous System

Laeth Nasir, MBBS
Professor
Department of Family Medicine
University of Nebraska Medical Center
Omaha, Nebraska
12. Musculoskeletal Problems

Michael L. O'Dell, MD, MSHA
Chair and Program Director
Department of Family Medicine
North Mississippi Medical Center Family
Medicine Residency;
Chair
Department of Family Medicine
North Mississippi Medical Center
Tupelo, Mississippi
13. Dermatologic Problems

Joseph E. Scherger, MD
Professor
Department of Family
and Preventive Medicine
University of California
San Diego, California
8. Respiratory Problems

Joann E. Schaefer, MD
Associate Professor
Department of Family Medicine
Creighton University Medical Center
Omaha, Nebraska
7. Cardiovascular Problems

Michael R. Spieker, MD
Associate Clinical Professor
Department of Family Medicine
University of Washington
Seattle, Washington;
Staff Physician
Department of Family Medicine
Naval Hospital Bremerton
Bremerton, Washington
9. Gastrointestinal Problems

Robert B. Taylor, MD
Professor
Department of Family Medicine
Oregon Health Sciences University
School of Medicine
Portland, Oregon
1. Principles of the 10-Minute Diagnosis

*P*rimary care physicians and other healthcare providers, residents, and students often face the challenge of diagnosing conditions for patients on the basis of undifferentiated presenting complaints or concerns. Pressures from payers of medical care to increase clinical efficiency while maintaining high-quality care has made the effective use of time in the clinic very important to primary care practitioners.

Taylor's 10-Minute Diagnosis Manual, 2nd ed., has been specifically designed to support the busy practitioner in the process of diagnosing patient problems in this environment.

The Manual is organized around common presenting symptoms, signs, and laboratory and imaging findings, and each chapter serves as a stand-alone, concise, clear, and easily read information source for the area covered. The Manual works well at the point of care and fits inside the lab coat pocket.

The editors are pleased to include in this new edition the latest information and clinical evidence in addition to changes in clinical practice since the first edition was published. While adding this new content, the editors of the 2nd edition have made every effort to maintain the excellent readability and utility that Dr. Taylor and the authors and editors of the 1st edition were able to achieve.

All the authors and editors of the 2nd edition hope that *Taylor's 10-Minute Diagnosis Manual* is useful to you while you care for patients.

For the authors and editors,

Paul M. Paulman, MD
Omaha, Nebraska
Lead Editor

PREFACE TO THE FIRST EDITION

The 10-Minute Diagnosis Manual is intended to be a quick-reference source for the primary care clinician faced with a diagnostic problem such as headache, fatigue, anemia, or jaundice. The book is structured in the same way in which we arrive at a diagnosis, starting not with a disease label, but with a chief complaint or, perhaps, an unexpected clinical finding. Chapter topics were selected because they occur commonly in the primary care setting or because they are likely to be first encountered by the primary care clinician. These topics include symptoms (e.g., dizziness), physical abnormalities (e.g., splenomegaly), and laboratory determinations (e.g., proteinuria). The chapters in the book are about diagnosis, and therapy is mentioned only if it might be relevant to diagnosis, such as the response of an inflamed joint to colchicine.

The "10-minute" premise of the book is based on studies showing that 10-minute office visits are the norm in primary care today.[1] Even with longer duration visits, the time devoted to diagnosis—and not to therapy, procedures, patient education, and so forth—is likely to be about ten minutes. Also, to the degree possible in a quick-reference guide, authors have presented information using an evidence-based approach.[2] For more on the book's premise and approach, see Chapter One.

Chapters are of a uniform length that is convenient for rapid reading during a patient care session, and each chapter is organized according to six major headings: Approach, History, Physical Examination, Testing, Diagnostic Assessment, and References.

I am grateful to the 18 section editors and to the 139 contributing authors. I also thank the following individuals who assisted with the development and production of this book: Coelleda O'Neil and Victoria Brown of the Department of Family Medicine of the Oregon Health Sciences University, Executive Editor Richard Winters and Developmental Editor Michelle LaPlante of Lippincott Williams & Wilkins, and Production Editor Emily Lerman.

I hope that you will find this book a useful guide to commonly encountered symptoms and signs, and that you will reach for this book first when you need help with diagnosis during a busy practice day.

Robert B. Taylor, MD
Portland, Oregon

---

[1] Stange KC, Zyzanski SJ, Jaen CR. Illuminating the "black box": a description of 4454 patient visits to 138 family physicians. *J. Fam Pract* 1998; 46:377–389.

[2] Rosser WW. Application of evidence from randomized controlled trials to general practice. *Lancet* 1999; 353:661–664.

ACKNOWLEDGMENTS

The editors of *Taylor's 10-Minute Diagnosis Manual*, 2nd edition, would like to acknowledge the work and contributions of the section editors and chapter authors who provided excellent manuscripts. We also thank the editing and production staff at Lippincott Williams & Wilkins: it was truly a pleasure to work with you on this book. The editors are grateful to Dr. Robert Taylor for editing the first edition: it provided an excellent template from which to work.

Special thanks to Sarah Bryan without whose help, organizational talent, and hard work this book would never have been published.

TAYLOR'S 10-MINUTE DIAGNOSIS MANUAL

SYMPTOMS AND SIGNS IN THE
TIME-LIMITED ENCOUNTER

Second Edition

Principles of the 10-Minute Diagnosis
Robert B. Taylor

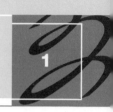

1

PRINCIPLES OF THE 10-MINUTE DIAGNOSIS
Robert B. Taylor

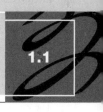

*T*en minutes for diagnosis? Really?

Yes, really!

If only we had 90 minutes to perform a diagnostic evaluation, as we did as third-year medical students on hospital rotations. Or, if we had even 30 minutes for diagnosis, as I recall from internship. But those days are gone. Today—as clinicians practicing in the age of evidence-based, cost-effective health care—office visits are of much shorter duration than in years past. For example, in a recent study of 4,454 patients seeing 138 physicians in 84 practices, the mean visit duration was 10 minutes (1). Another study of 19,192 visits to 686 primary care physicians estimated the visit duration to be 16.3 minutes (2). Even when the total visit duration exceeds 10 minutes, the time actually devoted to diagnosis—and not to greeting the patient, explaining treatment, doing managed care paperwork, or even the patient's dressing and undressing—is seldom more than 10 minutes.

So, if you and I generally have only 10 minutes per office visit for diagnosis, we need to be focused, while remaining medically thorough and prudent. Actually, such an approach is possible and is how experienced clinicians tend to practice. The following are some practice guidelines to the 10-minute diagnosis (*Dx10*). And, to illustrate, let us consider a patient: *Joan S., a 49-year-old married woman, in your office for a first visit, whose chief complaint is severe, one-sided headaches that have become worse over the past year.* (For a more complete approach to the diagnosis of headache, see Chapter 2.7.)

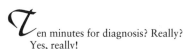 SEARCH FOR DIAGNOSTIC CUES THROUGHOUT THE CLINICAL ENCOUNTER

Note how the patient relates to the staff, takes off a jacket, and sits in the examination room. How does the patient begin to describe the problem and what does he or she seem to want from the visit? Who accompanies the patient to the office and who seems to do the talking?

Be sure to use "tell me about" open-ended questions. The inexperienced clinician moves early to closed-ended "Yes" or "No" questions, but the veteran *Dx10* clinician has learned that using narrow questions too early can lead to misleading conclusions, which are in the long run, at the least, wasteful of time and, at worst, dangerous. An example would be attributing chest pain inappropriately to gastroesophageal reflux disease because the patient has a past history of esophageal reflux and responds affirmatively to questions about current heartburn and intolerance to spicy foods.

Watch the facial reaction to issues discussed. Tune in to hesitation and evasive answers and be willing to follow these diagnostic paths, which may lead to otherwise hidden problems such as drug abuse or domestic violence. *In the case of Joan S., does she answer questions readily or does she seem evasive when addressing some topics, such as family concerns or her home life?*

THINK "MOST COMMON" FIRST

I remind medical students of the time-honored aphorism that "the most common problems occur most commonly." When working with a patient, the physician develops diagnostic hypotheses early in the encounter. When faced with a patient with headache, we should initially consider tension headache and migraine rather than temporal arteritis. Of course, the *Dx10* clinician thinks of special concerns, such as the possibility that the patient with headache might possibly have a brain tumor. The initial history seeks the characteristics and chronology of the symptoms. Then the clinician uses select questions that help rule in or out the diagnostic hypotheses: "What seems to precede the headache pain?" "Has the nature or the severity of your pain changed in any way?" The clinician also seeks important past medical, social, and family history: "What stress are you experiencing that may be influencing your symptoms?" "Does anyone else in your family have a headache problem?"

The physical examination should be limited to the body areas likely to contribute to the diagnosis, and a "full physical examination" is actually seldom needed. *Therefore, for our patient with recurrent headaches, Joan S., the* Dx10 *examination is likely to be limited to the vital signs, head, and neck, with a screening of coordination, deep tendon reflexes, and cranial nerve function. Examination of the chest, heart, and abdomen is unlikely to contribute to the diagnosis.*

Tests should be limited to those that will help confirm or rule out a diagnostic hypothesis or, later, those that would help make a therapeutic decision. For most patients with headache as a presenting complaint, no laboratory test or diagnostic imaging is needed.

Of course, the uncommon problem occurs *sometimes*. Occasionally, you will encounter the unexpected finding: the patient with headache having unanticipated unilateral deafness or the fatigued individual with an enlarged spleen. Stop and think when you note a cluster of similar unexpected findings; such alertness helped clinicians identify the Muerto Canyon virus as the cause of the 1993 outbreak of the hantavirus pulmonary syndrome in the southwestern United States and also the occurrence of primary pulmonary hypertension in patients using dexfenfluramine for weight control. A few times in your career you will have the opportunity to experience a diagnostic epiphany; the *Dx10* clinician will seize this opportunity by staying alert for the unexpected diagnostic clue.

 USE ALL AVAILABLE ASSISTANCE

In addition to your professional knowledge, experience, and time, your diagnostic resources include your staff, the patient and his or her family, and the vast array of medical reference sources available.

Your office and hospital staff can be valuable allies in determining the diagnosis. Important clues may be offered when the patient calls for an appointment or when being escorted to the examination room. If a patient remarks to the receptionist or nurse that his chest pain is "just like my father had before his heart attack" or if another wonders if her heartburn could be related to her 15-year-old daughter's misbehavior, the staff member should ask the patient's permission and then share the information with the physician.

The patient and the family generally have some insight into the cause of symptoms such as fatigue, diarrhea, or loss of appetite. In a study of patient's differential diagnosis of cough, Bergh found that while physicians considered a mean of 7.6 diagnostic possibilities, patients reported a mean of 6.5 possibilities, with only 2.8 possibilities common to both (3). *Joan S. and perhaps her family, may offer diagnostic suggestions that you have not strongly considered; also, these other hypotheses represent concerns that should eventually be addressed to provide reassurance. For example, might Joan be in the office today chiefly because an old friend has recently been diagnosed with brain cancer and she has become concerned about the significance of her own headaches?*

 CONSIDER THE PSYCHOSOCIAL ASPECTS OF THE PROBLEM

To continue the case of the patient with headache, a migraine diagnosis is incomplete if it fails to include the contribution of marital or job stress to the symptoms of family event cancellations, trips to the emergency room, and large pharmacy bills for sumatriptan injections, as well as the impact on others. No diagnosis of cancer or diabetes is complete without considering the impact on the patient's life and the lives of family members (4).

The *Dx10* clinician will be especially wary of the *International Classification of Diseases, Ninth Edition,* (ICD-9) diagnostic categories, which facilitate statistical analysis and managed care payments, but which lack the richness of narrative and also the personal and family context. For example, compare "diabetes mellitus, uncomplicated, ICD-9 code 250.00" with "type 2 diabetes mellitus in an elderly patient with poor diet, marginal retirement income, and isolation from the family."

Failure to consider the psychosocial aspects of disease invites an incompletely understood or even a missed diagnosis: how many instances of child abuse have been overlooked as busy emergency room physicians care for childhood fractures without also exploring the cause of the injury and the home environment?

When eliciting a medical history from Joan S., it will be important to learn the current stresses at work and at home, and how she thinks her life would be different if the headaches were gone.

 SEEK HELP WHEN NEEDED

Today, health care, including diagnosis, must be "evidence based" and not grounded in anecdote or even in your "years of clinical experience." The evidence is, of course, the vast body of medical knowledge, including research reports and meta-analyses found in clinical journals (5), on the World Wide Web (6), and in reference books such as *The 10-Minute Diagnosis Manual. When thinking about Joan S., you might search the literature for recent articles on the approach to migraine headaches.*

Help is also available from colleagues. Consider a consultation when you have a diagnosis that is somehow not "satisfying." A personal physician in a long-term relationship with a patient can develop a blind spot, and the diagnosis may be apparent only to someone taking a fresh look. What may be needed at such a time is a rethinking of the problem—almost the antithesis of continuity.

Help can be available from the same-specialty colleague down the hall or from a subspecialist.

 THINK IN TERMS OF A CONTINUALLY EVOLVING DIAGNOSIS

You do not always need to make the definitive diagnosis on the first visit; in fact, such an approach tends to foster prolonged visits, excessive testing, overly biomedical diagnoses, and high-cost medicine without adding quality. When faced with an elusive diagnosis, the best test is often the passage of time and a follow-up visit. For example, we all know that headaches are often influenced by stressful life events. Yet, a new patient may not be ready to share his or her personal, often embarrassing, burdens, and it is only when a trustful relationship has been established that the clinician learns about the abusive spouse, the pregnant teenager, or the impending financial disaster.

It is often useful to use the descriptive, categorical diagnosis and seek the definitive diagnosis over time. Examples include the teenage girl with chronic pelvic pain, the young adult with cough for 3 months, the middle-aged person with loss of appetite, and the older person with fatigue or insomnia. Sometimes, on an initial visit, this approach is the only reasonable option.

The *Dx10* clinician will be careful not to "fall in love" with the initial diagnosis and realize that the depressed patient losing weight might also have cancer and that it is too easy to attribute all new symptoms to a known diagnosis of menopause or diabetes mellitus. *If Joan S.'s headaches fail to respond as expected over time, you may wish to reconsider your original diagnosis and perhaps seek further testing that would have seemed excessive on the initial visit. For example, might the "1-year" duration of increased severity merit imaging if a favorable response to initial therapy does not occur?*

In your daily practice, use the time saved in the steps described here to consider and reconsider your diagnoses—as you review chart notes, read medical journals, search medical web sites, and see the patient in follow-up visits. The *Dx10* clinician will remain open to rethinking the patient's diagnostic problem list. In the end, patience and perseverance—often measured in 10-minute aliquots over time—will yield an insightful, biopsychosocially inclusive, and clinically useful diagnosis.

References

1. Stange KC, Zyzanski SJ, Jaen CR. Illuminating the black box: a description of 4454 patient visits to 138 family physicians. *J Fam Pract* 1998;46:377–389.
2. Blumenthal D, Causino N, Chang YC. The duration of ambulatory visits to physicians. *J Fam Pract* 1999;48:264–271.
3. Bergh KD. The patient's differential diagnosis: unpredictable concerns in visits for cough. *J Fam Pract* 1998;46:153–158.
4. Taylor RB. Family practice and the advancement of medical understanding: the first 50 years. *J Fam Pract* 1999;48:53–57.
5. Richardson WS, Wilson MC, Guyatt GH, et al. User's guide to the medical literature: how to use an article about disease probability for differential diagnosis. *JAMA* 1999;281:1214–1219.
6. Hersh W. A world of knowledge at your fingertips: the promise, reality, and future directions of on-line information retrieval. *Acad Med* 1999;74:240–243.

Undifferentiated Problems
Richard H. Hurd

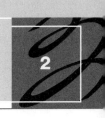

2

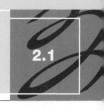

ANOREXIA
2.1
Michael D. Schooff

I. BACKGROUND. Anorexia is prolonged diminished appetite or appetite loss. This common symptom is to be differentiated from the eating disorder anorexia nervosa, which is often simply called *anorexia.* Anorexia may or may not be associated with weight loss. It is almost always a result of one or more underlying causes.

II. PATHOPHYSIOLOGY

A. General mechanisms. Although the exact mechanisms by which the body regulates appetite and body weight have yet to be fully determined, modern research is providing more and more information on the subject. The hypothalamus is believed to regulate both satiety and hunger, leading to homeostasis of body weight in ideal situations. The hypothalamus interprets and integrates a number of neural and humoral inputs to coordinate feeding and energy expenditure in response to conditions of altered energy balance. Long-term signals communicating information about the body's energy stores, endocrine status, and general health are predominantly humoral. Short-term signals, including gut hormones and neural signals from higher brain centers and the gut, regulate meal initiation and termination. Hormones involved in this process include leptin, insulin, cholecystokinin, ghrelin, polypeptide YY, pancreatic polypeptide, glucagonlike peptide-1, and oxyntomodulin (1). Alterations in any of these humoral or neuronal processes can lead to anorexia.

B. Etiology. Table 2.1.1 lists some causes of anorexia. These causes can be divided into four categories: pathologic, pharmacologic, psychiatric, and social.

1. Pathologic causes may be acute, such as appendicitis or other surgical emergencies, or chronic, such as heart or renal failure or malignancies. Pathologic causes rarely present without other signs or symptoms in addition to anorexia.

2. Pharmacologic causes include substances taken and those recently discontinued. Substances of abuse, such as alcohol, tobacco, narcotics, marijuana, and stimulants, can affect appetite. Prescription and over-the-counter medications, as well as dietary supplements, can lead to anorexia.

3. Psychiatric illnesses are sometimes more difficult to find than the other categories, requiring time and a high index of suspicion. Anorexia may be the result of a primary eating disorder, such as anorexia nervosa, or other illnesses, such as depression, personality disorders, schizophrenia, and bipolar disorders (2).

4. Social factors often affect appetite. Bereavement, stress, and loneliness may cause anorexia. Moving from one's home, loss of ability to shop for food or prepare meals, and lack of finances may also result in appetite changes (3).

III. EVALUATION

A. History. A careful history is key to determining the cause of anorexia in most patients.

1. History of present illness. The first step is to understand the exact nature of the anorexia. Is the problem a loss of desire to eat or a loss of appetite with maintained desire? Is it truly associated with appetite, or is it related to early satiety, difficult or painful swallowing, abdominal symptoms that follow eating, loss of pleasure or satisfaction with eating, or loss of ability to prepare a meal? What does the patient think the underlying problem is? Are the symptoms constant or do they fluctuate? Are there any coexisting emotional problems? Has the patient lost weight, and if so, how much?

TABLE 2.1.1   Etiology of Anorexia

Pathologic	Pharmacologic (taking or discontinuing)	Psychiatric	Social
Neoplasms	Tobacco	Depression	Bereavement
Lymphoma	Alcohol	Anxiety	Stress
Colon cancer	Caffeine	Personality disorders	Loneliness
Lung cancer	Amphetamines	Schizophrenia	Change of location
Stomach cancer	Marijuana	Eating disorders	Inability to shop for food
Endocrine disorders	Antihistamines	Obsessive-compulsive disorder	Inability to prepare meals
Diabetes mellitus	Anticonvulsants	Bipolar disorder	Insufficient finances
Addison's disease	Antidepressants	Dementia	
Hyponatremia	Ephedrine	Delirium	
Hypercalcemia	Chromium	Psychosis	
Hypothyroidism	Xanthenes		
Zinc deficiency	Antibiotics		
Infectious diseases	Digitalis		
Viral hepatitis	Morphine		
HIV	Codeine		
Tuberculosis	Meperidine		
Intestinal protozoa	Aspirin		
Chronic diseases	NSAIDs		
Anemia	Clonidine		
COPD	Chemotherapeutics		
Renal failure	Sedatives		

Heart failure
Parkinson's disease
Alzheimer's dementia
Multiple sclerosis
Cirrhosis

Inflammatory disorders
Pancreatitis
Inflammatory bowel disease
Peptic/duodenal ulcer
Cholelithiasis
Appendicitis
GERD/esophagitis
Lupus erythematosus

Others
Pain
Fever
Impaired sense of smell
Impaired sense of taste
Poor dentition
Dysphagia/odynophagia
Irritable bowel syndrome
Pregnancy

HIV, human immunodeficiency virus; NSAIDs, nonsteroidal anti-inflammatory drugs; COPD, chronic obstructive pulmonary disease; GERD, gastroesophageal reflux disease.

2. **Past medical history.** Is there any history of previous eating disorders, psychiatric conditions, or chronic medical conditions?
3. **Medications and habits.** What medications is the patient taking? What medications has the patient recently discontinued? Does the patient take any over-the-counter medications, dietary supplements, or herbal products? Does the patient use alcohol, tobacco, or illicit drugs?
4. **Social history.** Eating is a very social function in most cultures. Stress, bereavement, troubles with relationships, loneliness, and guilt can all lead to anorexia. Who does the patient live with? Is food available in the home? Is the patient capable of shopping and preparing meals (e.g., mobility, vision, and cognitive capacity)? Are there financial concerns?
5. **Review of systems.** A general review of systems should be performed, with focus on gastrointestinal (e.g., difficult or painful swallowing, nausea, abdominal pain or bloating, diarrhea or constipation, and rectal bleeding), psychiatric (e.g., depression and anxiety), and neurologic (e.g., mental status and recent head injury) systems. A diet history, either retrospective or prospective, through the use of a food diary, is often helpful.

B. **Physical Examination**
1. **General appearance.** Does the patient look healthy or ill? Is there fever or tachycardia, suggestive of a systemic illness? Carefully measure the patient's weight and compare to previous recordings.
2. **Head, eyes, ears, nose, and throat (HEENT).** Look carefully for poor dentition, oral lesions, difficult swallowing, lymphadenopathy, and thyroid abnormalities.
3. **Cardiorespiratory system.** Examine for arrhythmias, chronic obstructive pulmonary disease, and signs of heart failure, such as jugular venous distension or rales.
4. **Gastrointestinal system.** Listen for abnormal bowel sounds. Examine for tenderness, rigidity, ascites, and hepatomegaly. Rectal examination, including guaiac testing, should be performed.
5. **Skin.** Jaundice, skin tracks, cyanosis, lanugo, hyperpigmentation, and turgor should be noted.
6. **Neurologic and psychological systems.** Examine the functions of cranial nerves, including smell and taste. Look for focal or generalized weakness, gait or balance disturbances, or movement disorders. Assess the patient's functional capacity and mental status. Assess for anxiety, depression, dementia, delirium, and psychosis.

C. **Testing.** As in all areas of medicine, diagnostic studies should be guided by the history and physical examination. Tests to consider in anorexia include a complete blood count, electrolytes panel, hepatic panel, and albumin. When assessing nutritional status, measuring prealbumin level may be preferred over albumin level in acute cases of anorexia because prealbumin is the earliest marker of changes in nutritional status (4, 5). Chest x-ray and tuberculosis testing can be helpful in some cases, as might esophagogastroduodenoscopy, colonoscopy, and abdominal computed tomography or ultrasonography. Less commonly ordered tests include human immunodeficiency virus, thyroid-stimulating hormone and thyroid hormone, viral hepatitis panel, and urine protein, and testing for toxicology and drugs of abuse.

IV. **DIAGNOSIS.** Although the causes of anorexia are numerous and span the biopsychosocial spectrum, a thoughtful evaluation will generally reveal the underlying cause(s) of the loss of appetite, and specific interventions can then be instituted.

References
1. Murphy KG, Bloom SR. Gut hormones in the control of appetite. *Exp Physiol* 2004;89:507–516.
2. Garfinkel PE, Garner DM, Kaplan AS, et al. Differential diagnosis of emotional disorders that cause weight loss. *Can Med Assoc J* 1983;129(9):939–945.

3. Morley JE. Anorexia in older persons: epidemiology and optimal treatment. *Drugs Aging* 1996;8(2):134–135.
4. Beck FK, Rosenthal TC. Prealbumin: a marker for nutritional evaluation. *Am Fam Physician* 2002;65:1575–1578.
5. Lab Markers of Malnutrition. Accessed at *Family Practice Notebook.com* (http://www.fpnotebook.com/PHA48.htm) on 19 May 2005.

DIZZINESS
Richard H. Hurd

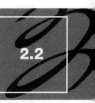

2.2

I. **BACKGROUND.** Dizziness is a rather imprecise term often used by patients to describe any of a number of peculiar subjective symptoms. These symptoms may include faintness, giddiness, light-headedness, or unsteadiness. True vertigo, a sensation of irregular or whirling motion, is also included in a patient's complaint of dizziness. Dizziness represents a disturbance in a patient's subjective sensation of relationship to space (1).

II. **PATHOPHYSIOLOGY**

A. **Etiology.** The causes of dizziness are numerous. It is helpful for the diagnostician to think in general categories of causes when searching for an etiology (see Table 2.2.1).

B. **Epidemiology.** Dizziness is the complaint in an estimated 7 million clinic visits in the United States each year (2,3). It is one of the most frequent reasons for referral to neurologists and otolaryngologists. The reasons for frequent referral of this usually benign condition are many. Ruling out potentially serious causes, including those of cardiac and neurologic origin, can be difficult. In addition, the fact that there is no

 TABLE 2.2.1   **Common Causes of Dizziness**

Peripheral vestibular[a]	Central vestibular[b]	Psychiatric[c]	Nonvestibular, nonpsychiatric[d]
Benign positional vertigo	Cerebrovascular disease[e]	Hyperventilation	Presyncope
Labrynthitis	Tumors[f]	—	Disequilibrium
Meniere's disease	Cerebellar atrophy	—	Medications
Other[g]	Migraine	—	Metabolic disturbances
—	Multiple sclerosis	—	Infection
—	Epilepsy	—	Trauma
—	—	—	Unknown causes[h]

[a] Encompasses 44% of patients.
[b] Accounts for 11% of dizziness cases.
[c] Causes make up 16% of the diagnosis.
[d] Accounts for 37% of the diagnosis.
[e] Stroke or transient ischemic attack and dehydration comprise the largest part of this group.
[f] Usually acoustic neuroma.
[g] Includes drug-induced, ototoxicity, and nonspecific vestibulopathy.
[h] A significant part of this subset and a significant part of all cases of dizziness.

specific treatment for many of the causes of dizziness leads to frustration for both the patient and the physician.

III. EVALUATION

A. History. It is extremely important, and can be very difficult, to get the patient to describe exactly what they mean when complaining of dizziness. A description of the attack, context, length, duration, and frequency is important. Any precipitating factors should be explored. Concurrent symptoms such as nausea, headache, chest fluttering, or tinnitus can help to direct the clinician to a cause. Any new or medication changes should be inquired about.

B. Physical examination. The physical examination, although thorough, is often focused on a specific system based on the history. It is seldom diagnostic in itself, but is more often confirmatory.

1. Vital signs including orthostatic blood pressures begin the examination.
2. A neurologic examination must be completed.
3. A cardiovascular examination including the heart for murmur or arrhythmia and carotid arterial auscultation should be completed.
4. An otoscopic examination to assess infection and nystagmus examination including gaze, Dix-Hallpike's maneuvers, and head shaking are important.
5. An observation of gait to assess cerebellar function is also a part of the examination.

C. Testing. It is obvious that there is no laboratory or imaging study directly related to dizziness. Instead, these types of studies are dictated by the etiology that the clinician feels is most likely. They are more to confirm a diagnosis than to actually make it.

1. Tests might include complete blood count, electrolytes, appropriate drug levels, and thyroid levels.
2. Imaging studies such as magnetic resonance imaging might be indicated if the concern of tumor is high.
3. A hearing test as well as maneuvers carried out in a tilt-chair to test labyrinth function may be of value.

D. Genetics. There does not appear to be any genetic predisposition to dizziness.

IV. DIAGNOSIS

A. Differential diagnosis

1. The differential diagnosis of dizziness includes all of those conditions mentioned in the preceding text that cause true dizziness (Table 2.2.1). It also includes many other conditions that cause patients to feel abnormal in some vague way, causing them to complain of dizziness. Psychologic conditions such as anxiety, depression, panic disorder, or somatization may all cause a patient to complain of dizziness. Cardiac arrhythmias, ischemic or valvular heart disease, vasovagal, anemia, or postural hypotension are some of the conditions leading to cerebral hypoperfusion, and therefore, presyncope.
2. Degenerative changes in the elderly may affect the vestibular apparatus, vision, or proprioception, all of which may be interpreted as dizziness. Finally, peripheral neuropathy or cerebellar disease may also be confused with dizziness.

B. Clinical manifestations. The clinical manifestations of dizziness are as varied as those entities included in both the etiologic and the differential diagnosis sections. The fact that dizziness is more often a symptom of some other condition than a separate diagnosis leads to a wide variety of manifestations that the clinician must decipher.

References

1. M. Bajorek. Night sweats. In: Taylor R., ed. *The 10-minute diagnosis manual.* Philadelphia, PA: Lippincott Williams & Wilkins, 2000:31–33.
2. Kroenke K, Hoffman R, Einstadter D. How common are various causes of Dizziness? A critical review. *South Med J* 2000;93(2):160–168, Table 2, P7.
3. Sloane PD. Dizziness in primary care: results from the National Ambulatory Medical Care Survey. *J Fam Pract* 1989;29:33–38.

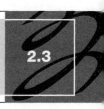

EDEMA
Roger Massie
2.3

I. BACKGROUND. Edema is defined as a clinically apparent increase in the interstitial fluid volume that may expand by several liters before the abnormality is evident (1).

XI. PATHOPHYSIOLOGY

  A. Etiology. The etiology is multifactorial, revolving around the intricate balance of capillary blood and oncotic pressures, tissue pressures, capillary permeability, and lymphatic flow. A change in any of these factors can offset the extravascular fluid balance and result in edema formation (2).

  B. Epidemiology. The epidemiology of edema in the United States is unknown.

XII. EVALUATION

  A. History. The following factors are pertinent to the establishment of the etiology of edema.

   1. Onset: gradual or sudden
   2. Site of the edema
   3. History of recurrence or chronicity
   4. Color, warmth, induration, sensitivity, and/or pain
   5. Associated dyspnea or orthopnea
   6. Associated fever or chills
   7. Medications such as nonsteroidal antiinflammatories, calcium channel blockers, α-blockers and β-blockers, corticosteroids
   8. Endocrine diseases: hypothyroidism, Cushing's disease
   9. Prolonged dependent position
   10. Pregnancy
   11. Increased sodium chloride intake
   12. Trauma: ecchymosis, abrasions

  B. Physical examination. A complete or focused examination should be performed, depending on information obtained from the history. Special attention should be paid to whether the edema is generalized or localized (see Table 2.3.1). Vital signs should be noted with special attention to an elevated temperature, decreased oxygen saturation, tachypnea, and/or tachycardia. Mental status changes reported by the patient or the patient's family should be noted. Neck vein distension should be evaluated. It is necessary to listen carefully for a gallop in the heart rhythm. Crackles in the lungs should also be noted. Ascites and hepatosplenomegaly should

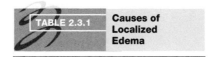

TABLE 2.3.1	Causes of Localized Edema

- Injury
- Local allergic reactions
- Arthritis/joint inflammations
- Insect stings/venomations
- Venous thrombosis or occlusion
- Surgical interruption of veins or lymphitis
- Angioedema
- Idiopathic
- Physiologic (e.g., dependent pedal edema)
- Infections

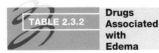

TABLE 2.3.2	Drugs Associated with Edema

Nonsteroidal anti-inflammatory drugs
Antihypertensive agents
Direct arterial/arteriolar vasodilators
   Minoxidil
   Hydralazine
   Clonidine
   Methyldopa
   Guanethidine
Calcium channel antagonists
   Adrenergic antagonists
Steroid hormones
   Glucocorticoids
   Anabolic steroids
   Estrogens
   Progestins
Cyclosporine
Growth hormone
Immunotherapies
   Interleukin-2
   OKT3 monoclonal antibody

From Braunwald E, ed. Edema. In: *Harrison's principles of internal medicine*, 15th ed. New York, NY: McGraw Hill; 2001:217–222.

be evaluated. It should be noted whether the edema is generalized or localized, whether it is pitting or nonpitting, and whether there is coloration if a painful sensation is present. The findings on physical examination should be very helpful in determining the etiology of the edema.

  C. Testing. The following tests should be entertained and/or ordered depending on the history and physical examination: complete blood count, urinalysis, thyroid-stimulating hormone, comprehensive metabolic profile including albumin and liver function tests, congestive heart failure peptide, chest x-ray, electrocardiogram, computed tomography, magnetic resonance imaging, venous Doppler study, and venograms.

XIII. DIAGNOSIS. For the differential diagnosis of drug-induced edema, see Table 2.3.2.

References
1. Braunwald E, ed. Edema. In: *Harrison's principles of internal medicine*, 15th ed. New York, NY: McGraw-Hill, 2001:217–222.
2. Terry, M., O'Brien, S., Kerstein, MD. Lower-extremity edema: evaluation and diagnosis. *Wounds* 10(4):11–124:1998.

FALLS
Kenneth D. Peters

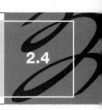

2.4

I. **BACKGROUND.** Falls are most common at age extremes. In children older than 1 year of age, injuries are the number one cause of death. Falls account for 25% of these deaths. Bike injuries account for 68% of falls in children from 5 to 14 years of age (1). In patients older than 65 years of age, the incidence of falls is 30%; in those older than 80 years of age, it is >50%. Accidents are the fifth leading cause of death in patients 65 years of age and older, and falls account for two thirds of these deaths. Of elderly patients hospitalized for falls, only 50% are alive 1 year later (2).

II. **PATHOPHYSIOLOGY.** Factors that contribute to falls need to be identified and evaluated for preventive measures to be taken. Children fall from heights; elderly fall from level surfaces.

A. **Children and adolescents.** Falls from heights over 3 feet and falls of infants younger than 1 year of age result in increased risk of skull fracture and intracranial bleeding. Emergent evaluation is needed in cases of loss of consciousness, behavioral changes, seizures, or ongoing vomiting.

B. **Falls in the elderly.** One half of the falls are secondary to accidents, including factors affecting stability. The other half of the falls are secondary to medical disorders (see Table 2.4.1). If syncope occurred with a fall, it must be determined whether the cause is cardiac or noncardiac (see Table 2.4.2) (Chapter 2.12). Cardiac mortality in falls related to syncope at 1 year is 20% to 30%, whereas noncardiac mortality is <5% (3). There is a strong association between falls and nursing home placement in the elderly; furthermore, specific individualized interventions help prevent falls (4). The risk of hip fracture in the frail elderly can be reduced with the use of an anatomically designed external hip protector (5).

III. **EVALUATION**

A. **History**

1. **History of the fall.** An interview of a witness to the fall is essential. This may identify any seizure activity, loss of consciousness, and method of fall. Ask what the patient was doing prior to the fall, including occurrence with positional changes or after voiding, eating, or constipation. Are there associated palpitations implying arrhythmia? Did the patient have a fall or syncope during exercise, which may indicate a cardiac cause? Is there any confusion that is new or changed from the past that suggests central nervous system trauma or seizure? Was urine or bowel incontinence present? Questions concerning home and risk factors should be raised (Table 2.4.1).

2. **Past history.** Explore coexisting illness that may have contributed to the fall (Table 2.4.1). A family history of sudden death can imply arrhythmias. Furthermore, inquire about any history of prior falls.

B. **Physical examination.** This should include:

1. Assessment of vital signs, including heart rate and rhythm, orthostatic blood pressure changes, temperature, and respiratory rate.

2. A general body survey for any evidence of trauma.

3. Examination of the eye (funduscopic, visual acuity, and fields), mouth (tongue lacerations), neck (bruits), lung (congestive heart failure or infection), and cardiovascular (murmurs and rhythm).

4. A neurologic examination that includes mental status, evaluation of balance, gait, mobility, and tests for peripheral neuropathy.

5. The "get up and go test" (rise from a chair, walk 10 feet, return, and sit down), which is a simple rapid way of assessing general condition and musculoskeletal and neurologic status (6).

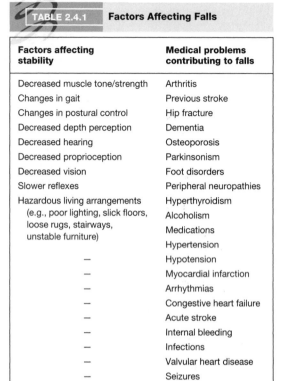

TABLE 2.4.1 Factors Affecting Falls

Factors affecting stability	Medical problems contributing to falls
Decreased muscle tone/strength	Arthritis
Changes in gait	Previous stroke
Changes in postural control	Hip fracture
Decreased depth perception	Dementia
Decreased hearing	Osteoporosis
Decreased proprioception	Parkinsonism
Decreased vision	Foot disorders
Slower reflexes	Peripheral neuropathies
Hazardous living arrangements (e.g., poor lighting, slick floors, loose rugs, stairways, unstable furniture)	Hyperthyroidism
	Alcoholism
	Medications
	Hypertension
—	Hypotension
—	Myocardial infarction
—	Arrhythmias
—	Congestive heart failure
—	Acute stroke
—	Internal bleeding
—	Infections
—	Valvular heart disease
—	Seizures

C. Testing

1. **Clinical laboratory tests.** Most blood tests are of low yield and should be done to confirm clinical suspicion. An electrocardiogram is useful in the elderly to rule out arrhythmia, atrioventricular block, prolonged QT syndrome, or ischemia. A diagnosis of the cause of the fall can be obtained in 50% to 60% of cases based on history, physical, and electrocardiographic study (7).

2. **Diagnostic imaging.** Skull x-ray (fracture) and computed tomography studies to detect intracranial bleeding are recommended in all infants younger than 1 year of age or if the fall was from >3 feet. Also consider imaging with any loss of consciousness, evidence of head trauma, behavioral changes, seizure disorder, ongoing vomiting, or focal neurologic deficits.

3. Other testing to consider includes echocardiogram (valvular heart disease), electroencephalogram (seizure), carotid ultrasound (bruits), carotid sinus massage (if suggested by history), and tilt table testing (if a vasovagal cause of fall is considered). Ambulatory cardiac monitor for sudden infrequent falls.

IV. DIAGNOSIS. A fall by an elderly individual frequently requires a home visit to evaluate factors contributing to falls and to correct unsafe conditions (Table 2.4.1). Symptoms of cardiac disease can occur with exertion or straining. Cardiac arrhythmias tend to be sudden without warning, although once in a while, patients can complain of palpitations. Noncardiac causes include the vasovagal reaction where the patient generally complains of dizziness or lightheadedness prior to a fall, often with changes in position or when upright. These can be associated with sweating and nausea.

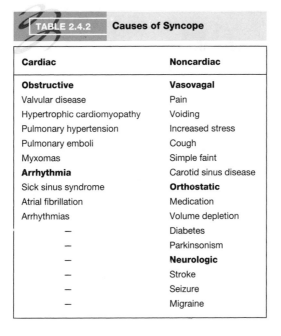

Cardiac	Noncardiac
Obstructive	**Vasovagal**
Valvular disease	Pain
Hypertrophic cardiomyopathy	Voiding
Pulmonary hypertension	Increased stress
Pulmonary emboli	Cough
Myxomas	Simple faint
Arrhythmia	Carotid sinus disease
Sick sinus syndrome	**Orthostatic**
Atrial fibrillation	Medication
Arrhythmias	Volume depletion
—	Diabetes
—	Parkinsonism
—	**Neurologic**
—	Stroke
—	Seizure
—	Migraine

Orthostatic noncardiac causes have gradual onset and resolution. These are most often associated with medications, including antihypertensives, sedatives, anxiolytics, antidepressants, hypoglycemics, psychotropics, histamine$_2$ blockers, alcohol, over-the-counter cold medicines, and medications with extended half-lives. Neurologic noncardiac events can usually be diagnosed by history and physical examination. A psychiatric cause for falls is less likely, but one should be suspicious in cases of frequent symptoms with no injury.

For the differential diagnosis, refer to Tables 2.4.1 and 2.4.2.

References
1. Gruskin KD, Schutzman SA. Head trauma in children younger than 2 years: are there predictors for complications? *Arch Pediatr Adolesc Med* 1999;153:15–20.
2. Steinweg KK. The changing approach to falls in the elderly. *Am Fam Physician* 1997;56:1815–1824.
3. Wiley TM. A diagnostic approach to syncope. *Resid Staff Physician* 1998;44:2947.
4. Tinetti ME, Williams CS. Falls, injuries due to falls, and the risk of admission to a nursing home. *New Engl J Med* 1997;337(18):1279–1284.
5. Kannus P, Parkkari J, Niemi S. Prevention of hip fracture is elderly people with use of a hip protector. *New Engl J Med* 2000:343(21):1506–1513.
6. Albert S, David R, Alison M. Comprehensive geriatric assessment. In: William H, Edwin B, John B, et al. eds. *Principals of geriatrics*, 3rd ed. New York, NY: McGraw-Hill, 1994: Chapter 17:206.
7. Hupert N, Kapoor WN. Syncope: a systemic approach for the cause. *Patient Care* 1997;31:136–147.

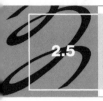

FATIGUE
Amy K. Jespersen

I. BACKGROUND
   A. General considerations. Fatigue is a very common complaint in the primary care office. It may be the primary reason a patient seeks care or a secondary complaint. We are all bothered by fatigue at some point in time. However, for millions of patients each year, it becomes bothersome enough to seek medical attention. True fatigue needs to be distinguished from weakness and from excessive somnolence secondary to sleep disturbances. Fatigue lasting less than a month is considered acute. If symptoms last more than a month, fatigue is considered prolonged.
   B. Definitions
   1. Chronic fatigue is diagnosed when symptoms last >6 months. The Center for Disease Control and Prevention has defined chronic fatigue syndrome (CFS) as profound fatigue of 6 months duration that presents with four of the following eight symptoms:
      a. Impairment in short-term memory or concentration
      b. Sore throat
      c. Tender lymphadenopathy
      d. Myalgias
      e. Multijoint pain
      f. Headaches of a new type, pattern, or severity
      g. Unrefreshing sleep
      h. Postexertional malaise lasting >24 hours (1)
   2. Idiopathic chronic fatigue is diagnosed if a patient has been fatigued for >6 months, but does not meet the other criteria for CFS.

II. PATHOPHYSIOLOGY
   A. Etiology. Some of the common causes of CFS are listed in Table 2.5.1. Fatigue may be due to medical disorders, psychiatric disease, or lifestyle factors. In some cases, a cause is never determined. Fatigue that persists for several months or years is more likely to have a psychiatric etiology, whereas a shorter duration of fatigue is more likely to have a medical explanation (2). If a medical cause of fatigue is present, it is usually identifiable on the initial history, physical and laboratory testing (3).
   B. Epidemiology. The true incidence of profound fatigue is unknown. It has been estimated that over 7 million office visits per year are for complaints of fatigue (3). The true gender predilection is also unknown, however, women present to the physician's office twice as often as men. Patients younger than 45 years of age are more likely to present for fatigue than patients older than 45 years of age (2).

III. EVALUATION
   A. History
   1. A detailed history and review of systems should be performed. The onset, duration, and degree of fatigue should be explored, along with any possible precipitating events. Specific attention should be given to sleep patterns, daytime somnolence, or sleep apnea symptoms.
   2. The patient's exercise habits, caffeine intake, and drug or alcohol use should be explored, and medications should be reviewed.
   3. A psychiatric history to evaluate symptoms of depression or anxiety should be obtained. Lifestyle issues such as stress at home or in the work place, childcare responsibilities, shift work, or changing work schedules should be addressed.
   B. Physical examination. A thorough physical examination should be performed. Vital signs should be carefully noted. Attention should be given to the presence of pallor, muscle weakness, goiter, lymphadenopathy, and body habitus. A psychiatric

TABLE 2.5.1	Common Causes of Fatigue	
Medical conditions	**Psychiatric disorders**	**Lifestyle factors**
Hypothyroidism	Major depressive	Sleep deprivation
Anemia	disorder	Marital discord
Cardiomyopathy	Bipolar disorder	Job stress
COPD	Alcoholism/substance	Caring for young
Morbid obesity	abuse	children
Sleep disorders	Anxiety	Altering work schedule
Medication side effects	Somatoform disorders	
β-Blockers		
Centrally acting		
α-Blockers		
Antihistamines		
Antidepressants		
Subacute infections		
Viral infections		
(CMV, EBV, HIV)		
Bacterial endocarditis		
Malignancy		
Fibromyalgia		

COPD, chronic obstructive pulmonary disease; CMV, cytomegalovirus; EBV, Epstein-Barr virus; HIV, human immunodeficiency virus.

evaluation for signs of depression, anxiety, or other mental illness should be performed. In older adults, a mental status exam to evaluate cognitive function may be appropriate.

C. Testing
  1. Initial laboratory testing should be limited to:
   a. Complete blood count
   b. Comprehensive metabolic profile
   c. Thyroid-stimulating hormone
   d. Erythrocyte sedimentation rate
   e. Urine analysis
  2. Other tests may be indicated by the history or physical examination:
   a. Antinuclear antibody
   b. Rheumatoid factor
   c. Monospot
   d. Chest x-ray
   e. Colonoscopy
   f. Sleep study
  3. Screening tests appropriate for age and gender should be performed.
IV. DIAGNOSIS. Fatigue is a very commonly encountered complaint. In most cases, a thorough history, physical and a limited number of ancillary tests reveal a more precise diagnosis. Fatigue is rarely the only presenting symptom in cases of malignancy or connective tissue disease. Studies have shown that among patients with fatigue, approximately 40% have an underlying medical diagnosis, approximately 40% have a psychiatric diagnosis, and 12% have both medical and psychiatric explanations for their fatigue. Approximately 8% of patients have no discernible diagnosis (2). If undiagnosed fatigue persists for >6 months and meets the other criteria for CFS, that diagnosis is applied. If the other criteria for CFS are not met, the term idiopathic chronic fatigue is used. Fatigue that cannot be attributed to a medical or psychiatric diagnosis is often thought to be due to lifestyle factors.

References
1. Centers for Disease Control and Prevention. *Chronic fatigue syndrome*, accessed at National Center for Infectious Diseases (www.cdc.gov/ncidod/diseases/cfs/index.htm) on 13 May 2005.
2. Morrison JD. Fatigue as a presenting complaint in FP. *J Fam Pract* 1980;10:795–801.
3. Epstein KR. The chronically fatigued patient. *Med Clin North Am* 1995;79:315–327.

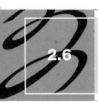

FEVER
Michael D. Schooff

I. **BACKGROUND.** Fever is an elevation in the core body temperature above the individual's normal range that occurs in conjunction with an increase in the hypothalamic temperature set point. Fever is defined as a core body temperature of 38°C (100.4°F). Hyperthermia is an elevated body temperature without a change in the hypothalamic setting. Hyperpyrexia, a medical emergency, is defined as a temperature over 41.1°C (106.0°F).

II. **PATHOPHYSIOLOGY**

A. **Mechanisms of temperature control.** Body temperature is controlled by the hypothalamus, which receives inputs from both the peripheral nerves and from the temperature of the blood supplying the area. Normal body temperature is maintained across environmental variations through the regulation of heat production from metabolic activity (mostly of the muscles and liver) and heat dissipation from the skin and lungs. It is widely held that normal body temperature is 37.0°C (98.6°F), but several studies have shown that average temperatures in healthy adults range from 30.0°C to 37.2°C (86.0°F–99.0°F) with averages 36.4°C to 36.8°C (97.5°F–98.2°F) and 99th percentile 37.5°C to 37.7°C (99.5°F–99.9°F) (1,2).

B. **Temperature measurement.** How the temperature is taken can affect the result. Rectal temperature is considered the closest approximation to core temperature. Sublingual temperatures are felt to be fairly reliable, and generally measure 0.6°C (1.0°F) lower than rectal temperatures. Axillary and tympanic measurements are less reliable, with axillary temperatures ranging from 0.25°C to 0.85°C (0.4°F–1.5°F) lower than rectal measurements, and tympanic measurements ranging from 1.3°C (2.3°F) lower than rectal to 0.7°C (1.3°F) higher (3,4).

C. **Temperature variation.** Normal body temperature varies by an average of 0.5°C (0.9°F) throughout the day, with the lowest temperature early in the morning and peak in the mid afternoon. Other factors that influence normal body temperature include age, race, physical activity, postprandial state, pregnancy or ovulation, endocrine disorders, clothing, and ambient temperature and humidity.

III. **EVALUATION**

A. **History.** A detailed history is essential to establishing the cause of fever. The history should include the following components:

1. Complete review of systems as well as past medical problems
2. Previous surgeries, with attention to any implanted materials or devices
3. Medications, supplements, and other drugs used
4. Recent and remote travel
5. Exposure to ill individuals
6. Exposure to animals or insects
7. Occupation
8. Ingestion of any questionable foods or substances
9. Family history of unusual illnesses

B. **Physical examination.** Careful physical examination should be performed.
   1. Temperature and other vital signs should be measured accurately. Heart rate, blood pressure, and respiratory rate normally increase in the face of fever. Bradycardia may be a sign of atypical infections. Hypotension may be a sign of systemic sepsis.
   2. An examination of all organ systems and body areas should be performed, with emphasis given to the skin, lymphatics, heart, lungs, and nervous system. In addition, genital and rectal examinations should be performed regardless of gender.
C. **Testing.** Diagnostic testing should be guided by the history and physical examination.
   1. When the source of the fever is unclear, helpful laboratory tests include white blood cell count with differential, urinalysis with microscopic examination and culture if results are abnormal, and aerobic and anaerobic blood cultures.

TABLE 2.6.1   Potential Causes of Fever of Unknown Origin

Infectious diseases	Collagen vascular diseases	Malignancies	Medications	Other
Tuberculosis	Still's disease	Lymphoma	Carbamazepine	Granulomatous diseases
Occult abscess	Temporal arteritis	Leukemia	Phenytoin	Pulmonary embolus
Osteomyelitis	Polyarteritis nodosa	Hypernephroma	Antihistamines	Venous thrombosis
Endocarditis	Rheumatic fever	Other solid tumors	Methyldopa	Endocrine disorders
Sinusitis	Systemic lupus erythematosus	Atrial myxoma	Allopurinol	Factitious fever
HIV (late stage)	Rheumatoid arthritis	Colon cancer	Sulfonamides	Cerebrovascular accident
Q fever	Polymyalgia rheumatica	Hepatoma	Cephalosporins	Alcoholic hepatitis
Tropheri	—	—	Isoniazid	Cirrhosis
Brucella	—	—	—	—
Mycoplasma	—	—	—	—
Chlamydia	—	—	—	—
Histoplasmosis	—	—	—	—
Legionella	—	—	—	
Bartonella	—	—	—	
HACEK	—	—	—	
Amebic hepatitis	—	—	—	
Medical device infections	—	—	—	

HACEK, *Haemophilus* species (*H. parainfluenzae*, *H. aphrophilus*, and *H. paraphrophilus*), *Actinobacillus actinomycetemcomitans*, *Cardiobacterium hominis*, *Eikenella corrodens*, and *Kingella* species.

  2. A chest radiograph and abdominal imaging (computed tomography or ultrasound) may be helpful if the history and physical examination suggest a pulmonary or abdominal infection.

  3. If the source of the fever remains undetermined after these common tests have been performed, other tests to consider include the human immunodeficiency virus serology, rapid plasma reagin, rheumatoid factor, antinuclear antibody, sedimentation rate or C-reactive protein, serum chemistries and enzymes, tuberculosis skin testing, examination of the spinal fluid, and technetium-labeled bone scan.

IV. DIAGNOSIS

  A. Acute febrile illness. In the outpatient setting, most fevers are associated with an acute illness and are caused by self-limited viral infections, such as upper respiratory tract infections or acute gastroenteritis. These infections usually resolve in 7 to 10 days and require only supportive and symptomatic therapy. Common bacterial infections requiring antibiotic therapy include streptococcal pharyngitis, cellulitis,

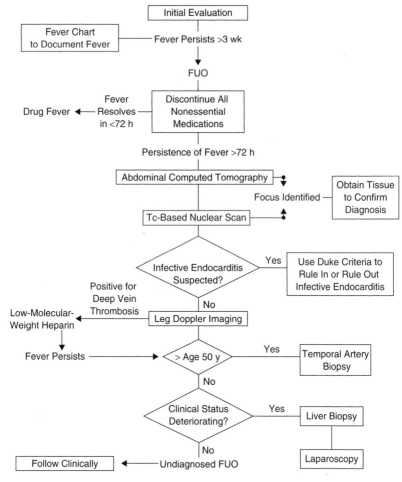

Figure 2.6.1. Approach to the evaluation of fever. FUO, fever of unknown origin.

urinary tract infections, pneumonia, acute exacerbation of chronic bronchitis, and bacterial sinusitis. A careful history and physical examination, supported by selected diagnostic tests should lead to a specific diagnosis in almost all of these cases.

B. Fever in the elderly. Infections in the elderly often do not result in the same signs and symptoms as in younger patients. While some elderly patients may fail to mount a febrile response to some infections, febrile elders are more likely to have a bacterial illness than are their younger counterparts. A careful search for an infection should be undertaken for older individuals with fever, signs or symptoms of an infection (e.g., cough, urinary frequency), or a change in their appetite, behaviors, physical abilities, or mental status. Common sites of infections in the elderly include the skin, lungs, and the urinary system.

C. Postoperative fever. Common causes of fever in the postoperative period can be categorized by how soon after surgery the fever develops. Fever in the first 2 days after surgery is often caused by atelectasis of the lungs. Urinary tract infections, pneumonia, and infections of intravascular access sites commonly present on postoperative days 3 through 5. Fevers beyond the fifth day after surgery should lead one to consider wound infections or abscesses.

D. Fever of unknown origin (FUO). Numerous definitions of FUO exist, but most include a fever documented on several different days over 2 or 3 weeks, with no diagnosis found following repeated physical examinations and routine diagnostic tests. Diseases that may cause FUO are listed in Table 2.6.1. One approach to evaluating the patient with FUO is shown in Figure 2.6.1. The underlying etiology is eventually found in over 90% of FUO cases. Historically, the most common cause of FUO was infection, followed by malignancies, and then rheumatologic diseases. In more recent studies, rheumatologic causes have surpassed malignancies as the second most common cause of FUO. FUO is much more likely to be caused by an unusual presentation of a common disease than a common presentation of an unusual disease (5).

References

1. Mackowiak PA, Wasserman SS, Levine MM. A critical appraisal of 98.6 degrees F, the upper limit of the normal body temperature, and other legacies of Carl Reinhold August Wunderlich. *JAMA* 1992;268:1578–1580.
2. Leckie T. *Normal temperature in the elderly.* Last modified 22 June 2004. Accessed at BestBETs: Best Evidence Topics (www.bestbets.org/cgi-bin/bets.pl?record=00774) on 15 May 2005.
3. Ridell A, Eppich W. *Should tympanic temperature measurement be trusted?* Last modified 19 February 2003. Accessed at BestBETs: Best Evidence Topics (www.bestbets.org/cgi-bin/bets.pl?record=00340) on 15 May 2005.
4. Craig JV, Lancaster GA, Williamson PR, et al. Temperature measured at the axilla compared with rectum in children and young people: systemic review. *BMJ* 2000;320:1174–1178.
5. Mourad O, Palda V, Detsky AS. A comprehensive evidence-based approach to fever of unknown origin. *Arch Intern Med* 2003;163:545–551.

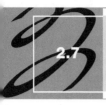

HEADACHES
Kenneth D. Peters

I. **BACKGROUND.** Headache is one of the 20 most frequent reasons that cause patients to visit primary care providers in the United States. In a study of 20,468 patients, migraine headache, one of the common causes of recurrent headache, occurred one or more times yearly in 17.6% of women and in 5.7% of men (1).

II. **PATHOPHYSIOLOGY.** In the evaluation of a recurrent headache, the important tasks are to categorize the headache type with as much precision as possible and to eliminate potentially serious causes.

    A. Headache types. Basically, two types of recurrent headaches are seen: primary headaches and headaches caused by other illnesses (see Table 2.7.1).

    B. Special concerns. These include a brain tumor, intracranial bleed, meningitis, or other serious causes. In primary care patients with "headache" as a presenting symptom, the risk of serious intracranial pathology is <1% (2). Generally, such patients have a history of a new-onset or worsening headache pattern or an abnormal neurologic finding, which might include a seizure.

III. **EVALUATION**

    A. History

        1. Characteristics of the headache. What is the type of pain, its location, its duration, and its intensity? What symptoms precede or accompany the pain? Does anything trigger the headache or make the pain better or worse? Inform the patient about a typical headache from beginning to end.

           a. Foods that trigger migraine include alcohol, aged cheese, chocolate, and aspartame.

           b. Approximately 20% to 30% of migraineurs report an aura, typically visual in nature.

           c. Patients with cluster headache report unilateral temporal headache, occurring generally once daily, usually in the evening and associated with ipsilateral nasal stuffiness and conjunctival injection.

           d. Patients with chronic daily headache (CDH) experience it at least 10 to 15 days/month and usually report heavy use of relief drugs.

           e. Red flags that might suggest intracranial pathology include a loss of consciousness, persistent visual loss, seizures, staggering, or hearing loss.

        2. Chronology of the headache. Most primary headaches recur periodically for years, with only subtle changes over time. If the headache is becoming worse, the cause may be psychosocial stressors, medication overuse, or evolving intracranial pathology (Table 2.7.1). Ask women whether the headache seems related to

TABLE 2.7.1	Types of Recurrent Headache With Selected Examples

Primary headaches: tension-type, migraine, cluster, other

Secondary headaches (*associated with*): brain tumor, vascular abnormality, hypertension, infection, chronic daily HA[a], substance withdrawal, temporal arteritis, neuralgia, sinus HA, metabolic disorders, other

---

[a]Chronic daily HA is classified as a secondary HA because it typically presents as a "rebound headache" in a migraineur who overuses analgesics.
HA, headache.

menses. Past and current medication use and how they affect the headache can be important clues to headache severity and how the patient may respond to the treatment.

3. **Family history.** Migraine headaches often exhibit a familial pattern; the causes of secondary headaches generally do not. Tension headache can represent a family pattern of reacting to stress.

4. **Psychosocial aspects of the headache.** What does the patient believe is the cause of the headache? What life events might be playing a role? How does the patient's family react to the headache? Ask: "If you did not have the headache, how would your life be different?" The key to the management of recurrent primary headaches often lies in the responses to these questions, which can reveal unanticipated stressors, secondary gain, or family discord.

5. **Other information.** Important data includes the use of tobacco, alcohol, or caffeine; response to exercise, a history of head trauma; exposure to toxic fumes or chemicals. Have there been symptoms of fever, or fatigue? Ask about depression, which is often seen in migraineurs. Generally, supratentorial space occupying lesions cause neurologic sequelae and seizures, whereas infratentorial lesions generally cause headache, malaise, nausea, and stiff neck. Allodynia is a common finding in chronic migraines (3).

B. **Physical examination**

1. **A focused physical examination.** This should include vital signs (notably blood pressure) and an examination of the scalp; eyes, including funduscopic examination; ears; nose; paranasal sinuses; throat; and neck. A screening neurologic examination, including cranial nerves, coordination (finger-to-nose test), and deep tendon reflexes, is sufficient in most instances. In the migraineur, the examination findings should be all normal in the absence of a current headache; a positive finding warrants further testing.

2. **Other physical examination maneuvers.** These are appropriate if the medical history suggests specific secondary headache causes: palpation of the superficial temporal arteries (temporal arteritis), audiometry (acoustic neuroma), transillumination of the paranasal sinuses ("sinus headache"), or checking for nuchal rigidity plus Kerning's and Brudzinski's signs (meningeal irritation).

C. **Testing**

1. **Clinical laboratory tests.** For most patients with recurrent headache, no blood, urine, or other clinical laboratory tests are needed. Laboratory tests that might be suggested by the clinical history and the physical examination include erythrocyte sedimentation rate (temporal arteritis), hematocrit or thyroid studies (fatigue), cerebrospinal fluid examination (meningeal irritation), and white blood count with differential (systemic infection).

2. **Diagnostic imaging.** In most instances, diagnostic imaging is not needed. In one study, 350 patients with a chief complaint of headache, regardless of the complaint headache, of the presence or absence of neurologic signs, were referred for computed tomography (CT) scan. Only 2% had clinically significant CT findings, and all patients with significant CT findings had abnormal physical examination findings or unusual clinical symptoms (4).

   a. Diagnostic imaging may be indicated in patients with atypical headache patterns, a history of seizures, or focal neurologic signs or symptoms (5). New-onset and "worst ever" headaches are significant complaints (i.e., atypical headache patterns).

   b. Despite the greater cost, magnetic resonance imaging provides the best imaging for the detection of brain tumors and most other chronic pathologic causes of headache that can be detected by imaging.

   c. More recent developments in imaging technology can help differentiate benign and malignant lesions and to more precisely define the anatomy (e.g., single-proton emission CT scan and magnetic resonance angiography) (3).

IV. **DIAGNOSIS.** The key to the diagnosis of headache is the clinical history. A history of an aching, bitemporal headache that is associated with stress and that waxes and wanes is a typical tension headache. Migraine is characteristically a one-sided headache, throbbing in nature, often associated with nausea and vomiting, frequently accompanied by photophobia and sonophobia, and lasting 4 to 12 hours, perhaps longer. It may be "with aura" (common migraine) or "without aura" (common migraine), with the latter seen in 70% to 80% of migraineurs. Cluster headache is a strictly one-sided, recurring headache that chiefly affects men, and that occurs in "clusters" of 1 to 2 months of episodes. An increasing number of patients have CDH, often with virtually constant discomfort; many CDHs are the result of "transformed migraine" following daily analgesic use, especially codeine derivatives (6).

Because recurrent headache is caused, at least in part, by life stresses and because it also causes personal and family stress, the diagnostic assessment is incomplete until this complex relationship has been adequately explored over a series of visits.

References

1. Stewart WF, Lipton RB, Celentano DD, et al. Prevalence of migraine headache in the United States. *JAMA* 1992;267:64–69.
2. Becker L, Iverson DC, Reed FM, et al. Patients with new headache in primary care: a report from ASPN. *J Fam Pract* 1988;27:41–47.
3. Silberstein SD, Headache diagnosis and management. *56th Annual Meeting*, San Francisco, CA: American Academy of Neurology, April 24, 2004–May 1, 2004.
4. Mitchell CS, Osborn RE, Grosskreutz SR. Computed tomography in the headache patient: is routine evaluation, really necessary? *Headache* 1993;33:83–86.
5. The utility of neuroimaging in the evaluation of headache in patients with normal neurologic examinations: summary statement. Report of the Quality Standards Subcommittee of the American Academy of Neurology *Neurology* 1994;44:1353–1354.
6. Silberstein SD, Lipton RB, Sliwinski M. Classification of daily and near daily headaches: field trials of revised IHS criteria. *Neurology* 1997;49:638–639.

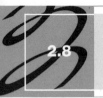

HYPERSOMNIA

Jennifer J. Buescher

I. **BACKGROUND.** Hypersomnia, also known as excessive daytime sleepiness (EDS), is defined by a need to sleep during daytime hours and the ability to fall asleep in situations during which alertness is desired (1). EDS should be differentiated from generalized fatigue and nonspecific tiredness, as patients often use the terms interchangeably. Generalized fatigue is a problem of decreased physical energy, muscle exhaustion, and possibly poor concentration and memory, whereas hypersomnia is the problem of falling asleep at inappropriate or undesired times.

II. **PATHOPHYSIOLOGY**

A. **Etiology.** Hypersomnia can be a primary sleep disorder, but is more commonly secondary to disorders that disrupt normal sleep patterns. Poor quality sleep may be caused by behavioral routines, environmental disturbances, medical and psychological disorders, or insomnia.

B. **Epidemiology.** EDS is a common problem, affecting between 5% and 15% of the general adult population (2), and as many as 58% of psychiatric patients (3). The prevalence of narcolepsy is thought to be approximately 0.05%, although epidemiologic studies vary greatly depending on the country of origin and the definitions of the disease.

III. **EVALUATION.** The evaluation of hypersomnia should include an investigation for intrinsic, extrinsic, and circadian rhythm sleep disorders, as well as medical and psychiatric diseases that are associated with sleepiness. Intrinsic causes of daytime sleepiness, including primary sleep disorders, are relatively uncommon as compared to extrinsic causes and circadian rhythm disorders (misalignment of sleep patterns with local time) (1).

A. History and review of systems. Generalized fatigue should be differentiated from daytime sleepiness in which one experiences head sagging, eyelid drooping, and short periods of sleep at inappropriate times (1). A history of sleep attacks (suddenly falling asleep in dangerous situations) or episodes of cataplexy (sudden and transient loss of muscle strength) can be particularly dangerous and highly suggestive of a diagnosis of narcolepsy (1, 3). A full review of systems often highlights other medical and psychiatric disorders that may be causing daytime sleepiness. Abrupt symptom onset should heighten concern for central nervous system tumors and ischemic stroke.

    1. Sleep patterns. A thorough discussion of the patient's sleep pattern should include details about bedtime and wake time, nighttime awakenings, eating habits prior to sleep, work patterns, and the sleep behavior of bed partners and other members of the household.

    2. Medication history. Medications that induce somnolence or interrupt the normal sleep cycle are listed in Table 2.8.1.

B. Physical examination. The physical examination is most useful in the evaluation of medical and psychological disorders that may be causing sleepiness. Patients with intrinsic, extrinsic, and circadian rhythm sleep disorders are likely to have a normal physical examination.

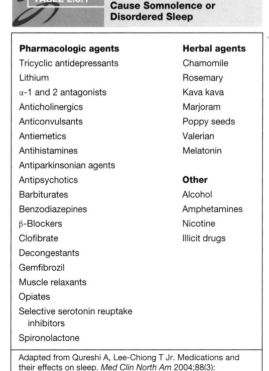

TABLE 2.8.1 Substances That Can Cause Somnolence or Disordered Sleep

Pharmacologic agents	Herbal agents
Tricyclic antidepressants	Chamomile
Lithium	Rosemary
α-1 and 2 antagonists	Kava kava
Anticholinergics	Marjoram
Anticonvulsants	Poppy seeds
Antiemetics	Valerian
Antihistamines	Melatonin
Antiparkinsonian agents	
Antipsychotics	**Other**
Barbiturates	Alcohol
Benzodiazepines	Amphetamines
β-Blockers	Nicotine
Clofibrate	Illicit drugs
Decongestants	
Gemfibrozil	
Muscle relaxants	
Opiates	
Selective serotonin reuptake inhibitors	
Spironolactone	

Adapted from Qureshi A, Lee-Chiong T Jr. Medications and their effects on sleep. *Med Clin North Am* 2004;88(3): 751–766.

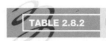

| TABLE 2.8.2 | Differential Diagnosis of Hypersomnia |

Intrinsic disorders (1, 2)	**Extrinsic disorders (2, 4)**

Narcolepsy with or without cataplexy
Posttraumatic hypersomnia
Obstructive sleep apnea
Restless legs syndrome
Periodic limb movement disorder
Parkinson's disease
Idiopathic hypersomnia
	Alcohol (decreases sleep latency and
	   causes rebound arousal in the middle of
	   the sleep cycle)
	Environmental factors causing poor sleep
	   (e.g., snoring spouse, loud noises)
	Sleep deprivation

Circadian rhythm sleep disorders (3)	**Medical and psychiatric diagnoses (2)**

Jet lag type
Delayed sleep phase type (more common in
   adolescents and young adults, usually very
   late bed times and late or midday wake
   times)
Advanced sleep phase type (more common in
   older adults, early bed time and early wake
   time)
Shift work type
	Alcoholism and substance abuse
	Alzheimer's disease and other dementias
	Anxiety disorders
	Chronic obstructive pulmonary disease
	Depressive disorders
	Gastroesophageal reflux
	Hypothyroidism
	Menopausal symptoms, "hot flashes"
	Obstructive sleep apnea
	Panic disorders
	Paroxysmal nocturnal dyspnea
	Central nervous system abnormalities
	   (rare)

    C. Testing. Intrinsic sleep disorders are best evaluated using a multiple sleep latency test (MSLT) and/or an overnight polysomnograph (1, 3). A sleep latency of <5 minutes is considered pathologic sleepiness (1, 3). The polysomnogram can detect excessive limb movement, sleep disordered breathing, apnea, and hypoxia (1).

IV. DIAGNOSIS
    A. Differential diagnosis. The differential diagnosis for hypersomnia is listed in Table 2.8.2.
    B. Clinical manifestations. Hypersomnia may present with significant fatigue, trouble with work or school performance, marital or relationship problems, accidents or personal injury (particularly with narcolepsy), and can be the first sign of dementia or other neurologic disorders.

References
1. Silber M, Krahn L, Morgenthaler T. *Sleep medicine in clinical practice.* London: Taylor & Francis, 2004.
2. Roth T, Kryger MH, Dement WC. *Principles and practice of sleep medicine,* 3rd ed. Philadelphia, PA: WB Saunders, 2000.
3. Doghramji K. Assessment of excessive sleepiness and insomnia as they relate to circadian rhythm sleep disorders. *J Clin Psychiatry* 2004;65(Suppl 16):17–22.
4. Qureshi A, Lee-Chiong T Jr. Medications and their effects on sleep. *Med Clin North Am* 2004;88(3):751–766.

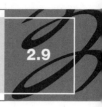

INSOMNIA
Jennifer J. Buescher

2.9

I. BACKGROUND. Insomnia is defined as a *persistent difficulty initiating and/or maintaining sleep* (1). Insomnia can be a primary syndrome; however, insomnia is more commonly a secondary symptom to underlying environmental, medical, or psychiatric disorders.

II. PATHOPHYSIOLOGY

 A. Etiology. Insomnia is caused by intrinsic disorders of the sleep-wake cycle and extrinsic factors affecting the quality or the timing of sleep. Depression, anxiety, and trauma can trigger insomnia, and over the years a perpetual cycle of poor sleep can continue even after the trigger is treated or removed (psychophysiological insomnia) (2). Poor sleep hygiene, a disruptive sleep environment, alcohol-dependence, and chronic use of hypnotics can also cause insomnia (2). Circadian rhythm disturbances (misalignment of sleep patterns with local time) (1) can present with the primary symptom of insomnia. Finally, many medical and psychiatric disorders can cause or be associated with insomnia.

 B. Epidemiology. As many as 33% of the general adult population report symptoms of insomnia, and between 9% and 21% report insomnia with serious daytime consequences (3). Insomnia is more prevalent in women and increases in prevalence with increasing age (4).

III. EVALUATION

 A. History. A thorough history should focus on determining the cause and duration of insomnia. Precipitating events such as emotional trauma, illness, stress, and prescription or other drug use should be explored with the patient and his or her bed partner.

  1. Sleep patterns. A thorough discussion of the patient's sleep pattern and the sleep patterns of other members of their household should include the timing and the content of evening meals, bedroom environment (temperature, noise, comfort of bed), work schedules, and sleep schedules (including daytime napping).

  2. Review of systems. The review of systems should pay special attention to common medical and psychologic problems that are associated with insomnia.

  3. Medications. Table 2.9.1 lists medications that can cause insomnia.

 B. Physical examination. The physical examination should focus on associated medical conditions associated with insomnia. In primary insomnia, the physical examination is likely to be normal.

 C. Testing. Laboratory and diagnostic testing is infrequently useful in the diagnosis of primary insomnia. Asking the patient to keep a 7 to 14 day sleep diary may help in determining extrinsic factors causing insomnia (4, 5). Polysomnography can assist in the diagnosis of some sleep disorders, including sleep apnea, restless leg syndrome and periodic limb movement disorder.

 D. Genetics. Fatal familial insomnia is a rare prion disease that tends to run in families. In general, insomnia is not assumed to be genetically inherited (2).

IV. DIAGNOSIS

 A. Differential diagnosis (see Table 2.9.2). The differential diagnosis of insomnia includes primary sleep disorders as well as medical, psychiatric, and environmental disturbances.

 B. Clinical manifestations. Insomnia can cause significant functional impairment, difficulty in work or school, and marital or relationship problems. Chronic sleep loss from untreated insomnia can cause fatigue-related accidents at work or while driving, job loss, decreased productivity, major depression, and suicidal

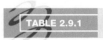

TABLE 2.9.1	Drugs that Cause Insomnia

Prescription drugs	**Nonprescription drugs**
Methylphenidate	Caffeine
Theophylline	Stimulant diet pills
Albuterol	Nicotine
Quinidine	Illicit drugs (e.g., cocaine,
Pemoline	amphetamines)
Dextroamphetamine	—
Pseudoephedrine	—
Phenylephrine	—
Phenylpropanolamine	—
Selective serotonin reuptake	—
inhibitors	—

Modified from Eddy M, Walbroehl GS. Insomnia. *Am Fam Physician* 1999;59(7):1911–1916,1918.

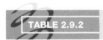

TABLE 2.9.2	Differential Diagnosis of Insomnia

Primary insomnia	**Extrinsic sleep disorders**
Psychophysiologic insomnia	Environmental sleep disorder (adverse
Sleep related disordered breathing	sleep environment)
Sleep apnea	Alcohol-dependent insomnia
Loud snoring	Hypnotic-dependent insomnia
Hypnosia	Illicit drug use
Asthma	**Associated medical and psychiatric**
Circadian rhythm sleep disorders	**conditions**
Jet lag type	Alzheimer's and other dementia
Delayed sleep phase type (more common in	Anxiety disorders
adolescents and young adults, usually very	Asthma
late bed times and late or midday wake	Chronic obstructive pulmonary disease
times)	Depressive disorders
Advanced sleep phase type (more common in	Gastroesophageal reflux
older adults, early bed time and early wake	Hyperthyroidism
time)	Mania
Shift work type	Nocturia
Environmental disruptions	Restless leg syndrome
Loud noises	Pain, acute, or chronic
Bed partner with sleep disorder	Parkinson's disease
Uncomfortable or unsafe sleeping conditions	Periodic limb movement disorder

Modified from Eddy M, Walbroehl GS. Insomnia. *Am Fam Physician* 1999;59(7):1911–1916,1918 and Silber M, Krahn L, Morgenthaler T. *Sleep medicine in clinical practice* London: Taylor & Francis; 2004.

ideation (3). Individuals with insomnia may present with generalized fatigue or daytime sleepiness, and a careful history can help elucidate possible underlying problems of insomnia.

References

1. Espie CA, Morin CM. *Insomnia a clinical guide to assessment and treatment.* 2003.
2. Silber M, Krahn L, Morgenthaler T. *Sleep medicine in clinical practice* London: Taylor & Francis, 2004.
3. Schenck CH, Mahowald MW, Sack RL. Assessment and management of insomnia. *JAMA* 2003;289(19):2475–2479.
4. National Heart, Lung, and Blood Institute Working Group on Insomnia. Insomnia: assessment and management in primary care. *Am Fam Physician* 1999;59(11):3029–3038.
5. Eddy M, Walbroehl GS. Insomnia. *Am Fam Physician* 1999;59(7):1911–1916,1918.

NAUSEA AND VOMITING
Jennifer J. Buescher

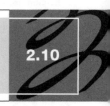

2.10

I. **BACKGROUND.** Nausea is a "vague, intensely disagreeable sensation of sickness or 'queasiness' that may or may not be followed by vomiting and is distinguished from anorexia" (1). Vomiting is the active and forceful expulsion of gastric contents.

II. **PATHOPHYSIOLOGY**

    A. **Etiology.** Nausea is a subjective symptom experienced in many of the disorders that also cause vomiting. Vomiting can result from the stimulation of one of four neurologic processes: (a) vagal and splanchnic fibers in the viscera, stimulated by distention, inflammatory irritation, or infection, (b) vestibular system fibers mediated through muscarinic cholinergic and histamine H_1 receptors, (c) higher central nervous system (CNS) centers where sights, sounds, or emotions can trigger vomiting, and (d) a chemoreceptor trigger zone within the brain that is rich in opioid, serotonergic, and dopamine receptors triggered by toxins, hypoxia, acidosis, radiation therapy, uremia, and chemotherapy (1).

    B. **Epidemiology.** Nausea and vomiting are common symptoms and frequently seen in outpatient, inpatient, and emergency settings.

III. **EVALUATION**

    A. **History.** A thorough history should discuss sleep habits, the onset and frequency of vomiting, the symptoms of other family members, and the relationship of nausea and vomiting to meals or types of food.

        1. A review of systems should specifically address associated anorexia, weight loss, abdominal pain, gastrointestinal (GI) symptoms, and neurologic symptoms. Vomiting prior to breakfast is more common in pregnancy, alcohol overuse, uremia, and increased intracranial pressure (1). Vomiting of undigested food one or more hours after meals should raise concern for gastric outlet obstruction or gastroparesis, whereas vomiting immediately after a meal is more common with psychogenic vomiting and bulimia (1).

        2. Many medications can induce nausea and/or vomiting, including nonsteroidal anti-inflammatory drugs, opiates, antibiotics, calcium channel blockers, anticonvulsants, antiparkinsonian agents, nicotine, β-blockers, digoxin, antiarrhythmics, alcohol, and chemotherapeutic agents (1,2).

    B. **Physical examination.** The physical examination should evaluate for acute dehydration and signs of infection. The abdominal exam should attempt to localize pain and evaluate for peptic ulcer disease, gallbladder disease, liver disease, or an acute abdomen.

  C. Testing. In severe acute or persistent vomiting, a flat and upright abdominal radiograph can help rule out GI obstruction or a perforated viscous (1). Barium radiography, an upper GI series, or abdominal computed tomography may be helpful in the diagnosis of gastric outlet obstruction or gastroparesis (1). Concerns for intracranial lesions should prompt computed tomography or magnetic resonance imaging of the brain. Based on the clinical assessment, blood tests, liver function, amylase, pregnancy testing, hepatitis testing, or a metabolic profile may be appropriate. For acute gastroenteritis that is not complicated by dehydration, laboratory tests are not necessary.

IV. DIAGNOSIS

  A. Differential diagnosis. The diagnosis of acute nausea and vomiting can often be made on clinical history alone (3). Chronic symptoms may be more difficult to diagnose and may require laboratory and diagnostic testing. Table 2.10.1 lists the differential diagnosis of nausea and vomiting.

  B. Clinical manifestations. Most patients with nausea and vomiting do not seek medical consultation and their disease is self-limiting (2). Persistent or severe nausea and vomiting can lead to severe weight loss, hypokalemia and other electrolyte disturbances, dehydration, and metabolic alkalosis (1, 3).

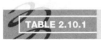 **TABLE 2.10.1**   Differential Diagnosis of Nausea and Vomiting

Infections
Viral: self-limiting
Bacterial: *Staphylococcus aureus,*
  Escherichia coli, Bacillus cereus,
  Clostridium perfringens, and
  Campylobacter, Helicobacter, Shigella,
  Salmonella, Vibrio organisms
Hepatitis A or B
Meningitis, encephalitis
Peritonitis: spontaneous bacterial
  peritonitis, appendicitis, perforated
  viscus
Pyelonephritis
Gastrointestinal irritation
Nonsteroidal anti-inflammatory drugs
Alcohol
Gastroesophageal reflux disease
Esophagitis
Obstruction
Gastric outlet obstruction: malignancy, gastric
  volvulus, peptic ulcer disease, pyloric
  stenosis (infants)
Small intestine obstruction: adhesions,
  volvulus, Crohn disease, hernia
Colon obstruction: tumors, constipation,
  obstipation

Dysmotility
Gastroparesis: diabetic, postviral,
  postvagotomy
Small intestine: scleroderma, amyloidosis
Vestibular and central nervous
system disorders
Labyrinthitis
Ménière's syndrome
Migraine headache
Motion sickness
Tumors: causing increased ICP
Intracranial hemorrhage (increased ICP)
Other
Acute pancreatitis
Adrenocortical crisis
Bulimia
Cholecystitis, choledocholelithiasis
Diabetic ketoacidosis
Nephrolithiasis
Pancreatitis
Psychogenic vomiting
Pregnancy
Uremia
Medications
Chemotherapy, radiation therapy
Postoperative nausea and vomiting

ICP, intracranial pressure.
Modified from McQuaid K. Alimentary tract. In: Tierney LJ, McPhee S, Papadakis M, eds. *Current medical diagnosis & treatment 2005.* New York, NY: McGraw-Hill; 2005.

References
1. McQuaid K. Alimentary Tract. In: Tierney LJ, McPhee S, Papadakis M, eds. *Current medical diagnosis & treatment 2005*. New York, NY: McGraw-Hill, 2005.
2. Spiller RC. ABC of the upper gastrointestinal tract: anorexia, nausea, vomiting, and pain. *Br Med J* 2001;323(7325):1354–1357.
3. American Gastroenterological Association. Medical position statement: nausea and vomiting. *Gastroenterology* 2001;120(1):261–263.

NIGHT SWEATS
Richard H. Hurd

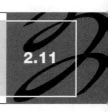

2.11

I. BACKGROUND. Night sweats are drenching sweats that require a change of bedding (1).

II. PATHOPHYSIOLOGY

   A. Etiology. Night sweats that are caused by fever represent a separate entity and are discussed in Chapter 2.6. Night sweats are likely to be an autonomic response to some physical or emotional condition, representing a rather nonspecific symptom that should prompt the clinician to seek a specific cause.

   B. Epidemiology. One study of approximately 800 patients in the practices of several primary care physicians indicated that about 10% were bothered to some degree by night sweats. Seventy percent of patients affected reported some trouble, 20% a fair amount of trouble, and 10% a great deal of trouble (2).

III. EVALUATION

   A. History

   1. It is helpful to characterize night sweats by determining the onset, frequency, exacerbations, and remissions of symptoms (3). The clinician must thoroughly explore any risk of exposure to infectious causes of night sweats. This history must include questions about behaviors that put the patient at risk of human immunodeficiency virus (HIV)-related infections, sexually transmitted diseases, hepatitis, and tuberculosis. Explorations of travel and occupational exposures should be carried out.

   2. The state of concurrent medical conditions must be determined. Changes in treatment modalities that are both physician driven as well as those initiated by the patient may be a causative factor for night sweats. All the patient's current and recently discontinued medications must be determined.

   3. A thorough review of the systems may point the clinician toward a primary disease that includes night sweats as a symptom. Psychologic factors that might precipitate night sweats in healthy individuals should be discussed.

   4. Interviewing the sleeping partner is an important source of information that must not be neglected. A history of snoring or apneic episodes may point to sleep apnea that has been reported to be a common cause of night sweats (4).

   B. Physical examination. The fact that night sweats in the absence of any other identifiable cause constitute a physically benign condition makes it imperative that a complete physical examination be carried out in an effort to determine the presence of any concurrent condition. The history may direct the physician toward a more detailed examination of a specific organ system; however, the knowledge that the cause may be multifactorial must be remembered, and no part of the physical examination should be neglected.

   C. Testing. The choice of laboratory tests is guided by the history. For those patients with known medical conditions, appropriate tests for exacerbations should be

	Causes of Night Sweats				
Malignancy	**Infectious**	**Endocrine**	**Rheumatologic**	**Drugs**	**Other**
Lymphoma	Human immun-odeficiency virus	Hyperthyroidism	Rheumatoid arthritis	—	Sleep apnea
Leukemia	Tuberculosis	Ovarian failure	Lupus	—	Gastroesophageal reflux disease
Other malignancy	Endocarditis	Diabetes mellitus	Juvenile rheumatoid arthritis	—	Angina
	Lung infections	Endocrine tumors	Temporal arteritis	—	Anxiety
	Other infection			—	Pregnancy
					Overbundling
					Extreme heat

carried out. The tests might include a complete blood count to assess the status of the infection, erythrocyte sedimentation rate, Hb A_{Ic}, and a C-reactive protein. A history of exposure might suggest an HIV test, a hepatitis panel, or a purified protein derivative skin test for tuberculosis. Thyroid function testing in individuals identified as at risk should also be carried out. Special testing may be required in individuals with travel-related exposure.

D. Genetics. There is not a reported familial cause of primary night sweats.

IV. DIAGNOSIS

A. Differential diagnosis. The diagnosis of night sweats is largely historical. See Table 2.11.1.

B. Clinical manifestations. Night sweats are most frequently a manifestation of an underlying illness. As such, the manifestation is most often a part of a much larger symptom complex. The diagnosis centers on discovering the underlying disease entity. When no cause is evident, watchful waiting is useful in an attempt to let the cause become more evident (5).

References

1. Smetana GW. Diagnosis of night sweats. *JAMA* 1993;70:2502–2503.
2. Mold JW, Roberts M, Aboshady H. Prevalence and predictors of night sweats, day sweats, and hot flashes in older primary care patients. *Am Fam Med* 2004;2(5):391–397.
3. Bajorek Mark. Night sweats, In: Robert Taylor, ed. *The 10-minute diagnosis manual.* Philadelphia, PA: Lippincott Williams & Wilkins, 2000:31–33.
4. Duhon DR. Night sweats: two other causes. *JAMA* 1994;271:1577.
5. Chambliss ML. Frequently asked questions from clinical practice. What is the appropriate diagnostic approach for patients who complain of night sweats? *Arch Fam Med* 1999;2:168–169.

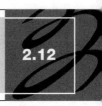

SYNCOPE
Roger Massie
2.12

I. **BACKGROUND.** Syncope is defined as a *transient loss of consciousness* with an inability to maintain a postural tone that is followed by spontaneous recovery. The term syncope excludes seizures, coma, shock, or other states of altered consciousness (1).

II. **PATHOPHYSIOLOGY**

   A. **Etiology.** Cardiac causes include vascular disease, cardiomyopathy, arrhythmias, or valvular dysfunction. Noncardiac causes include vasovagal response to pain, dehydration with orthostasis, situational syncope, dysfunction, although neurovascular causes are rare. Alternatively, the etiology may be unknown.

   B. **Epidemiology.** Syncope is a prevalent disorder, accounting for 1% to 3% of emergency department visits and up to 6% of hospital admissions each year in the United States (1). In the United States, the data from the Framingham study demonstrates a first occurrence rate of 6.2 cases/1,000 patient/year. Three percent have recurrences, and approximately 10% have a cardiac etiology (1).

III. **EVALUATION.** A thorough history and physical examination have been shown to establish the cause in up to 45% of patients. A 12-lead electrocardiogram (ECG) provides another 5% to 10% yield. However, after this initial examination, syncope remains unexplainable in 34% to 47% of patients (2).

   A. **History**

   1. A detailed account of the episode by the patient and from any person witnessing the episode is very important. Specifically, information about activity prior to the syncopal episode, including position or change in position, precipitating factors such as fatigue, alcohol consumption, strong emotions, hunger, and a warm environment should be elicited. Also, questions concerning prior dizziness, nausea, diaphoresis, chest pain, dyspnea, visual changes, headache, and focal neurologic changes should be asked. Finally, the patient and/or witness should be asked to estimate the total time of the syncopal episode.

   2. Past medical history should include a complete list of medications, whether they are prescription drugs, over-the-counter medications, street drugs, vitamins, and/or health supplements. In addition, the usual inquiry relating to disease states such as hypertension, coronary artery disease, diabetes mellitus, prior stroke, deep vein thrombosis, and anemia should be made. Also, if the patient is a woman of childbearing age, the possibility of pregnancy should be determined.

   3. It is important to specifically inquire about a family history of sudden death, heart disease, and diabetes mellitus, especially in first-degree relatives.

   B. **Physical examination.** A complete physical examination is always necessary when a patient presents with syncope. Vital signs including mental status should be obtained. Syncope as a presenting complaint always necessitates a head to toe examination; specifically looking for previous or present trauma, cardiac, pulmonary, abdominal, and/or neurologic abnormalities. Also, a rectal examination should be performed along with a test for occult blood.

   C. **Testing.** If a syncopal patient presents to the emergency department, an immediate finger stick blood sugar and/or ECG should be obtained, even as vital signs are taken. Then a complete blood count, comprehensive metabolic profile, cardiac enzymes, and a chest x-ray should be obtained. Later tests or conditions to consider if indicated by the history and the physical examination are:

   1. A test for pulmonary embolus or abdominal aortic aneurysm.

   2. A head-up tilt-table test which is useful for confirming autonomic dysfunction safety and can generally be arranged to be done as an outpatient.

   3. An electroencephalogram to be obtained if a seizure is suspected.

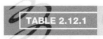

TABLE 2.12.1 Differential Diagnosis of Syncope	
Cardiac	**Noncardiac**
Bradydysrhythmia	Hypoglycemia
Cardiac myxoma	Orthostasis
Cardiac outflow obstruction	Drug toxicities–stimulants (amphetamines, cocaine)
Dysrhythmias	Antidepressants
Hypertrophic subaortic stenosis	β-Blockers
Paroxysmal supraventricular tachycardia	Calcium channel blockers
Paroxysmal ventricular tachycardia	Antidysrhythmics
Prolonged QT syndrome	Adrenal insufficiency and crisis
Sick sinus syndrome	Vasomotor
Aortic dissections	Dehydration
Atrial fibrillation	Hypovolemia whether due to hemorrhage or other factors
Heart blocks	Carotid sinus syncope
Myocardial infarction	Cough (post-tussive) syncope
Pulmonary embolism	Defecation syncope
	Micturition syncope
	Hyperventilation
	Migraine headache
	Narcolepsy
	Panic attacks
	Seizure disorders

IV. DIAGNOSIS. The differential diagnosis of syncope is presented in Table 2.12.1.

References

1. Hongo RH, Goldschlager N. *Evaluating patients with unexplained syncope* MED-SCAPE, 11/2004.
2. Morag R. *emedicine.com—Syncope excerpt* June 2005.

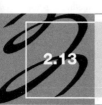

WEIGHT LOSS
2.13
Amy K. Jespersen

I. **BACKGROUND.** Unintentional weight loss is generally considered to be significant when greater than 5% of body weight is lost over a period of 6 months or less. It is often associated with increased morbidity and mortality especially among the elderly. Perceived weight loss should be verified before initiating a workup, because 50% of patients with perceived weight loss do not have true weight loss. Of patients with confirmed weight loss, an explanation is generally found in 75% of cases. In 25% of patients an explanation is never found. If a physical cause is present, it is usually discovered within 6 months (1–3).

II. **PATHOPHYSIOLOGY.** The various conditions that cause unintentional weight loss do so through one or more of the following mechanisms: inadequate caloric intake, excessive metabolic demands, or loss of nutrients through urine or stool. Other conditions that cause weight loss include:

A. Malignant conditions. Cancer is often the patient's or physician's greatest fear. Malignancy is the cause for unintentional weight loss in 16% to 36% of cases (1–3). Although any cancer can cause weight loss, the more common malignancies to consider are gastrointestinal (GI), leukemia or lymphoma, lung, ovarian, and prostate cancers.

B. Benign medical conditions. Many chronic medical conditions can cause anorexia, nausea, diarrhea, or postprandial symptoms which discourage the patient from eating. Medical conditions may also necessitate limiting salt, fat, or sugar in the diet, leaving the patient less inclined to eat.

   1. GI disorders account for the most common physical cause of weight loss affecting approximately 17% of patients (4). These include:

      a. Peptic ulcer disease/gastroesophageal reflux disease

      b. Inflammatory bowel disease

      c. Hepatitis, cholestasis

      d. Pancreatitis

      e. Atrophic gastritis

      f. Constipation.

   2. Cardiac diseases, especially congestive heart failure.

   3. Respiratory diseases, such as chronic obstructive pulmonary disease.

   4. Renal disease.

   5. Neuromuscular disorders may affect the ability to swallow. These include:

      a. Scleroderma

      b. Polymyositis

      c. Systemic lupus erythematosus.

   6. Endocrine disorders can increase metabolic rate or cause nutrient loss. These include:

      a. Hyperthyroidism

      b. Diabetes mellitus

      c. Other causes, such as pheochromocytoma, panhypopituitarism, adrenal insufficiency, and hyperthyroidism.

   7. Infection, especially tuberculosis, fungal disease, subacute bacterial endocarditis, and any prolonged febrile illness can decrease appetite and increase metabolic demand. Human immunodeficiency virus infection is a special consideration with patients having multiple causes for weight loss.

   8. Neurologic conditions (e.g., dementia, Parkinson's disease, stroke) can cause weight loss secondary to apathy, decreased appetite, or difficulty swallowing.

   9. Medications can cause anorexia, nausea, abdominal pain, or diarrhea, or inhibit gastric emptying.

C. Psychiatric causes. These are responsible for weight loss in 10% to 20% of patients (1–3).

   1. Depression is the most common psychiatric cause.

   2. Substance abuse, especially alcoholism, and bereavement are other causes.

D. Social and age related causes. These include the following:

   1. Financial hardship.

   2. Diminished sense of taste and smell.

   3. Functional inability to shop or prepare food.

   4. Poor dentition.

III. EVALUATION

A. History. A detailed history should be obtained from the patient and caregivers if applicable. Special attention should be given to the types and quantity of food consumed; alcohol use; history of cigarette smoking (current and remote); exercise patterns; medications; presence of nausea, vomiting, diarrhea, early satiety, difficulty swallowing; history of GI illnesses or previous abdominal surgery; cardiac history; respiratory history; history of kidney disease; depressive symptoms; social situation, including financial resources; and functional ability to shop for groceries and prepare meals.

B. Physical examination

   1. Document weight and compare it to previous weights.

   2. Perform a thorough physical examination, paying special attention to an oral examination, especially dentition; a respiratory examination; a cardiac examination; a GI examination; a psychologic examination; and an evaluation of cognitive function, especially if the patient is elderly.

C. Testing. Extensive undirected laboratory testing is not indicated and is rarely helpful.

   1. Initial laboratory tests should include:

     a. Complete blood count

     b. Comprehensive metabolic profile

     c. Thyroid-stimulating hormone

     d. Urinalysis

     e. Fecal occult blood testing.

   2. Other laboratory tests as indicated by history or physical examination may include:

     a. Chest x-ray, which may be helpful, especially with a history of cigarette smoking, or a new or different cough or dyspnea.

     b. Appropriate age and gender based screening (e.g., mammography, colonoscopy).

     c. Other tests as indicated by history (e.g., upper GI endoscopy).

IV. DIAGNOSIS. Diagnosis of weight loss is made by verifying that a loss of more than 5% of body weight has occurred. A thorough history and physical examination and directed laboratory and ancillary tests result in an explanation approximately 75% of the time. Malignancy is the cause of weight loss in 16% to 36% of cases. Psychiatric causes, usually depression, is the cause in 10% to 20% of the cases. An organic cause other than malignancy is present in 30% to 50% of cases. Twenty-five percent of the time no identifiable cause is found. If a physical cause is responsible, but not identified on initial workup, it usually becomes evident within 6 months (4).

References

1. Marton KE, Sox HC Jr, Krupp JR. Involuntary weight loss: diagnostic and prognostic significance. *Ann Intern Med* 1981;95:568–574.
2. Rabinovitz M, Pitlik SD, Leifer M, et al. Unintentional weight loss. A retrospective analysis of 154 cases. *Arch Intern Med* 1986;146:186–187.
3. Thompson MP, Morris LK. Unexplained weight loss in the ambulatory elderly. *J Am Geriatr Soc* 1991;39:497–500.
4. Huffman GB. Evaluating and treating unintentional weight loss in the elderly. *Am Fam Physician* 2002;65:640–650.

Mental Health Problems

Jim Medder

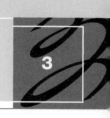

3

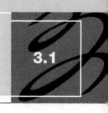
ANXIETY

Layne A. Prest

3.1

I. BACKGROUND. The experience of anxiety is ubiquitous in society. Anxiety can be part of an adaptive or protective response to threat (e.g., the fight-freeze-flight response) or a natural reaction to physical and emotional stress, but it can also be debilitating and a serious health concern. At its core, anxiety is a complex bio-psychosocial-spiritual experience that requires comprehensive assessment and treatment. Undiagnosed anxiety disorders contribute to inappropriate or overutilization of healthcare resources, but as many as 80% of the individuals with anxiety disorders can be significantly helped through appropriate treatment.

II. PATHOPHYSIOLOGY

A. Etiology. Many factors contribute to both the development and experience of anxiety. These include genetic/neurologic predisposition, family history, acute and chronic stressors, resources for coping, comorbid conditions, and overall physical health. Extreme anxiety responses, known as *anxiety disorders*, are often comorbid with mood disorders or other chronic health conditions (e.g., coronary artery disease, cancer). These disorders usually include debilitating physical and emotional symptoms and may be due, at least in part, to primary medical problems such as hyperthyroidism or hypoxia. Consequently, anxious patients present to the emergency room or primary care setting with complaints that can be difficult to assess and diagnose.

B. Epidemiology. According to the National Institute of Mental Health (NIMH), 19 million Americans experience an anxiety disorder at any one time. Estimates of the prevalence of the various anxiety disorders vary from study to study but generally are as follows: generalized anxiety disorder (GAD)—4 million, 2.8% (women twice as likely as men); obsessive compulsive disorder—3.3 million, 2.3% (equally common among men and women); panic disorder—2.4 million, 1.7% (women twice as likely); posttraumatic stress disorder—5.2 million, 3.6% (women more likely than men); social anxiety disorder—5.3 million, 3.7% (equally common among men and women); and specific phobia—6.3 million, 4.4% (women twice as likely as men). The various anxiety disorders affect approximately 10% of primary care patients (1).

III. EVALUATION

A. History

1. Patients with anxiety disorders frequently describe experiencing physical symptoms such as chest pain, dizziness, palpitations, fatigue, shortness of breath, sweating, muscle aches or tension, or a variety of gastrointestinal complaints. Common psychologic symptoms can include shakiness, nervousness, fear of dying or going crazy, or a sense of unreality or detachment from oneself.

2. Some patients attribute their anxiety to their physical symptoms ("Of course, I was anxious. I thought I was having a heart attack"). Consequently, the assessment of anxiety disorders should include the nature, frequency, and duration of the preceding symptoms and the extent to which the symptoms have impacted the individual's life and activity.

3. The patient should also be asked about precipitants of the symptoms, including stressors, medications (e.g., stimulants), and other drug use (e.g., caffeine, cocaine).

4. Questions about the patient's general medical condition are also appropriate.

B. Physical examination. As with all patients, those whose clinical picture is suspected of including a significant component of anxiety should be examined carefully.

The extent of the physical examination should be dictated by the patient's personal health and medical history.

1. The examination may include the following: blood pressure (hypertension, hypovolemia), cardiovascular (angina, arrhythmia, congestive heart failure, valvular heart disease), respiratory (chronic obstructive lung disease, pulmonary embolism, pneumonia), and neurologic (tumor, encephalopathy, vertigo).

2. Patients frequently present with nervous agitation, intermittent eye contact, somewhat pressured speech, and, in the primary care context, a worried focus on the somatic concerns described in the preceding text.

C. **Testing.** Useful laboratory tests include serum calcium (hypocalcemia), hematocrit (anemia), and thyroid-stimulating hormone (hyperthyroidism/hypothyroidism). Depending on the clinical scenario, an exercise stress test to evaluate chest pain or other tests to rule out organic causes (such as drug screen, oximetry (hypoxia), glucose (hypoglycemia), and electrolytes) may be useful as well.

IV. DIAGNOSIS

A. Differential diagnosis

1. GAD is characterized by persistent and excessive worry about a number of issues on most days for a period of at least six months. GAD usually begins by early adulthood, is exacerbated by situational stressors, and usually involves a combination of psychologic and physical symptoms.

2. Panic disorder, with or without agoraphobia, presents with recurrent panic attacks—discrete episodes of anxiety involving shortness of breath, fear of dying, impending doom or losing control, pounding heart, sweating, chest pain, paresthesias, trembling, and nausea. The panic attacks may be provoked by identifiable stressors or situations but often seem to "come out of the blue." Individuals with panic disorder may be so fearful of being in a situation in which they have another panic attack and are unable to escape that they develop agoraphobia (an intense fear of being in open or crowded places, which often contributes to the individuals being reluctant to leave the perceived safety of their home).

3. Acute stress disorder (ASD) and Posttraumatic stress disorder (PTSD) are characterized by reexperiencing (through recollections, flashbacks, nightmares) an extremely traumatic and possibly life-threatening experience (e.g., rape, murder, motor-vehicle accident, war), followed by hyper-arousal, panic, depressed mood, sleep disturbance, and hyper-vigilance. The individual usually attempts to avoid these memories or the chance of being in danger again through numbing, dissociation, repression, and behavioral changes. The main distinction between ASD and PTSD is the duration of symptoms (i.e., in PTSD symptoms last longer than one month).

4. Specific phobia is excessive anxiety provoked by exposure to a specific feared object or situation. Common phobias include fear of animals or insects, natural environment (e.g., heights, storms, water), blood-injection-injury, or situations (e.g., tunnels, bridges, elevators, flying, driving).

5. Social phobia is an excessive anxiety provoked by exposure to social or performance situations and unfamiliar individuals or surroundings. As a result, individuals with social phobia avoid these types of situations.

6. Obsessive-compulsive disorder is characterized by obsessions that cause anxiety (e.g., germs on hands) and compulsions (behaviors aimed at reducing the anxiety such as hand-washing). The obsessions usually fall into one or more of the following categories: infection/contagion, safety, religiosity, sexuality, death/dying, orderliness.

7. Adjustment reaction with anxious features is a condition in which a patient experiences significant anxiety in reaction to a specific stressor such as a major life event or interpersonal conflict. To qualify for this diagnosis, the level of anxiety should be assessed as being more than expected under the circumstances. In addition to these conditions, the clinician should investigate the possibility of mood, substance abuse, and other psychiatric disorders (2).

B. **Clinical manifestations.** Most anxious patients present in the primary care setting with a primary focus on their bodies and somatic symptoms rather than "their minds." But inevitably there is a significant component of worry, fear, apprehension, and so on in the background. Because an exclusive focus on physical complaints (e.g., chest pain, dizziness) can obscure the diagnosis, it is important to ask patients about their psychologic state, living situation, and current stressors, as well as evaluate them for underlying medical issues.

References

1. American Anxiety Disorders Association. Silver Spring, MD. Available at: www.adaa. org, accessed on July 20, 2005.
2. American Psychiatric Association. *Diagnostic and statistical manual of mental disorders*, 4th ed. Washington, DC: American Psychiatric Association, 1994.

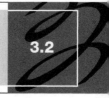

DEPRESSION
W. David Robinson

3.2

I. BACKGROUND

A. Definition. Depression is an illness that affects the mind, body, mood, thoughts, and relationships. It is not just unhappiness but an overwhelming sense of sadness and physical decline that has potential far-reaching deleterious effects.

B. Cost. Depression costs the United States billions of dollars annually in lost productivity and direct medical costs. Health service costs are 50% to 100% greater for depressed patients compared to patients without depression. These increased costs are due to higher medical utilization and not due to speciality mental health care (1). Depression also contributes to impaired concentration, failure to advance in education and vocational endeavors, increased substance abuse, impaired or lost relationships, and increased risk of suicide (2).

II. PATHOPHYSIOLOGY

A. Etiology. The biopsychosocial model is an effective way to conceptualize the etiology of anxiety and depression because the factors that create anxiety and depression are varied. The interplay between the biologic, psychological, and social aspects of the particular patient should be assessed to determine the etiology of the disease.

1. Biologic. There is ample information suggesting that genetics plays a role in the development of mood disorders. Studies related to twins have shown that the rate of mood disorders in identical twins is 67% to 76% but only 19% in fraternal twins (3). Women are at least twice as likely to suffer from depression as men. Individuals with a family history of mood disorders are at a higher risk of developing a disorder themselves. Other important biological factors include comorbidities or depression as a result of medical problems and abuse of substances, which may be either the cause or the symptom of the depression.

2. Psychological. Individuals who are continually under a great deal of stress, have a negative outlook on life, or a passive temperament are more likely to suffer from a mood disorder. These individuals often engage in cognitive distortions, including unrealistic expectations, overgeneralizing adverse events, personalizing negative or difficult events, and overreacting to stressors. Behaviorally, individuals who are continually under stress often believe that any action on their part would be futile, and therefore they continue to repeat self-defeating or problematic behaviors or do nothing at all (learned helplessness).

3. Social. There are many social influences that are related to mood disorders. These include difficult marriages, divorce, problems with children, family and community violence, and economic difficulties. Many individuals do not have the social resources (e.g., friendships, family, community) or buffers that aid in coping (e.g., spirituality).

B. **Epidemiology.** Depression is one of the most common conditions seen in primary care. Reliable estimates suggest that depressive symptoms are present in approximately 70% of patients who visit primary care providers with approximately 15% to 20% of these patients suffering from major depression (4). The prevalence of major depression is two to three times higher in general medical practice than in the overall population. However, physicians often underdiagnose patients with depression. Even among patients correctly diagnosed, most patients with depression still do not receive treatment concordant with recommended guidelines. Further, patient adherence to the recommended treatment plan is low (5).

III. EVALUATION

A. **History.** To be diagnosed with major depression, an individual must have experienced over the same two-week period five or more symptoms and must have depressed mood and/or anhedonia. The mnemonic SIGECAPS highlights the symptoms of a major depressive episode:

1. **S**leep disturbance—early morning awakenings or restless sleep
2. **I**nterest—little interest in activities they used to enjoy (anhedonia)
3. **G**uilt—feeling guilty or worthless
4. **E**nergy—feeling tired or fatigued
5. **C**oncentration—impaired concentration and/or indecisiveness
6. **A**ppetite—weight change and/or changes in their normal eating patterns (eating less or more than usual)
7. **P**sychomotor disturbance—any psychomotor agitation or retardation
8. **S**uicidal thoughts—recurrent thoughts of death, suicidal ideation, and suicide attempt.

B. **Physical examination.** Any patient with depression severe enough to warrant treatment should have both a general screening physical examination (paying particular attention to signs of anemia and endocrinopathies [e.g., hypothyroidism]) and a careful screening neurologic examination. Depression is also often a symptom of many medical conditions that are related to depressive disorders (e.g., cardiovascular disease, multiple sclerosis, cancer, thyroid disorders, acquired immunodeficiency syndrome, endocrine changes).

C. **Testing.** Laboratory tests should be ordered on the basis of the history and examination findings (e.g., complete blood count for anemia, thyroid-stimulating hormone for thyroid disorders).

1. Multiple screening instruments can be used to detect depression (i.e., Zung, Beck depression inventory). A relatively new screening tool that has been found to be efficient and effective in determining depression severity is the Patient Health Questionnaire-9 (PHQ-9) (6). The PHQ-9 is a screening questionnaire chosen because of the ease of administration, scoring, and its high sensitivity/specificity. The PHQ-9 is a 9-question form that addresses all the symptoms of major depression (6). Questions are answered using a 4-point-Likert scale (0 = not at all and 3 = nearly everyday). Scores of 5 to 9 are associated with mild depression, and scores of 10 or above are associated with moderate or severe depression (7).

2. The U. S. Preventive Services Task Force (8) recommends screening adults for depression in clinical practice. A quick two question screen for depression can be used to identify individuals at risk: over the past two weeks have you (a) felt down, depressed, or hopeless? and (b) felt little interest or pleasure in doing things? If an individual answers yes to one or both of these, he/she should be further evaluated for depression.

IV. DIAGNOSIS

A. **Differential diagnosis**

1. In addition to the medical conditions related to depression discussed earlier, each individual suspected of depression should also be screened for anxiety disorders, alcohol and drug abuse, suicidality, homicidality, and domestic violence or perpetration of abuse.

2. There are many types of depressive disorders. It is important to distinguish the specific type of disorder so as to most effectively recommend treatment options.
   a. Major Depressive Disorder is present when the individual has two or more major depressive episodes.
   b. Dysthymic Disorder is characterized by at least two years of low-grade depression
      (does not meet the criteria for a major depressive episode).
   c. Depressive Disorder Not Otherwise Specified is used when the individual does not meet criteria for other depressive conditions, but depressive features exist.
   d. Bipolar I Disorder is characterized by one or more manic episodes and is usually accompanied by major depressive episodes. It is important to rule out mania in individuals who are depressed because psychopharmalogical treatment of depression can make individuals with Bipolar disorder become manic. Manic episodes must include at least three of the following symptoms lasting for a period of at least seven days:
      i. inflated self-esteem or grandiosity
      ii. decreased need for sleep
      iii. more talkative than usual or pressure to keep talking
      iv. flight of ideas or subjective experience of thoughts racing
      v. distractibility
      vi. increase in goal-directed activity (socially, at work, or sexually) or psychomotor agitation
      vii. excessive involvement in pleasurable activities that have a high potential for painful consequences (e.g., spending, gambling, sexual indiscretions).
   e. Bipolar II Disorder is characterized by one or more major depressive episodes and at least one hypomanic episode (lasting at least four days). Hypomanic episodes use the same criteria as manic episodes, but hypomania does not cause marked impairment in social or occupational functioning or require hospitalization.
   f. Cyclothymic Disorder is characterized by at least two years of numerous periods of low-grade depression and hypomanic symptoms.
   g. Mood Disorder Due to a General Medical Condition and Substance-Induced Mood Disorder are characterized by a mood disturbance caused by the direct physiological consequence of either a general medical condition or substance use, respectively.
   h. Seasonal Affective Disorder, Grief Reaction, and Adjustment Disorder with Depressed Mood are other disorders that are caused by the time of the year, response to loss, and response to a significant change (e.g., divorce), respectively.

B. Clinical manifestations
   1. Depression does not often present in a primary care setting by the patient complaining of depressed mood. More likely the patient will discuss the symptoms of depression (e.g., fatigue, insomnia, gastrointestinal upset). It is therefore important for the physician to not only attend to the physical complaints but also probe into the emotional symptoms (e.g., dysphoria, anhedonia).
   2. The treatment of depressive disorders is important. On the basis of the biopsychosocial model, treatment modalities that address the biologic, psychological, and social aspects of the individual difficulties have been found to be the most effective. Creating a treatment plan tailored to the individuals' needs, including addressing the use of psychotherapy (cognitive-behavioral or interpersonal), marital therapy, medication, and exercise, have been found to be most effective.

References
1. Henk HJ, Katzelnick DJ, Kobak KA, et al. Medical costs attributed to depression among patients with a history of high medical expenses in a health maintenance organization. *Arch Gen Psychiatry* 1996;53(10):899–904.

2. Pincus HA, Pettit AR. The societal costs of chronic major depression. *J Clin Psychiatry* 2001;62(S6):5–9.
3. Papolos D, Papolos J. *Overcoming depression*, 3rd ed. New York: HarperCollins, 1997.
4. Montano CB, Montano MB. *A new paradigm for treating depression in the primary care setting. Medical Education Collaborative*, at: http://www.medscape.com, accessed on October 10, 2004.
5. Young AS, Klap R, Sherbourne CD, et al. The quality of care for depressive and anxiety disorders in the United States. *Arch Gen Psychiatry* 2001;58(1):55–61.
6. Kroenke K, Spitzer RL, Williams JBW. Validity of a brief depression severity measure. *J Gen Intern Med* 2001;16(9):606–613.
7. The MacArthur Initiative on Depression and Primary Care. Tool Kit, at: http://www.depression-primarycare.org, accessed on July 22, 2005.
8. U. S. Preventive Services Task Force. Screening for depression: recommendations and rationale. *Ann Intern Med* 2002;136(10):760–764.

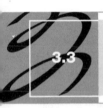

SUICIDE RISK

Heath A. Grames

3.3

I. BACKGROUND. Suicide is ranked as the 11th leading cause of death in the general US population and the 3rd leading cause of death for adolescents and young adults from age 15 to 24 years (1). Although the risk of suicide can be difficult to assess and predict because of the number of factors that contribute to such a decision, an understanding of the risk factors and assessment questions may prevent this tragic event. Many patients visit their primary care provider (PCP) some months before attempting suicide (2). If the red flags of suicidal ideation are present and recognized by the PCP, an opportunity is created for positive intervention to prevent suicide attempts.

II. PATHOPHYSIOLOGY

A. Etiology. Suicide is a topic that receives much attention through media and other platforms of discussion—perhaps because suicide is often viewed as a moral decision that is contrary to many religious and societal values. However, for many individuals who attempt or commit suicide, their quality of life (physical, emotional, and/or spiritual) has become so depleted that they may see no other options. Many factors contribute to a low level of quality of life and, therefore, the decision to take one's own life. Both physical and psychiatric disorders are recognized as being among these factors. Physical contributors include chronic illness and changes in neurotransmitters (i.e., serotonin) (1). Psychiatric disorders include major depression, substance abuse, schizophrenia, panic disorder, and borderline personality disorder (3). Other factors include a history of suicide attempts by the individual or close relatives and friends, violence at home, history of physical or sexual abuse, ownership of a firearm, history of family mental illness, a recent crisis (i.e., loss of income, divorce), illness, and old age. In addition, hopelessness, hostility, negative self-esteem, and isolation have been identified as suicide risk factors in adolescents (4).

B. Epidemiology. The most current data on suicide rates posted by the National Institute of Mental Health (NIMH) from 2001 show that 30,622 individuals died by suicide in the United States that year. To put this in perspective, this is higher than the number of individuals who died by homicide by a ratio of three to two and twice as many as those who died from complications from human immunodeficiency virus/acquired immunodeficiency syndrome. The highest risk population for committing suicide is white men age 85 and over (54 deaths by suicide per

100,000), which is five times greater than the general population (10.7/100,000). Among children, adolescents, and young adults, the latter are at slightly greater risk of committing suicide (12/100,000) than the national average. Among all age-groups, men are more likely to commit suicide than are women (4:1), but women are reported to have made more suicide attempts. White men are most likely to commit suicide, accounting for 73% of all deaths by suicide. Firearms are the most common mode of suicide by both men and women (1).

III. EVALUATION. One of the best precautions a PCP can take to assess for suicidal risk is completing a brief history with patients, asking about the previously mentioned risk factors. Although it is not necessary to exhaustively interview all patients, everyone who has any suicide risk factors should be queried about these issues.

A. History. Patients rarely talk to their PCPs about suicidal thoughts or past attempts. In fact, patients rarely bring up issues that may reveal risk factors for suicide (e.g., depression) without being asked directly. Instead, they often discuss the physical manifestations such as headaches, muscle pain, and insomnia. To assess for suicidal ideation, the PCP must ask patients specific questions to uncover their intentions. Patients at greater risk for suicidal ideation or attempts should be assessed for current thought of harming themselves. This can be done easily as part of an assessment for depression such as the Patient Health Questionnaire-9 (PHQ-9) (5) or by simply asking the patients if they are experiencing thoughts of harming themselves. Some PCPs may feel hesitant to ask such a direct question pertaining to suicide for fear that they may be planting an idea in a patient who is already struggling. However, no research has suggested that a patient may kill himself or herself simply because of being asked about thoughts of suicide. On the contrary, at-risk patients must be asked about suicidal thoughts and behavior so that appropriate measures can be taken.

B. Assessment

1. If patients have thoughts of suicide and a plan for the same, the PCP should determine how serious the individual is about carrying out the plans of suicide and the time frame for the suicide attempt. *Level of seriousness* in carrying out suicide plans can be assessed by asking patients if they have told other individuals of the plan to commit suicide and the details of the plan and by asking patients directly how serious they are about actually harming themselves. Also, the PCP should distinguish between a realistic and unrealistic plan to commit suicide. A *realistic* plan refers to a plan where the individual has the access and means to complete a suicide such as a patient who threatens to overdose on a medication that may have been prescribed. An *unrealistic* plan refers to a plan that is based on unlikely or impossible means of fulfilling suicidal desires. For example, a patient may state that he wants to shoot himself but does not own a gun, does not know someone who owns a gun, cannot purchase a gun, and does not consider other more realistic means of suicide to which he has access. Although this patient merits concern and in need of a suicide management plan, he may be in less immediate danger than the patient who has developed a realistic and accessible means to end his life. Determining if the plan is realistic or not gives insight into how likely the individual is to commit suicide.

2. To determine the *suicide attempt time frame*, patients should be asked when they plan to attempt suicide and estimate how likely they are to attempt suicide before the next visit to the physician. The answer to these questions should carry weight in determining the level of management. For example, a patient may be very depressed, state a realistic plan of suicide, and offer little reason to live but then say that he will not attempt until his three-year-old child has graduated from high school. Although this individual should receive help, he may not be in immediate danger for suicide.

C. Risk. On the basis of your assessment, a patient's *level of risk* is determined. For example, a patient who reports that she has had thoughts that she would be better off dead, or even of actually harming herself, but says she has never nor will ever attempt suicide due to personal and religious beliefs and because of family commitments, is different from the patient who reports that he owns firearms, has attempted suicide in the past, and can give no reason for living. Patients may be classified as being in *minimal, moderate, or severe risk*, and the treatment should be in direct relationship to how the patient is classified.

1. The *minimal* risk category includes patients who have experienced thoughts of self harm but have no specific plan, no history of past attempts, and who state that they would not actually attempt suicide. These are patients who can offer reasons to continue living or at least are active with the PCP in developing a safety plan.

2. *Moderate* risk patients include individuals who have considered a suicide plan (which may or may not be realistic), but say that they do not think they could actually harm themselves. Moderate risk patients may have made attempts in the distant past but are willing to create a safety plan and explore reasons to live.

3. *Severe* risk patients have a specific plan that is realistic and state that they will attempt suicide or will not commit to a no–suicide contract, even for a short duration. These individuals may or may not have a history of past attempts but are at greater risk if they have attempted in the past.

IV. DIAGNOSIS. If a patient responds that they are considering suicide, the suicide assessment becomes the primary focus of the medical appointment. A full assessment and creating a safety plan or admission to the hospital may take as little as ten minutes, or it may take more, depending on staff training and treatment accessibility.

References

1. National Institute of Mental Health. *In harm's way: suicide in America*. Revised ed. [Brochure]. Bethesda, MD: US Department of Health and Human Services, 2003.
2. Murphy GE. The physician's responsibility for suicide. I. An error of commission. *Ann Intern Med* 1975;82:301–304.
3. Gliatto MF, Rai AK. Evaluation and treatment of patients with suicidal ideation. *Am Fam Physician* 1999;59:1500–1506.
4. Rutter PA, Behrendt AE. Adolescent suicide risk: four psychological factors. *Adolescence* 2004;39:295–302.
5. The MacArthur Initiative on Depression and Primary Care. Tool Kit, at: http://www.depression-primarycare.org, accessed on July 25, 2005.

Problems Related to the Nervous System

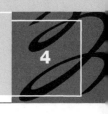

4

Michael A. Myers

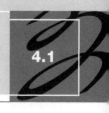

ATAXIA
Robert R. Rauner

4.1

I. BACKGROUND. Ataxia is the loss of the ability to coordinate muscular movement.

II. PATHOPHYSIOLOGY

A. Etiology. Ataxia is caused by the dysfunction of the cerebellum and its afferent and efferent pathways. Ataxia has a broad list of causes, including:

1. Drugs, such as alcohol, barbiturates, lithium, or chemotherapeutic drugs
2. Toxins, such as mercury, solvents, lead, gasoline, or glue
3. Infections, such as coxsackievirus, human immunodeficiency virus (HIV), *Legionella*, Lyme disease, or varicella
4. Nutritional conditions, such as vitamin B_1, B_{12}, or E deficiency
5. Endocrine conditions, such as hypothyroidism
6. Vascular conditions, such as cerebellar infarction or hemorrhage
7. Hereditary conditions, such as Friedreich's ataxia, ataxia telangiectasia, or Machado-Joseph (SCA-3)
8. Neoplastic conditions, such as cerebellar glioma, metastatic tumors, or paraneoplastic syndromes
9. Congenital conditions, such as Chiari or Dandy-Walker malformations (1).

B. Epidemiology. Friedreich's ataxia is the most common cause of hereditary ataxia, constituting about half of hereditary ataxias. The incidence of Friedreich's ataxia is approximately 1 to 2 per 50,000 in the United States (2).

III. EVALUATION

A. History. The history should include time of onset of the development of ataxia, whether it is symmetric or asymmetric, and whether it is focal or diffuse. A gradual onset with symmetric and bilateral symptoms suggests a biochemical, immune, metabolic, or toxic cause. Focal and asymmetric ataxias with other symptoms such as headaches and cranial nerve palsies suggest a cerebellar mass. The history should also include questioning regarding medications that can cause ataxia (e.g., lithium), exposure to toxins (e.g., mercury), and history of ethanol intake. The age of onset can be helpful in differentiating some of the hereditary ataxias. The patient should be questioned about recent or chronic infections because there are several that can cause ataxia (e.g., varicella, Lyme disease, or HIV).

B. Physical examination. The examination should include an evaluation of the type of ataxia. The patient's speech should be observed for difficulties such as dysarthria or scanning speech. The patient's gait should be observed. Eye movements should be examined for nystagmus or cranial nerve palsies. The patient's movements should be evaluated for tremor, loss of proprioception, weakness, loss of fine motor control, spasticity, rigidity, bradykinesia, and dystonia. In addition, the history and physical examination should search for other problems that can mimic ataxia from cerebellar causes, such as vertigo from vestibular disease, or difficulties in gait that are actually due to leg weakness (1,2).

C. Testing

1. Computed tomography or magnetic resonance imaging (MRI) of the brain (preferably MRI) to evaluate for causes such as a neoplasm, hemorrhage, or infarction. This should be done as soon as possible, because some causes may be surgical emergencies (e.g., mass effect leading to brain stem herniation).
2. Many other causes may be discovered by laboratory testing. Possible tests include thyroid-stimulating hormone, vitamin B_1 and vitamin B_{12} levels, HIV,

53

rapid plasma reagin, Lyme, and toxicology. Antibodies to Yo, Ri, and PCD may be present in paraneoplastic syndromes. In children, screening for inherited metabolic disorders may be warranted.

3. Lumbar puncture may be helpful for diagnosing causes such as multiple sclerosis, viral cerebellitis, and other infections. An electroencephalogram may reveal seizure-related ataxia (1).

D. Genetics. There is a long list of hereditary ataxias. The most common of these is Friedreich's ataxia. The hereditary ataxias are subdivided by the mode of inheritance. The most common are autosomal recessive (e.g., Friedreich's ataxia). Autosomal dominant ataxias are classified by a sequential numbering system (e.g., SCA-3 which is most common in the United States). There are also X-linked and mitochondrial forms of hereditary ataxias (2).

IV. DIAGNOSIS

A. Differential diagnosis. Ataxia has diverse causes, ranging from toxins (e.g., mercury), infections (e.g., Lyme disease), and neoplasms to hereditary degenerative causes (e.g., Friedreich's ataxia) (1). Friedreich's ataxia usually starts before 25 years of age. It most commonly presents with lower extremity symptoms including gait disturbances, diminishing reflexes, and loss of proprioception. Other symptoms (which can occasionally be presenting symptoms) include dysarthria, scoliosis, nystagmus, and foot deformities. Approximately 25% of patients have hypertrophic cardiomyopathy and 10% have diabetes mellitus (1, 2).

B. Clinical manifestations. The speed of the onset and the type of symptoms (symmetric vs. focal) can be very helpful in diagnosing the cause of ataxia.

1. A common example of acute symmetric ataxia is alcohol intoxication with its clumsiness, slurred speech, unbalanced gait, nystagmus, and inaccurate finger-to-nose testing. An acute and symmetrical onset would lead a clinician to suspect drugs, toxins, or infection. Examples of more chronic symmetrical ataxias include hypothyroidism, paraneoplastic disorders, inherited disorders, or vitamin B_{12} deficiency.

2. A rapid but focal onset would lead a clinician to suspect vascular or infectious causes. For example, the sudden onset of right-sided clumsy movements, the inward gaze of the right eye, and a headache would lead one to suspect a right-sided (cerebellar symptoms are ipsilateral) mass in the posterior fossa such as a hemorrhage or abscess.

3. A slower onset of focal or asymmetric findings would lead one to suspect neoplasms, multiple sclerosis, vascular lesions, or congenital malformations (1).

References

1. Rosenberg RN. Ataxic disorders. In: Braunwald E, Hauser SL, Fauci AS, eds. *Harrison's principles of internal medicine*, 15th ed New York, NY:. McGraw-Hill, 2001:2406–2412.
2. Bressman SB, Saunders-Pullman RJ, Rosenberg RN. Hereditary ataxias. In: Rowland LP, ed. *Merritt's neurology*, 11th ed New York, NY:. Lippincott Williams & Wilkins, 2005:783–797.

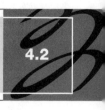

COMA
Robert R. Rauner

4.2

I. BACKGROUND. Coma is a sustained period (>1 hour) of unconsciousness that is distinguished from sleep by the inability to arouse the patient (1,2).

II. PATHOPHYSIOLOGY. Coma is a nonspecific manifestation of central nervous system (CNS) impairment that may be due to any number of insults. There is a large differential of possible causes that may be subdivided into focal (e.g., stroke) versus nonfocal (e.g., hypoxia), traumatic versus nontraumatic, or CNS versus systemic causes. The end result is that there is a global dysfunction of both the cerebral hemispheres or the ascending brain stem and diencephalon activating systems (2).

III. EVALUATION. The history and physical examination can often elicit the potential causes of coma.

    A. History. After ensuring the stability of the airway, breathing, and circulation (ABCs), it is essential to gather pertinent history from friends, family members, and any medical personnel. A sudden loss of consciousness would suggest causes such as intracerebral hemorrhage, seizure, cardiac arrhythmias, or drug overdose. A slower progression implies a much larger list of differential diagnoses.

    B. Physical examination. The examination should pay particular attention to the following:

        1. Motor responses. Are there any purposeful movements? Is there withdrawal from pain? Any posturing? Are the movements symmetric? Asymmetry may imply a structural lesion or a more focal cause. Flexor or extensor posturing implies an impairment of the cerebral hemispheres possibly from metabolic causes, brain stem lesions, or transtentorial herniation. Patients with flexor posturing generally have a better prognosis.

        2. Respiration. Is there a respiratory effort? If so, what pattern (Cheyne-Stokes, cluster breathing, hyperventilation)? Cheyne-Stokes respiration is more likely with transtentorial herniation, upper brain stem lesions, or metabolic causes. Cluster breathing may be associated more with posterior fossa lesions or elevated intracranial pressure. Hyperventilation is more likely due to metabolic acidosis, hepatic encephalopathy, or analgesic drugs.

        3. Pupillary response. Are the pupils equal? Are they reactive? Anisocoria implies a structural cause. Pinpoint pupils may be from pontine hemorrhages or drug toxicity. Fixed dilated pupils may follow anoxic or ischemic injury.

        4. Eye movements. Are the eyelids open? Does the patient blink? Do eye movements conjugate or do they deviate? Do the eyes move with the passive movement of the patient's head (oculocephalic or doll's eye maneuver) (1)?

        5. Temperature. Is it low, normal, or elevated? Low temperature would suggest drug intoxication, hypoglycemia, hypothyroidism, or environmental exposure (3). A fever suggests infectious causes, heat stroke, neuroleptic malignant syndrome, status epilepticus, or anticholinergic overdose (2).

    C. Testing. The imaging of the head using either a computed tomography (CT) scan or a magnetic resonance imaging (MRI) should be done as quickly as possible to rule out structural causes and to guide emergent treatment (e.g., hemorrhage or herniation). Laboratory testing should include an arterial blood gas, a complete blood count, a comprehensive metabolic profile, toxicology (including ethanol, commonly abused drugs, acetaminophen, and salicylates), ammonia, and lactate. Blood and cerebrospinal fluid should also be cultured. An electroencephalogram (EEG) should be performed to look for unrecognized seizures. The EEG can also give clues to the cause and the prognosis (2).

IV. DIAGNOSIS

A. Differential diagnosis. The differential diagnosis of coma is broad but is usually established based on history, physical, laboratory findings, EEG, and imaging. The differential diagnosis, subdivided based on normal versus abnormal CT scan or MRI, includes:

1. Normal CT scan or MRI
   a. Drugs/overdose: alcohol, sedatives, opiates
   b. Metabolic: anoxia, electrolyte disturbances, glucose abnormalities, thyroid disorders, hepatic coma
   c. Severe infections: pneumonia, meningitis, encephalitis, sepsis
   d. Shock
   e. Seizure-related conditions
   f. Severe hypothermia or hyperthermia
   g. Concussion.
2. Abnormal CT scan or MRI
   a. Hemorrhage or infarction
   b. Infection: abscess, empyema
   c. Brain tumor
   d. Traumatic injuries
   e. Others (3).

B. Clinical manifestations. The patient lacks self-awareness and makes no purposeful movements. Vital signs, including the ability to maintain respiratory function may be impaired; so, immediate attention to ensuring stable ABCs is essential. Coma must be distinguished from other similar clinical entities such as vegetative state, catatonia, severe depression, neuromuscular blockade, or akinesia plus aphasia (1, 2).

References

1. Burst JCM. Coma. In: Rowland LP, ed. *Merritt's neurology*, 11th ed. Philadelphia, PA: Lippincott Williams & Wilkins, 2005:20–28.
2. Michelson DJ, Ashwal S. Evaluation of coma and brain death. *Semin Pediatr Neurol* 2004;11(2):105–118.
3. Ropper AH. Acute confusional states and coma. In: Braunwald E, Hauser SL, et al. eds. *Harrison's principles of internal medicine*, 15th ed. Philadelphia, PA: McGraw-Hill, 2001:132–140.

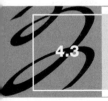

4.3 DELIRIUM
Les Veskrna

I. BACKGROUND. According to the American Psychiatric Association's *Diagnostic and Statistical Manual of Mental Disorders*, Fourth Edition (DSM-IV-TR) (1), delirium has the following key features: disturbance of consciousness with a reduced ability to focus, sustain, or shift attention; change in cognition or the development of a perceptual disturbance that is not better accounted for by a preexisting, established, or evolving dementia; disturbance developing over a short period of time (usually hours to days), and tending to fluctuate during the course of the day; evidence from the history, physical examination, or laboratory findings that the disturbance is caused by the direct physiologic consequence of a general medical condition, substance intoxication or withdrawal, a medication side effect or toxin exposure, or a combination of these factors.

II. PATHOPHYSIOLOGY

A. Etiology. The neurobiologic mechanism of delirium is poorly understood, because it is not a disease but a syndrome with multiple disparate causes. The causes of delirium can be categorized according to whether they are predisposing or precipitating factors. The most common predisposing factors are advanced age and dementia. Other risk factors include immobility and functional dependence, sensory impairment, dehydration, malnutrition, and alcoholism. Nearly any acute systemic illness or medical condition may precipitate delirium in a susceptible patient. The common causes are listed in Table 4.3.1.

B. Epidemiology. Variation in case identification and sample bias make estimates of the prevalence and incidence of delirium difficult to determine. Clinicians often fail to recognize delirium, although it is one of the most common mental disorders encountered in patients with medical illnesses, especially those who are critically ill or elderly. Most studies of mixed hospital inpatient populations report prevalences of 10% to 20%.

III. EVALUATION

A. History. Determining that a cognitive impairment or perceptual disturbance is not due to a preexisting or progressing dementia or other mental disorder requires knowledge of the patient's baseline mental status, and level of functioning. If this is not known, information should be sought from family, friends, and other care providers. Because it is difficult or impossible to obtain a history from a confused or uncooperative patient, important clues as to the cause of delirium may also be elicited from these historical sources (recent febrile illness, recent trauma, history of drug abuse or alcoholism) and a careful review of the medical history. Because drug toxicity accounts for a significant percentage of all cases of delirium, clinicians should not neglect considering over-the-counter drugs, drugs belonging to other family members, drugs prescribed by other physicians, or illicit drugs. Because the features of delirium fluctuate during the course of the day, a review of nursing notes, especially from the evening and night shifts, can be very helpful for discovering or documenting changes in consciousness and cognition.

B. Physical examination. The examination must focus on two issues: (i) confirming that delirium is present, and (ii) uncovering the medical illness that has likely caused the delirium. A comprehensive examination is often difficult in a confused and uncooperative patient. Clinicians should perform a focused examination guided by the history and context, keeping in mind the multifactorial nature of delirium.

C. Testing. The history and physical examination should guide most of the diagnostic investigation. First-line investigations should include electrolytes, complete blood count, urinalysis, liver and thyroid function tests, glucose, creatinine, calcium, chest x-ray, and electrocardiogram. Blood gas determinations are often helpful. Drug levels can be obtained when appropriate, but the clinician should be aware that delirium can occur even with therapeutic levels. The following diagnostic tests may be indicated when a cause of delirium is not apparent after the initial evaluation: urine and blood toxicology screen, syphilis serology, human immunodeficiency virus antibody, autoantibody screen, vitamin B_{12} level, head computed tomography or magnetic resonance imaging, a lumbar puncture with cerebrospinal analysis, and electroencephalogram testing.

IV. DIAGNOSIS

A. Differential diagnosis. The most common issue in the differential diagnosis is whether the patient has dementia rather than delirium, has delirium only, or a delirium superimposed on a preexisting dementia. Careful attention to the key features (disturbed consciousness, change in cognition or perceptual disturbance, acute onset, and fluctuating course) should readily distinguish delirium from dementia and other primary psychiatric disorders such as depression, psychosis, or mania. Nonconvulsive status epilepticus and several lobar or focal neurologic syndromes (Wernicke's aphasia, transient global amnesia, Anton's syndrome, frontal lobe tumors) can result in features that may overlap with those of delirium.

B. Clinical manifestations. Engaging in conversation with a patient in delirium can be difficult because he or she may become easily distracted, unpredictably switch from subject to subject, or persevere with answers to a previous question. In more advanced cases of delirium, the patient may be drowsy or lethargic. Cognitive changes may include memory impairment (most commonly short-term

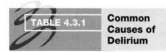

TABLE 4.3.1   Common Causes of Delirium

Anemia
Hypoxemia
   Congestive heart failure
   Chronic obstructive pulmonary disease
   Shock
Infections
   Pneumonia
   Septicemia
   Meningitis
   Urinary tract infection
Central nervous system disorders
   Cerebrovascular accidents
   Seizures or postictal state
   Head trauma
   Increased intracranial pressure
Withdrawal from substances
   Alcohol
   Benzodiazepines
   Opiates
Metabolic disorders
   Renal failure, fluid/electrolyte disorder
   Acid–base disorders
   Endocrinopathy
   Hepatic failure
   Hyperglycemia or hypoglycemia
   Thiamine deficiency
Other
   Fecal impactions
   Bladder catheterization
   Urinary retention
   Physical restraints
Medications
   Psychotropic drugs
   Drugs with anticholinergic effects
      Tricyclic antidepressants
      Diphenhydramine
Benztropine

memory), disorientation (usually to time and place), difficulty with language or speech (dysarthria, dysnomia, dysgraphia, or aphasia), and perceptual disturbances (illusions, hallucinations, or misperceptions). The patient may be so inattentive and incoherent that it may be difficult or impossible to assess cognitive function. Other associated features of delirium may include sleep disturbance or a reversal of the night-day sleep-wake cycle, hypersensitivity to light and sound, anxiety, anger, depressed affect, and emotional lability. Because of confusion, disorientation, and agitation, patients with delirium may harm themselves by climbing over bedrails or pulling out their intravenous line or Foley catheter.

Reference
1. American Psychiatric Association. *Diagnostic and statistical manual of mental disorders*, 4th ed, Text Revision. Washington, DC: American Psychiatric Association, 2000.

DEMENTIA
Christian Kyle Haefele

4.4

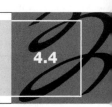

I. **BACKGROUND.** Dementia is characterized by memory impairment along with the loss of other cognitive functions. Cognitive deficits may include difficulty with language (aphasia), common motor tasks (apraxia), the identification of common objects (agnosia), or complex and abstract thinking (executive functioning). These deficits must be severe enough that social behavior or independent living is impaired (1).

II. **PATHOPHYSIOLOGY**

A. **Etiology.** Dementia is a syndrome rather than a disease, so etiology and pathophysiology can vary greatly. Most of the common dementias are progressive, but some are due to reversible causes.

1. Alzheimer's disease (AD) is multifactorial. There is both a familial predisposition and some evidence that AD has a significant vascular component, because there are many risk factors for progression in common with vascular dementia (2).

2. Vascular dementia can be due to multiple infarcts or small vessel disease.

3. Dementia syndromes can be found in connection with other degenerative neurologic diseases such as Parkinson's disease with dementia (PDD), frontotemporal dementia (FTD), Lewy body dementia (LBD), Huntington's disease and progressive supranuclear palsy (PSP).

4. Infectious diseases such as neurosyphilis, acquired immunodeficiency syndrome dementia, and Creutzfeldt-Jacob disease (CJD) can present with dementia. However any infection, such as urinary tract infection, can cause a patient with diminished reserve to decompensate and present with dementia.

5. Other dementias are found with metabolic diseases such as Gaucher's disease or with toxins such as alcohol-related dementia.

6. Normal pressure hydrocephalus is a potentially reversible dementia, which is characterized by the triad of dementia, gait instability, and urinary incontinence.

7. Other reversible dementias can be due to a variety of medical conditions such as hypothyroidism or vitamin B_{12} deficiency. Dementia can be due to electrolyte imbalance, hypoglycemia, hepatic, or renal dysfunction, hypoxia due to cardiac or pulmonary disease, depression, drugs, or trauma.

B. **Epidemiology**

1. The most common chronic dementia syndrome in the elderly is AD, accounting for an estimated 50% to 60% of dementias or over four million Americans (3).

2. Chronic dementia is due to vascular dementia in about 15% to 20% of cases. The other neurodegenerative dementias are less common (3).

3. Reversible dementias are more likely to be found in younger patients and may have a rapid onset measured in days or weeks rather than months or years.

III. EVALUATION

A. History and physical examination. The history and physical findings make the diagnosis or help direct the workup of a potentially reversible dementia. A Mini-Mental State Examination (MMSE) (see Chapter 4.5), complete neurologic examination, and depression screen should be performed. A referral for formal neuropsychologic testing may be considered in patients who are difficult to evaluate because of a language barrier, suspected psychiatric diagnosis, education level, or upon request.

B. Testing

1. The American Academy of Neurology (AAN) recommends routine testing only for vitamin B_{12} deficiency and hypothyroidism as causes of dementia (4).

2. Other laboratory tests that may be helpful if clinically indicated due to a suspected medical condition contributing to dementia, include complete blood count, urinalysis, lipid panel, coagulation studies, comprehensive metabolic panel, toxicology, human immunodeficiency virus, Lyme disease titer, or Venereal Disease Research Laboratory test. A lumbar puncture is not routinely recommended.

3. A noncontrast head computed tomography or magnetic resonance imaging is recommended for initial evaluation. Positron emission tomography, single-photon emission computed tomography, and other imaging are investigational and are not recommended (4).

C. Genetics. The most studied genetic marker for dementia is apolipoprotein E epsilon 4 associated with AD. The AAN guidelines currently recommend against routine testing for any genetic markers for dementia syndromes except for specific cerebrospinal fluid proteins found in cases of suspected CJD (4).

IV. DIAGNOSIS

A. Differential diagnosis. Any reversible dementias should be considered. The diagnosis of chronic dementia syndromes is based mainly on clinical manifestations.

1. The diagnosis of AD is clinically based on a slowly progressive dementia not due to other diseases, and not exclusively during a period of delirium.

2. A stroke syndrome or sudden or stepwise deterioration may suggest vascular dementia.

3. Findings of Parkinson's disease may indicate PDD or LBD. In PDD the motor features are most prominent, whereas in LBD the main features are sleep disturbance, syncope, falls, and hallucinations.

4. In FTD, also known as Pick's disease, patients have socially inappropriate uninhibited behavior or personality changes, but memory may be fairly well maintained.

5. Patients with PSP have downward gaze abnormalities and frequent falls.

6. Pseudodementia is common with depression, as well as with other psychiatric diagnoses.

B. Clinical manifestations. Dementia, whether mild, or advanced, often presents as a complaint from family. If a patient presents with the complaint of memory loss, it is important to consider depression, factitious disorders such as malingering, mild cognitive impairment, or normal age related cognitive decline (see Chapter 4.5). A high index of suspicion, a good history from those who know the patient well, and following serial examinations and MMSE scores help make the diagnosis.

References

1. American Psychiatric Association. *Diagnostic and statistical manual of mental disorders*, 4th ed. Washington, DC: APA Press, 1994.
2. Sadowski M, Pankiewicz J, Scholtzova H, et al. Links between the pathology of Alzheimer's disease and vascular dementia. *Neurochem Res* 2004;29(6):1257–1266.
3. Adelman AM, Daly MP. Initial evaluation of the patient with suspected dementia. *Am Fam Physician* 2005;71(9):1745–1750.
4. Knopman DS, DeKosky ST, Cummings JL, et al. Practice parameter: diagnosis of dementia (an evidence-based review): report of the quality standards subcommittee of the American Academy of Neurology. *Neurology* 2001;56(9):1143–1153.

MEMORY IMPAIRMENT
Christian Kyle Haefele

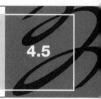

4.5

I. **BACKGROUND.** Memory impairment refers to the inability to learn new information or recall previously learned information. It can be a component of delirium when accompanied by an altered level of consciousness (see Chapter 4.3) or a component of dementia in patients with disturbances in behavior, other cognitive functions, and independence (see Chapter 4.4). There is a normal cognitive decline with aging that consists of a stable mild memory loss and a decline in the rate of processing new information. This normal cognitive decline does not progress to the point of affecting daily function.

II. **PATHOPHYSIOLOGY**

A. **Etiology**

1. Memory disorders without delirium or dementia are called *amnestic disorders*. They are usually due to the effects of other medical conditions, medications, toxins, or drugs of abuse (1). Often there is a period of delirium that precedes amnestic disorders. For example, infectious encephalitis and alcohol use can both cause an initial period of delirium followed by memory problems, which remain after the level of consciousness has returned to normal.

2. Memory disturbance can be caused by physical trauma such as head injury or emotional trauma, which may cause a rare, but dramatic presentation with one of the dissociative psychiatric disorders, such as a conversion reaction or fugue state (1).

3. Mild cognitive impairment (MCI) is the term used for memory loss that is more than is usual with normal aging, but does not meet the criteria for dementia. MCI is characterized by increasing difficulty with memory and progressive decline, while maintaining other cognitive functions and activities of daily living (2). As the definitive criteria for this term improves, it may become a more useful clinical predictor of progression to dementia.

B. **Epidemiology.** It is difficult to quantify the prevalence of MCI because the criteria are not uniform, and many patients may not seek professional care. Patients with MCI may progress to dementia at a rate that is four times higher than that of normal peers, although there are limited studies to help identify who is likely to progress (3). The prevalence of pure amnestic syndromes depends on the etiology, but they are not as common as dementias, which are discussed in Chapter 4.4.

III. **EVALUATION**

A. **History.** The history should initially focus on ruling out dementia and delirium. Careful drug history must include over-the-counter medicines, which may have central nervous system side effects. It is important to obtain corroborating history from family also. Patients with dementia are often brought in by relatives who are concerned about their function, but the patients have poor insight into their own deficits. These patients are different from patients with normal age related cognitive decline, MCI, or depression who will often complain about their own forgetfulness.

B. **Physical examination.** A complete physical examination, including a neurologic examination, should be performed.

1. A Mini-Mental State Examination (MMSE) takes only a few minutes to perform. It can help identify memory deficits as well as discern non-memory cognitive problems, which aids in differential diagnosis (4). Patients with depression may score well or may show poor effort rather than give incorrect answers. Patients with dissociative disorders may be able to score well as their memory loss may only be for a specific time or situation. If cognitive deficits other than memory are found, dementia must be strongly considered. A score of 24/30 points or greater is considered normal, but may be adjusted for age or educational level. A copy of the

MMSE and a discussion of the scoring norms as they relate to age and education level is available on-line at http://www.aafp.org/afp/20010215/703.html (5).

2. Instructions for performing the MMSE:

   a. **Orientation to time.** First, ask the patient the day, date, month, year, and season. The maximum score is 5.

   b. **Orientation to place.** Second, ask the patient what building, town, county, state, and country they are in. The maximum score is 5.

   c. **Memory registration.** Say the name of three objects (e.g., cup, flag, door), and ask the patient to repeat them. If they miss any, continue until they are able to repeat the words so that recall can be tested later. The maximum score of 3 is based on the first trial.

   d. **Attention.** Ask the patient to spell the word "world" backwards or to subtract 7 from 100 serially backwards (stop after five answers). The maximum score is 5.

   e. **Memory recall.** Ask the patient to remember the three objects from the registration portion of the test. The maximum score is 3.

   f. **Language**

      i. **Agnosia.** Show the patient a pencil and ask them to identify the object. The maximum score is 2.

      ii. **Aphasia.** Ask the patient to repeat the phrase "no ifs, ands, or buts." Any mistake or starting over on the first try scores 0. The maximum score is 1.

      iii. **Aphasia.** Write the phrase "close your eyes" on a blank sheet of paper. Ask the patient to read and obey the command. The maximum score is 1.

      iv. **Apraxia.** Ask the patient to follow a 3-step command. "Pick up this paper with your right hand, fold it in half, and place it on the floor." The maximum score is 3.

      v. **Agraphia.** Ask the patient to write a sentence. It must have a subject and a verb and make sense. The maximum score is 1.

   g. **Visual-spatial awareness.** Ask the patient to copy a set of interlocking pentagons. All ten angles must be present, and one angle of each figure should intersect with the other figure. The maximum score is 1.

C. **Testing.** There are no specific laboratory tests for memory impairment. Any tests should be used to confirm or rule out suspected medical causes of amnestic disorders. If early dementia or delirium is suspected, the workup can be found in Chapters 4.3 or 4.4.

D. **Genetics.** A family history may uncover a predilection for substance abuse, depression, or a dementia syndrome. There are no specific genetic tests for disorders of memory impairment. Genetic testing is investigational for a number of dementia syndromes including Alzheimer's dementia, but none is currently recommended for clinical use.

IV. DIAGNOSIS

A. **Differential diagnosis**

   1. Normal age related cognitive decline does not progress over time to impair daily function. Ask about the onset and course of the problem and follow serial cognitive function testing when in doubt.

   2. Dementia syndromes include memory impairment, but must also affect other cognitive functions to the extent that activities of daily living are progressively impaired (see Chapter 4.4).

   3. Delirium must be considered if the patient's level of consciousness is affected (see Chapter 4.3).

   4. Pseudodementia is seen with depression. Patients may show poor effort on cognitive testing as opposed to incorrect answers. A formal depression screen may be helpful.

   5. Malingering or factitious disorder may present as memory impairment in the right social or work setting. Formal cognitive testing may reveal inconsistent deficits.

B. **Clinical manifestations.** Memory impairment most commonly presents with a patient complaining of normal age related cognitive decline or MCI if it is progressive. Memory loss may persist after an identified illness, trauma, or intoxication. A patient will rarely present with a dissociative disorder in which specific memories are lost, whereas cognitive testing usually remains normal.

References

1. American Psychiatric Association. *Diagnostic and statistical manual of mental disorders*, 4th ed. Washington, DC: APA Press, 1994.
2. Winblad B, Palmer K, Kivipelto M, et al. Mild cognitive impairment–beyond controversies, towards a consensus: report of the International Working Group on Mild Cognitive Impairment. *J Intern Med* 2004;256(3):240–246.
3. Ganguli M, Dodge HH, Shen C, et al. Mild cognitive impairment, amnestic type: an epidemiologic study. *Neurology* 2004;63:115.
4. Folstein MF, Folstein SE, McHugh PR. "Mini-mental state": a practical method for grading the cognitive state of patients for the clinician. *J Psychiatr Res* 1975;12:196–198.
5. Santacruz KS, Swagerty D. Early diagnosis of dementia. *Am Fam Physician* 2001;63(4): 620–626.

PARESTHESIA AND DYSESTHESIA
Robert R. Rauner

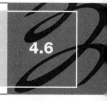

4.6

I. **BACKGROUND.** Paresthesia is a skin sensation, such as burning, prickling, itching, or tingling, with no apparent physical cause. Dysesthesia is defined as either the impairment of sensation, especially that of touch, or a condition in which an unpleasant sensation is produced by ordinary stimuli.

II. **PATHOPHYSIOLOGY**

A. **Etiology.** Paresthesias and dysesthesias are due to dysfunction of the nervous system that can occur anywhere along the pathway of sensation between the cortex and the sensory receptor. Dysfunction can be related to either lack of function (e.g., numbness due to carpal tunnel syndrome) or excess function (e.g., pain from postherpetic neuralgia) (1).

B. **Epidemiology.** The most common source of paresthesia is peripheral neuropathy. The most common causes in the United States are diabetes and alcoholism. Other common causes include hypothyroidism, vitamin B_{12} deficiency, postherpetic neuralgia, and nerve entrapments such as carpal tunnel syndrome (2).

III. **EVALUATION**

A. **History.** The history should include time of onset, duration, and location. Past medical history should be obtained for illnesses that can cause paresthesias or dysesthesias (e.g., diabetes, human immunodeficiency virus [HIV], hypothyroidism, rheumatoid arthritis). Social history may reveal substance abuse (e.g., alcoholism, or intravenous drug use, which would raise the suspicion of HIV) or occupational exposures (e.g., exposure to lead or mercury). In addition, occupational history may reveal an occupation at risk for repetitive motion injuries at work (e.g., a transcriptionist who would be at higher risk for carpal tunnel syndrome). Family history may disclose a hereditary neuropathy (2).

B. **Physical examination.** The patient should have a complete physical examination, paying particular attention to the sensory portion of the neurologic examination. Complicating the physical examination is the fact that the examiner must rely on the patient's subjective response to the examination. The examination should test for pain (using a pin or needle), light touch (using a cotton-tipped swab or wisp of cotton), vibration (using a tuning fork), temperature, and position sense (performed with the eyes closed). The examination should delineate the distribution of abnormal sensation as this may be enough to establish a diagnosis. The patient may be asked to map the affected area. Other aspects of the neurologic examination should include testing of muscle strength and reflexes. Muscle wasting may be noted (1,2). Flexion of the patient's neck (Lhermitte's sign) causing electric shocklike pain in the back or extremities may be present in patients with multiple sclerosis, cervical spinal cord disease, or vitamin B_{12} deficiency.

  C. Testing. Initial laboratory work-up should include complete blood count, renal function, fasting serum glucose, vitamin B_{12} level, urinalysis, thyroid-stimulating hormone, and erythrocyte sedimentation rate. Further laboratory testing might include folate, the Venereal Disease Research Laboratory or rapid plasma reagin test, antinuclear antibody, serum immunoelectrophoresis, purified protein derivative, and blood levels of heavy metals (e.g., lead) (2,3). Electromyography and nerve conduction testing are often helpful in delineating either the anatomic source of the neuropathy (e.g., carpal tunnel syndrome) or the systemic cause (e.g., paraneoplastic syndromes) (3). Radiologic studies such as computed tomography or magnetic resonance imaging may be indicated for specific causes, such as a suspected lumbar disc herniation.

  D. Genetics. There are several hereditary causes of neuropathies. These include Charcot-Marie-Tooth disease, Denny-Brown's syndrome, and familial amyloidotic polyneuropathy (2).

IV. DIAGNOSIS

  A. Differential diagnosis. The differential diagnosis of paresthesias and dysesthesias is broad (see Table 4.6.1).

  B. Clinical manifestations. The cause of paresthesias and dysesthesias can frequently be determined by examination. Distal sensory loss is the most common and is frequently due to metabolic or toxic causes such as diabetes, alcoholism, vitamin B_{12} deficiency, or heavy metal exposure. Some causes, such as diabetes or alcoholism, can have various clinical patterns. Diabetes most commonly causes a symmetric distal sensory loss, but can also cause multifocal neuropathies, autonomic neuropathies, or even symmetrical proximal motor neuropathies (3).

   Most nerve entrapments are distinguished by an examination consistent with their nerve distribution (e.g., loss of sensation of the fifth finger and adjacent half of the

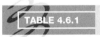

TABLE 4.6.1   **Causes of Paresthesia and Dysesthesia**

Endocrine	Diabetes, hypothyroidism, acromegaly
Nutritional	Vitamin B_{12}/folate deficiencies
Toxic	Chemotherapy, heavy metals, chronic overdose of pyridoxine, alcohol, medications such as nitrofurantoin
Connective tissue disorders	Polyarteritis nodosa, rheumatoid arthritis, lupus
Entrapment syndromes	Carpal and cubital tunnel syndromes, thoracic outlet syndrome, lateral femoral cutaneous syndrome, tarsal tunnel syndrome, spinal disc herniations
Trauma	
Central nervous system	Cerebrovascular accident, tumors
Infectious	Syphilis, Lyme disease, postherpetic neuralgia, human immunodeficiency virus, leprosy
Malignancy	Paraneoplastic syndromes from small cell carcinoma of the lung and cancers of the breast, ovary, and stomach
Miscellaneous	Guillain-Barré syndrome, multiple sclerosis, critical illness polyneuropathy (2,3)

fourth finger in ulnar neuropathies, which are usually caused by compression at the cubital tunnel in the elbow).

Dermatomal distributions would point to either a radiculopathy or postherpetic neuralgia. Neuropathies involving the cranial nerves are rare, but may be caused by Guillain-Barré syndrome, diabetes, HIV, or Lyme disease (3).

References

1. Asbury AK. Numbness, tingling, and sensory loss. In: Braunwald E, Hauser SL, et al. eds. *Harrison's principles of internal medicine*, 15th ed. New York, NY: McGraw Hill, 2001:128–132.
2. McKnight JT, Adcock BB. Paresthesias: a practical diagnostic approach. *Am Fam Physician* 1997;56(9):2253–2260.
3. Poncelet AN. An algorithm for the evaluation of peripheral neuropathy. *Am Fam Physician* 1998;57(4):755–760.

SEIZURES
Les Veskrna

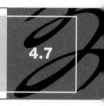

4.7

I. **BACKGROUND.** A seizure is the manifestation of a transient, uncontrolled, synchronous discharge of a population of neurons in the cerebral cortex. Some seizures occur as a symptom during the course of an acute neurologic or medical illness; they do not recur after the underlying disorder has resolved. Epilepsy is a chronic disorder characterized by recurrent seizures that are typically unprovoked and unpredictable.

II. **PATHOPHYSIOLOGY**

A. **Etiology.** Most cases of epilepsy are idiopathic. Some causes of epilepsy can be a result of trauma, tumors, perinatal encephalopathy, congenital brain malformations, inborn errors of metabolism, genetic syndromes, central nervous system infections, stroke, and neurodegenerative disorders. Epilepsy tends to have age patterns that reflect underlying causes. A higher proportion of epilepsy in children is idiopathic or due to congenital brain malformations or developmental neurologic disorders than in older age-groups. The older the patient, the more likely it is that the cause is a cerebrovascular, neurodegenerative, or neoplastic disorder. The following medical disorders are known to cause nonepileptic seizures: hypocalcemia, hyponatremia, disorders of porphyrin metabolism, cerebral anoxia, nonketotic hyperglycemia, and advanced renal failure. High fever, drug reactions, and withdrawal states can also cause seizures.

B. **Epidemiology.** The prevalence of epilepsy is in the range of 5 to 10 per 1,000. Age-specific incidence rates have changed, with a decrease in younger age-groups and an increase in persons older than 60 years (1).

III. **EVALUATION**

A. **History.** Care should be taken to elicit risk factors for seizures pertinent to the patient's age (including a family history of seizures), possible seizure precipitants (medication, alcohol or drugs of abuse, sleep deprivation, strong emotion or stress, intense exercise, flashing lights, fever, or menses), and the clinical features, setting, chronology, and duration of the seizure. In many cases, information about the seizure must be obtained from a witness because the patient may lose awareness or consciousness. The following questions are especially important in determining the etiology of the seizure:

1. Was there an aura?
2. Was there a fall or injury?
3. Was there a loss or impairment of consciousness?

4. Was there staring, eye blinking, vocalizations, or automatisms (repetitive purposeless movements such as lip smacking, chewing, or facial grimacing)?

5. Was there loss of bowel or bladder continence?

6. Was there rhythmic muscular jerking and/or rigidity?

7. Was there a postictal period?

B. Physical examination. The examination is usually normal in patients with epilepsy but occasionally some signs of trauma, an underlying systemic or neurologic disorder, or stigmata of chronic alcoholism may be evident. Additionally, it is important to look for cutaneous manifestations of some genetic disorders (facial nevus flammeus of Sturge-Weber syndrome, adenoma sebaceum of tuberous sclerosis, or *café au lait* macules and cutaneous neurofibromas of neurofibromatosis).

C. Testing. Laboratory studies in adults and children should be ordered on the basis of suggestive historical or clinical findings. In children with a first simple febrile seizure (<10 minutes, isolated, generalized), laboratory testing should be directed toward identifying the cause of the fever. Studies that may be appropriate for evaluation of a first seizure include a complete blood count, glucose, electrolytes, calcium, magnesium, renal, liver and thyroid function tests, and drug and heavy metal toxicology screening (if there is a question of substance abuse or possibility of exposure).

1. A lumbar puncture should be performed if there is a concern about meningitis or encephalitis or if the patient is immunocompromised. The American Academy of Pediatrics suggests that a lumbar puncture be "strongly considered" when a febrile seizure occurs in an infant younger than 12 months of age or all children on prior antibiotic treatment, "considered" in infants 12 to 18 months of age, and "recommended" if meningeal signs are present in infants older than 18 months of age (2). If increased intracranial pressure is suspected, the lumbar puncture should be preceded by computed tomography (CT) scan or magnetic resonance imaging (MRI) of the head.

2. An electroencephalogram (EEG) is essential in the evaluation of epileptic seizures. An abnormal EEG may confirm the diagnosis but a normal or nonspecifically abnormal EEG does not rule out epilepsy. Sleep deprivation and provocative measures such as hyperventilation and photic stimulation may increase the yield of an EEG.

3. Neuroimaging is often necessary to rule out a structural lesion of the brain. A brain MRI is more sensitive than a CT scan; however, the latter may be appropriate in emergency situations or if an MRI is unavailable or contraindicated. An EEG and neuroimaging need not be performed in the evaluation of an otherwise neurologically healthy child with a simple febrile seizure.

IV. DIAGNOSIS

A. Differential diagnosis. A variety of events, either physiologic or psychogenic, can often be mistaken as seizures. These include syncope, complex migraines, breath-holding spells, transient ischemic attacks, sleep disorders (parasomnias, narcolepsy), transient global amnesia, movement disorders, and psychiatric disorders (panic attacks, anxiety with hyperventilation, dissociative states, psychogenic seizures).

B. Clinical manifestations. The clinical expression of a seizure depends on the location and extent of propagation of the discharging neurons.

1. Partial seizures. A partial (focal) seizure begins in a localized area of the cortex. Partial seizures are subdivided into *simple* partial or *complex* partial seizures based on the impairment of consciousness (no impairment in simple partial seizures). The signs and symptoms of a partial seizure depend on the cortical region involved and may range from a subjective perception (aura) to motor, autonomic, somatosensory, or psychic phenomena. A complex partial seizure implies spread of the seizure discharge to allow impairment of consciousness. Patients with complex partial seizures usually exhibit automatisms or some other complex motor activity that is not directed or purposeful. A simple partial seizure may evolve into a complex partial seizure, and both may evolve into a generalized seizure.

2. Generalized seizures. A generalized seizure involves both the cerebral hemi-spheres at the onset. Generalized seizures begin with an abrupt loss of con-sciousness (except myoclonic seizures). Subdivisions of generalized seizures are based mainly on the presence or absence and character of ictal motor manifes-tations: absence (eyelid fluttering, no loss of postural tone, staring), tonic-clonic (muscular rigidity followed by rhythmic muscular jerking), tonic, clonic, atonic (sudden collapse due to loss of postural tone), myoclonic (sudden, brief muscle contractions affecting any group of muscles).

References

1. Sander JW. The epidemiology of epilepsy revisited. *Curr Opin Neurol* 2003;16(2):165–170.
2. American Academy of Pediatrics. Practice parameter: the neurodiagnostic evaluation of the child with a first simple seizure. *Pediatrics* 1996;97(5):769–772; discussion 773–775.

STROKE
Ronald D. Craig

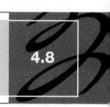

4.8

I. **BACKGROUND.** Stroke is defined as an acute neurologic deficit that lasts more than 24 hours. Events lasting <24 hours are referred to as transient ischemic attacks (TIAs).

II. **PATHOPHYSIOLOGY**
   A. **Etiology.** Stroke is caused by occlusive vascular disease 85% of the time and hemorrhagic vascular disease 15% of the time.
   B. **Epidemiology.** Risk factors for stroke include uncontrolled hypertension, hyper-lipidemia, tobacco smoking, cardiac disease, coagulopathies, diabetes mellitus, and hormone therapy. Stroke is the third most common cause of death (1) and the most common acute neurologic event in the United States.

III. **EVALUATION (2, 3)**
   A. **History.** Historical factors of note include:
      1. Acute onset of symptoms
      2. Unilateral change in motor control, vision, gait, strength, or sensation
      3. Other neurologic disorders such as migraine, systemic lupus, vasculitis
      4. Sudden onset of unusual headache
      5. Presence of one or more risk factors
   B. **Physical examination.** Physical findings include:
      1. Alteration of mental status and/or consciousness
      2. Slurred or inappropriate speech, aphasia
      3. Hemiparalysis, hemiparesis
      4. Altered sensation
      5. Visual field defect, diplopia, nystagmus
      6. Hypertension
      7. Cardiac dysrhythmia
      8. Dizziness, ataxia
      9. Vascular tenderness to palpation, temporal and carotid arteries
   C. **Testing.** Studies and laboratory tests include:
      1. Computed tomography (CT) scan of the head to identify hemorrhage. Other imaging studies are undergoing clinical evaluation
      2. Complete blood count, with platelet count, comprehensive chemistry panel, prothrombin time, partial thromboplastin time for underlying diseases and baseline if thrombolytic or anticoagulant therapy is anticipated

3. Special studies such as toxicology screen, antiphospholipid antibodies, protein S and C, antithrombin III, and others if indicated by history or physical examination
4. Electrocardiogram to help diagnose dysrhythmias or preceding myocardial infarction
5. Echocardiogram to visualize structural defects or mural thrombi. Transesophageal echocardiography may possibly be appropriate
6. Carotid/intracranial Doppler studies to find occlusive vascular disease or source of artery to artery emboli

IV. DIAGNOSIS

A. Differential diagnosis. The differential diagnosis of stroke includes aberrant migraine, seizure disorder, metabolic disorders, psychogenic condition (hysterical conversion reaction, hyperventilation), and tumor with hemorrhage.

B. Clinical approach. With the availability of thrombolytic therapy, the urgency of making a rapid diagnosis has become more critical. Getting the patient to a medical care facility as quickly as possible is very important. A history and physical examination should be completed as quickly as is practical, with special attention to the neurological examination. Quantitative assessment of strength and function on the affected side should be documented for comparison with subsequent examinations. Clinical improvement in the first couple of hours would favor a TIA or a more localized stroke. After the initial history and physical examination, laboratory studies can be ordered and a noncontrast head CT scan can be obtained to rule out hemorrhage provided the patient is clinically stable enough. Appropriate interventions to control blood pressure, seizures, and cardiac dysrhythmias should proceed concomitantly with the evaluation.

References

1. CDC FASTATS: www.cdc.gov/nchs/fastats/stroke.htm, 2005
2. American Heart Association Stroke Outcome Classification. Executive summary. *Circulation* 1998:97:2474–2478.
3. Harrison's Online: Part 15. Neurological disorders. Section 2. Diseases of the Central Nervous system. Chapter 349. Cerebrovascular diseases.

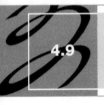

4.9 TREMORS
Ronald D. Craig

I. BACKGROUND. Tremors, which represent the most common type of movement disorder, are abnormal, involuntary, rhythmical movements (1,2). They all stop during sleep.

II. PATHOPHYSIOLOGY. Tremors are of three basic types: rest, postural, and kinetic.

A. Rest tremors. These occur when the limb muscles are not activated and diminish with activity. They occur slowly in disease states such as Parkinson's disease, multiple systems atrophy, and supranuclear palsy, whereas they occur rapidly or suddenly in toxin or drug-induced and psychogenic states, including those brought on by phenothiazines, metoclopramide, and anxiety. Rest tremors have a relatively slow oscillation frequency.

B. Postural tremors. They are also referred to as essential, physiologic, benign, and familial tremors. They are usually gradual in onset. Benign causes include the essential/physiologic tremor, and acute causes include toxic drug and alcohol withdrawal, stimulant use, and metabolic states such as hyperthyroidism and stress reactions. Postural tremors are maximal with the limb maintained against gravity, are reduced by rest, and are not enhanced during voluntary movement.

C. Kinetic tremors. Simple kinetic tremor has variable frequency and does not change with purposeful movement. Intention tremor has a low frequency that increases with directed movement. Etiology includes cerebellar lesions from causes such as stroke, tumor, multiple sclerosis, and drugs such as lithium and alcohol. Isometric tremor has a medium frequency and occurs with muscle contraction against a stationary object. Task-specific tremors occur only with specific tasks such as writing and sewing.

III. EVALUATION. The history and physical examination remains the most valuable tool for the evaluation of a tremor.

A. History. A detailed history should include:

1. Duration, progression, and aggravating and ameliorating factors. Relationship to stressful events is particularly useful in evaluating for psychogenic causes

2. Family history of neurologic and metabolic disorders

3. Medication history to include alcohol, tobacco, and illicit drug use. Over-the-counter drug use such as decongestants, weight loss preparations, and herbal products should be elicited, because many people believe them to be free of side effects.

B. Physical examination. This should begin with observation with the patient at rest during the interview. The examination should document the following:

1. Relative frequency (fast or slow) and amplitude (fine or coarse) of the tremor as well as symmetry and the effect of position, rest, and actions

2. Affected body parts (e.g., head, hands, arms, legs, feet)

3. Any related findings such as tachycardia, hypertension, exophthalmia, thyromegaly, abnormal skin pigmentation, muscle rigidity, cog wheeling, and hyper-reflexiveness or hyporeflexiveness.

C. Testing. Testing should be directed by the history and physical examination. Generally, a comprehensive metabolic panel with tests of liver, kidney, thyroid functions, blood glucose, and complete blood count are appropriate for most tremors.

1. Computed tomography or magnetic resonance imaging may be indicated in cerebellar tremors.

2. Cerebrospinal fluid analysis, including immuniglobulin G (IgG) analysis, may be necessary if multiple sclerosis is suspected.

3. Appropriate drug and alcohol screens are indicated by the history and physical examination.

4. Positron emission tomography and single photon emission computed tomography are undergoing clinical usefulness trials.

IV. DIAGNOSIS. The most critical step is to differentiate benign tremors from those with more ominous consequences. Treatment is based on the classification of the tremor. Therapeutic trials of drugs such as β-blockers may be useful in differentiating some types of tremor.

References

1. McGraw-Hill's Access Medicine, Harrison's Online. Part 2. Cardinal manifestations and Presentation of Diseases. Section 3. Nervous System Dysfunction. Chapter 21. Weakness, Disorders of Movement and Imbalance. Movement Disorders.

2. Sharon Smaga MD. Tremor. *Am Fam Physician* 2003;68(8):1545–1552.

Eye Problems

Shou Ling Leong

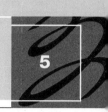

5

BLURRED VISION

Norman Benjamin Fredrick

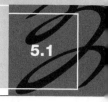

5.1

I. BACKGROUND. Blurred vision is the most common visual complaint (1). "Blurred vision is the loss of sharpness of vision and the inability to see small details" (2).

II. PATHOPHYSIOLOGY

A. Etiology. The causes of blurred vision range from mild to potentially catastrophic. Most causes involve the orbit (anterior and posterior segments); although a number of extraocular causes must be considered (medication, cerebrovascular event, sarcoidosis, herpes simplex).

B. Epidemiology. Certain age-related eye disorders such as macular degeneration, cataracts, and temporal arteritis may cause blurred vision. In younger patients, blurred vision is often acquired through trauma, occupational exposures, and infections.

III. EVALUATION

A. History. Careful attention should be paid to the rapidity of the onset, associated eye pain, and whether the blurring is unilateral or bilateral. Blurred vision that worsens at night may indicate a cataract (3). Intermittently blurred vision may be caused by excess tearing, allergies, uncontrolled diabetes, acute glaucoma, transient ischemic attacks, cerebrovascular insufficiency, and multiple sclerosis (4). Other important factors include a family history of eye disorders (macular degeneration, glaucoma), any work exposures (chemicals), medications (such as corticosteroids, antibiotics), and past medical history (diabetes, hypertension) (5).

B. Physical examination. The physical examination should include the following elements:

1. Careful documentation of visual acuity (corrected and uncorrected) is important to monitor the progression of the disease. If the patient is unable to discern letters on the Snellen eye chart, the examiner should determine the extent of acuity impairment by testing the distance from the patient's eyes at which the patient can first see the examiner's fingers.

2. Visual field testing may indicate an underlying stroke (homonymous field defect) or retinal detachment (quadrant or hemispheric loss of vision).

3. Ocular muscle involvement may be detected by testing the cardinal positions of the orbit through range of motion.

4. Conjunctival erythema and discharge should be noted. The corneal light reflex should be symmetric and sharp; fluorescein staining should be performed to evaluate for the evidence of trauma, ulcers, or herpetic lesions. The anterior chamber (space between the cornea and the iris) should be evaluated with a penlight for blood (hyphema) and pus (hypopyon).

5. In up to 20% of the cases, *pupillary examination* may be the only clue to serious underlying pathology. Using a penlight, the abnormalities of pupillary size or shape (the pupils should be symmetric; a unilateral miotic pupil may indicate iritis) or color (black is normal) may be detected. Other findings may include cataracts, ruptured globes (with eccentric pupils), and optic nerve disease (afferent papillary defect—paradoxical papillary dilatation in response to light).

6. Direct ophthalmoscopy may reveal an abnormal red reflex that suggests a hemorrhage, cataract, or retinal detachment. Papilledema warrants further evaluation.

C. Testing. An elevated sedimentation rate may suggest a diagnosis of temporal arteritis. Computed tomography is appropriate to evaluate blurred vision following trauma, or when there is concern for mass effect (1).

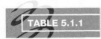

TABLE 5.1.1	Causes of Blurred Vision

	Painless		Painful	
	Sudden onset	**Gradual onset**	**Sudden onset**	**Gradual onset**
Unilateral	Vitreous hemorrhage, macular degeneration, retinal detachment, retinal-vein occlusion, amaurosis fugax, cataracts	Cataracts, "dry" macular degeneration, tumor	Corneal abrasion, infection or edema, uveitis, traumatic hyphema, acute glaucoma, temporal arteritis, optic neuritis, orbital cellulitis	Rare
Bilateral	Poorly controlled diabetes, medications (anticholinergics, cholinergics, corticosteroids), migraines, psychological trauma	Cataracts, macular degeneration, medications (hydrochloroquine, ethambutol, digoxin toxicity), optic chiasm mass, fatigue, refractive errors (myopia, hyperopia, astigmatism, presbyopia); incorrect eyewear	Trauma, chemical spill, welder's exposure	Rare (sarcoidosis, collagen vascular disease)

Compiled from Shingleton BJ, O'Donoghue MW. Primary care: blurred vision. *N Engl J Med* 2000;343(8): 556–562.

D. Genetics. Macular degeneration, glaucoma, collagen vascular diseases, diabetes, and multiple sclerosis (optic neuritis) are potentially heritable conditions.

IV. DIAGNOSIS

    A. Differential diagnosis. (see Table 5.1.1)

    B. Clinical manifestations. A careful history and physical examination often limit the differential diagnosis. Conditions that require immediate ophthalmologic referral include acute glaucoma, retinal detachment, vitreous hemorrhage, retinal-vein occlusion, herpes simplex infection, and orbital cellulitis.

References

1. Shingleton BJ, O'Donoghue MW. Primary care: blurred vision. *N Engl J Med* 2000; 343(8):556–562.
2. Hart JA. Diplopia. *Medline plus encyclopedia*. Medline Plus.com (http://www.nlm.nih.gov/medlineplus/ency/article/003029.htm), 2004.
3. Pavan-Langston D. *Manual of ocular diagnosis and therapy*. Philadelphia, PA: Lippincott Williams & Williams, 2002.
4. WrongDiagnosis.com. Blurred vision. *Wrongdiagnosis symptoms* (http://www.wrongdiagnosis.com/sym/blurred_vision.htm#possible), 2003.
5. Vaughan DG, Asbury T, Riordan-Eva P. *General ophthalmology*. New York, NY: McGraw-Hill Medical, 2003.

CORNEAL FOREIGN BODY
Peter R. Lewis

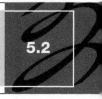

5.2

I. BACKGROUND. Macroscopic and/or microscopic material from the external environment may lodge in the cornea—the anterior and transparent part of the eye that overlies the anterior chamber and is continuous with the sclera.

II. PATHOPHYSIOLOGY

    A. Etiology. Commonly involved materials include sand, dirt, leaves, and other organic materials in the environment and additional occupational exposure to materials such as metal shavings or glass particles.

    B. Epidemiology. Among symptomatic patients, a corneal foreign body represents a common cause of eye-related complaints for adult and pediatric patients presenting to primary care physicians, ophthalmologists, and emergency departments (1). The frequent association between a corneal foreign body and occupational or leisure-time exposure highlights the eminently preventable nature of this condition with protective eyewear (2).

III. EVALUATION

    A. History. A patient with a corneal foreign body is frequently self-evident by history. "Foreign-body" sensation, pain, photophobia, and lacrimation are commonly associated patient complaints. The patient frequently notes redness in the eye (see Chapter 5.6). Decreased vision may be reported. Individuals with corneal foreign bodies who are victims of significant industrial accidents, motor vehicle trauma, or gunshot wounds may be unable to communicate or may primarily complain of pain at sites of more substantial injury. Tetanus immunization status should be determined in these patients. By contrast, some patients with corneal foreign bodies may have no symptoms. A history of metal grinding or welding should raise the clinician's suspicion for an asymptomatic foreign body; this is an important detail to consider for the patient undergoing magnetic resonance imaging (MRI).

    B. Physical examination. If the injury is clearly confined to the eye, a comprehensive ocular examination should commence with gross inspection to evaluate for asymmetry in the periorbital region, conjunctiva, cornea, and pupils. A sufficiently large foreign body may be visible by gross inspection with a penlight on physical examination. Magnification should be used, including a slit lamp, where available. The eyelids should be everted, because foreign bodies may lodge in multiple locations. A funduscopic examination should also be performed.

        1. A topical anesthetic may be required. Visual acuity should be determined before the use of any topical anesthetic. Altered visual acuity may be due to a corneal foreign body interfering with the visual axis, and may be associated with penetrating ocular trauma.

        2. Screening for a corneal infiltrate or hyphema (blood in the anterior chamber) is necessary. The presence of a rust stain is highly suggestive of a metallic foreign body.

        3. Fluorescein staining and examination with cobalt-blue light or Wood's lamp should be used to search for an associated corneal abrasion (3). A vertically oriented corneal abrasion suggests the presence of an associated foreign body in the upper tarsal region.

    C. Testing. For patients with suspected associated penetrating foreign body, computed tomograph or ultrasound may be required. An MRI should be avoided in the setting of a suspected or a confirmed metallic foreign body.

IV. DIAGNOSIS. In the event of serious and/or multiple injuries, an expedited and detailed trauma survey should be conducted and plans made for ambulance transport to the closest emergency department. Severe corneal trauma related to a foreign body, especially in children, may require examination under general anesthesia in the operating room by an ophthalmologist. Other reasons for prompt ophthalmologic referral include corneal infiltrate (increased association with infection), corneal laceration, hyphema, and any suspicion for a penetrating injury. For the patient suitable for evaluation in the outpatient setting, the differential diagnosis for anterior eye pain includes corneal ulceration, keratitis (including that caused by shingles), cluster or migraine headache, and glaucoma.

References
1. Shields T, Sloane PD. A comparison of eye problems in primary care and ophthalmology practices. *Fam Med* 1991;23:544.
2. Work Loss Data Institute. *Eye.* Corpus Christi, TX: Work Loss Data Institute, Available online at National Guideline Clearinghouse–www.guideline.gov/summary/summary.aspx?view_id=1&doc_id=6559, 2004.
3. Wilson SA, Last A. Management of corneal abrasions. *Am Fam Physician* 2004;70(1): 123–128.

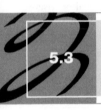

5.3 DIPLOPIA
Norman Benjamin Fredrick

I. **BACKGROUND.** Diplopia means double vision. Patients complain of seeing the same view as two overlapping images (1). The images may be horizontal, vertical, or diagonal to one another (2).

II. **PATHOPHYSIOLOGY**

 A. **Etiology.** Diplopia occurs when the scene before the patient is sent as two different images to the visual cortex. The normal mapping process cannot occur and the brain perceives two overlapping images. There are two main types of diplopia: monocular and binocular. Monocular diplopia implies a problem with only one of the eyes. These are often refractive abnormalities and disorders of the globe itself (i.e., cornea, lens, retina) (1). Binocular diplopia is primarily due to disorders of ocular motility (i.e., either the muscles or the innervation of the ocular muscles). Monocular diplopia is readily distinguished from binocular diplopia by the fact that the diplopia persists despite covering the unaffected eye (1).

 B. **Epidemiology.** Patients primarily complaining of diplopia are adults. Children younger than 10 years of age tend to compensate for visual disturbances by suppressing one of the images. Binocular diplopia is more common than monocular diplopia.

III. **EVALUATION**

 A. **History.** Standard history is required with an emphasis on the following points:

 1. Distinguishing between double vision and blurry vision is important. Patients complain of seeing two images with diplopia.

 2. Most complaints of diplopia are due to a binocular abnormality arising from in-coordination of the ocular muscles. Asking whether the images are side-by-side, vertical to each other, or diagonal to each other may help determine which ocular muscle group is involved. Complaints of vertical diplopia (which includes diagonal diplopia) are due to muscle groups associated with the cranial nerves (CNs) III and IV. The abnormality may stem from these nerves or, more distally, from the muscles themselves (i.e., myasthenia gravis, muscle entrapment). Complaints of horizontal diplopia indicate an abnormality with the lateral/medial rectus muscles and/or CN VI (binocular vertical diplopia).

3. A sudden onset of diplopia may suggest a vascular etiology.
4. A history of any instigating events such as facial trauma, sinus infection, or migraine headache may provide important diagnostic information.
5. The review of symptoms should include questions about a history of fever, headache, sinus congestion, and associated neurologic complaints.
6. A family history of thyroid disorders, myasthenia gravis, or diabetes may suggest an autoimmune cause.
7. Other significant past medical history includes diabetes (retinopathy, third CN palsy), hypertension, and underlying vascular diseases (2).
8. Ask the patient whether the symptom improves with gazing in a certain direction. If the gaze improves (although it is unlikely to resolve), the cause is usually due to a neuromuscular problem or a mechanical restriction (1).

B. Physical examination. The examination should include:
1. **Observation.** Look for any evidence of strabismus (malalignment of the globes as indicated by an abnormal corneal light reflex), cataracts, corneal abnormalities such as scars, evidence of cellulitis, eyelid ptosis (myasthenia gravis, CN III palsy), eyelid retraction (thyroid ophthalmopathy), or periorbital ecchymoses (trauma). If the patient's head is being held at a tilt, consider a lesion involving the superior oblique muscle (and its corresponding CN VI).
2. **Auscultation.** Listen over the closed eye for a carotid cavernous fistula bruit.
3. **Palpation.** Palpate for a step-off or any tenderness to suggest a periorbital fracture.

C. Testing. The following office-based testing should be considered:
1. Visual acuity should include testing the patient's uncorrected and corrected vision.
2. Cover test—cover each eye sequentially. If the diplopia persists when one eye is covered (i.e., the diplopia persists with just one eye open) the patient has monocular diplopia. Monocular implies an abnormality of just one eye (the "bad" eye). When the offending eye is covered, the diplopia resolves. When the good eye is covered, the diplopia persists. If the patient's vision returns to normal when either the left or right eye is covered, the patient has binocular diplopia. This is an extremely useful test to help narrow the causes of diplopia (see Fig. 5.3.1). Further evaluation for the causes of monocular diplopia can be focused on the abnormal eye (2).
3. Visual acuity with a pinhole is most helpful for patients who have monocular diplopia. If the offending eye is covered with a pinhole, the visual acuity in that eye often improves. This points to a problem with refraction (3).
4. Range of ocular movements and visual field testing—these tests may be used to further narrow the differential diagnosis. In orbital trauma, for example, entrapment (or contusion) of the inferior rectus and/or the inferior oblique muscles or their nerves may worsen the diplopia (4).
5. Pupillary evaluation may reveal asymmetric pupils. Consider a CN III palsy.

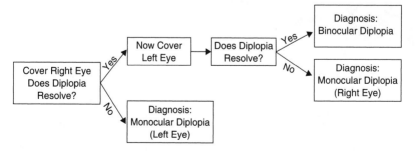

Figure 5.3.1. The diplopia cover test.

6. An abnormal corneal reflex indicates a problem with the alignment of the globes themselves. This produces a binocular diplopia (although not exclusively). Further imaging, such as with a computed tomography (CT) scan or a magnetic resonance imaging (MRI; with contrast) may be warranted (2).

7. If an ocular muscle group is suspected in binocular diplopia, a Parks 3-step test is used to determine the particular muscles. Consult an ophthalmology text, or see references 2 and 3.

8. Fatigability of ocular muscles suggests myasthenia gravis.

9. Consider a CT scan or an MRI of the skull and orbits if there is concern for mass, fracture, increased intracranial pressure, sinus disease, or vascular abnormality. A Tensilon test may be ordered if myasthenia gravis is suspected.

IV. DIAGNOSIS

A. Differential diagnosis. The differential diagnosis for diplopia, which can often be substantially narrowed based on the history and the physical examination, is broken into two main groups—monocular and binocular diplopia.

1. **Causes of monocular diplopia.** Corneal distortions (scars, keratoconus), multiple openings in the iris, cataract, lens displacement (e.g., Marfan's syndrome), advanced astigmatism, pseudophakos (artificial intraocular lens) subluxation, vitreous abnormalities, retinal conditions, contact lens complication, intraocular foreign body, herpes zoster ophthalmicus, orbital cellulitis, orbital fracture (floor, medial wall), orbital tumors (rhabdomyosarcoma), arteriovenous malformations (carotid cavernous fistula).

2. **Causes of binocular diplopia.** Nerve palsies (abducens, oculomotor, trochlear), migraine headache, myasthenia gravis, thyroid ophthalmopathy, mononeuritis multiplex (CN VI—abducens), diabetic CN III palsy (normal pupil, headache, or pain around the orbit), diabetic palsies (CN IV or V).

B. Clinical manifestations. Diplopia may cause difficulty with depth perception, especially with balance, and activities such as driving or operating machinery. Patients with diplopia should not perform these activities (2).

References

1. Vaughan DG, Asbury T, Riordan-Eva P. *General ophthalmology.* New York, NY: McGraw-Hill Medical, 2003.
2. Wessels I. Diplopia. *Medline plus encyclopedia* (http://www.nlm.nih.gov/medlineplus/ency/article/003029.htm). 2004.
3. Brazis PW, Lee AG. Binocular vertical diplopia. *Mayo Clin Proc* 1998;73:55–66.
4. Webb LA. *Manual of eye emergencies.* Philadelphia, PA: Butterworth-Heineman, Bartley, 2004.

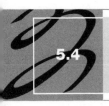

5.4 NYSTAGMUS
Peter R. Lewis

I. BACKGROUND. Nystagmus is an involuntary, rhythmic oscillation of one or both eyes in any or all fields of gaze. It may be continuous or intermittent. Nystagmus can be classified into two basic types, jerk (the more common classification) and pendular.

A. Jerk nystagmus. This consists of an initial slow phase, followed and named for the direction (upbeat, downbeat, horizontal, torsional, or mixed) by the corrective saccade or fast phase ("jerk") in the opposite direction.

B. Pendular nystagmus. This consists of smooth back and forth ("pendular") movement (horizontal, vertical, torsional, or mixed) of the eye(s).

II. PATHOPHYSIOLOGY. The appropriate development, function, and integration of the visual/oculomotor and vestibular systems are required for optimal focus and tracking of visual objects (1). Nystagmus may be associated with abnormalities of central or peripheral origin in this complex neurologic network, although in many instances a precise cause may not be identified (2). Any form of vision loss may be associated with nystagmus. Extreme-gaze evoked nystagmus is effectively physiologic, occurring in approximately one half of the population.

A. Etiology. Jerk or pendular nystagmus may be characterized as being either congenital/infantile or acquired.

1. Congenital/infantile nystagmus is most commonly associated with underlying sensory (efferent) visual abnormalities. It may not become evident until several months of age. If no efferent defect is identified the nystagmus is judged to be idiopathic, presumably due to a defect in the oculomotor complex.

2. Acquired nystagmus that develops later in life is more likely to be neuropathologic and associated with a life-threatening disorder.

a. Two forms of acquired nystagmus when seen in the young are noteworthy.

i. Opsoclonus is characterized by repetitive, irregular, and multidirectional ("dancing eyes" or saccadomania) eye movements, opsoclonus may be associated with cerebellar or brain stem disease, postviral meningitis, or neuroblastoma.

ii. Spasmus nutans is the rare triad of head turn (torticollis), nystagmus, and head bobbing. The nystagmus can be monocular or binocular and dissociated; of low amplitude and high frequency; and with horizontal or vertical pendular movements. It most commonly develops between 6 months to 3 years in otherwise healthy children. This usually resolves between the ages of 2 and 8 years. Of note, an identical clinical picture can be produced by a glioma of the optic chiasm or nearby structures.

b. Acquired forms of nystagmus that occur more commonly in adults include the following:

i. Seesaw nystagmus, in which the movements are pendular. One eye rises and rotates inward, whereas the other descends and rotates outward. This is frequently seen with lesions of the optic chiasm or third ventricle, as may occur with a parasellar mass (e.g., craniopharyngioma or pituitary adenoma).

ii. Downbeating nystagmus, in which the fast phase beats down and may be associated with a lesion of the cervicomedullary junction at the level of the foramen magnum. Arnold-Chiari malformation and spinocerebellar degeneration are the most common causes. Oscillopsia (the intermittent or constant sensation of the environment moving back and forth) may be present.

iii. Upbeating nystagmus, in which the fast phase beats up and is of large or small amplitude. The associated lesion commonly involves the brain stem or vermis of the cerebellum as occurs in stroke, tumor, or degeneration.

iv. Convergence—retraction nystagmus, which is marked by the convergence of the eyes with jerk nystagmus and the retraction of the globe on upgaze, eyelid retraction, limitation in upgaze, and large unreactive pupils. This is caused by midbrain abnormalities.

v. Periodic alternating nystagmus, in which the fast phase occurs in one direction with a head turn for 60 to 90 seconds, and then reverses direction with an intermediate "neutral zone." This can be seen with vestibulocerebellar disease (stroke, multiple sclerosis, spinocerebellar degeneration), severe bilateral visual loss (optic atrophy, dense vitreous hemorrhage), or it can be congenital.

vi. Gaze-evoked nystagmus, which is a type of jerk nystagmus that appears only when the eyes look to the side. Pathologic forms are most commonly seen with alcohol or other central nervous system (CNS) depressants. Cerebellar brain stem disorders can also be associated with this type of nystagmus.

    vii. Vestibular nystagmus, which is caused by the dysfunction of the inner ear, auditory nerve, or the central nuclear complex. Peripheral vestibular disease (e.g., labyrinthitis, Ménière's disease, neuronitis, vascular ischemia, trauma, or drug toxicity) produces unidirectional jerk nystagmus with a fast phase opposite the lesion that is usually horizontal. Common associated symptoms include vertigo, tinnitus, hearing loss, and vomiting. Central (nuclear) disease (e.g., demyelinating disorder, tumor, trauma, or stroke), by contrast, is characterized by unidirectional or bidirectional nystagmus that may be purely horizontal, vertical, or rotatory and is characteristically toward the side of the lesion. Vertigo, tinnitus, and deafness are mild, if present, and symptoms are not relieved with eye fixation as in peripheral disease.

    viii. Torsional nystagmus, which is usually constant and due to an associated midbrain (e.g., pons, medulla) lesion involving the vestibular nuclei as may occur in stroke or multiple sclerosis. The nystagmus may be superimposed on horizontal or vertical nystagmus and directed toward or away from the side of the associated lesion.

    ix. Dissociated nystagmus, in which nystagmus in one eye is different from the other. This is seen in posterior fossa lesions. If an abduction nystagmus is present with an internuclear ophthalmoplegia, consider multiple sclerosis with a lesion involving the medial longitudinal fasciculus.

B. Epidemiology. Precise data regarding the prevalence of nystagmus are unavailable.

III. EVALUATION

A. History. Age of onset, self-identified precipitants, time course, associated symptoms, family history of visual impairment and/or associated neurologic disorders, and functional impairment should be elicited from the patient or parent. In children, it is necessary to inquire about a history of prematurity and related visual impairment(s). Blurred vision, if present, is characteristic of an acquired nystagmus. Vertigo implies vestibular disease. Associated weakness, numbness, or loss of vision may be suggestive of multiple sclerosis. A history of medication and substance use is important. Medications that can induce nystagmus (usually downbeat or upbeat) include lithium, barbiturates, phenytoin, salicylates, and benzodiazepines. Nystagmus may also be seen with phencyclidine use. Acute alcohol intoxication can produce a gaze-evoked nystagmus, as does the chronic alcohol-induced thiamin deficiency common to Wernicke's encephalopathy.

B. Physical examination. This should begin with a developmental assessment followed by a visual examination. Loss of established visual acuity is typically worse in acquired nystagmus. The ability to track moving objects with the head in a fixed position (optokinetic reflex) takes a number of months to mature and typically fails to develop in congenital nystagmus. The direction, plane, and amplitude of the eye movement should be characterized. It is necessary to evaluate any cause of poor vision that may contribute to the nystagmus. Aniridia (absence of iris) or iris transillumination as seen in albinism should be sought. Congenital cataracts or corneal opacities have poor red reflexes. It is important to analyze the optic nerve to assess for hypoplasia or atrophy. Latent nystagmus (seen only when one eye is covered—the basis of the screening "cover-uncover" test) is present in infantile strabismus (3). Altered head position and head bobbing may be associated with congenital nystagmus and spasmus nutans. If benign paroxysmal positional vertigo is suspected, the Dix-Hallpike's maneuver may be performed in an effort to reproduce the patient's symptoms (4). A complete neurologic assessment should be performed. Appropriate neurology and ophthalmology consultation(s) should be requested as indicated.

C. Testing. Urine drug screening for alcohol or barbiturates should be considered when significant gaze-evoked nystagmus is observed. Serum drug levels of phenytoin or lithium should be obtained as indicated. Additional blood tests to be considered include vitamin B_{12}, magnesium, and toxoplasmosis and/or human immunodeficiency virus serologies. If a CNS infection is suspected (e.g., herpes simplex), then cerebrospinal fluid analysis is indicated. Magnetic resonance imaging (MRI) (as seen in the subsequent text) should be obtained before the lumbar puncture. Ocular albinism can be associated with a bleeding disorder secondary to platelet dysfunction (Hermansky-Pudlak syndrome), or white blood cell dysfunction with increased susceptibility to infection and lymphoma (Chédiak-Higashi syndrome). Respectively, a bleeding time and a polymorphonuclear leukocyte function test should be ordered. Urinary vanillylmandelic acid should be obtained in a patient with opsoclonus to look for the by-products of a neuroblastoma.

  D. Genetics. Variable patterns of inheritance have been associated with congenital nystagmus (5). Certain autosomal dominant ataxias are associated with downbeat nystagmus. Symptoms usually begin in late adulthood.
IV. DIAGNOSIS
  A. Differential diagnosis. Other involuntary ocular oscillations include:
    1. Oculogyric crisis consists of nonrhythmic, sustained, and irregular eye deviations. This is seen in phenothiazine (e.g., prochlorperazine) toxicity.
    2. Ocular bobbing is characterized by fast, conjugate, downward movement of the eye, followed by a slow drift to the primary position of gaze. This is seen in comatose patients with large pontine lesions (e.g., hemorrhage, stroke, or tumor). Obstructive hydrocephalus or metabolic encephalopathy can also cause this type of eye movement.
    3. Superior oblique myokymia is characterized by small unilateral, vertical, and rotatory movements of one eye. Symptoms of oscillopsia worsen when looking downward and inward. This is usually benign and self-limited, but has been noted with multiple sclerosis.
    4. Nystagmus may occur with essential head tremor, and may be extinguished by fixing the head position or by utilizing a β-blocker.
  B. Clinical manifestations. The clinical manifestations of nystagmus were discussed in section **II.A.** Because many forms of nystagmus localize to the posterior fossa or are associated with a demyelinating disorder, an MRI is the imaging modality of choice if the cause is otherwise not identified. In a patient with opsoclonus, an abdominal computed tomography (CT) scan or an MRI should be done to look for neuroblastoma involving the adrenal glands. An abdominal ultrasound or a CT scan is needed to evaluate the kidneys in aniridia, because there is a significant incidence of associated Wilms' tumor.

References
1. Leigh RJ, Zee DS. *The neurology of eye movements*, 3d ed. Oxford: Oxford University Press, 1999.
2. Serra A, Leigh RJ. Diagnostic value of nystagmus: spontaneous and induced ocular oscillations. *J Neurol Neurosurg Psychiatry* 2002;73(6):615–618.
3. Simon JW, Kaw P. Commonly missed diagnoses in the childhood eye examination. *Am Fam Physician* 2001;64(4):623–628.
4. Swartz R, Longwell P. Treatment of vertigo. *Am Fam Physician* 2005;71(6):1115–1122.
5. Gottlob I. Nystagmus. *Curr Opin Ophthalmol* 2001;12(5):378–383.

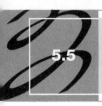

PAPILLEDEMA
Peter R. Lewis

I. **BACKGROUND.** Papilledema is an optic disc swelling produced by increased intracranial pressure. It may be detected in the asymptomatic pediatric or adult patient during the course of a screening funduscopic examination with a non–life-threatening cause. Conversely, it may be identified in initially asymptomatic or gravely symptomatic patients (including pregnant women) as a marker of a life-threatening condition such as subarachnoid hemorrhage, meningitis, or brain tumor (1).

II. **PATHOPHYSIOLOGY**

A. **Etiology.** True papilledema is always associated with increased intracranial pressure. The most often cited causes include trauma, primary or metastatic intracranial tumor, aqueductal stenosis (as is seen in certain types of congenital hydrocephalus), pseudotumor cerebri (idiopathic intracranial hypertension; frequently misdiagnosed as migraine headache) (2), subdural hematoma, subarachnoid hemorrhage, arteriovenous malformations, brain abscess, meningitis, encephalitis, and sagittal sinus thrombosis.

B. **Epidemiology.** Most patients with papilledema are adults. Many of the causes of papilledema (e.g., subarachnoid hemorrhage and cancer) are more common with advancing age. Pseudotumor cerebri is characteristically discovered in overweight adolescent women. Individuals with immunosuppression (e.g., human immunodeficiency virus [HIV]/acquired immunodeficiency syndrome, chemotherapy, chronic prednisone therapy) are at heightened risk of central nervous system (CNS) infections (e.g., meningitis, encephalitis, and brain abscess) that may be associated with papilledema.

III. **EVALUATION.** The history and physical examination are tailored to the age, setting, and urgency of the patient presentation. Patients with an acute and rapid increase in intracranial pressure with associated papilledema may be moribund and comatose, requiring emergent and expedited assessment and care. In less dramatic presentations, patients present with nonspecific symptoms (e.g., headache; see in the subsequent text) (1) that sparks a search, initially on the basis of the history and physical examination, for associated intracranial pressure and its cause. Alternatively, the search for clues to the presence and the cause of increased intracranial pressure only begins subsequent to the discovery of papilledema during the course of a screening funduscopic examination.

A. **History.** In the symptomatic patient, headache, nausea, vomiting, diplopia, focal weakness, fever, neck stiffness, and/or photophobia, and/or fleeting loss of vision (obscurations)—especially with the head in dependent positions—raise the index of suspicion for increased intracranial pressure. Parents of infants or children may report increased head size or decreased alertness. After probing patient complaints and associated symptoms, determine the presence or risk factors for vascular disease (including prior stroke), cancer, trauma, or immunosuppression. A thorough medication and drug use history should also be obtained. A family history of conditions related to increased intracranial pressure should be elicited.

B. **Physical examination**

1. This commences with vital signs, including blood pressure and visual acuity. Rarely is a decrease in visual acuity seen in association with increased intracranial pressure; if present, it typically suggests other causes (e.g., vein occlusion, anterior ischemic optic neuropathy, or optic neuritis—as seen in the subsequent text).

2. Additional features of a detailed ophthalmologic examination, including funduscopic assessment, should be obtained. Sixth nerve palsies show limited lateral

gaze and may be associated with horizontal diplopia, whereas third nerve palsies demonstrate a limitation in medial gaze, elevation, and depression. Regarding the funduscopic examination in the asymptomatic patient, it is necessary to take care to first determine if there is true disc edema or only pseudopapilledema (this may well require consultation with an ophthalmologist). Pseudopapilledema is optic nerve head elevation caused by hyaline deposition ("drusen") within the optic nerve head itself, and is reported to be more common in whites (3). There is no associated increased intracranial pressure or CNS pathology. When true papilledema is present, it is typically bilateral. Disc edema produces an obscuring of the blood vessels' margins. Tiny splinter hemorrhages are seen in and around the optic nerve. Spontaneous venous pulsations (SVPs) should be sought. If SVPs are present, there is normal intracranial pressure. Prominent retinal hemorrhages suggest malignant hypertension or central retinal vein occlusion (as seen in the subsequent text).

   3. A complete head and neck examination to check for neck stiffness, temporal artery tenderness, pain in and around the eyes, and sinus tenderness is also important. Thorough vascular and neurologic examinations are indicated. Measure head circumference in infants and young children; check for bulging or prematurely closed fontanels in the former group.

C. Testing. If true papilledema is found, laboratory testing and clinical imaging should be directed at determining the cause and the severity of the associated increased intracranial pressure. Suggested laboratory tests include sedimentation rate, C-reactive protein, and white blood count if CNS infection is suspected. Serologies for HIV, syphilis, and herpes should be obtained as indicated. A lumbar puncture for the measurement of opening pressure and a cerebrospinal fluid (CSF) examination to evaluate for evidence of meningitis, tumor, or hemorrhage should be performed only after ruling out a compressive lesion with a computed tomography (CT) scan or magnetic resonance imaging (MRI). If true papilledema is suspected by the primary care clinician and/or confirmed in consultation with an ophthalmologist, then diagnostic imaging is mandatory. A CT scan with and without contrast should be ordered. If the CT scan is inconclusive, an MRI will be particularly helpful in imaging brain stem and cerebellar lesions, which can obstruct CSF flow in children and adults. An MRI angiography may be required to identify a related vascular abnormality. A CT scan is the preferred technique to image acute intracranial bleeding. An ultrasound of the optic disc may be used if the diagnosis of pseudopapilledema is uncertain.

D. Genetics. Many of the underlying conditions associated with papilledema have genetic contributions.

IV. DIAGNOSIS

A. Differential diagnosis. Disc swelling without increased intracranial pressure may be caused by the following conditions:

   1. Optic neuritis. An afferent pupillary defect exists along with decreased vision and pain on extraocular movement. Color vision will be decreased in this normally unilateral condition. It may be seen with multiple sclerosis.

   2. Malignant hypertension. (of essential or secondary causes, including severe preeclampsia). Blood pressure is markedly elevated. The eye findings are characteristic: bilateral prominent disc edema, flame hemorrhages that extend peripherally, and cotton wool spots (see Chapter 7.8).

   3. Central retinal vein occlusion. This is characterized by a unilateral disc swelling with very prominent flame and blot hemorrhages, without increased blood pressure.

   4. Anterior ischemic optic neuropathy. This may be due to arteritis (e.g., temporal/"giant cell") presenting with headache, stiff neck, temporal tenderness, jaw claudication, elevated sedimentation rate, and severe visual loss in one eye followed by visual loss of the other eye in 60% of the cases. When arteritis is absent, typically no symptoms are present except decreased vision. Associated conditions include systemic hypertension, diabetes mellitus, or collagen vascular disorders.

5. **Infiltration of the optic nerve.** Tuberculosis granuloma, leukemic infiltrate, sarcoidosis, and metastatic disease are the more common examples of infiltrative processes. The infiltration can be unilateral or bilateral and can lead to rapid loss of vision. Radiation therapy can be helpful to preserve vision.

6. **Leber's hereditary optic neuropathy.** This usually affects men in the second or third decade and is characterized by unilateral progressive loss of vision with disc swelling.

7. **Diabetic papillitis.** It is an ischemic infarction to the nerve in advanced diabetics. This is often bilateral and causes mild disc elevation (see Chapter 14.1).

B. **Clinical manifestations.** Chronic papilledema can result in optic atrophy (with decreased optic nerve swelling) and progressive visual (initially peripheral) loss that may progress to frank blindness. Such patients should be followed with serial perimetry by an ophthalmologist.

References

1. Clinch CR. Evaluation of acute headaches in adults. *Am Fam Physician* 2001;63(4): 685–692.
2. Brazis PW, Lee AG. Elevated intracranial pressure and pseudotumor cerebri. *Curr Opin Ophthalmol* 1998;9(6):27–32.
3. Giovannini J, Chrousos G. *Papilledema.* eMedicine www.emedicine.com/oph/topic187. htm, accessed on August 2, 2005.

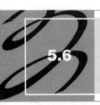

5.6 PUPILLARY INEQUALITY
David C. Holub

I. **BACKGROUND.** Anisocoria is defined as an inequality of pupillary size (diameter).

II. **PATHOPHYSIOLOGY**

A. **Etiology**

1. The pupil is a hole or aperture in the iris that permits the passage of light through to the retina. There are two muscles within the iris that control pupillary size. The *sphincter pupillae* is a circular muscle that controls pupillary constriction, or miosis. The *dilator pupillae* is a radial muscle that controls pupillary dilation, or mydriasis.

2. The pupillary constrictor is innervated by fibers from the parasympathetic autonomic nervous system. These fibers originate in the midbrain and travel to the Edinger-Westphal nucleus in the dorsal midbrain, and then with the cranial nerve (CN) III (the oculomotor nerve) through the cavernous sinus to the orbit. They diverge from the CN III to synapse in the orbit with the ciliary ganglion. Postganglionic short ciliary nerves then innervate the pupillary constrictor muscle. Lesions at any anatomic site along this pathway lead to pathologic mydriasis (1).

3. The pupillary dilator muscle is innervated by fibers from the sympathetic autonomic nervous system. These neurons originate in the hypothalamus, descend through the brain stem to the C8-T2 lateral horn, and then travel with the cervical sympathetic trunk to the superior cervical ganglion. Postganglionic long ciliary nerves travel with the internal carotid artery until the superior orbital fissure, where they diverge and continue to the dilator pupillae muscle. These fibers both stimulate the dilator pupillae and inhibit the pupillary constrictor and ciliary muscles. They also innervate the levator palpebrae muscle, and therefore contribute to eyelid elevation. Lesions at any anatomic site along this pathway lead to pathologic miosis (1).

B. Epidemiology. Physiologic anisocoria is common, affecting perhaps as much as 20% of normal individuals. The difference in pupillary size is small, usually <1 mm (2).

III. EVALUATION

A. History. In most patients, anisocoria is discovered incidentally; presenting symptoms are relatively uncommon. It is necessary to inquire about ocular symptoms such as pain, redness, tearing, or photophobia. Any past history of eye disease, injury, surgery, or medications should be elicited.

B. Physical examination. The pupils should be examined in both dim and bright lights, assessing both direct and consensual pupillary light reflexes. An afferent pupillary defect (Marcus Gunn pupil) permits a consensual light reflex, but no pupillary constriction or paradoxical pupillary dilation to direct light. In an efferent pupillary defect, pupillary constriction to both direct and consensual light reflexes is absent.

1. The critical first step in assessing a patient with anisocoria is to determine which is the abnormal pupil (i.e., is one pupil abnormally constricted or is one pupil abnormally dilated?). It is necessary to examine the pupillary responses in both bright and dim lighting. The pupil that does not dilate in dim light or constrict in bright light is the abnormal one.

2. Extraocular movements should be tested. In patients with third nerve palsy, the affected eye shows outward deviation during primary gaze. It is able to come to midline only with attempts at inward gaze, and downward gaze leads to inward rotation.

C. Testing. Computed tomography or magnetic resonance imaging is valuable for suspected intracranial mass lesions or bleeding. Angiography is indicated for suspected cerebral aneurysm or carotid dissection. Obtaining chest radiography for occult lung malignancy is reasonable in patients with Horner's syndrome.

IV. DIAGNOSIS

A. Differential diagnosis

1. The differential diagnosis of miosis includes Horner's syndrome, unilateral anterior uveitis, Lyme disease, or syphilis.

2. The differential diagnosis of mydriasis includes palsy of or damage to CN III, Adie's pupil, the use of certain medications (with anticholinergic effects), and acute angle closure glaucoma.

B. Clinical manifestations

1. Pathologic miosis may be caused by a lesion or disease state that affects any anatomic site from the brain to the pupil itself. Horner's syndrome is the triad of miosis with ptosis and ipsilateral facial anhidrosis (variably present depending on the level of the lesion). It is caused by damage to the cervical thoracic sympathetic fibers. A brain stem stroke may lead to these findings. Disease of the internal carotid artery, such as dissection, may also interrupt the signals normally carried by these nerves. Horner's syndrome also frequently occurs due to tumors that compress these nerve fibers. These may include parotid gland tumors, carotid body tumors, lymphoma with enlarged cervical adenopathy, mediastinal tumors, or apical lung tumors (typically in the superior sulcus). Direct trauma can also damage the sympathetic nerve fibers (3). Miosis may also be caused by unilateral ocular disease such as anterior uveitis, in which inflammation leads to the development of adhesions (synechiae) between the iris and the anterior lens capsule. Lyme disease and neurosyphilis may involve the eye as well, leading to an Argyll Robertson pupil—an irregular pupil that reacts poorly to light but normally to accommodation.

2. Pathologic mydriasis is typically caused by disease states that affect the oculomotor nerve (CN III) and thereby the parasympathetic fibers that travel with this nerve. Other clinical manifestations of a third nerve palsy include abnormalities of ocular movement and ptosis. Neurologic diseases such as multiple sclerosis may cause third nerve palsy. Nerve compression can occur from vascular phenomena (posterior communicating artery aneurysm), increased intracranial pressure due to head trauma with bleeding, or an intracranial mass. In the comatose patient with head trauma, a temporal lobe herniation compressing the

midbrain may also lead to unilateral mydriasis. Unilateral mydriasis may also be an isolated finding in Adie's pupil, caused by damage to the ciliary ganglion through infection, ischemia, or trauma. Patients are typically women, 20 to 50 years of age, and usually asymptomatic. They present with anisocoria, diminished or absent light reflexes (both direct and consensual), and an exaggerated and prolonged (tonic) pupillary constriction during accommodation.

  3. Unilateral pharmacologic mydriasis may occur with anticholinergic medications.

  4. Acute angle closure glaucoma is a crucial consideration in the evaluation of unilateral mydriasis. Patients present with eye pain, redness, and visual impairment. An examination reveals a fixed, mid-dilated pupil, and elevated intraocular pressure.

References

1. Mosenthal W. *A textbook of neuroanatomy.* London: Parthenon Publishing, 1995.
2. Eggenberger E. *Anisocoria.* http://www.emedicine.com/oph/topic160.htm, accessed on July 2005.
3. Bardorf C. *Horner's syndrome.* http://www.emedicine.com/OPH/topic336.htm, accessed on July 2005.

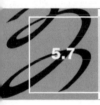

5.7   RED EYE
David C. Holub

I. BACKGROUND
  A. The red eye is one of the most common ocular complaints encountered in primary care. Although many causes of the red eye are benign, some are true emergencies. Failure to act accordingly may pose an immediate threat to the patient's vision.

  B. Anatomically, almost any structure in the eye or its surrounding tissues may manifest with redness.

II. PATHOPHYSIOLOGY
  A. Etiology. The primary causes of a red eye are infection or trauma to the various anatomic structures of the eye. Occasionally, connective tissue disease or a primary ocular disease can also manifest with a red eye. Causes include the following:

    1. Scleritis is an inflammation of the sclera, the fibrous outer envelope of the eye.

    2. Episcleritis is an inflammation of the connective tissue that lies between the sclera and the conjunctiva.

    3. Conjunctivitis is an inflammation of the conjunctiva, the mucous membranes that line the anterior surface of the eye and the posterior surface of the eyelid.

    4. Blepharitis is an inflammation of the eyelid, which may appear red.

    5. A **hordeolum** is a superficial inflammatory granuloma of the eyelid that develops acutely from an obstruction of the ocular sebaceous glands (Zeis or meibomian glands).

    6. A **chalazion** manifests similarly, but is a deeper-seated granulomatous obstruction of these glands.

    7. Acute dacryocystitis results from an obstruction and secondary infection of the lacrimal system.

    8. Iritis or **anterior uveitis** involves an inflammation of the middle part of the eye (iris and ciliary body).

    9. Keratitis occurs when the cornea, the transparent outer covering of the anterior eye, becomes infected or is injured traumatically, resulting either in a **corneal abrasion** or a **corneal foreign body.**

    10. Hyphema, or hemorrhage into the anterior chamber, which also results from trauma, may manifest with visible redness if the amount of bleeding is significant. Even relatively minor trauma may lead to a **subconjunctival hemorrhage,** evident as a prominent red area in the normally white sclera.

   11. Acute angle closure glaucoma leads to a rapid rise in intraocular pressure and may manifest as redness along with ocular pain, visual loss, headache, and nausea.

   12. Contact dermatitis, atopic dermatitis, periorbital cellulitis, or **orbital cellulitis** cause the skin and soft tissues surrounding the eye or involving the eyelid to become inflamed or infected.

   B. Epidemiology. Conjunctivitis is the most common eye complaint in the United States, accounting for 30% of all acute ocular complaints (1).

III. EVALUATION

   A. History. An assessment of the red eye begins with questions regarding its location (unilateral, bilateral, or unilateral spreading to bilateral), onset (sudden or gradual), duration (acute, subacute, or chronic), inciting factors (such as trauma), and associated signs and symptoms. Ocular pain, swelling, photophobia, or disturbances in visual acuity are frequently signs of a more emergent condition. Other associated symptoms may include crusting, discharge, itching, burning, tearing, dry eyes, or a foreign body sensation. Systemic symptoms such as fever, headache, abdominal pain, nausea/vomiting, rhinorrhea, or cough should be elicited. A past history of similar ocular complaints is important. The patient should be asked about the use of contact lenses or eye drops. The past medical history may include certain systemic diseases that produce ocular involvement, such as syphilis, inflammatory bowel disease, and some collagen vascular diseases (sarcoidosis, ankylosing spondylitis, reactive arthritis, rheumatoid arthritis, and Sjögren's syndrome). There may also be a history of allergic or atopic disorders such as asthma, eczema, or allergic rhinitis.

   B. Physical examination

   1. The physical examination of the eye should always begin with an assessment of visual acuity with a wall-mounted or handheld Snellen's eye chart. Visual acuity should always be measured either with the patient's corrective lenses or through pinhole testing. Visual disturbances owing solely to refractive error improve with the use of lenses or pinhole testing. Visual impairment due to organic eye disease does not.

   2. Once this has been completed, a significant portion of the physical examination can then be easily accomplished in the primary care office setting without specialized equipment. A visual *inspection* of the eye and its surrounding soft tissues is essential to determine where the redness is located anatomically (i.e., sclera, conjunctiva, anterior chamber, eyelid, or periorbital tissues). Other notable findings include the presence of any lid swelling or crusting, purulent discharge, tearing, erythema or swelling of the periorbital tissues, or proptosis. Vesicular skin lesions near the eye suggest a herpes infection, which can have severe consequences on any infected structures within the eye. A palpation of the globe and surrounding soft tissues for firmness or tenderness should then be performed. A limitation of or tenderness with extraocular movements should be assessed. Eyelid eversion should be carried out to look for retained foreign bodies. Finally, a pupillary examination should be undertaken to assess size, shape, and reactivity.

   3. Further examination of the eye requires both the appropriate equipment and the skill to use this equipment and interpret the findings correctly. Although this is feasible in the primary care setting, clinicians should obtain ophthalmologic consultation at this time if needed.

   4. A slit lamp examination should be performed to assess for abnormalities of the anterior chamber, such as the presence of red or white blood cells or visible floating particulate matter (flare). The slit lamp is a more precise method for measuring anterior chamber depth than lateral visual inspection of the eye with a penlight. The cornea, with the application of fluorescein staining and the cobalt blue light source on the slit lamp, can be assessed for abrasion, ulceration, or a foreign body. Some patients may be unable to tolerate this examination due to pain or photophobia. In this instance, a topical anesthetic such as tetracaine may be applied to the eye.

5. The measurement of intraocular pressure is important in the evaluation for acute angle closure glaucoma. This can be accomplished with a Schiötz tonometer in the primary care setting. In the ophthalmologist's office, a gonioscopy or the measurement of the angle between the iris and cornea, can also be performed.

6. A funduscopic examination should be undertaken, ideally after pupillary dilatation has been effected through the installation of a mydriatic solution. As pupillary dilatation can precipitate an attack of acute angle closure, it is essential that this diagnosis be excluded prior to attempting this. Under direct ophthalmoscopy, the cornea, lens, and vitreous humor can be assessed for pathology.

C. **Testing.** Relatively few studies are useful in the differential diagnosis of the red eye. Cultures of purulent discharge are occasionally helpful if bacterial conjunctivitis is suspected. Blood cultures and a complete blood count with differential are prudent in cases of suspected orbital cellulitis. Workup for rheumatologic disease may be considered in patients with iritis, episcleritis, or scleritis. Imaging studies are rarely of value (2).

IV. DIAGNOSIS

A. **Differential diagnosis.** Given the potential severity of some of the causes of red eye, the primary care physician's first priority is to determine if immediate intervention or ophthalmologic referral is warranted. The most serious causes of the acute red eye that need to be ruled out include acute angle closure glaucoma, hyphema, orbital cellulitis, acute keratitis, corneal ulcer, scleritis, and iritis/uveitis. Less serious causes include conjunctivitis, lid disorders, and subconjunctival hemorrhages.

B. **Clinical manifestations**

1. **Acute angle closure glaucoma** presents with severe unilateral eye pain and blurry vision, often accompanied by visual halos, headache, abdominal pain, and nausea and vomiting. The physical examination reveals a shallow anterior chamber either by penlight or slit lamp examination, partially dilated pupils that respond poorly to light, firmness of globe on palpation, and elevated intraocular pressure on tonometry (3).

2. **Scleritis** typically presents with pain, tearing, photophobia, and decreased visual acuity. Visible swelling accompanies the redness. Discharge is typically absent. Fifty percent of the cases are bilateral.

3. **Iritis** or **uveitis** usually presents as blurred vision, pain, and photophobia affecting a single eye. Discharge is typically absent, although occasionally patients may have watery discharge. Physical examination reveals a sluggishly reactive pupil with pain and photophobia on both direct and consensual pupillary testing. Slit lamp examination also reveals proteinaceous or cellular matter in the anterior chamber (flare).

4. **Keratitis** commonly presents with severe eye pain, photophobia, and blurry vision. A slit lamp examination with fluorescein staining identifies any disruption in the corneal epithelium. Owing to its serious nature, this must be regarded as a corneal infection until proven otherwise.

5. **Hyphema** may be preceded by a history of ocular trauma. Vision is impaired only with a large quantity of blood in the anterior chamber. Physical examination shows visible blood on slit lamp examination, a dilated pupil, and elevated intraocular pressure.

6. **Orbital** or **periorbital cellulitis** presents with visible erythema, swelling, warmth, and tenderness of the skin and soft tissues surrounding the eye. The eyelid may be involved. Orbital cellulitis, a more serious infection, may manifest with fever, proptosis, and abnormalities of vision or pupillary response. Extraocular movements may also be limited. These findings are absent in periorbital cellulitis.

7. **Conjunctivitis** is the most common cause of eye redness and may be bacterial, viral, or allergic in etiology. Allergic conjunctivitis usually begins bilaterally,

as opposed to infectious conjunctivitis, which often begins unilaterally and is then spread to the other eye due to manipulation by the patient. Itching and tearing are common. A discharge is ubiquitous—clear or watery in allergic or viral etiologies but purulent in bacterial cases. Allergic conjunctivitis may be accompanied by other allergic symptoms or physical examination findings. Although cultures of purulent discharge are often negative, it is virtually impossible to clinically distinguish between viral and bacterial conjunctivitis. Therefore, either cultures or empiric treatment with topical antibiotics is warranted. Notable exceptions to the typically benign course of infectious conjunctivitis are cases of gonococcal and chlamydial conjunctivitis. A history of exposure to genital secretions is critical, as the course of the illness and the treatment differs significantly.

8. **Episcleritis** appears similar to simple conjunctivitis. The redness may be deeper and more localized than seen in conjunctivitis. Discharge is typically absent (1).

9. **Blepharitis** presents as redness, crusting, and often as a swelling of the eyelid. It commonly occurs in combination with conjunctivitis, a **hordeolum** (with associated eyelid tenderness and possibly a visible abscess), or a **chalazion** (without associated eyelid tenderness or abscess).

10. **Dacryocystitis** presents with unilateral redness, swelling, and tenderness over the lacrimal sac, which is located in the inferonasal quadrant of the eye. This condition is seen almost exclusively in children and in patients over the age of 40.

11. **Corneal abrasions, ulcerations**, and **foreign bodies** manifest with a foreign body sensation, eye pain, and tearing. An examination with a slit lamp under fluorescein reveals dark green staining in areas where the corneal epithelium has been disrupted. Lid eversion is essential to search for retained foreign bodies. As stated in the preceding text, corneal infections must first be excluded.

12. **Subconjunctival hemorrhage** appears as a localized reddish discoloration of the sclera due to minor trauma (including sneezing or coughing).

References

1. Silverman MA, Bessman E. *Conjunctivitis.* http://www.emedicine.com/emerg/topic110.htm, accessed on July 2005.
2. Farina GA, Mazarin G. *Red eye evaluation.* http://www.emedicine.com/oph/topic267.htm, accessed on July 2005.
3. Beers MH, Berkow R, eds. *The Merck manual of diagnosis and therapy*, 17th ed. West Point, PA: Merck & Co, 1999.

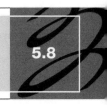

SCOTOMA
David C. Holub

5.8

I. BACKGROUND. A scotoma is a focal area of visual loss in the patient's visual field. Patients commonly refer to a scotoma as a "blind spot." Scotomata may be further categorized in several different ways.

A. A scotoma may be classified by its location in the visual field. A **central scotoma** occurs at the point of fixation and causes significant and immediately noticeable visual impairment to the patient. A **paracentral scotoma** occurs near the point of fixation and is also usually noticeable to the patient. A **peripheral scotoma** occurs away from the point of fixation in the periphery of the visual field. Peripheral scotomata may be asymptomatic and only discovered on visual field testing performed for a different reason.

B. A **positive scotoma** manifests as a black spot in the patient's visual field. A **negative scotoma** manifests as a blank spot in the patient's visual field. Patients are nearly always aware of positive scotomata, but negative scotomata may only be detected during an ophthalmologic examination.

C. An **absolute scotoma** indicates a complete loss of visual perception, whereas a **relative scotoma** involves diminished but not absent light perception in the affected area. A **color scotoma** defines diminished or lost color vision only.

D. The term scintillating scotoma has come into common usage by both patients and clinicians, typically in the context of a migraine with aura. This is something of a misnomer, because scintillations and scotomata are distinct visual phenomena. That they frequently occur together in a migraine with aura has led to the origin of this term.

II. PATHOPHYSIOLOGY

A. Etiology. Everyone has a physiologic scotoma at the optic disk, the site where the optic nerve enters the retina. Diseases that affect the optic nerve may cause an enlargement of this scotoma to the point that it interferes with vision. This manifests as a central scotoma. Diseases that affect the macula may also present with central scotoma as a prominent symptom. Peripheral scotomata result from disease processes that affect the retina. Table 5.8.1 lists the common causes of both central and peripheral scotomata.

B. Epidemiology. The incidence of scotoma varies depending upon the associated disease state. The strongest association is with optic neuritis. Sixty percent of patients with scotoma due to optic neuritis will eventually develop multiple sclerosis (1).

III. EVALUATION

A. History. Patients with a central scotoma report a visual field defect as a primary complaint. Elucidating the exact type of scotoma, as outlined in the definitions in the preceding text, is important in anatomically localizing the lesion responsible for the scotoma. A focused history should assess for other visual disturbances such as diminished visual acuity or diminished color vision, and ocular pain. Neurologic symptoms may be found in patients with multiple sclerosis. Systemic symptoms may indicate an underlying connective tissue disease or vasculitis. The past medical history may include known neurologic or connective tissue diseases or vasculitis. A history of current and past medications is very important. Certain medications such as chloroquine/hydroxychloroquine, isoniazid, ethambutol, digitalis glycosides, and possibly amiodarone can be directly toxic to the retina or optic nerve (2). Immune suppressant medications can predispose to infections such as cytomegalovirus retinitis. A human immunodeficiency virus (HIV) infection can also predispose the patient to these infections. A history of risk factors for HIV infection should be obtained. A history of ingestion or exposure to toxins such as lead, methanol, or ethylene glycol should be obtained (2). Certain dietary practices or poor nutrition may lead to thiamine or vitamin B_{12} deficiency.

B. Physical examination

1. No ocular physical examination should be undertaken for any condition without first performing a test of visual acuity. This may be done with a handheld or wall-mounted Snellen eye chart. Once visual acuity has been documented, the rest of the eye examination may be undertaken.

2. Color vision should be tested with pseudoisochromatic plates (Ishihara plates are most commonly used). Diminished color vision is common in optic nerve disease.

3. Pupillary testing is important, because the presence or absence of a relative afferent pupillary defect is helpful in diagnosing or excluding unilateral optic neuritis. A relative afferent pupillary defect is also known as a Marcus Gunn pupil. The testing is performed in a dimly lit room with the patient's eyes fixated on a distant object. The examiner shines a bright light into the asymptomatic eye and should observe bilateral pupillary constriction due to the consensual light reflex. The examiner then swings the flashlight across the nasal bridge to the affected eye. If there is optic nerve dysfunction in the affected eye, the pupil paradoxically dilates due to the inadequate transmission of direct light

TABLE 5.8.1	Causes of Central and Peripheral Scotomata	
Cause	**Optic nerve/macula**	**Retina**
Ocular disease	Primary open-angle glaucoma	Retinal detachment
	Age-related macular degeneration	
Neurologic disease	Optic neuritis (secondary to multiple sclerosis)	
	Optic neuritis (idiopathic)	
Vascular disease	Temporal arteritis	Retinal vasculitis
		Retinal artery occlusion
		Retinal vein occlusion
Rheumatologic disease	Sarcoidosis with ocular infiltration	
Endocrine disease	Thyroid ophthalmopathy	Diabetic retinopathy
Infectious disease	Ocular syphilis	Cytomegalovirus retinitis
Malignancy	Optic nerve glioma	
	Optic nerve sheath meningioma	
	Intracranial tumor with optic nerve compression	
	Paraneoplastic syndromes	
Nutritional deficiency	Thiamine deficiency	
	Vitamin B_{12} deficiency	
Toxin exposure	Lead exposure	Chloroquine toxicity
	Methanol exposure	
	Ethylene glycol exposure	
	Ethambutol toxicity	
	Isoniazid toxicity	
	Digitalis toxicity	
	Amiodarone toxicity	
	Nutritional amblyopia (due to chronic tobacco or alcohol use)	

stimulation to the brain. In patients with systemic disease causing bilateral optic neuritis, an afferent pupillary defect may be absent (3).

4. A funduscopic examination is best performed after pupillary dilatation. A pale or white optic disk indicates optic neuritis. Retinal hemorrhages or exudates or retinal vasculature abnormalities may be visualized.
5. After the ocular examination is complete, a general physical examination including a complete neurologic examination should be undertaken.
6. Visual field analysis is critical in the evaluation of scotoma. Primary care clinicians seldom have the office equipment to perform this testing properly. Visual field testing by confrontation or by tangent screen examination is inadequate; patients should be referred to an eye specialist for testing with the appropriate equipment.

C. Testing. There is no role for untargeted diagnostic studies in the evaluation of scotoma. The selection of appropriate laboratory and radiographic studies should arise from the history and physical examination findings, including formal visual field testing. Blood tests such as antinuclear antibodies, rheumatoid factor, or levels of angiotensin-converting enzyme should be ordered if there is a clinical suspicion for a vasculitis or connective tissue disease. Temporal arteritis requires urgent diagnosis and an erythrocyte sedimentation rate should be ordered immediately when this is suspected. Serum vitamin B_{12} and red blood cell folate levels are indicated in patients with bilateral central scotoma. Serologic testing for syphilis or HIV is indicated in patients with risk factors for these infections. Thyroid function tests are appropriate in patients with ocular or systemic physical examination findings that suggest thyrotoxicosis. Serum lead levels should be measured in patients with a history of occupational or domestic lead exposure. In patients with suspected multiple sclerosis, a lumbar puncture should be considered to obtain cerebrospinal fluid for analysis of myelin basic protein and oligoclonal bands. Magnetic resonance imaging (MRI) with gadolinium is both sensitive and specific for optic neuritis. An MRI may also be useful in establishing a diagnosis of multiple sclerosis or in visualizing intracranial tumors. Some central nervous system tumors, such as optic nerve sheath meningioma, are also well visualized by computed tomography with contrast. Again, tests should be deferred unless there is a significant pretest clinical suspicion for these conditions, based on the patient's history and physical examination findings.

IV. DIAGNOSIS

A. Differential diagnosis. The approach to scotoma begins with classifying central versus peripheral scotomata. Central scotomata are attributable to optic nerve or macular disease. Peripheral scotomata are caused by retinal disease.

B. Clinical manifestations. Scotoma presents with a visual field defect as the primary complaint. Patients with retinal diseases and glaucoma have few, if any, symptoms, except for vision loss. Patients with multiple sclerosis may also present with symptoms such as gait abnormalities, speech difficulties, difficulties with bowel and/or bladder control, weakness, or paresthesias. Jaw claudication and headache are seen in temporal arteritis. Sarcoidosis may cause fever, arthralgias, lymphadenopathy, or skin lesions.

References

1. Riordan-Eva P. Eye. In: Tierney LM, McPhee SJ, Papadakis MA, eds. *Current medical diagnosis and treatment*, 44th Ed. New York: Lange Medical Books, 2005:166.
2. Zafar A, Sergott RC. *Toxic/nutritional optic neuropathy.* http://www.emedicine.com/oph/topic750.htm, accessed on July 2005.
3. Ing E. *Neuro-ophthalmic examination.* http://www.emedicine.com/oph/topic643.htm, accessed on July 2005.

Ear, Nose, and Throat Problems

Frank S. Celestino

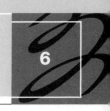

6

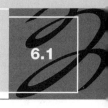

HALITOSIS
Mark D. Andrews

I. BACKGROUND. Halitosis (fetor oris) refers to unpleasant or offensive odors emitted in the expired air. It may merely be a social handicap related to poor oral hygiene or oral cavity disease. Rarely, it can represent a marker of more serious systemic illness requiring diagnosis and treatment (1). The Greeks and Romans wrote about bad breath and it was discussed in the Jewish Talmud. Today, oral malodor has been stigmatized, giving rise to a commercial market for mouth fresheners exceeding $900 million annually (2). Despite this publicity, patients only seek help rarely and are generally unaware of the problem, although it can severely affect personal relations.

II. PATHOPHYSIOLOGY

A. Etiology. Physiologic halitosis, such as with eating onions and garlic or with morning breath, is temporary. These odors are reversible, transient, and responsive to traditional oral hygiene practices (3). In contrast, pathologic halitosis is more intense and not easily reversible. It may arise from similar mechanisms but results more frequently from regional or systemic pathology, leading to persistent odors that ultimately require treatment (1–3).

Persistent halitosis (usually noted by individuals around the patient) is more severe than physiologic halitosis. The important task initially is to categorize the halitosis as either localized to the oral cavity or originating systemically. In 80% to 90% of patients, halitosis is due to bacterial activity from disorders of the oral cavity, and in the remainder of patients, the condition is attributed to nonoral or systemic sources. Volatile sulfur compounds arising through the microbial degradation of amino acids are the presumed source of most offending odors. Bad breath may originate from the following areas: oral cavity—85% to 88%, nasal passages—8%, tonsils—3%, and other sites—2% to 3% (4). In addition, the causes of halitosis can be subcategorized into pathologic and nonpathologic types.

1. Nonpathologic causes

a. Morning breath is due to decreased salivary flow overnight associated with increased fluid pH, elevated gram-negative bacterial growth, and volatile sulfur compounds production (3).

b. Xerostomia of any cause (e.g., sleep, diseases, medication, mouth breathing, and especially age-related declines in salivary quantity and quality) can contribute to halitosis.

c. Missed meals can lead to halitosis secondary to decreased salivary flow and the absence of the mechanical action of the food on the tongue surface to wear down filiform papillae.

d. Tobacco or alcohol can be a contributing cause of halitosis.

e. Metabolites from ingested food (onions, garlic, alcohol, pastrami, and other meats) are absorbed into the circulation and then excreted through the lungs.

f. Medications such as anticholinergic drugs can cause xerostomia, especially in the elderly. Other agents include amphetamines, psychiatric drugs, antihistamines, decongestants, narcotics, antihypertensives, anti-parkinsonian agents, chemotherapy, and radiation therapy.

2. Pathologic causes

a. Local oropharynx. Chronic periodontal disease and gingivitis are common sources through the promotion of bacterial overgrowth. In their absence, the most likely oral source is the posterior dorsum of the tongue with posterior nasal drainage being a frequent contributing factor to local bacterial overgrowth. Stomatitis and glossitis caused by systemic disease, medication, or vitamin deficiencies can lead to trapped food particles and desquamated tissue. An improperly cleaned prosthetic appliance can be a local contributor, as can primary pharyngeal cancer. Other conditions associated with parotid dysfunction (e.g., viral and bacterial infections, calculi, drug reactions, systemic conditions including Sjögren's syndrome) are also important. Tonsils infrequently cause halitosis (found in 7% of the population), even with crypt tonsillitis. These may alarm patients but are usually asymptomatic and not associated with any pathology.

   b. Gastrointestinal tract. Gastrointestinal sources occasionally contribute to intermittent bad breath. Potential sources include gastroesophageal reflux disease, gastrointestinal bleeding, gastric cancer, malabsorption syndromes, and enteric infections.

   c. Respiratory tract. Chronic sinusitis, nasal foreign bodies or tumors, postnasal drip, bronchitis, pneumonia, bronchiectasis, tuberculosis, and malignancies may cause halitosis.

   d. Psychiatric. Halitophobia is imaginary halitosis associated with psychiatric disorders (3).

   e. Systemic sources include diabetic ketoacidosis (sweet, fruity, acetone breath), renal failure (ammonia or "fishy" odor), hepatic failure ("fetor hepaticus"—a sweet amine odor), high fever with dehydration, and vitamin or mineral deficiencies leading to a dry mouth.

B. Epidemiology. The prevalence of halitosis is not known, but many individuals worry about it. In one study, 20% of adults worried about bad breath, when little was measured (5). Approximately 25% of individuals seeking help for halitosis may be halitophobic or suffering from pseudohalitosis (4).

III. EVALUATION

A. History. Focus on the characteristics of the bad breath, although the patient is often unable to describe his or her condition accurately because of olfactory desensitization. Is the odor transient or constant? Constant odor suggests chronic systemic disease or serious disorders of the oral cavity. What are the precipitating, aggravating, or relieving factors? Ask about smoking habits, diet, drugs, dentures, mouth breathing, snoring, hay fever, and nasal obstruction. Because the therapy for halitosis of oral origin, beyond the limitation of aggravating factors, is proper oral hygiene and vigorous tongue brushing, an evaluation of the patient's tooth brushing and flossing regimen is imperative.

B. Physical examination. This should be undertaken with an emphasis on the oral cavity, particularly looking for ulceration, dryness, trauma, postnasal drainage, infections, inflamed cryptic tonsils, or neoplasms. Techniques for localizing the odor source (systemic vs. oral cavity) include:

   1. Seal the lips and blow air through the nose. If a fetid odor is noted, this is suggestive of a systemic source. If an odor is only noted from the nose, then a nasal source is likely.

   2. Pinch the nose with the lips closed. Hold respiration and exhale gently through the mouth. Odors detected in this fashion generally are local in origin.

   3. If a similar odor is noted from both sources then a systemic source may be suspected.

C. Testing. For most patients, clinical laboratory testing and diagnostic imaging are unnecessary, and should only be pursued on the basis of specific findings indicated by the history and physical examination. The Schirmer's test may be useful in identifying xerophthalmia and associated xerostomia seen with Sjögren's syndrome and some other rheumatologic conditions (Chapter 12.1). If indicated, radiologic studies and imaging procedures of the sinuses, thorax, and abdomen may be used to identify infectious processes and neoplasms.

IV. DIAGNOSIS

A. Differential diagnosis. The key is a thorough history and focused physical examination to distinguish local oral from systemic processes (see section **II.A.**). Because 80% to 90% of all malodorous conditions can be traced to oral causes, simple maneuvers can be diagnostically helpful in excluding the likelihood of more distant or complex systemic sources.

B. Clinical manifestations. In addition to fetid odor, there may be ulceration, dryness, trauma, postnasal drainage, infections, inflamed cryptic tonsils, or neoplasms.

References

1. Replogle WM, Keebe DK. Halitosis. *Am Fam Physician* 1996;53:1215–1223.
2. Spielman AI, Bivona P, Refkin BR. Halitosis: a common oral problem. *N Y State Dent J* 1996;62:36–42.
3. Rosenberg M. The science of bad breath. *Sci Am* 2002;286(4):58–65.
4. Ben-Aryeh H, Horowitz G, Nir D, et al. Halitosis: an interdisciplinary approach. *Am J Otolaryngol* 1998;19:8–11.
5. Knaan T, Cohen D, Rosenberg M. Predicting bad breath in the non-complaining population. *Oral Dis* 2005;11:105 (abstract).

HEARING LOSS

Mark P. Knudson

6.2

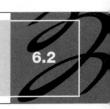

I. **BACKGROUND.** Hearing is the complex set of events in which sound waves are converted to electrical impulses, transmitted to the brain, and interpreted as sound. Any interruption in this set of events results in hearing loss.

II. **PATHOPHYSIOLOGY**

　A. Etiology. Causes of hearing loss can be divided into three categories (1, 2): conductive hearing loss (CHL), sensorineural hearing loss (SNHL), and mixed hearing loss (MHL). CHL results from the obstruction of the canal, the derangement of the tympanic membrane (TM), or the increased impedance in the middle ear (effusion) or ossicles (otosclerosis). SNHL may reflect defects in the inner ear or cochlea, the eighth cranial nerve, or the central nervous system. MHL involves a conduction impairment complicating a sensorineural impairment.

　B. Epidemiology. Approximately 28 million Americans have documented hearing loss. At birth, 1 in 1,000 newborns have profound hearing loss, with an equal number having moderate hearing loss affecting speech (3). Among individuals older than 65 years of age, 7% to 8% report hearing loss; nevertheless, more than twice that number have evidence of hearing loss if screened (4). As many as 50% of Americans have evidence of hearing loss by the time they reach 75 years of age. Subgroups at higher risk of hearing loss include those individuals in a variety of occupations (military veterans, firefighters, factory workers), and in many recreational activities (loud music, target shooting) (1, 2).

III. **EVALUATION**

　A. History. Although patients rarely present with a complaint of decreased hearing, most have no specific hearing concern. Instead they present with depression, confusion, social isolation, or poor job performance, which may be caused or complicated by hearing impairment. Family members note abnormal, slow, or overly loud answers, a sudden tendency to monopolize or disrupt conversation, or to tilt the head in conversation. CHL is often of sudden onset but of a mild degree. Complete occlusion or rapid collection of fluid in middle ear causes an abrupt change in hearing. SNHL can be abrupt and severe (stroke, idiopathic, trauma), or gradual (Ménière's syndrome, acoustic neuroma, hypothyroidism). CHL often affects the quality of hearing first. Described as muffled "like a head in a drum," the patient may lose high frequency and voice discrimination; however, they are still capable of detecting subtle sounds. SNHL, when not associated with tinnitus, can have good quality but diminished hearing usually more profound than CHL.

B. Physical examination

1. A simple hearing challenge may confirm hearing loss or detect significant hearing asymmetry. Ask the patient to cover one ear and try to detect soft sounds such as the tick of a watch, the scratching of two fingers rubbed together, or a softly whispered voice. Inspect the canal and TM to rule out the obvious causes of CHL. Cerumen impaction is a remarkably common and easily corrected cause of hearing loss. Pneumatoscopy to check for the normal movement of the TM helps rule out perforation, atelectasis, eustachian tube dysfunction, stiffened TM, ossicular disruption, and middle ear effusion.

2. The Weber's test is commonly employed with a vibrating tuning fork placed on the top of the head. The patient is asked to describe the sound heard and perceives the sound to be louder in the affected ear in CHL, because the background noise is absent on that side. The sound in the unaffected ear is perceived as louder in SNHL. The Rinne's test is conducted with the vibrating tuning fork placed on the mastoid, and the patient detects bone conduction (BC). The tuning fork is removed when the patient can no longer hear the sound. Then the tuning fork is held next to the ear to test for air conduction (AC). In an individual with normal hearing, AC is significantly better than BC. CHL reduces AC and has little effect on BC.

C. Testing

1. Laboratory testing. An audiogram performed at several frequency responses may detect individuals who are at risk of hearing loss. Although the sensitivity is good (93%–95%), the poor specificity (60%–74%) can result in many false-positive findings (3). Audiography may be performed to detect pure tone loss or for speech detection. Pure tone testing documents the number of decibels heard at a given frequency. Unfortunately, it describes nothing about the ability to discriminate language. On the other hand, speech detection estimates the impairment of actual language function better, but requires a more cooperative and attentive patient.

Auditory-evoked response detects the electroencephalographic stimulation caused by repetitive sounds and can be useful in the obtunded, uncooperative, or very young patient.

2. Imaging. Computed tomography (CT) scan may be used in the setting of traumatic loss of hearing, as it is fast, less expensive than magnetic resonance imaging (MRI), and is able to detect acute bleeding and abnormalities within the petrous ridge where fractures can affect hearing (4). A CT scan is also useful in detecting CHL caused by tumors, middle ear anomalies, myringosclerosis, and cholesteatoma. An MRI is used in patients with SNHL. An MRI with gadolinium is superior to a CT scan in identifying multiple sclerosis or vascular infarcts. In addition, acoustic neuromas and labyrinth disorders, often too small to be seen with a CT scan, may be detected with an MRI (4).

D. Genetics. Since the first hearing related gene was isolated in 1992, several hundred genetic loci that contribute to hearing loss have been isolated (1). This genetic hearing loss can be syndromic (30%) or nonsyndromic. More than 400 syndromes have been identified, most resulting in CHL or MHL that occurs early in life. The genes that cause nonsyndromic hearing loss are usually inherited in an autosomal recessive manner, and the majority result in SNHL due to cochlear defects. Although common forms of adult hearing loss such as otosclerosis and Ménière's disease are not linked to a specific gene defect, they follow a genetic pattern of inheritance (3).

IV. DIAGNOSIS

A. Differential diagnosis. Common causes of SNHL include acoustic neuroma, multiple sclerosis, hypothyroidism, vertebrobasilar insufficiency, or stroke, Ménière's syndrome, drug toxicity, and idiopathic hearing loss. CHL is most frequently caused by cerumen impaction, perforation of the TM, middle ear effusion, atelectasis, and otosclerosis. In addition, a variety of tumors (e.g., squamous cell cancer, exostoses, or cholesteatoma) can cause CHL. MHL may be secondary to presbycusis, medications, and noise-induced hearing loss.

B. Clinical manifestations. Adult patients with CHL typically present with sudden onset of partial (often high frequency) hearing loss, at times associated with external ear symptoms. Patients with SNHL present more insidiously; however, they often progress to more complete and profound hearing loss. As a result, screening is critical to detect and treat these patients when possible (5).

References
1. Isaacson JE. Differential diagnosis and treatment of hearing loss. *Am Fam Physician* 2003;68:1125–1132.
2. Weber P, Klein A. Hearing loss. *Med Clin North Am* 1999;83:125–137.
3. Aggarwal R, Saeed SR. The genetics of hearing loss. *Hosp Med* 2005;66:32–36.
4. Maggi S, Minicuci N, Martini A, et al. Prevalence rates of hearing impairment and co-morbid conditions in older people: the Veneto Study. *J Am Geriatr Soc* 1998;46:1069–1074.
5. Shapiro YB, MacLean CH, Shekelle PG. Screening and management of adult hearing loss in primary care: scientific review. *JAMA* 2003;289(15):1976–1985..

HOARSENESS
L. Gail Curtis

6.3

I. **BACKGROUND.** Hoarseness is a change in normal voice quality and is caused by an abnormal flow of air past incompletely apposed vocal cords. It is the most common symptom of laryngeal disease. Hoarseness occurs early in the process of laryngeal disease and can be readily diagnosed in primary care settings. Because cancer of the larynx has usually been present for 6 months before a diagnosis is made (1, 2), the recognition and prompt evaluation of hoarseness is paramount.

II. **PATHOPHYSIOLOGY**
   A. Etiology. Four broad etiologic categories account for most vocal changes (2–5):
   1. **Inflammation or edema of the larynx.** Infection (especially viral laryngitis), gastrointestinal reflux, allergies, exposure to irritants (tobacco, alcohol, toxic fumes), voice abuse, aspiration
   2. **Processes affecting position or approximation of the vocal cords.** Vocal polyps or nodules, contact ulcers, granulomatous disease (sarcoid, fungal, syphilitic, autoimmune), neoplasms (hemangioma, papilloma, squamous cell carcinoma)
   3. **Malfunction of the larynx.** Intubation, trauma, nerve damage (recurrent laryngeal or vagal) from tumors, surgery, aging changes (atrophy, bowing)
   4. **Systemic processes.** Hypothyroidism, rheumatoid arthritis, Parkinson's disease, multiple sclerosis, acromegaly, myasthenia gravis, and psychogenic/psychiatric

   B. Epidemiology. Laryngeal cancer is rare in patients younger than 50 years of age. Children with hoarseness must be evaluated for juvenile papillomatosis (2,5). Certain lifestyles and occupations lead to hoarseness and development of vocal nodules. Smoking and alcohol are well-known laryngeal irritants and carcinogens. Patients with reflux, nasal allergies, sinusitis, prior surgery (thyroid), and hypothyroidism are more likely to present with hoarseness. Laryngitis, voice abuse, and vocal cord nodules are among common causes of hoarseness.

III. EVALUATION

A. History. Ask patients about the circumstances preceding the onset, the mode of onset, duration, and consistency of the hoarseness. The voice of patients with myasthenia gravis becomes hoarser as the day progresses. Intermittent symptoms argue against a fixed lesion. Prominent morning symptoms that improve through the day suggest nocturnal gastroesophageal reflux disease (GERD) (Chapter 9.6). A history of indigestion, heartburn, or regurgitation suggests reflux laryngitis from GERD. Question whether talking exacerbates the hoarseness. Ask about pain, dysphagia, or trouble mounting an adequate respiratory force. Pain is a late phenomenon in carcinoma but is prominent in viral or reflux laryngitis. Chronic cough, sputum production, or sinus problems points to postnasal drainage. Specific inciting events—upper respiratory infections, sore throats, fevers, myalgias, fatigue, or other infectious exposures (tuberculosis)—need to be explored. Exposure to environmental irritants such as dust, fire, smoke, or noxious fumes should be investigated. A smoking and alcohol history is critical. Any history of intubation, prior neck surgery, or neck mass should be noted. Information about voice use and possible abuse should be obtained. Does the patient raise his or her voice over crowds or machinery or by yelling? Does his or her profession involve voice overuse or abuse?

B. Physical examination

1. Listen to the patient's voice to evaluate voice quality (1). No specific features of hoarseness are definitively diagnostic, but the voice is harsh when turbulence is created by the irregularity of the vocal cords, as in laryngitis or a mass lesion. A raspy voice suggests cord thickening caused by edema or inflammation; a breathy voice indicates poor vocal cord position or approximation; and a high, shaky, or soft voice is most probably caused by the malfunction of the larynx (1, 2). Examine the scalp, neck, thyroid gland, cervical nodes, ears, nose, sinuses, and oral cavity. Tender neck adenopathy suggests infection, whereas painless enlargement may imply malignancy (Chapters 15.1 and 15.2). If no diagnosis is obvious from the history and physical examination, the visualization of the larynx is recommended, especially if the hoarseness is of more than 2 to 3 weeks' duration (5). Using one of the techniques described in the subsequent text, carefully inspect the posterior nasopharynx, tongue, lymphoid tissue, and entire larynx. Perform vocal maneuvers while directly observing vocal cord movement. Assess for mucosal and cartilaginous lesions, edema, erythema, and excess mucus; the latter finding suggests prominent allergies. Edematous vocal cords and glottis with hyperemia suggests GERD or laryngitis.

2. Techniques for laryngeal visualization include the following:

a. Indirect laryngoscopy is performed by placing a laryngeal mirror (warmed to prevent fogging) against the soft palate while grasping the tongue with gauze. A bright light source is focused on the laryngeal mirror to reveal an image of the larynx. This technique, although simple, can prove difficult due to a strong tongue or gag reflex.

b. Flexible nasopharyngolaryngoscopy provides an excellent view of the larynx and avoids the problems noted in the preceding text. The scope is passed intranasally after topical anesthesia is applied (e.g., 2% lidocaine gel). The larynx is visualized while the patient swallows and phonates.

c. Video-assisted rigid laryngoscopy is superior to all other examination methods but is reserved for consultant use when diagnosis remains uncertain (5).

C. Testing. Thyroid function is the only routine blood testing recommended, unless dictated by features of the history or physical examination. If indicated, magnetic resonance imaging is the modality of choice to assess the extent of serious laryngeal or neck disease (5).

IV. DIAGNOSIS

A. Differential diagnosis. The key to diagnosis is a thorough history combined in most cases with the visualization of the larynx. Hoarseness of less than 2 weeks duration is considered acute and is usually self-limited. Chronic hoarseness (>2–3 weeks duration) suggests a more serious cause and a laryngeal examination is critical (2–5).

B. Clinical manifestations. Most causes of hoarseness are benign (1–3). Some laryngeal lesions have a pathognomonic appearance (1, 2). Vocal polyps are benign and result from chronic voice abuse or direct trauma. They occur on the anterior portion of one vocal cord. Vocal nodules result from poor voice use (e.g., singers, preachers), and always occurs at the junction of the anterior and middle third of the vocal cords bilaterally. Contact ulcers present as bilateral ulcerations at the tips of the laryngeal cartilages and are the only common lesions other than cancer that cause throat pain. Leukoplakia presents as a raised, white plaque at the anterior extremity of one vocal cord. It is usually premalignant, related to alcohol use or smoking, and needs to be biopsied. Laryngeal cancer produces early changes in voice quality and is the most serious cause of hoarseness. It presents as persistent hoarseness with a lesion in the hypopharynx, glottis, or supraglottis. Any suspicious lesion seen on laryngoscopy should be biopsied.

References
1. Rosen CA, Anderson D, Murry T. Evaluating hoarseness. *Am Fam Physician* 1998;57: 2775–2782.
2. Garrett CG, Ossoff RH. Hoarseness. *Med Clin North Am* 1999;83:115–123.
3. Banfield G, Tandon P, Solomons N. Hoarse voice: an early symptom of many conditions. *Practitioner* 2000;244:267–271.
4. Simpson BC, Fleming DJ. Medical and voice history in evaluation of dysphonia. *Otolaryngol Clin North Am* 2000;33(4):719–730.
5. Van der Goten A. Evaluation of patients with hoarseness. *Eur Radiol* 2004;14:1406–1415.

NOSEBLEED

Douglas G. Browning and Chad Ezzell

6.4

I. BACKGROUND. Nosebleed, or epistaxis, is a common otolaryngologic problem, defined as the loss of blood from the mucous membranes lining the nose, usually from a single nostril.

II. PATHOPHYSIOLOGY

  A. Etiology. Epistaxis results from an interaction of factors that damage the nasal epithelial (mucosal) lining and vessel walls. The causative factors or processes include:

    1. Environmental. Dry air, cold ambient temperature

    2. Local. Accidental or self-inflicted trauma, infection, allergies, foreign body, anatomic abnormalities (deviated septum), iatrogenic (surgery), neoplasms

    3. Systemic. Hypertension, platelet and coagulation abnormalities, blood dyscrasias, disseminated intravascular coagulation, renal failure, alcohol abuse

    4. Drugs affecting clotting. Aspirin, nonsteroidal anti-inflammatory drugs, warfarin, heparin, ticlopidine, dipyridamole

    5. Other drugs. Nasal steroids, thioridazine, anticholinergics (drying)

    6. Hereditary. Hemophilia, von Willebrand's disease, hereditary hemorrhagic telangiectasia (Osler-Weber-Rendu)

    7. Idiopathic. Cold, dry air increases cases of epistaxis as demonstrated in countries with seasonal climates where hospital admissions for nosebleed increase significantly during the winter months (1). Regarding the importance of anatomic abnormalities, a study of recurrent epistaxis showed that 81% of patients had septal deviation versus 31% of the control group (2). Although hypertension is often associated with epistaxis, studies have had conflicting results and the relationship has yet to be confirmed (3) (Chapter 7.8).

B. **Epidemiology.** As many as 15 per 10,000 individuals require physician care annually for epistaxis, and 1.6/10,000 require admission to the hospital for a persistent nosebleed. Most cases occur in patients younger than 10 years of age, and the incidence decreases with age (4).

III. EVALUATION

A. **History.** Initial history should include onset, duration, whether one or both nostrils are affected, and the quantity (number of soaked towels). A detailed history exploring the possible precipitating factors (see section **II.A.**) should be taken. It is also important to inquire about chronic medical conditions that could be contributory, including a history of blood dyscrasias, hypertension, liver disease, and alcohol use. In children with epistaxis with unilateral nasal discharge or foul odor, be alert to the possibility of an intranasal foreign body.

B. **Physical examination.** The blood supply to the nose arises from the internal maxillary and facial arteries through the external carotid artery and the anterior and posterior ethmoid arteries through the internal carotid. The anteroinferior septum (Little's area) is supplied by a confluence of both systems known as "Kiesselbach's plexus." Little's area is a common site of epistaxis because it is ideally placed to receive environmental irritation (cold, dry air, cigarette smoke), and is easily accessible to digital trauma. Fortunately, this area is easy to access and treat. However, as approximately 10% of nosebleeds originate from a posterior nasal source (4), it can be far more difficult to identify a source of epistaxis in this area. Providing effective treatment for obstinate bleeding in this area may also be more uncomfortable for the patient and more formidable for the health provider.

1. When examining the patient with epistaxis, first assess the vital signs for hypotension, orthostasis, and hemodynamic instability. After examining the face for any obvious signs of recent injury, it is important to visualize as much of the nasal vestibule as possible. It is imperative to keep the patient's head upright, for if he or she tilts backward, only the roof of the nasal cavity is seen. The nasal speculum should be held in a horizontal position to allow an optimal view of the nasal septum, which is the site of most bleeding.

2. Visualization of the bleeding can be performed by the direct illumination of the area or sometimes more easily by indirect illumination using a head mirror. Suction may be needed to remove clots, fresh blood, or mucus to visualize the bleeding. Direct nasopharyngoscopy with endoscopy (using a topical anesthetic such as Cetacaine or lidocaine gel) may be necessary, especially if the source of the bleeding is extremely posterior. Topical vasoconstrictors such as phenylephrine or oxymetazoline can be useful in decreasing the rate of bleeding in order to visualize the area (and may sometimes help achieve long-term cessation of the bleeding).

3. Depending on the patient's history, a more general examination may be needed with a focus on the skin to look for petechiae, telangiectasias, hemangiomas, and ecchymoses (Chapter 15.3).

C. **Testing**

1. **Laboratory tests.** If bleeding is minor and not recurring, no testing is needed. For vigorous bleeding or recurrent epistaxis, order a complete blood count (CBC) with platelet count, bleeding time, prothrombin time, partial thromboplastin time, and possibly blood type and crossmatch for hypovolemic shock or severe anemia. Testing the stools for occult blood may help assess chronicity. The CBC can detect blood dyscrasias as well as anemia. An elevated bleeding time may imply aspirin use, von Willebrand's disease, and many platelet-based bleeding disorders. Coagulation times can be elevated in coagulation factor diseases, but more often than not, they implicate liver disease.

2. **Imaging.** Sinus radiographs or a limited computed tomography of the sinuses may also be considered if concern exists for benign neoplasms or malignancy. Rarely, angiography may also be indicated for diagnosing (and treating) vascular lesions.

D. Genetics. Epistaxis is the presenting complaint in four of five cases of the rare, hereditary hemorrhagic telangiectasias (Osler-Weber-Rendu disease) (3).

IV. DIAGNOSIS

A. Differential diagnosis. For persistent or recurrent nosebleeds, it is important to look further for the underlying cause of the problem by performing a careful history and evaluating the problem with expedient laboratory evaluations, appropriate imaging, or further consultation when necessary to rule out more malignant causes. Rare causes of epistaxis include potentially life-threatening posttraumatic pseudoaneurysm of the internal carotid artery. This entity presents from days to weeks after initial trauma to the base of the skull with a classic triad of unilateral blindness, orbital fractures, and massive epistaxis. Finally, although the obstruction of air movement is the most common presenting symptom of intranasal neoplasms, patients may also present with epistaxis and/or nasal pain (5).

B. Clinical manifestations. Bleeding from one or both nostrils occurs, with associated frequent swallowing and sensation of fluid in the back of the nose and/or throat.

References

1. Tomkimon A, Bremmer-Smith A, Craven C, et al. Hospital epistaxis admissions and ambient temperature. *Clin Otolaryngol* 1995;20:239–240.
2. O'Reilly BJ, Simpson DC, Dharmeratnam R. Recurrent epistaxis and nasal septal deviation in young adults. *Clin Otolaryngol* 1996;21:82–84.
3. Herkner H, Laggner A, Mullner M, et al. Hypertension in patients presenting with epistaxis. *Ann Emerg Med* 2000;35(2):126–130.
4. Middleton PM. Epistaxis. *Emerg Med Australas* 2004;6(5–6):428–440.
5. Dykewicz MS. Rhinitis and sinusitis. *J Allergy Clin Immunol* 2003;111(Suppl 2): S520–S529.

PHARYNGITIS
Richard W. Lord

6.5

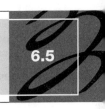

I. BACKGROUND.
Pharyngitis, commonly called sore throat (ST), is an inflammatory process of the pharynx that can be caused by viral or bacterial pathogens, and occasionally both. ST is one of the most common reasons for adults and children to seek care from a primary care physician (1). Although the differential diagnosis of ST includes such entities as epiglottis, peritonsillar abscess, Ludwig angina, and gastroesophageal reflux, the most common cause in immunocompetent individuals is acute pharyngitis. Acute pharyngitis is a frequent reason for antibiotic prescriptions although the most common causes are viral (2). The inappropriate use of antibiotics can have negative consequences for individual and public health. Therefore, it is important for physicians to develop an approach for identifying those individuals with pharyngitis caused by group A α-hemolytic streptococcus (GABHS).

II. PATHOPHYSIOLOGY

A. Etiology. Only a small minority (10%–20%) of patients with ST are infected with GABHS (3–5). However, to minimize the potential adverse effects of inappropriate antimicrobial therapy, it is important to identify GABHS infection accurately because it is the only commonly occurring form of pharyngitis for which antibiotic therapy is definitively indicated (2, 3). The early identification and treatment of GABHS helps prevent rheumatic fever, provide symptomatic relief, reduces suppurative complications, and decreases infectivity (3, 4). Table 6.5.1 lists the different causes of pharyngitis (3–5).

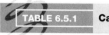

Cause	Percent of cases
Viral	50%–80%
Group A α-hemolytic streptococcus	5%–30% (mean 15% in adults)
Epstein-Barr virus	1%–10%
Chlamydia pneumoniae	2%–5%
Mycoplasma pneumoniae	2%–5%
Neisseria gonorrhoeae	1%–2%
Acute human immunodeficiency virus	Rare
Other bacteria, fungi, parasites	Rare
Referred pain (dental)	Rare
Noninfectious causes	Rare

TABLE 6.5.1   **Causes of Acute Pharyngitis**

B. Epidemiology. Pharyngitis is the sixth most common reason for seeing a physician, and accounts for approximately 5% of all primary care office visits (1). Data show that the probability of GABHS pharyngitis in primary care peaks between 5 and 15 years of age (3–5). Infectious mononucleosis (IM) as a cause of ST peaks between 15 and 30 years of age (3–5).

Transmission occurs mostly by hand contact with nasal discharge rather than by contact with oral secretions (4, 5). Symptoms typically occur 48 to 72 hours later. Most pharyngitis is self-limited and lasts 7 to 10 days. If pharyngitis lasts for longer than 3 weeks, noninfectious causes should be considered. Although pharyngitis can occur at anytime during the year, there is a peak in the winter and spring.

III. EVALUATION. The goal of the evaluation is to differentiate those patients who are likely to have an infectious cause of pharyngitis and need laboratory testing, and those who have noninfectious causes. History, physical examination, and appropriate diagnostic laboratory tests are used to accomplish this goal.

A. History

1. The onset and duration of the ST can help differentiate infectious from noninfectious causes. Typically, the onset of infectious causes is abrupt and lasts for 7 to 10 days. Often with noninfectious causes, the onset of symptoms is unclear and often persists for more than 3 weeks.

2. Associated symptoms can also give clues to the cause of the ST. Fever, cough, headache, and other constitutional symptoms are the hallmarks of an infectious etiology. Symptoms of allergies, heartburn, and depression point to noninfectious causes. Any history of seasonal allergies, trauma, malignancy, radiation therapy, inhalation, ingestion, or thyroid dysfunction point to noninfectious causes.

3. If infection is believed to be the cause of the ST, the focus is then on trying to differentiate GABHS from other bacterial and viral causes. Classically, GABHS pharyngitis is severe and of acute (<1 day) onset, and accompanied by fever (temperature >101°F [38.33°C]), painful swallowing, tender anterior cervical adenopathy, and myalgias, but not by cough or rhinitis. Headache, nausea, vomiting, and abdominal pain may be seen as well, especially in children. Conversely, the gradual onset of mild ST accompanied by rhinorrhea, cough, hoarseness, conjunctivitis, or diarrhea in an afebrile patient speaks strongly for a viral cause. Despite these broad generalizations, classic symptom complexes alone are neither sensitive nor specific enough to rely on for judging the need for antibacterial treatment (2–5).

B. Physical examination. The physical examination should include assessing vital signs (especially temperature) and examining the head, eyes, ears, nose, throat, neck, and skin. Findings classically associated with GABHS infection include palatal petechiae, intense ("beefy red") tonsillopharyngeal erythema with exudates, tender anterior cervical adenopathy, and a scarlatiniform rash. Conversely, the absence of these features, along with the presence of rhinitis, hoarseness, conjunctivitis, stomatitis, discrete ulcerative lesions, or a typical viral exanthem points toward a viral cause. In IM, the classic features of GABHS are often combined with posterior cervical or generalized lymphadenopathy and hepatosplenomegaly. However, once again, none of these physical findings in and of themselves have sufficiently high sensitivity and specificity to rely on for accurate diagnosis (3–5). An abdominal examination is dictated either by gastrointestinal symptoms or by the presence of severe fatigue with posterior cervical adenopathy (suggesting IM). A cough or a fever should lead to a pulmonary examination. A cardiac examination is important for toxic-appearing patients.

C. **Testing.** The two tests typically used in the diagnosis of pharyngitis are the throat culture (TC) and the rapid streptococcal antigen detection test (RSADT).

   1. The sensitivity of an appropriately obtained (vigorously swabbing both tonsils and posterior pharynx) TC is 90% to 95% (3–5). Unfortunately, the TC does not reliably distinguish between an acute GABHS infection and a streptococcal carrier state with concomitant viral infection. A negative TC does permit the withholding of antimicrobial therapy (i.e., specificity = 0.99) (3–5).

   2. Although methods vary, RSADTs do have high degrees of specificity (92%–95%) (3–5). Their sensitivity in routine clinical practice is low (60%–85%) (3–5). Therefore, in the past the recommendation had been to follow up a negative antigen test with a backup TC. Newer guidelines (2) have been developed that base treatment decisions only on the RSADTs. A study of 30,000 patients over 2 years did not find a difference in sequelae from using only RSADTs for decision making. RSADTs suffer the same limitation as TCs in the presence of carrier states.

   3. Streptococcal antibody titers are of no immediate value in the diagnosis of acute GABHS pharyngitis. If IM is suspected, a complete blood count and heterophil antibody testing can reliably confirm the diagnosis if the patient is in the second week of illness.

   4. Generally, no other testing is needed unless a serious suppurative sequela is suspected (e.g., retropharyngeal abscess), in which case radiologic imaging should be pursued.

IV. DIAGNOSIS

A. Differential diagnosis

   1. Recent guidelines (2–5) have called for the use of specific criteria to estimate the probability of diagnosing GABHS. One popular set, the Centor criteria (2), includes the following: tonsillar exudates, tender anterior cervical lymphadenopathy, and absence of cough and history of fever. The positive predictive value of three or four of these criteria is 40% to 60%. The absence of three or four of these criteria has a negative predictive value of 80% (2, 4). The following principles are put forth in these guidelines.

      a. Clinically, screen all adult patients with pharyngitis using the Centor criteria.

      b. Do not test or treat patients with none or only one of these criteria.

      c. For patients with two or more criteria, the following options have been defined.

         i. Test patients with two, three, or four of the criteria and treat only those with positive RSADTs.

         ii. Test patients with two or three criteria and treat those with positive RSADTs or those with four criteria.

         iii. Do not use any diagnostic tests and only treat patients with three or four criteria.

      d. Do not perform follow-up TCs on patients with negative RSADTs when the sensitivity is >80%.

   2. Other scoring systems have also been developed that incorporate the patient's age generalizing the use of these to children and adults (5). This system gives

1 point for each of the Centor criteria present, and then adds 1 point for age less than 15 years, 0 points for age 15 to 45 years, and −1 for age greater than 45 years. This guideline recommends the following strategy: 0–1 points, no treatment or testing; 1–3 points, treat those with positive RSADTs; 4–5 points, treat empirically.

   3. The goal of these scoring systems is to help reduce the overuse of antibiotics in treating pharyngitis. Studies estimated that clinical screening could decrease inappropriate antibiotic use by 88% (2, 4).

   4. Although obtaining RSADTs and confirmatory TCs is still an appropriate option, simply trying to use clinical judgment without a clinical prediction rule is not. Continued research in this area will help define the most appropriate method of diagnosis.

B. Clinical manifestations. The primary manifestation is throat and anterior neck pain accompanied by some degree of painful swallowing. Other symptoms, depending on the underlying etiology, may include fever, nausea, vomiting, fatigue, rash, ear pain, and even abdominal discomfort. Signs may range from minimal or no pharyngeal erythema and exudate to severe suppurative findings, including marked cervical adenopathy. Tonsillar abscess formation causes swelling and deviation of the soft palate with malodorous breath.

References

1. Woodwell DA, Cherry DK. *National ambulatory medical care survey:* 2002 summary. Hyattsville, MD: National Center for Health Statistics; *Adv Data* 2004;346:1–44.
2. Cooper RJ, Hoffman JR, Bartlett JG, et al. Principles of appropriate antibiotic use for acute pharyngitis in adults. *Ann Emerg Med* 2001;37:711–717.
3. Bisno AL. Acute pharyngitis. *N Engl J Med* 2001;344(3):205–211.
4. Institute for Clinical Systems Improvement (ICSI). Acute pharyngitis: clinical guideline, May 2005 update, at http://www.icsi.org, accessed on July 25, 2005.
5. Vincent MT, Celestin N, Hussain AN. Pharyngitis. *Am Fam Physician* 2004;69:1465–1470.

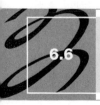

6.6 RHINITIS
Gail S. Marion

I. BACKGROUND. No universal definition or classification exists for rhinitis—a common presenting symptom. Rhinitis implies inflammation of the nasal mucosa but can also refer to a constellation of rhinopathy symptoms, including mucous drainage, stuffiness, sneezing, and itching.

II. PATHOPHYSIOLOGY

   A. Etiology

   1. Allergic. Seasonal, perennial (50% of cases)

   2. Infection. Acute versus chronic, bacterial versus viral (20%–40% of cases)

   3. Nonallergic perennial rhinitis. Eosinophilic, noneosinophilic

   4. Miscellaneous. Foreign body, nasal polyp, septal deviation, neoplasm, enlarged adenoids, or tonsils, recent head trauma (with cerebrospinal fluid leak), autonomic, vasomotor rhinitis

   5. Drug-induced. Oral contraceptives, hormone replacement therapy, antihypertensives, ophthalmic β-blockers, local decongestants (rhinitis medicamentosum), aspirin and nonsteroidal anti-inflammatory drugs, cocaine

   6. Atrophic rhinitis. Extensive surgery

7. **Physical/chemical exposures.** Occupational, pollution, gustatory, dry air, bright light
8. **Associated with a systemic disorder.** Hypothyroidism, pregnancy, acquired immunodeficiency syndrome, systemic lupus, rheumatoid arthritis, Sjögren's syndrome, primary mucous, or ciliary defect, cystic fibrosis, antibody deficiency, granulomatous disease.

B. **Epidemiology.** Rhinitis currently affects about 40 million Americans, with annual costs to society of more than $15 billion dollars (1,2). Although rhinitis is considered a minor complaint and is frequently left untreated, proper evaluation and treatment improves health outcomes and the quality of life for patients (3,4). An important example is the increasing evidence that aggressive allergic rhinitis management improves the management of asthma because the nose serves as a filter for inhaled air (3,5). Rhinitis is an important cause of morbidity; it can cause fatigue, headache, cognitive impairment, and other systemic symptoms (4).

III. **EVALUATION.** Evaluation of rhinitis requires determining whether the symptoms are caused by (a) allergy, (b) infection, (c) anatomic defect, (d) serious systemic illness, or (e) some combination of these.

A. **History.** What are the specific symptoms (i.e., stuffiness, itching, clear or purulent drainage)? Are the symptoms unilateral or bilateral? Allergy and infection produce bilateral nasal complaints, whereas most rhinitis relating to the structural problems of the nose is unilateral. When did the symptom(s) begin? Ask what the patient believes causes the symptoms. How often and when do the symptoms occur? Do they predominate at certain times of the year? What other symptoms are associated? What makes the symptoms better or worse? Associated complaints (e.g., frank fatigue, irritability, depression, or chest symptoms) tend to point to untreated allergic causes, systemic disease, or drug-induced illness. Include questions about atopic disease, upper respiratory allergies, asthma, nasal surgery, and prescription medication use. Address tobacco (personal or secondary exposure), alcohol or recreational drug use, over-the-counter medication, herbal remedies, and pets in the home. Are there suspected environmental irritants? Is there a family history of allergies or other relevant systemic diseases?

B. **Physical examination.** A general inspection of the patient frequently offers clues to the cause. "Allergic shiners" (infraorbital, bluish discoloration of the skin) or a crease at the lower part of the nose from repeated rubbing are common physical findings of allergic rhinitis. Evaluate vital signs (especially temperature) and the ears, nose, and throat, including an examination for lymphadenopathy and thyroid disease. A competent examination of nasal passages requires a nasal speculum (a 4–5 mm ear speculum on a handheld otoscope is acceptable for children), and a good light source. Carefully place the nasal speculum vertically into each vestibule. Insert a handheld otoscope light source through the speculum to survey for nasal patency, mucosal color (pale, red, or bluish), the degree and the location of edema, presence and type of nasal drainage (thin, clear, thick, purulent, unilateral, or bilateral), anatomic deformities (bone spurs, septal deviation), and the presence of polyps or other masses. If swollen nasal turbinates block the view, apply a short-acting decongestant spray, then reexamine in 10 minutes. An evaluation of the posterior portion of the nose is often suboptimal with a nasal speculum and light source. A flexible nasopharyngoscope permits the examination of the structures between the nasal vestibule and the larynx (1). Assess the lungs and the skin for signs of atopic disease (wheezing or eczema). If systemic illness is suggested after focused examination, a thorough multisystem exam is necessary.

C. **Testing.** The most common causes of rhinitis do not require additional testing to initiate effective treatment. A microscopic examination of nasal secretions can be performed to help define uncertain allergic or bacterial causes of rhinitis, although most primary care clinicians often leave these tests to an otolaryngologist because these are usually done to clarify less common causes of rhinitis (3). Referral is indicated if doubt exists, if serious pathology is suspected or found, if physical examination is difficult secondary to nasal obstruction, or if the symptoms do not improve with treatment. If an anatomic abnormality or sinus pathology is suspected, limited computed tomography of the sinuses is recommended (1,2,5).

IV. DIAGNOSIS

A. Differential diagnosis. To distinguish between allergic and nonallergic rhinitis, focus on the symptoms of sneezing, clear drainage, postnasal drip, itching, nasal congestion, generalized sinus pressure, specific irritants or allergens, and family and personal history of atopy and allergy. Next, consider seasonal, perennial, or geographic relationships. The presence of blue or pale boggy turbinates with clear drainage suggests an allergic process. A physical examination should confirm the patient's story and help identify any anatomic defects or systemic disease. Several follow-up visits may be necessary to assess, treat, and educate patients with allergic rhinitis and to confirm any need for further evaluation or treatment by an otolaryngologist or allergist (4).

B. Clinical manifestations. Purulent nasal drainage implies an infectious cause, whereas clear discharge suggests a noninfectious cause. Viral infection produces whitish to pale yellow drainage with associated symptoms of generalized head or body aches, nasal congestion, and sneezing. Bacterial infection results in yellow or green drainage with focal sinus pain, upper teeth complaints, and possibly fever. Look for edematous, erythematous turbinates. Other less common infectious sources (fungal or parasitic) should be suspected if treatment fails or if the patient has a suggestive medical or travel history (5).

References
1. Fornadley JA. The stuffy nose and rhinitis. *Med Clin North Am* 1999;83:211–224.
2. Bachert C. Persistent rhinitis—allergic or nonallergic? *Allergy* 2004;59:11–15.
3. Hadley JA. Evaluation and management of allergic rhinitis. *Med Clin North Am* 1999;83:13–25.
4. Dykewicz MS, Fineman S, Skoner DP, et al. Diagnosis and management of rhinitis: complete guidelines of the joint task force on practice parameters in allergy, asthma and immunology. *Ann Allergy Asthma Immunol* 1998;81:478–518.
5. Benninger MA, Anon JB, Mabry RL. The medical management of rhinosinusitis. *Otolaryngol Head Neck Surg* 1997;117:S41–S49.

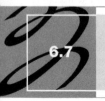

6.7 STOMATITIS
John G. Spangler

I. BACKGROUND.
Stomatitis, generally referred to as lesions in the mouth, represents a broad category of oral mucosal infections, inflammatory conditions, and other oral lesions. Because of possible malignancy, persistent lesions require definitive diagnosis.

II. PATHOPHYSIOLOGY

A. Etiology. Causes include the following: (i) premalignant or malignant lesions to tobacco or alcohol use (leukoplakia, erythroplasia, and oral cancer); (ii) human immunodeficiency virus (HIV)-related lesions (e.g., Kaposi's sarcoma, oral hairy leukoplakia); (iii) infections that may be bacterial (e.g., necrotizing ulcerative gingivitis), viral (e.g., herpes simplex virus (HSV), hand-foot-and-mouth disease), or fungal (e.g., thrush, angular cheilitis); (iv) ulcerative and erosive conditions (e.g., recurrent aphthous ulcers, Behçet's disease, autoimmune disorders); (v) traumatic and irritant lesions (chronic cheek biting, chemical exposures, burns from hot food); and (vi) drug-related eruptions (Stevens-Johnson syndrome, chemotherapy-associated mucositis).

B. Epidemiology. Oral lesions are more common in the adult population than tension headaches, phlebitis, or arthralgias. In a mass screening of more than 23,000 adults, the 30 most common lesions accounted for 93% of all oral lesions (1).

III. EVALUATION

A. History. The history should describe the lesion and the potential risk factors for its etiology. Describe the onset: was it abrupt, suggesting an infection, or insidious, suggesting an inflammatory or neoplastic origin? Are there associated signs and symptoms? Many oral infections are associated with pain, malaise, and fever. Behçet's disease has associated ocular and genital lesions, whereas other autoimmune diseases such as systemic lupus erythematosus (SLE) or ulcerative colitis may have systemic symptoms (2, 3). Describe the lesions: are they painful or painless? Infections, inflammatory lesions, and aphthous ulcers are usually painful (3), whereas premalignant and malignant lesions may be painless (2, 4). Are there vesicles or bullae? Pemphigoid and pemphigus may cause bullae and/or ulcers. HSV starts as vesicular lesions and then ulcerates. Varicella zoster lesions can occur in the mouth (3, 4). Did vesicles precede the lesions suggesting HSV or was there ulceration without vesicles, suggesting aphthous ulcers (3)? Are the lesions that will not wipe off the mucosa white? Leukoplakia, a premalignant lesion, is white, and will not wipe off. Any coexisting red component, called *erythroplasia*, greatly increases the malignant potential of the lesion (2, 4). Lichen planus also produces a striated white lesion, usually on the buccal mucosa (3). Where are the lesions? HSV tends to occur on periosteally bound mucosa (gingiva, hard palate), whereas recurrent aphthous ulcers occur on nonperiosteally bound mucosa (buccal, lip, or tongue mucosa) (3). The floor of the mouth under the tongue, the lateral aspects of the tongue, the retromolar regions, and the soft palate are worrisome areas for malignancy to develop (4), but malignancy can occur anywhere.

Past medical history is also important. Systemic inflammatory conditions such as SLE or lichen planus can produce oral ulcerations. Recurrence suggests aphthous ulcers and HSV. Dentures increase the susceptibility to denture stomatitis or angular cheilitis, both caused by *Candida* species (2–4). HIV increases the likelihood of oral hairy leukoplakia, Kaposi's sarcoma, and severe oral candidiasis. Exposure to individuals with similar symptoms suggests enteroviral infections such as herpangina and hand-foot-and-mouth disease. Medications such as sulfonamides and many other drugs can cause Stevens-Johnson syndrome, whereas chemotherapy for the treatment of cancer can produce severe mucositis. Social history should focus on alcohol and tobacco use, exposures to oral irritants, and sexual activity, including oral-genital sexual contact.

B. Physical examination

1. Head, eyes, ears, nose, throat (HEENT). Based on the history, a focused physical examination of the HEENT is necessary. Look for signs of trauma. Examine the conjunctiva and nasal mucosa for inflammatory changes or ulcerations. Evaluate the patient for coexisting upper respiratory signs and symptoms such as rhinorrhea, sinus tenderness to palpation, and otitis media. Inspect facial skin for vesicles from HSV or varicella zoster or other lesions such as ecchymoses, a malar rash, or a viral exanthem. Look for facial asymmetry. Varicella zoster can cause facial nerve paralysis, called the *Ramsey Hunt syndrome*. Evaluate preauricular, postauricular, and cervical lymph node chains. Finally, evaluate the oral cavity, documenting the size, location, and appearance of the lesion.

2. Additional physical examination. Based on the results of the HEENT examination, additional physical examination might include: (i) pulmonary examination for viral pneumonitis or findings in autoimmune diseases; (ii) abdominal and rectal examination for Crohn's disease or ulcerative colitis; (iii) genitourinary examination for mucosal ulcers in Behçet's disease and Stevens-Johnson syndrome, as well as for signs of syphilis or gonorrhea; (iv) a skin examination looking for viral exanthems, drug eruptions, lichen planus, pemphigus, pemphigoid, and SLE; and (v) a musculoskeletal examination for signs of SLE, Reiter's syndrome, or other autoimmune diseases.

C. Testing

1. Clinical laboratory testing should be guided by the history and physical findings. A potassium hydroxide wet mount is useful in the diagnosis of candidiasis. Viral and bacterial cultures can be obtained from swabs of oral lesions, but viral cultures are usually more helpful than bacterial cultures. Darkfield microscopy can be performed from swabs of syphilis chancres or plaques. Cytologic scrapings of premalignant or malignant lesions, prepared in a manner similar to a Papanicolaou smear, are not a substitute for a biopsy of suspected oral neoplasia (2–4). A new brush has been developed to sample mucosal lesions down to the basement membrane (OralCDx, CDx Laboratories, Suffern, New York).

2. Diagnostic imaging is indicated only in selected cases such as coexisting sinus disease ("mini" sinus computed tomography [CT] scan), coexisting neck mass or lymphadenopathy suspicious for malignant disease (head and neck CT scan), suspected metastatic disease (chest x-ray, CT scan of the head, abdomen, and chest), or trauma (cervical spine series, cranial CT scan, dental Panorex films). If HSV is suspected, cranial magnetic resonance imaging (MRI) may be useful. A chest x-ray is indicated in suspected viral or autoimmune pneumonitis or in secondary bacterial pneumonia. If a severe lip laceration has occurred, plain films can help rule out mandibular condylar fractures or tooth fractures.

D. Genetics may play a role in the susceptibility to aphthous ulcers, and autoimmune disorders.

IV. DIAGNOSIS

A. Differential diagnosis of stomatitis includes lesions in the six categories listed in section **II.A.** The diagnosis depends on the synthesis of the key historical and physical examinations, as well as the laboratory and imaging elements. **All oral ulcers that do not heal, as well as white or reddish-white lesions that do not resolve in 2 weeks, need a biopsy to rule out malignancy (2–4).**

B. Clinical manifestations. Stomatitis manifests as lumps, ulcerations, or discolored patches that may be painful, or painless depending on the underlying pathology.

References

1. Bouquot JE. Common oral lesions found during a mass screening examination. *J Am Dent Assoc* 1986;112(1):50–57.
2. Silverman S. *Oral cancer*, 4th edn. Hamilton, OH: BC Decker, 1998.
3. Bruce AJ, Rogers RS, III. Acute oral ulcers. *Dermatol Clin* 2003;21:1–15.
4. Porter SR, Leao JC. Review article: oral ulcers and its relevance to systemic disorders. *Aliment Pharmacol Ther* 2005;21:295–306.

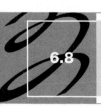

6.8 TINNITUS
Sara Neal

I. BACKGROUND. Tinnitus has been described as "ear noise" and consists of sounds heard by the patient with no sound source external to the body. Although there are infinite variations, patients usually describe ringing, buzzing, clicking, whistling, cricket-like, hissing, or humming sounds (1).

II. PATHOPHYSIOLOGY

A. Etiology. Tinnitus is not a disease but an indication of some other ongoing process, whether pathologic or benign. The first step in determining the etiology is to define the type of sound heard and any relationship to the pulse or respiration. These answers subdivide tinnitus into two general categories—objective and subjective

(1–3). Subjective tinnitus, which is far more common, is heard only by the patient. Objective tinnitus can be heard through a stethoscope placed over the head and neck structures near the patient's ear (3).

1. **Objective (vibratory, pseudotinnitus).** These sounds are often synchronous with the pulse. They are real sounds, mechanical in origin, and can be heard by the examiner as well as the patient. Sources, either vascular or muscular, include:

   a. **Venous hum** is due to eddy currents in the jugular vein. The patient is more aware of the noise when there is a concurrent conductive hearing loss.

   b. **Arteriovenous malformations** can be found between the occipital artery and the transverse sinus.

   c. **Myoclonus** of nearby structures, most commonly the palate, the stapedius muscle, and the tensor tympani. These are usually asynchronous with the pulse.

   d. **A patulous or abnormally patent eustachian tube** can cause chronic or inter-mittent tinnitus. Sometimes related to respirations, it is frequently described as a "hissing" sound.

2. **Subjective (nonvibratory).** This type is more common, but has a less easily definable etiology than vibratory types. Its causes can be divided into various subcategories (1, 3).

   a. **Otologic.** Noise-induced hearing loss, presbycusis, otosclerosis, otitis, im-pacted cerumen, sudden deafness, Ménière's disease.

   b. **Neurologic.** Head injury, whiplash, multiple sclerosis, acoustic neuroma, and other cerebellopontine angle tumors.

   c. **Infectious.** Otitis media, sequelae of Lyme disease, meningitis, syphilis.

   d. **Drug-related.** See section **III.A.5.**

   e. **Metabolic.** Thyroid disease, hyperlipidemia, vitamin B_{12} deficiency, zinc deficiency.

   f. **Psychogenic.** Depression, anxiety, fibromyalgia.

   g. **Other.** Temporomandibular joint dysfunction, other mandibulodental disor-ders.

B. **Epidemiology.** In the United States, approximately 9% of individuals older than 65 years of age and 1% of individuals younger than 45 years of age experience tinnitus (4). Whites are more frequently affected than blacks, and the prevalence in the South is almost twice that in the Northeast (4). Approximately one-fourth of patients who experience tinnitus have significant symptoms that impact their life, especially because the condition is so frequently associated with hearing loss (1). Special attention should be paid to patients presenting with unilateral tinnitus, associated vertigo, unilateral sensorineural hearing loss, and eye inflammation.

III. EVALUATION

A. **History.** Important features of the history should include (1, 3, 5):

1. **Date of tinnitus onset** particularly any relation to an illness or change in drug regimen.

2. **a detailed description of the tinnitus** may help subdivide it into objective and subjective sources. Are there any exacerbating or ameliorating factors? An asso-ciation with respirations or pulse points to a vibratory source. Positional change, such as lowering the head between the knees (causing venous engorgement) can point toward a patulous eustachian tube as the mechanism for the tinnitus. Variation with respiration or distortions of one's own voice may also indicate the eustachian tube. Is the sound constant or episodic, unilateral or bilateral? Was the onset sudden or gradual? What are the pitch and loudness of the sound? Is there associated hearing loss, vertigo, or pain? Is there evidence of other conditions (see section **II.A.**) that are associated with tinnitus? What else affects tinnitus—background noise, alcohol, stress, or sleeplessness? Is there a history of exposure to loud noise, ear infections, otologic surgery, head injuries, and use of ototoxic drugs? Are there any adverse effects of the tinnitus? How does tinnitus affect daily life and the ability to function?

3. **Fluctuation of symptoms.** Fluctuating symptoms are commonly associated with Ménière's disease (endolymphatic hydrops).

4. **History of noise exposure or hearing loss.** Noise-induced hearing loss usually causes high-pitched tinnitus, whereas Ménière's disease usually produces a lower pitched sound. Also, conductive hearing loss due to cerumen impaction, otitis media, or otosclerosis may heighten awareness of internal vibratory sounds such as a venous hum or myoclonus. Presbycusis, or degeneration within the organ of Corti, is frequently seen in the elderly. It is associated with a downsloping high frequency hearing loss and a high-pitched tinnitus.

5. **Medication history.** Many drugs have been associated with tinnitus (1, 3). The list includes salicylates, caffeine, aminoglycosides, alcohol, quinidine, non-steroidal anti-inflammatory drugs, carbamazepine, loop diuretics, cisplatin, vincristine, levodopa, propranolol, and aminophylline. Some hormonal preparations have also been indicated as has the postpartum state.

6. **Significant weight loss** can be associated with a patulous eustachian tube.

7. **Concurrent medical conditions** to be considered include hypertension, diabetes mellitus, thyroid disorders, hyperlipidemia, and infection. Arteriovenous sounds are heightened by increased cardiac output. Vascular disease can lead to ischemia of the auditory organs, including the cortex. Neural impulses can be affected by neuropathic conditions such as diabetes.

8. **Psychiatric disturbances** can affect sound perception. Anxiety or depressive disorders may heighten the awareness of internal auditory sounds. In turn, tinnitus may exacerbate these underlying conditions as well. Auditory hallucinations must be ruled out by history.

B. **Physical examination.** This should focus on the head, ears, eyes, nose, throat, cardiovascular, and neurologic systems. Assess vital signs and perform a complete ear examination, including an evaluation for the obstruction of the external auditory canal. Look for tympanic membrane landmarks, tympanic pulsations, and signs of tumor. Auscultate the external auditory canal for transmitted sounds and use tuning forks to assess air and bone conduction (Weber and Rinne testing). Observe the neck for thyroid masses and auscultate for thyroid or carotid bruits. Evaluate extraocular movements, speech discrimination, and the integrity of the central nervous system (gait, equilibrium, sensation). If appropriate, include an evaluation of mood, affect, and perception (e.g., hallucinations).

C. **Testing.** Most patients with tinnitus do not need blood or urine testing (1, 3, 5). If indicated by history and physical examination, consider thyroid function tests, electrolytes, lipids, sedimentation rate, toxicology, syphilis serology, and rheumatologic screening (5). An audiogram to assess sensorineural hearing loss should always be performed. A tympanogram may reveal pulsations consistent with the heart rhythm or respirations. Plain radiographs are rarely useful. An evaluation for neoplasm, especially an acoustic neuroma, is best performed with magnetic resonance imaging, which also delineates eighth nerve lesions and cortex damage. Auditory brain stem-evoked responses can be helpful as well, especially in consideration of cortex lesions (5). An angiogram may be necessary to examine vasculature near the inner ear.

D. **Genetics.** To date there is no evidence that tinnitus has a genetic or familial cause.

IV. **DIAGNOSIS**

A. **Differential diagnosis.** The key to the diagnosis of tinnitus is determining if it is objective or subjective. Objective tinnitus should prompt a search for a structural source of the sound. Consider vascular complexes and muscular components close to the inner ear and the eustachian tube. Subjective tinnitus, although more common, has a less easily discerned etiology in most cases. Drug effects and hearing loss are the most common sources. Altered metabolic states such as diabetes, hyperthyroidism, or infection should then be considered. Evaluate for neurologic contributions, including acoustic neuroma, damage to the organ of Corti, or a brain lesion. Always keep in mind the possibility of psychiatric causes.

B. **Clinical manifestations.** Because only the patient hears tinnitus, there are no outward manifestations noted by others. The impact of tinnitus can be significant, however. Approximately one-fourth of tinnitus sufferers report an increase in symptoms over time.

References
1. Lockwood AA. Tinnitus. *N Engl J Med* 2002;347(12):904–910.
2. Moller AR. Pathophysiology of tinnitus. *Otolaryngol Clin North Am* 2003;36(2):249–266.
3. Crummer RW, Hassan GA. Diagnostic approach to tinnitus. *Am Fam Physician* 2004; 69(1):120.
4. Adams PF, Hendersot GE, Marano MA. National Center for Health Statistics. Current estimates from the National Health Interview survey. *Vtal Health Stat* 1999;200:81.
5. Schwaber MK. Medical evaluation of tinnitus. *Otolaryngol Clin North Am* 2003;36(2): 287–292.

VERTIGO
Frank S. Celestino

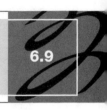

6.9

I. BACKGROUND

A. True vertigo is characterized by the illusion of movement—a feeling that the body or environment is moving. Patients often report rotation or spinning, although occasionally they describe a sensation of linear acceleration or tilting. This sensation often begins abruptly and, if severe, it is accompanied by nausea, vomiting, and staggering gait (1). Vertigo represents one of the four major symptom categories that account for patients' complaints of dizziness (2) (Chapter 2.2). The other three categories are:

1. **Presyncope.** This is a sensation of impending faint ("severe lightheadedness") and implies a temporary decrement of cerebral circulation. Common causes include postural hypotension, vasovagal reactions, cardiac arrhythmias, impaired cardiac output, and hypoglycemia.

2. **Disequilibrium.** This is a feeling of unsteadiness of gait or imbalance in the absence of any abnormal head sensation indicating a disturbance of the motor control system. Causes include alcoholism, drugs, cervical facet joint arthropathy, multiple sclerosis, and multiple neurosensory deficits (e.g., a combination of visual impairment, vestibular hypofunction, peripheral neuropathy, and medications).

3. **Other or atypical.** Patients often describe a vague or mild wooziness, lightheadedness, or heavy headedness, or a swimming or floating sensation. This category has a high association with psychologic disturbances such as anxiety, depression, and panic (2).

B. Careful interviewing allows the placement of patient complaints into one of the four categories, each implying certain pathophysiologic mechanisms and, therefore, specific differential diagnoses (1–3). The remainder of this chapter will primarily focus on evaluating patients with the complex symptom of true vertigo in an effort to determine specific underlying causes.

II. PATHOPHYSIOLOGY

A. Etiology. The vestibular system monitors the motion and position of the head in space by detecting angular and linear acceleration. The sensory receptors in the utricle and saccule detect linear acceleration, and it is the cristae of the semicircular canals that detect angular acceleration (head turning). Information from the peripheral receptors is relayed through the vestibular portion of the eighth cranial nerves to the brain stem nuclei, and portions of the cerebellum. Additional important connections are made with the ocular motor nuclei and spinal cord. True vertigo represents an asymmetry or imbalance of neural activity between the left and right vestibular nuclei. Abnormal activity in this system can arise either from peripheral lesions (labyrinth or vestibular nerve) or from central lesions (brain stem or cerebellum).

B. Epidemiology. The overarching complaint of "dizziness" accounts for 1% to 2% of all office visits, 7% of visits by patients older than 80 years of age, and 20% to 25% of all non–pain-related emergency department visits (1,2). In young adults (<30 years of age), psychologic causes account for most cases of dizziness, whereas vestibular lesions become more common in midlife. In the elderly, cerebrovascular and cardiac disorders, combined with multiple sensory deficits, outweigh simple vestibular causes. Approximately one-fourth of these dizziness-related visits are related to true vertigo (2). Therefore, most patients with dizziness have nonvestibular underlying processes. Of those with vertigo, central lesions are found in approximately 1% of all patients and 10% to 20% of elderly individuals (2). Dizziness and vertigo are usually benign, self-limited processes not associated with excess mortality, although some individuals suffer impaired quality of life because of recurrent or persistent symptoms.

III. EVALUATION

A. History. The patient's age, underlying comorbidities (especially hypertension, diabetes, heart disease, and psychiatric illness), and symptom classification category help limit the diagnostic possibilities. Further specificity is gained by eliciting the following:

1. **Temporal pattern.** Are the symptoms episodic or continuous? If episodic, how long do they last? Peripheral origin vertigo is often intermittent and of sudden onset compared with the usual, more gradual onset of central vertigo. A continuous history suggests central nervous system (CNS) pathology, drug or toxin effects, metabolic dysfunction, or psychiatric disease. Benign paroxysmal positional vertigo (BPPV) episodes last less than a minute; vertebrobasilar transient ischemic attacks last for several minutes up to an hour; Ménière's disease persists for 1 to 24 hours; and vestibular neuronitis or acute labyrinthitis continues for several days.

2. **Precipitating or exacerbating factors.** Has there been recent head trauma (implying perilymphatic fistula) or viral illness (labyrinthitis)? What is the relationship to sudden head movement or turning over in bed (BPPV), coughing or sneezing (perilymphatic fistula), postural changes (orthostasis), exercise (arrhythmias), foods (salty meals exacerbating Ménière's), walking and turning (multiple sensory deficits), micturition or pain (vasovagal reaction), and emotional upset (hyperventilation)?

3. **Associated symptoms.** Marked nausea, vomiting, diaphoresis, aural fullness, and recruitment (perception of sounds being too loud) are typical of peripheral vestibular disorders. Episodic vertigo associated with tinnitus and gradual (unilateral) hearing loss involving low frequencies preferentially suggests Ménière's disease. Asymmetric weakness, cranial nerve or cerebellar dysfunction, diplopia, numbness, or dysarthria suggests brain stem or CNS disease. Headache, scotomata, or tunnel vision points to migraine. Numbness or paresthesias may indicate neuropathy contributing to multiple sensory deficits (Chapter 4.6). A single, abrupt episode of severe vertigo with negative Dix-Hallpike (DH) testing (section **III.B.1**) that gradually subsides over days implies labyrinthitis (if hearing is affected), or vestibular neuronitis (if hearing is unaffected) (4). Mild vertigo with prominent tinnitus, unilateral hearing loss, and loss of corneal reflex is worrisome for an acoustic neuroma.

4. **Medications or toxins.** Many medications can cause "dizziness," although only a few (aminoglycosides, lead, mercury) cause vertigo. Assess toxin exposure by exploring job and recreational activities, including illicit drug use.

B. Physical examination. This emphasizes orthostatic vital signs, the eyes, ears, and neurologic and cardiovascular systems.

1. **Detection of nystagmus** is critical because it is the only objective sign of vertigo (3). Nystagmus can occur spontaneously or in response to changes in eye or body position. Peripheral vestibular disorders usually cause horizontal or rotatory nystagmus, whereas CNS pathology is reflected by vertical nystagmus—an ominous sign. In true vertigo caused by BPPV, DH maneuvers often confirm

the diagnosis (sensitivity 60%–90%, specificity 90%–95%) (5). The patient is moved rapidly from a sitting to a supine position with the head turned at a 30° angle, first to one side and then to the other. A positive DH test includes precipitation of vertigo, latency of onset by a few seconds, rotational nystagmus, resolution within a minute, and lessened symptoms and nystagmus with prolonged latency on repeated testing (i.e., fatigability) (3, 5). The lack of latency and fatigability characterize vertigo caused by serious central lesions.

2. **Neurologic examination** serves to detect brain stem or CNS pathology. It is important to focus on the patient's motor coordination and sensory function to detect the presence of an unsteady gait, past-pointing, ataxia, or abnormal Romberg test.

3. **Otoscopy** can detect otitis media or cholesteatoma. Nystagmus with vertigo following positive or negative pressure applied to the tympanic membrane (pneumatic otoscopy) suggests a perilymphatic fistula.

4. **Other provocative tests** (forced hyperventilation, vestibulo-ocular reflex testing, vigorous horizontal head shaking) are not routinely helpful and are best left to consultants.

C. **Testing**

1. **Clinical laboratory tests.** Most (80%–90%) patients need no laboratory testing (1–3). Audiometry is suggested if tinnitus or hearing loss is present. Blood tests are dictated by appropriate clinical indications only. Brain stem auditory-evoked responses can help detect multiple sclerosis or acoustic neuroma. Holter monitoring is indicated if arrhythmias are suspected. Specialized testing—posturography, rotational chair testing, electronystagmography—is best ordered by a consultant when the diagnosis remains unclear after initial evaluation.

2. **Diagnostic imaging.** Consider Doppler ultrasound for suspected transient ischemic attack and magnetic resonance imaging if CNS lesions are suspected.

D. **Genetics.** There are no significant genetic or familial influences related to vertigo.

IV. **DIAGNOSIS**

A. **Differential diagnosis.** Peripheral causes of vertigo (in approximate order of frequency in primary care) include BPPV, viral labyrinthitis or vestibular neuronitis (acute unilateral vestibulopathy), serous otitis, perilymphatic fistula, Ménière's disease, and drugs (alcohol, aminoglycosides) (2). Central causes of vertigo include vertebrobasilar transient ischemic attack, cerebellar infarction or neoplasm, demyelinating disease, brain stem infarction or neoplasm, cerebellopontine angle tumors, migraine, hyperventilation, seizures, spinocerebellar degeneration, and certain systemic disorders (infections, vasculitis, syphilis). The cervical spine is rarely the source of vertigo, either by osteoarthritic spur occlusion of the vertebral arteries or by proprioceptive overstimulation by facet joint arthropathy.

B. **Clinical manifestations.** The common features of vestibular dysfunction are vertigo, nystagmus, and postural instability. The clinician's chief task is to distinguish between usually benign peripheral causes and more ominous central processes by attending to the historical and physical examination characteristics outlined in section **III**. Central vertigo is associated with moderate nausea and vomiting, ataxia, neurologic signs and symptoms, rare hearing loss, and very slow compensation (3). Peripheral vertigo manifests combinations of severe nausea and vomiting, tinnitus, fluctuating hearing loss, milder postural imbalance, a lack of neurologic signs and symptoms, and rapid compensation.

References

1. Dieterich M. Dizziness. *The Neurologist* 2004;10:154–164.
2. Sloane PD, Coeytaux RR, Beck RS, et al. Dizziness: state of the art. *Ann Intern Med* 2001;134(9 Part 2):S823–S832.
3. Traccis S, Zoroddu GF, Zecca MT, et al. Evaluating patients with vertigo: bedside examination. *Neurol Sci* 2004;25(Suppl 1):S16–S19.
4. Balok RW. Vestibular neuritis. *N Engl J Med* 2003;348:1027–1032.
5. Parnes LS, Agrawal SK, Atlas J. Diagnosis and management of benign paroxysmal positional vertigo (BPPV). *CMAJ* 2003;169(7):681–693.

Cardiovascular Problems

Joann E. Schaefer

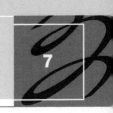

7

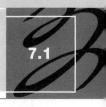

ATYPICAL CHEST PAIN
Thomas J. Hansen

7.1

I. **BACKGROUND.** "Typical" chest pain is pain that is typical of anginal pain. This pain is usually described as substernal, radiating to the left neck and arm, and is pressurelike or has a squeezing sensation. "Atypical" chest pain is defined as the absence of this typical presentation.

II. **PATHOPHYSIOLOGY.** Atypical chest pain can originate in any of the thoracic organs, as well as from extrathoracic sources (e.g., thyroiditis or panic disorder).

III. **EVALUATION.** The approach to the evaluation of acute chest pain, whether typical or atypical, should be to rapidly assess whether the pain is due to cardiac disease. Atypical chest pain does not rule out an acute myocardial infarction (AMI), especially in women (1), patients with diabetes, and the elderly, in whom an AMI may present in an atypical fashion. A clinical history of the chest pain and an electrocardiogram (ECG) should be obtained within 5 minutes after presentation (2). The ECG is critical for guiding initial therapy and decisions regarding diagnosis and treatment.

A. **History.** The clinical history should focus on the time of onset, the characteristic of the pain, the location (retrosubsternal, subxiphoid, diffuse), the frequency of the pain (constant, intermittent, acute onset), the duration of the pain, precipitating factors (exertion, stress, food, respiration, movement), the quality of the pain (burning, squeezing, dull, sharp, tearing, heavy), and any associated symptoms (shortness of breath, diaphoresis, nausea, vomiting, jaw pain, back pain, radiation, palpitations, weakness, fatigue).

Other pertinent questions include assessing risk factors for coronary artery disease (diabetes, smoking, hypertension, hypercholesteremia, family history), anorexia, anxiety, cough and/or wheezing, drug use, fever, previous history of deep vein thrombosis or pulmonary embolism, pain increased with recumbency or relieved by leaning forward, presence of a mass, lesion, or rash on the chest, previous history of cancer, pregnancy/postpartum, oral contraceptive use, or trauma, relationship of pain with eating, and syncopal or near-syncopal episodes.

B. **Physical examination.** The physical examination should include a rapid assessment of vital signs, as well as oxygen saturation and electrocardiographic evaluation. Following this, an examination of the chest should be performed. Cardiac examination should focus on pericardial rubs, systolic and diastolic murmurs, third or fourth heart sounds, and distended jugular veins. Auscultation of the lungs should focus on diminished breath sounds, a pleural rub, rales, rhonchi, and wheezes. Examination of the legs should focus on edema and poor perfusion of a limb, which may indicate an aortic dissection. Examination of the musculoskeletal system should focus on reproducible or localized pain. Examination of the skin should assess for lesions, masses, or rashes.

C. **Testing**

1. **Oxygen saturation.** Oxygen saturation below 92% may indicate a myocardial infarction, spontaneous pneumothorax, pulmonary embolism, or pneumonia. An arterial blood gas is warranted.

2. **ECG.** Always compare with an old ECG when available. The presence of T wave inversion is consistent with *myocardial ischemia*. ST elevation is consistent with *myocardial injury*, and ST depression is consistent with *subendocardial infarction*. A Q wave is diagnostic of a *myocardial infarction* (3). A *pulmonary embolism* is classically associated with the $S_1 Q_3 T_3$ pattern representing a large S wave in I, an ST depression in II, and a large Q wave in III with T wave inversion.

Sensitivity of this is less than 20%, however. *Acute pericarditis* demonstrates diffuse ST-segment elevation, in which the ST segment is flat or slightly concave, and PR depression.

3. **Other laboratory tests**
   a. **Comprehensive metabolic profile.** Used to detect metabolic abnormality as the cause of chest pain as well as abnormalities of the liver
   b. **Complete blood count.** Used to detect infection and inflammatory disorders
   c. **Creatine kinase-MB (CK-MB) and troponin.** High positive predictive value for an AMI if elevated but may be negative initially
   d. **D-dimer.** Sensitive but not specific for a pulmonary embolism
   e. **Liver function tests, amylase, *Helicobacter pylori*.** Used to determine a gastrointestinal etiology of the pain, such as liver distention, pancreatitis, gastric, or duodenal ulcers due to *H. pylori*
   f. **Toxicology screen.** Recommended if cocaine use is believed to be the cause of the chest pain
4. **Imaging studies**
   a. **Chest x-ray.** Useful in diagnosing pneumonia, pneumothorax, aortic dissection, acute pericarditis, and esophageal rupture
   b. **Ultrasound.** Helpful to diagnose pericardial, valvular disease, and to demonstrate cardiac wall motion abnormalities
   c. **Stress echocardiogram.** Used for stable patients who have been ruled out for infarction to determine if cardiac disease is present
   d. **Computed tomography.** Used to diagnose aortic dissection in stable patients and may identify pulmonary embolism or cardiac effusion

IV. **DIAGNOSIS**
   A. **Differential diagnosis.** The differential diagnosis for atypical chest pain includes:
      1. **Breast lesions.** Abscess, carcinoma, fibroadenosis, mastitis
      2. **Cardiovascular.** AMI, angina pectoris, aortic dissection, aortic valvular disease, hypertrophic cardiomyopathy, mitral valve prolapse, myocarditis, pericarditis, primary pulmonary hypertension, thoracic aortic aneurysm, neoplasm
      3. **Gastrointestinal disease.** Esophageal rupture, esophagitis, foreign body presence, gastric distention, gastritis, liver distention, Mallory-Weiss syndrome, pancreatitis, peptic ulcer disease, Plummer-Vinson syndrome, splenic infarct, subphrenic abscess, Zenker's diverticulum
      4. **Thyroid.** Thyroiditis
      5. **Psychogenic causes.** Anxiety, panic attack
      6. **Pulmonary disease.** Bronchitis, neoplasm, pleuritis, pneumonia, pulmonary hypertension, pulmonary embolism
      7. **Musculoskeletal disorder.** Bruised or fractured rib, cervical disc herniation, costochondritis, intercostal muscle cramp, intercostal myositis, pectoral strain, osteoarthritis, thoracic outlet syndrome
      8. **Neuralgia.** Herpes zoster, neurofibroma, neoplasm, tabes dorsalis (4)
   B. **Clinical approach.** Once a cardiac etiology for atypical chest pain has been eliminated, a careful history and physical examination usually yields a diagnosis. The aforementioned tests are useful in making the diagnosis and determining an appropriate treatment plan.

References

1. DeCara JE. Noninvasive cardiac testing in women. *J Am Med Womens Assoc* 2003 Fall, 58(4):254–263.
2. Lee TH, Goldman L. Evaluation of the patient with acute chest pain. *JAMA* 2000;342: 1187–1195.
3. Braunwald B, Fauci A, Kasper D, et al. eds. *Harrison's principles of internal medicine*, 15th ed, New York, NY: McGraw-Hill, 2001.
4. Adler SN, Gasbarra DB, Adler-Klein D, eds. *A pocket manual of differential diagnosis*, 4th ed. Philadelphia, PA: Lippincott Williams & Wilkins, 2000.

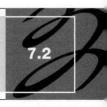

CHEST PAIN
Sanjeev Sharma

7.2

I. BACKGROUND. Chest pain accounts for approximately 5.6 million emergency department visits annually. It is second only to abdominal pain as the most common reason for an emergency department visit. More than 3 million patients are hospitalized yearly in the United States for chest pain. A standardized approach to addressing the management of these patients is essential, given the adverse consequences of missing a life-threatening condition.

II. PATHOPHYSIOLOGY. Cardiac pain is usually due to low perfusion to the myocardium through the coronary arteries that are completely or partially blocked by atherosclerotic plaque. This leads to tissue hypoxia, anaerobic metabolism, lactic acidosis, and abnormal prostaglandin secretion. Pain originating from the lungs or pleura is caused by the irritation or inflammation of the lungs and/or the pleura or diaphragm. Gastrointestinal pain arises from mucosal inflammation or structural abnormality, such as stricture or obstruction.

III. EVALUATION. The patient should be evaluated to determine the diagnosis and to formulate an immediate management plan. Priority should be given to rule out life-threatening cardiovascular causes. In patients with acute pain, the clinician must assess the patient's hemodynamic and respiratory status. If either is compromised, management should focus on stabilizing the patient.

    A. History. Questions should be asked about the exact location, quality, and nature of onset, duration, exacerbating factors, and radiation of pain. Radiation of pain to the left arm is common in myocardial ischemia. Pain of aortic dissection radiates between the scapulae. It is necessary to inquire about cardiac risk factors, including smoking, hypertension, diabetes mellitus, hyperlipidemia, and a family history of coronary artery disease (1).

    B. Physical examination. A rapid physical assessment of the patient should include a full set of vital signs, determination of the presence or absence of cyanosis, dyspnea and diaphoresis, examination of the neck, thorax, and abdomen, and palpation of the major peripheral arteries for the presence of and the characteristics of the pulse.

    C. Testing

        1. Laboratory tests. Pulse oximetry should be ordered to assess oxygen status. Cardiac enzymes, creatinine phosphokinase (CK, CK-MB) and troponin T or I should also be ordered in patients suspected of cardiac pain (2). C-reactive protein, brain natriuretic peptide, and serum myoglobin have been used in the management of patients with chest pain. The possibility of life-threatening cardiac pain cannot be excluded based upon a single negative value of any of these markers; three sets of cardiac enzymes should be used (3). A complete metabolic profile including liver function tests, amylase, and lipase should be ordered if a gastrointestinal cause is suspected (4).

        2. Electrocardiogram (ECG). An electrocardiogram (ECG) is essential. An ECG showing changes consistent with ischemia or infarction is associated with a high probability of acute myocardial infarction or unstable angina.

        3. Echocardiogram. This is helpful if valvular abnormality is suspected.

        4. Chest x-ray. Pulmonary diseases such as pneumonia, pleural effusion, and pneumothorax can be diagnosed. Widened mediastinum is seen in patients with aortic dissection.

        5. Computed tomography (CT) scan or magnetic resonance imaging. If the patient's history and examination are consistent with aortic dissection, these imaging studies should be performed to evaluate the aorta. A transthoracic echocardiogram can be performed to assess cardiac function.

6. **Ventilation–perfusion scan/spiral CT scan of the chest.** These are appropriate initial tests in patients with a history of venous thromboembolism or coagulation abnormality.
7. **Other testing.** If the patient with chest pain shows no evidence of life-threatening conditions, the clinician should focus on serious chronic conditions with the potential to cause major complications in the future; the most common of these is stable angina. Cost-effective and noninvasive tests for coronary disease such as exercise electrocardiography or stress echocardiography should

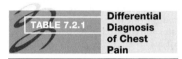

TABLE 7.2.1 Differential Diagnosis of Chest Pain

Cardiac
Ischemic disease
Acute myocardial infarction
Stable angina
Unstable angina
Myocarditis
Pericarditis
Valvular heart disease
Aortic stenosis
Mitral valve prolapse
Hypertrophic cardiomyopathy
Aortic dissection
Noncardiac
Pulmonary
Pneumonia
Pleuritis
Pulmonary embolism
Pleural effusion
Pneumothorax
Gastrointestinal
Esophageal spasm
Esophagitis/gastritis
Peptic ulcer disease
Gall stone
Musculoskeletal
Costochondritis
Muscle spasm
Cervical radiculopathy
Neurologic
Herpes zoster
Nerve root compression
Psychiatric
Anxiety state

be performed for low-risk patients. Gastrointestinal causes can be evaluated by endoscopy. As many as 10% of patients with chest pain may have emotional or psychiatric conditions. These patients should be appropriately evaluated by an expert (5).

IV. DIAGNOSIS. The differential diagnosis of chest pain is presented in Table 7.2.1.

References

1. Rich EC, Crowson TW, Harris IB. The diagnostic value of the medical history. *Arch Intern Med* 1987;147:1957.
2. Hamm CW, Goldmann BU, Heeschen C, et al. Emergency room triage of patients with acute chest pain by means of rapid testing for cardiac troponin T or troponin I. *N Engl J Med* 1997;337(23):1648–53.
3. Caragher TE, Fernandez BB, Jacobs FL, et al. Evaluation of quantitative cardiac biomarker point-of-care testing in the emergency department. *J Emerg Med* 2002;22(1):1–7.
4. Eslick GD, Fass R. Noncardiac chest pain: evaluation and treatment. *Gastroenterol Clin North Am* 2003;32(2):531–552.
5. Ho KY, Kang JY, Yeo B, et al. Non-cardiac, non-oesophageal chest pain: the relevance of psychological factors. *Gut* 1998;43(1):105–110.

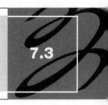

BRADYCARDIA   7.3
Mark D. Goodman

I. BACKGROUND. Bradycardia, which is defined as a heart rate less than 60 beats/minute, results from abnormalities in impulse formation or failure of conduction. It may or may not be a cause for concern. For the well-conditioned athlete, bradycardia may carry no underlying risk or morbidity, but for the patient with a cardiac or neurologic condition, bradycardia can be deadly.

The most important initial assessment is whether the slow heart rate is pathologic or innocent. In the presence of syncope, neurologic changes, myocardial ischemia/angina, fatigue, or dyspnea, one can safely assume that bradycardia adversely impacts health (1).

II. PATHOPHYSIOLOGY

    A. Etiology. Conditions that can manifest as bradycardia include exposure, electrolyte imbalance (hypokalemia), infection, hypoglycemia, hypothyroid/hyperthyroid, inferior wall myocardial infarction, cardiac ischemia, increased intracranial pressure, medications (e.g., β-blockers, calcium channel blockers, antiarrhythmics, lithium, digoxin), atrial fibrillation, long QT syndrome, and sick sinus syndrome. Reversible causes include profound bradycardia, which often develops in patients with obstructive sleep apnea and hypoxia, but may be eliminated with appropriate apnea treatment.

        1. Long QT syndrome

            a. This condition was first described in 1957 in a family with recurrent syncope and sudden death. Several different familial syndromes manifest as QT prolongation on an electrocardiogram (ECG), with a predilection for malignant ventricular arrhythmias and possible syncope or sudden death. If the presenting event is syncope, a clinical evaluation that includes an ECG almost always reveals the prolongation of the QT interval, the clinical hallmark of this disorder. Several drugs can prolong the QTc interval, and it is important to distinguish drug-induced QTc prolongation from the inherited form of long QT syndrome (2).

   b. Life-threatening cardiac events tend to occur under specific circumstances in a gene-specific manner: some during exercise, some with arousal/emotion, some at sleep/rest, and some with loud noises.

2. Sick sinus syndrome

   a. Sick sinus syndrome comprises a variety of conditions involving sinus node dysfunction (more common in the elderly). Multiple manifestations on ECG include sinus bradycardia, sinus arrest, sinoatrial block, and bradytachycardia syndrome, characterized by alternating periods of sinus bradycardia and supraventricular tachycardia. The mainstay of treatment is an atrial or dual-chamber pacemaker (3,4).

   b. Causes can include cardiomyopathies, collagen-vascular disease, ischemia, infarction, pericarditis, myocarditis, rheumatic heart disease, electrolyte disorders (especially hypokalemia or hypocarbia), and medications. The most common cause is idiopathic degenerative fibrotic infiltration. Coronary artery disease can coexist with sick sinus syndrome. The syndrome occurs in 1/600 cardiac patients older than 65 years and accounts for 50% of pacemaker placements in the United States.

B. Epidemiology. The incidence of bradycardia in the general population is unknown, but among cardiac patients and those older than 50 years, it is present in 0.6/10000 individuals. Peak incidence occurs in the sixth and seventh decade.

III. EVALUATION

A. History

   1. Symptoms. Elicit evidence of cardiac neurologic or respiratory compromise, such as dyspnea, palpitations, angina, decreased exercise tolerance, tachypnea, lightheadedness, or syncope.

   2. Cardiac risk factors. Inquire about family history, tobacco use, hyperlipidemia, diabetes mellitus, and hypertension.

   3. Underlying conditions. Are underlying bradycardia risk factors present? Ask about cardiomyopathies, alcohol dependence/misuse, rheumatic heart disease, and any other coexisting medical conditions.

   4. Medications. Bradycardia can be induced by digoxin, phenothiazine, quinidine, procainamide, β-blockers, calcium channel blockers, clonidine, lithium, and antiarrhythmic medications. β-Blocker bradycardia is especially common, because β-blockers are not only used for hypertension and angina prophylaxis, but also for migraine prevention, essential tremor, thyrotoxicosis, glaucoma, and anxiety. β-Blockade can also manifest as QT interval prolongation.

B. Physical examination. Resting pulse and blood pressure, temperature, and respiratory rate should be taken, and if there is concern for hypovolemia, blood pressure and pulse in both lying and standing positions (orthostatic evaluation). Cardiac auscultation follows the palpation of the thyroid gland, and the search for other evidence of thyroid disorder (skin, hair, eye proptosis). The presence or absence of pulses, and search for bruits and abdominal aneurysm should follow. Is edema present? Are lung fields clear? Is there jugular venous distention? Cyanosis?

C. Testing

   1. Obtain cardiac enzymes, congestive heart failure peptide, electrolytes, calcium and magnesium, thyroid-stimulating hormone, thyroxine, and triiodothyronine levels, as well as drug levels of digoxin and antiarrhythmics if indicated.

   2. Obtain an ECG, and if necessary an event monitor (for patients reporting rarer intermittent symptoms) or a Holter monitor (in those patients who report more frequent symptoms).

IV. DIAGNOSIS

A. Differential diagnosis. The different types of bradycardia include:

   1. Sinus bradycardia (5). Normal P-QRS-T sequence at a rate less than 60 beats/minute

   2. Sinus nodal block: a missing P wave. This can be incomplete, where the occasional sequence of P-QRS-T is lost, or complete, where P waves are completely absent, and QRS-T proceeds at a slow "escape" rate from the ventricular pacemaker.

3. **Sick sinus syndrome.** Generalized abnormality, as previously described, of cardiac impulse formation that can manifest as varying combinations of bradycardia and tachycardia
4. **First-degree atrioventricular (AV) block: common ECG finding.** The PR interval represents the conduction time from the sinus node through the atrium, AV node, and His-Purkinje system to the development of ventricular depolarization. Values over 0.2 qualify (by convention).
5. **Second-degree AV block.** This occurs when an organized atrial rhythm fails to conduct to the ventricle in a 1:1 ratio. There are several types, including the following:
   a. Mobitz type 1 (Wenckebach), in which the ECG shows a stable PP interval but a progressive increase in the PR interval until a P wave fails to conduct
   b. Mobitz type II, which is characterized by a stable PP interval with no measurable prolongation of the PR interval before an abrupt conduction failure
6. **Third-degree AV block: referred to as complete heart block.** Atrial and ventricular activity are independent of each other.
B. **Clinical approach.** There are few indications for intervention in patients with bradycardia who are truly asymptomatic. Where possible, and if symptoms or considerable cardiac risk is present, offending medications can be changed or reduced, underlying conditions (e.g., thyroid abnormalities) should be treated, pacing can be considered, and patient education and prevention strategies should be tried.

References
1. Mangrum JM, Dimarco JP. The evaluation and management of bradycardia. *JAMA* 2000;342(10):703–709.
2. Moss AJ. Long QT syndrome. *JAMA* 2003;289(16):2041–2044.
3. Roth B. *Beta-blocker toxicity eMedicine.* (www.emedicine.com) updated April 15, 2005
4. Adan V, Crown LA. Diagnosis and treatment of sick sinus syndrome. *Am Fam Physician* 2003;67(8):1725–1732.
5. Baustian GH, Hodgson JM. *Sinus bradycardia.* FIRSTConsult (www.firstconsult.com) updated May 19, 2005.

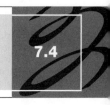

CARDIOMEGALY
Lou Ann McStay

7.4

I. **BACKGROUND.** Cardiomegaly is true enlargement of the heart beyond the upper limits of normal. This is a physical finding, not a specific disease. It is the result of other diseases and is almost always abnormal. Heart size is easily, rapidly, and most commonly determined radiographically by the cardiothoracic ratio (CTR). This is defined as the sum of the distances from the body midline (a vertical line through the spinous processes) to the furthest left and right heart borders, which is then divided by the widest thoracic diameter measured horizontally between the inner surfaces of the ribs. The CTR is normally 050 to 055 in adults and up to 06 in infants and children. The heart may therefore appear falsely enlarged due to abnormalities of the chest wall, or to radiographic technique.

II. **PATHOPHYSIOLOGY**
A. **Etiology.** Ventricular aneurysm and pericardial effusion can enlarge the cardiac silhouette. However, most cardiac enlargement is due to pressure overload and

muscle hypertrophy of one or more chambers of the heart, volume overload with dilation of cardiac chambers, or cardiomyopathy. As such, cardiomegaly is usually the result of other cardiovascular disorders (hypertension, ischemic or valvular heart disease, familial structural abnormalities) but can also be caused by systemic diseases (anemia, viral or rickettsial infections, bite or sting toxins, medications, hyperthyroidism, hypothyroidism, hyperparathyroidism, acromegaly, diabetes, autoimmune and infiltrative (amyloid) diseases, and metastases). In many cases, particularly with left ventricular hypertrophy, cardiomegaly is reversible with treatment of the underlying cause.

B. Epidemiology. Cardiomegaly can be an incidental finding when discovered early in the disease process. It can occur in children and young adults as a result of rheumatic heart disease, infections, or familial cardiomyopathies, where the presenting symptom may be sudden death from arrhythmias, often brought on by physical exertion, as in sports. Left ventricular mass is increased in obese adolescents (1). Due to the higher prevalence of ischemia and hypertension, most cases are in older adults.

III. EVALUATION

A. History. Past medical history may include congestive heart failure, coronary disease, hypertension, rheumatic fever, and systemic diseases. Family history may reveal hypertension, hyperlipidemia, or sudden death. Social history might include alcohol or substance abuse or an exposure to a cardiac toxin. System review could include fatigue, dizziness, dyspnea, angina, cough, edema, nocturia, and loss of weight with cardiac cachexia, as well as symptoms more specific to any systemic underlying disease.

B. Physical examination

1. Cardiac. Examination may note a chest deformity causing apparent cardiomegaly. Inspection may note a visible heave lateral to the midclavicular line. Palpation of the point of maximal impulse (PMI) below the fifth intercostal space and lateral to the midclavicular line is highly specific for left ventricular enlargement, in the absence of chest wall abnormalities. The PMI may be diffuse (2–3 cm) and may be weak in dilated cardiomyopathy, or it may be hyperdynamic in increased sympathetic states. The PMI may be nonpalpable with pericardial effusion. Peripheral pulses may be weak and pulsus alternans detectable with decreased left ventricular function. If the PMI cannot be appreciated by palpation, the location of the left border of the heart can be ascertained by dullness to percussion. Dullness beyond the midclavicular line and fifth intercostal space is abnormal. Heart murmurs of abnormal valves responsible for the cardiomegaly may be auscultated, as well as the regurgitant murmurs resulting from dilated chambers. Diminished heart sounds or friction rubs may be noted with pericardial disease. S_3 and S_4 gallops may be heard with heart failure resulting from the cardiomegaly. Arrhythmias are common with cardiomegaly. Hypertension, as a cause of cardiomegaly, may be present.

2. Extracardiac. Examination findings may relate to the underlying causes of cardiomegaly (e.g., autoimmune, infectious, and endocrine diseases, and alcoholism). The typical extracardiac findings of heart failure (cough, dyspnea, rales, wheezes, edema, hepatojugular reflux, jugular venous distension) resulting from the cardiomegaly may also be present.

C. Testing. Cardiomegaly is detectable by chest x-ray, electrocardiogram (ECG), and echocardiography. Serologic testing primarily identifies systemic causative disorders, and B-type natriuretic peptide increases with ventricular wall stretch (2).

1. A standard upright posterior–anterior chest x-ray with the 10th rib visible at full inspiration in a nonrotated position without chest deformity is useful for determining the CTR. However, 20% of echocardiogram-confirmed cases of cardiomegaly are not seen on chest x-ray (2). Determination of specific chamber enlargement by x-ray is most reliable with the left atrium, where enlargement projects it posteriorly and superiorly, resulting in increased cardiac density centrally, displacement of the left main bronchus superiorly giving it a more horizontal take-off, and a more readily visible, and curved, left atrial appendage. These findings are significant, because left atrial enlargement is associated with a poor prognosis and was the only identified independent predictor of mortality in a cohort of patients with ischemic cardiomyopathy (3).

2. The ECG is almost always abnormal with cardiomegaly, although the changes are often nonspecific. The voltage amplitude is often increased or the axis shifted. Atrial and ventricular arrhythmias are common, with atrial fibrillation occurring in 25% of patients with cardiomyopathy (4). Because lead V_1 is directly over the atria, this lead can best indicate atrial enlargement. A diphasic P wave in V_1 indicates atrial hypertrophy. In right atrial hypertrophy, the initial half of the wave is the largest segment. If the second half of the diphasic P wave in lead V_1 is larger or wider, there is left atrial hypertrophy. As lead V_5 is over the left ventricle, a tall R wave in V_5 indicates left ventricular hypertrophy. There may be ischemic changes noted on the ECG in cardiomegaly as well.

3. Echocardiography is the test of choice for a definitive diagnosis of cardiac enlargement. It can also yield useful information about systolic and diastolic function, wall hypertrophy, ischemic areas, aneurysms, pericardial effusion, and the heart valves.

D. **Genetics.** There are familial dilated as well as obstructive cardiomyopathies and a familial right atrial enlargement. Studies have indicated that the presence of certain gene alleles can modify the risk of cardiac hypertrophy (5). Many autoimmune and endocrine causes of cardiomegaly are known to be familial.

IV. DIAGNOSIS

A. **Differential diagnosis.** The differential diagnosis of cardiomegaly consists mainly in distinguishing true from factitious cardiomegaly due to suboptimal chest x-ray technique. Here the most important factor is an adequate inspiration revealing the 10th rib. Otherwise, the heart appears larger and more globular toward the left. Anterior–posterior films and portable chest x-rays, shot closer than the standard upright view, also falsely enlarge the heart. Supine views preclude adequate inspiration. Trunk rotation, scoliosis, and pectus excavatum can cause apparent cardiomegaly.

B. **Clinical manifestations.** An enlarged heart is less efficient in providing adequate blood flow to the body and itself. Therefore, clinical manifestations of cardiomegaly are primarily those of heart failure (e.g., dyspnea, dizziness, fatigue). Additional symptoms are arrhythmia, angina, and sudden death. Other manifestations are signs and symptoms particular to the specific disease causing the cardiomegaly.

References

1. Damias PG, Tritos NA. Increased left ventricular mass in obese adolescents. *Eur Heart J* 2005;26(2):201–202.
2. Sutter M, Diereks DB. New insights into decompensated heart failure. *Emerg Med* 2005:18–25.
3. Sabharwal N, Cemin R, Rajan K, et al. Usefulness of left atrial volume as a predictor of mortality in patients with ischemic cardiomyopathy. *Am J Cardiol* 2004;94(6):760–763.
4. Wenger NK, Abelman WH, Roberts WC. Cardiomyopathy and specific heart muscle disease. In: Hurst JW, ed. *The heart, arteries, and veins*, 7th ed. New York, NY: McGraw-Hill, 1990:1278–1347.
5. Dursanoglu D. ACE polymorphism in healthy young subjects. *Acta Cardiol* 2005;60(2): 153–158.

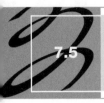

CONGESTIVE HEART FAILURE
Hemant K. Satpathy and Chhabi Satpathy

I. BACKGROUND. Heart failure (HF) is defined as a complex clinical syndrome resulting from any structural or functional cardiac disorder that impairs the ability of the ventricle to fill with or eject blood. Often, it is associated with features of vascular congestion. The term *heart failure* is more appropriate than congestive heart failure, because many patients with this disease may not show evidence of congestion, particularly when treated aggressively with diuretics. HF is a major public health problem in industrialized nations. It appears to be the only common cardiovascular condition that is increasing in prevalence and incidence in North America and Western Europe. Despite improvements in therapy, the mortality in patients with HF has remained unacceptably high, making early detection of susceptible individuals imperative (1).

II. PATHOPHYSIOLOGY

    A. Etiology

        1. Two interrelated processes, chamber remodeling and systolic dysfunction, play critical roles in HF, which may be systolic or diastolic. In patients with HF, approximately 70% have systolic dysfunction, 15% have diastolic dysfunction, and the remaining 15% have combined dysfunction. Systolic HF is associated with markedly dilated heart chamber with reduced wall motion and preserved filling. Diastolic HF is associated with a normal chamber size with normal emptying but impaired filling.

        2. Causes of HF differ depending on whether it is systolic or diastolic, left-sided or right-sided, or acute or chronic. Refer to Table 7.5.1 for the common causes of HF. In the United States and Western Europe, ischemic heart disease is responsible for 75% of all cases of HF followed by cardiomyopathy. The most common

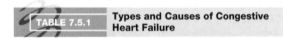

TABLE 7.5.1	**Types and Causes of Congestive Heart Failure**

Left ventricular systolic dysfunction

Causes include:

Ischemic heart disease, hypertension, alcohol toxicity, obesity, valvular disease (e.g., aortic stenosis), or chronic tachydysrhythmia

Preserved left ventricular systolic function

Causes include:

Transient systolic dysfunction due to acute myocardial ischemia

Left atrial hypertension due to high-output states (e.g., thyrotoxicosis), volume excess, or mitral stenosis

Left ventricular diastolic dysfunction due to hypertension, ischemia, aging, obesity, or sustained tachyarrhythmias

Miscellaneous disorders such as restrictive cardiomyopathy due to infiltrative diseases (e.g., amyloidosis), constrictive pericarditis and pericardial tamponade, and pure right-sided heart failure

cause of right-sided HF is left-sided HF. Other causes of right-sided HF include pulmonary hypertension, cor pulmonale, or dysfunction of right-sided valves (2).

B. Epidemiology

1. In evaluating patients with HF it is important to identify not only the underlying causes, but also the precipitating factors. Most common precipitating factors include inappropriate therapy (increased salt and water intake, noncompliance with medications, or taking nonsteroidal anti-inflammatory drugs), acute myocardial infarction, tachyarrhythmias, worsening of hypertension, pulmonary embolism, high-output states (anemia, pregnancy, thyrotoxicosis), cardiotoxins (e.g., alcohol, cocaine, antiarrhythmics, calcium channel blockers, β-blockers, antineoplastics), cardiac infections (myocarditis, endocarditis, pericarditis) and systemic illness (pneumonia, acute renal failure).

2. The national hospital discharge survey estimates that 4.8 million Americans have HF. Its prevalence is substantial and increases steeply with age. The prevalence in African-Americans is reported to be 25% higher than in Caucasians (3). This study was based on symptomatic HF, which considered only half of the participants with left ventricular dysfunction. There has been an increase in the prevalence of HF over time, secondary to aging of the population and improved treatment of valvular and coronary artery disease (4). The incidence of HF, like the prevalence, increases with age. In the Framingham Study, the incidence of HF approximately doubled over each successive decade of life. Diastolic failure has a better prognosis than systolic failure.

III. EVALUATION

A. History

1. This evaluation should include specific consideration of noncardiac diseases such as collagen-vascular diseases, bacterial or parasitic infection, thyroid excess or deficiency, and pheochromocytoma. A detailed family history should be obtained not only to determine whether there is familial predisposition to atherosclerotic disease, but also to identify relatives with cardiomyopathy, sudden unexplained death, conduction system disease, and skeletal myopathy. Twenty percent of cases of idiopathic dilated cardiomyopathy are familial.

2. Symptoms of HF belong to three broad groups. Dyspnea on exertion (DOE), orthopnea, and paroxysmal nocturnal dyspnea (PND) result from pulmonary congestion, and are the most specific symptoms of HF. Dyspnea is the most predominant symptom of HF, whereas orthopnea and PND occur in a more advanced stage of HF. Systemic vascular congestion causes peripheral edema, ascites, abdominal pain/fullness and nausea, whereas low cardiac output causes fatigue and change in mental status. Older patients with HF may not have DOE because of a sedentary baseline status. They often present with atypical symptoms such as dry cough, daytime oliguria with nocturia, and confusion.

B. Physical examination. In general, physical examination is more sensitive in detecting acute HF than chronic HF. In mild or moderately severe HF, the patient appears in no distress at rest except feeling uncomfortable when lying flat for more than a few minutes. In severe HF, the pulse pressure may be diminished, and the diastolic arterial pressure may be elevated. In severe acute HF, systolic hypotension may be present with cool, diaphoretic extremities, and Cheyne-Stokes respiration. There may be cyanosis in lips and nail beds and sinus tachycardia. Elevated systemic venous pressure may be reflected in the distention of the jugular veins, and when this pressure is abnormally high, characteristic abdominojugular reflex is seen. Third and fourth heart sounds are often audible but are not specific for HF, and pulsus alternans may be present. Other physical findings include pulmonary rales, cardiac edema (which is usually symmetric and dependant on HF, pitting in acute and brawny in chronic HF), hydrothorax, ascites, congestive hepatomegaly, occasional splenomegaly, jaundice, and cardiac cachexia.

C. Testing. While ordering laboratory tests for patients with HF, it is important to screen for diabetes, kidney disease, anemia, thyrotoxicosis, liver dysfunction, and electrolytes including calcium and magnesium. Screening for hemochromatosis may also be given a consideration. Serial monitoring of kidney function and electrolytes is needed at follow-up visits. Additional tests may be ordered when there is suspicion of certain diseases either causing or precipitating the HF, such as cardiac markers in the presence of chest pain. Although the sodium and potassium values are usually normal in these patients, hyponatremia and hyperkalemia could be associated with severe HF. These patients could have hypokalemia when treated aggressively with loop diuretics. Impaired liver function is often associated with hepatic congestion or cardiac cirrhosis.

1. *Brain natriuretic peptide (BNP)* is the most sensitive and specific indicator of all natriuretic peptides for ventricular disorders. It has been used more often of late in order to screen for HF, in addition to its role in prognosis and monitoring therapy. BNP is an independent predictor of high left ventricular end-diastolic pressure (LVEDP). Its release is proportional to ventricular volume expansion and pressure overload. A BNP cut point of 100 pg/mL distinguishes patients with HF from those without it. An elevated BNP on patients with clinical HF and normal systolic function in echo substantiates the diagnosis of diastolic heart dysfunction.

2. *Cardiac catheterization* with coronary arteriography may be considered in patients with HF, angina, and known or suspected coronary artery disease but without angina, who are candidates for revascularization.

3. *Chest x-ray* typically shows cardiomegaly, except in diastolic HF. Other x-ray findings of HF include pulmonary vascular redistribution, interstitial and alveolar pulmonary edema, and less often, cloudlike appearance with concentration of fluid around the hilum, giving butterfly or batwing appearance. Serial chest x-rays are not recommended for routine follow-up.

4. *Electrocardiography (ECG)* reveals atrial fibrillation in approximately 20% to 30% patients with HF. ECG may also show evidence of old infarction, left ventricular hypertrophy, left atrial enlargement, arrhythmias other than atrial fibrillation, low voltage, or bundle branch block.

5. *Echocardiography* is the single most effective diagnostic test in the evaluation of patients with HF. It is one of the fastest growing procedures in cardiology. In systolic HF, the ejection fraction is less than 40%, whereas in diastolic HF, the ejection fraction could be deceivingly normal. High LVEDP suggests diastolic HF. This also provides information about associated pericardial, myocardial, or valvular disease. Reassessment of HF is only needed in patients who had a change in clinical status or received treatment that might have had a significant effect on heart function.

6. Magnetic resonance imaging, radionuclide ventriculography, or endomyocardial biopsy is used for diagnosis or finding the cause of HF less often in clinical practice. Because of frequent comorbid lung disease, *pulmonary function* testing should be considered in older patients before dyspnea is attributable to HF.

References

1. Ho KK, Pinsky JL, Kannel WB. The epidemiology of HF: the Framingham Study. *J Am Coll Cardiol* 1993;22:6A–13A.
2. Nohria A, Lewis E, Stevenson LW. Medical management of advanced HF. *JAMA* 2002;287:628–640.
3. AHA. Heart & stroke statistical update. *Economic case of cardiovascular disease*. Dallas TX: AHA, 2001.
4. Cleland JG, Khand A, Clark A. The HF epidemic: exactly how big is it? *Eur Heart J* 2001;22:623–626.

HEART MURMURS, DIASTOLIC
Jelyn W. Lu

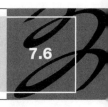

7.6

I. **BACKGROUND.** A diastolic heart murmur occurs during heart muscle relaxation starting with or after S_2 and ending before or after S_1 ($*S_2/\sim$murmur$\sim/S_1*$). Diastolic murmurs are typically due to the stenosis of the mitral or tricuspid valves, or the regurgitation of the aortic or pulmonary valves. The diastolic murmur should more often than not be considered pathological or associated with structural cardiac abnormalities and therefore, warrants further evaluation. These murmurs can be classified into four categories:

A. **Early diastolic murmur,** which starts with S_2 and peaks in the first third of diastole

B. **Mid-diastolic murmur,** which starts after S_2 and ends prior to S_1

C. **Late diastolic murmur,** which starts in the concluding part of diastole during atrial contraction and persists to S_1

D. **Continuous murmur,** which extends from systole into diastole. Such a murmur results from blood flow continuing from a high-pressure to a lower-pressure area (1).

II. **PATHOPHYSIOLOGY/EVALUATION/DIAGNOSIS**

A. **Early diastolic murmur**

1. **Aortic regurgitation (AR)**

a. **Pathophysiology.** Insufficient closing of the aortic valve leaflets, which can be caused by alteration or dilatation of the aortic root and ascending aorta. AR causes greater resultant end-diastolic left ventricular volume, resulting in a residual left ventricular dilatation and hypertrophy. Eventually, peripheral signs include the gradient between systolic and diastolic pressure increases (widened arterial pulse pressure), observable carotid pulse, suprasternal pulsations, rapid rise and fall of pulse ("water-hammer" pulse), flushing pulsations of nail beds (Quincke's pulse), "to-and-fro" murmur from slight stethoscope compression on the femoral artery (Duroziez's murmur), head bob with each pulse (de Musset's sign), and rapid ejection of large stroke volume ("pistol-shot" femoral artery sound) (2,3).

b. **Epidemiology.** More common in men than women; more common in adults older than 60 years, if associated with Marfan's syndrome, Ehlers-Danlos syndrome, autosomal recessive or X-linked inheritance, collagen-vascular diseases, there may be familial predisposition (3).

c. **Causes (2–4).** Rheumatic heart disease, congenital heart disease (bicuspid aortic valve, prolapsed aortic cusp with ventricular septal defect), collagen-vascular diseases (systemic lupus erythematosus), connective-tissue disease (Marfan's syndrome, Turner's syndrome, pseudoxanthoma elasticum, ankylosing spondylitis, Ehlers-Danlos syndrome, polymyalgia rheumatica), ascending aortic aneurysm, aortitis (syphilis, Takayasu's arteritis, granulomatous aortitis), cystic medial necrosis, Reiter's syndrome, myxomatous aortic valve, calcific changes in aortic valve, anorectic drugs or patients treated with dexfenfluramine or phentermine/fenfluramine, infective endocarditis, aortic dissection, trauma, hypertension, end-stage renal disease (transient murmur from fluid overload)

d. **History.** Is there a history of rheumatic fever (RF)? Check for recurrent strep throat, shortness of breath at rest (signs of cardiac decompensation), chest pressure during physical activity, palpitations (symptomatic arrhythmias), lower extremity swelling, trauma (risk of aortic dissection), intravenous drug use, recent dental work (risk of endocarditis), use of fenfluramine/dexfenfluramine (Fen-Phen) or other weight loss drugs, history of lens dislocation/long slender limbs (presence of Marfan's syndrome), sexually transmitted diseases (risk of syphilis), and lax joints (Ehlers-Danlos syndrome) (3).

e. **Diagnosis.** Decrescendo, "blowing" character, low intensity, high-pitched diastolic murmur at the left sternal border or over the right second intercostal space while the patient is sitting and leaning forward with breath held in deep expiration, radiating to the cardiac apex, increases with handgrip or squatting; can even present with a musical quality "diastolic whoop." A diastolic rumble at the ventricular apex is known as the *Austin Flint murmur* (1).

f. **Presentation.** Heart failure symptoms, exertional dyspnea, fatigue, paroxysmal nocturnal dyspnea, pulmonary edema, angina pectoris, atypical chest pain, elevated systolic and decreased diastolic blood pressure (3)

2. **Pulmonary regurgitation (PR)**

   a. **Pathophysiology.** Insufficient closure of the pulmonary valve leaflets

   b. **Causes.** Usually secondary to pulmonary hypertension. However, pulmonary regurgitation (PR) can also be caused by the idiopathic dilatation of the pulmonary artery, status postsurgery or post–balloon valvuloplasty, right-sided endocarditis, or congenital absence of the pulmonary valve.

   c. **Diagnosis.** Decrescendo, "blowing" character, high-pitched diastolic (Graham Steell) heard best over the left sternal border and left second and third intercostal space (vs. AR, which is heard in the right intercostals). The PR murmur increases with inspiration.

   d. **Presentation.** Right ventricular volume and pressure overload; a significant right ventricular heave, elevated jugular venous pressure (1, 3)

3. **Left anterior descending artery stenosis.** "Dock's murmur" is similar to that of AR and is caused by turbulent flow across the stenotic coronary arteries. Auscultate for murmur at the left second or third intercostal space and the left sternal border (1).

4. **S₃ gallop/ventricular gallop.** This can be heard as an early diastolic gallop. In children it is usually normal; however, in adults it is typically a sign of heart failure.

B. **Mid-diastolic murmur**

   1. **Mitral stenosis (MS)**

      a. **Pathophysiology.** Fibrosis and lack of mobility of the mitral valve leaflets, which causes an impediment in flow from the left atrium to the left ventricle, resulting in increased pressure in the left atrium, pulmonary vasculature, and right side of the heart

      b. **Epidemiology.** Predominately women

      c. **Causes.** RF, congenital disease, malignant carcinoid, methysergide therapy, systemic lupus erythematosus, rheumatoid arthritis

      d. **History.** Is there a history of RF (most common cause), breathlessness with exertion (most common symptom), palpitations (atrial fibrillation associated with mitral stenosis [MS]), travel history (RF is common in developing countries), and/or migraine medications (methysergide)?

      e. **Diagnosis.** Loud opening snap followed by a low-pitched diastolic rumble heard best at the apex while patient lying on left side; murmur increased with expiration

      f. **Presentation.** "Mitral facies" (vasoconstriction with resultant pinkish-purple patches on cheeks), heart failure symptoms (exertional dyspnea, edema), atrial fibrillation, chest pain, hoarseness from left atrial enlargement and compression of recurrent laryngeal nerve, fatigue (4).

   2. **Tricuspid stenosis**

      a. **Pathophysiology.** Fibrosis and lack of mobility of the tricuspid valve leaflets with resultant elevation of pressure in the right atrium and jugular veins; more common in mid-diastole when in atrial fibrillation (in normal sinus rhythm, murmur is late diastolic)

      b. **Causes.** Usually in association with MS, RF, carcinoid heart disease, right atrial myxoma (1)

      c. **Diagnosis.** Begins with a tricuspid opening snap and associated with a mid-diastolic rumble best auscultated at the left sternal border; murmur increases with inspiration (Carvallo's sign)

      d. Presentation. Can present with atrial fibrillation, right-sided heart failure, hepatomegaly, ascites, dependent edema.

   3. Atrial myxoma. This is the most common primary heart tumor consisting of a benign gelatinous growth. The growths can cause an obstruction of the mitral and tricuspid valves presenting with chest pain, dyspnea, edema, and syncope. Left atrial myxoma murmur is similar to that of MS (as right atrial myxoma is similar to tricuspid stenosis). Atrial myxoma murmurs can change with alterations of position and also present with the "tumor plop."

   4. Increased flow across the atrioventricular valve. This is otherwise known as a *flow murmur* (1).

  C. Late diastolic murmur

   1. Mitral stenosis. This murmur becomes a late diastolic murmur when atrial contraction increases the pressure and flow at the end of the diastole.

   2. Tricuspid stenosis. This late diastolic murmur occurs during sinus rhythm.

   3. Atrial myxoma. This murmur can also present in late diastole as well as mid-diastole.

   4. Left-to-right shunt

   5. Complete heart block. This is a short late murmur called *Rytand's murmur*.

   6. S_4/atrial gallop. This occurs from the resistance of atrial filling after an atrial contraction. It presents as a late diastolic atrial gallop that may be associated with myocardial disease, coronary artery disease, or hypertension, and increases sound with deep inspiration (1).

  D. Continuous murmur. This murmur begins in systole, peaks near S_2, and continues into all or part of the diastole.

   1. Patent ductus arteriosus. This continuous machinelike murmur is auscultated best at the left middle and left upper sternal border and second intercostal space with radiation to the back.

   2. Other causes of continuous murmurs. These include aortopulmonary window, shunts (through an atrial septal defect), arteriovenous fistulas, constriction of systemic/pulmonary arteries, coarctation of the aorta, "mammary soufflé" in pregnancy, venous hum, and pericardial friction rub (1).

III. LABORATORY TESTS

  A. The test of choice is echocardiography—transthoracic or transesophageal (better to test for endocarditis and evaluate vegetations).

  B. Other possible diagnostic tools include electrocardiogram, chest x-ray, cardiac catheterization, blood cultures, complete blood count with differential and erythrocyte sedimentation rate in suspected cases of endocarditis, radionuclide angiography when echocardiography is nonconclusive, aortogram for evaluation of aorta; chest computed tomography (to diagnose dissection), aortic magnetic resonance imaging (to diagnose dissection), exercise testing, tissue testing/DNA testing for genetic abnormalities, and serologic tests for collagen-vascular disease and syphilis (2, 4, 5).

References

1. Chatterjee Kanu. *Auscultation of cardiac murmurs. Up To Date*: online 13.2 (www. uptodate.com); updated on April 2005.
2. Cheitlin MD. Surgery for chronic aortic regurgitation: when should it be considered? *Am Fam Physician* 2001;64:1709–1714.
3. Scherger JE, O'Hanlon KM, Jones RC, et al. *Aortic regurgitation. FIRSTConsult* (http://www.firstconsult.com.cuhsl.creighton.edu/?type=med&id=01014202) Updated on Wednesday, June 25, 2005.
4. Cunningham R, Corretti M, Henrich W. *Valvular heart disease in patients with end-stage renal disease. Up to Date*: online 13.2. (www.uptodate.com); updated on April 2005.
5. Ferri FF, Saver DF, Hodgson JM, et al. *Mitral stenosis. FIRSTConsult* (http://www. firstconsult.com.cuhsl.creighton.edu/?type=med&id=01014231) Updated on Friday, May 27, 2005.

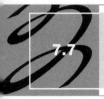

HEART MURMURS, SYSTOLIC
Carlos A. Prendes, Jr.

Systolic murmurs are a common finding during the physical examination. William James' advice is certainly applicable: "The art of being wise is the art of knowing what to overlook." The reality of today's healthcare system dictates judicious use of resources, so familiarity with commonly encountered systolic murmurs and an evaluation protocol aid in efficient, cost-effective use of medical imaging technology.

I. BACKGROUND. A heart murmur can be defined as turbulent flow through a valve or vessel. Murmurs arise with abnormal blood flow patterns. Several conditions may give rise to audible murmurs: fast flow through a normal valve (such as anemia or tachycardia), abnormal narrowing of a valve (aortic stenosis), flow into a dilated vessel (dilated aortic root), incompetent valves allowing backward flow (regurgitation [e.g., mitral regurgitation]), and persistent or acquired abnormal communications between heart chambers or arteries (ventricular septal defect) (1).

II. PATHOPHYSIOLOGY. Systolic murmurs are generally less likely to be significant than diastolic murmurs, however, they are also much more frequently encountered. Murmurs with certain characteristics may be safely documented and monitored, and others warrant urgent workup, as well as everything in between. Knowledge of common physical findings and their associated pathology aid in the prudent and efficient evaluation of new murmurs. Diastolic murmurs are never considered innocent and should always warrant investigation; they are addressed elsewhere in this volume (1,2).

III. EVALUATION

  A. History. A thorough and complete history is paramount when evaluating a previously unheard murmur.

    1. It is important to note any previous history of valvular disease, or congenital heart disease. A social history of intravenous drug use and tobacco abuse, and other high-risk behaviors should be documented. Past medical history of anemia, thyroid disorders, and pregnancy are notably associated with flow murmurs.

    2. Review of systems should include any complaints of dyspnea, dyspnea on exertion, diaphoresis, chest pain, palpitations, edema, exacerbating and relieving factors, as well as a timeline of symptoms and any progression. Other systemic complaints to address include weight loss, fevers and/or chills, new rashes, and easy fatigability.

    3. It is reasonable to *observe* murmurs that are not associated with subjective complaint or other physical findings such as a thrill. Generally they are midsystolic and have several possible etiologies; including, vibration of the pulmonary leaflets, pulmonic leaflets, or systemic arteries. Older patients may also have vibrations of the aortic cusps. Changes in the murmurs over time may warrant further workup, especially if associated with worsening of your patient's condition (2).

  B. Physical examination. Medical educators report their belief that teaching cardiac auscultation is of great importance; however, a nationwide survey presented in 1991 revealed less than half of internal medicine and cardiology programs offered any structured teaching of auscultation (3). Accuracy of the cardiac examination improves with structured teaching and repetition (4,5).

    1. Always begin with the vital signs and observing your patient for signs of distress.

    2. The cardiac examination involves auscultation at the five cardiac listening points, palpation of carotid and peripheral pulses, and description of the heart sounds. Murmurs are described by their location, loudness, and timing. It should also

TABLE 7.7.1	**Physical Examination Findings of Systolic Heart Murmurs**		
Systolic murmur	**Description**	**Maneuvers**	**Location heard**
Aortic stenosis	Midsystolic crescendo-decrescendo	Transmits to carotids, thrill with expiration	Right sternal border, second rib space
Tricuspid regurgitation	Pansystolic, plateau	Increases with inspiration	Lower left sternal border, heard below zyphoid process
Mitral regurgitation	Most common, holosystolic	Squatting may increase	Apex, radiates to axilla
Mitral valve prolapse	Late systolic, may hear click	Stand and inhale amyl nitrate	Apex, use diaphragm
Pulmonic stenosis	Midsystolic, diamond-shaped	Increases with inspiration, transmits to suprasternal notch	Left sternal border, second to third rib space
Ventral septal defect	Harsh holosystolic	Radiates to right sternal border	Apex to right sternal border
Hypertrophic cardiomyopathy	Harsh midsystolic, ejection murmur	Decreases with handgrip and squatting	Aortic area to Apex, does not radiate beyond heart

be noted if the murmur changes with inspiration/exhalation. A review of the listening posts and their associated murmurs is found in Table 7.7.1.

3. Murmurs should be graded according to volume and the absence or presence of a palpable thrill (1).

 a. **Grade I.** Faint and difficult to hear, which is easily missed and requires special effort to hear

 b. **Grade II.** Soft murmur more easily heard, especially with experience

 c. **Grade III.** A fairly loud murmur that is not associated with a thrill

 d. **Grade IV.** A loud murmur which is associated with a thrill

 e. **Grade V.** A louder murmur with a thrill, but a stethoscope is still required to hear it

 f. **Grade VI.** A murmur with a thrill that is so loud it can be heard before the stethoscope touches the chest.

C. **Testing.** Grade III/VI and higher murmurs, as well as murmurs associated with symptoms of cardiac disease should be referred for echocardiogram (2).

 1. Electrocardiography (ECG) is readily available and inexpensive. It provides useful information about the presence of ventricular hypertrophy, myocardial ischemia, prior infarct, and arrhythmias (2).

 2. Posteroanterior and lateral x-rays of the chest yield useful information about ventricular size, pulmonary congestion, and calcifications of the vasculature. They also may show findings consistent with congestive heart failure (CHF), chronic obstructive pulmonary disease, and/or pneumonia (2).

 3. Useful laboratory tests may include: complete blood count (anemia, infection, red blood cell destruction), thyroid-stimulating hormone (hypothyroidism/hyperthyroidism), blood culture (endocarditis), troponin I creatine kinase (CK)/CK-MB (markers of myocardial damage), and CHF peptide.

4. Transthoracic echocardiography is noninvasive, available, and yields important information by imaging cardiac structures and measuring flow rate and direction through cardiac valves.

5. Transesophageal echocardiography and cardiac catheterization are also available if the diagnosis is still uncertain after reviewing the transthoracic echocardiogram. These are invasive and expensive studies and not appropriate for initial workup of systolic heart murmurs without compelling evidence such as evidence of acute coronary syndrome.

IV. DIAGNOSIS

A. Systolic murmurs are commonly encountered during routine examination. Always maintain a high index of suspicion when auscultating cardiac sounds. Diligent attention to the patient's history and thorough physical examination often yields the information necessary for an accurate diagnosis, even before additional studies are obtained. If any doubt remains about what should be done next, remember Dr. Osler's advice "*Care more particularly for the individual patient than for the special features of the disease.*"

B. Several websites have been developed that may be useful for learning to recognize specific murmurs. Some include the following:

1. The Auscultation Assistant. http://www.wilkes.med.ucla.edu/inex.htm
2. Cardiac Auscultation. http://egeneralmedical.com/egeneralmedical/listohearmur.html
3. Virtual Stethoscope. http://sprojects.mmi.mcgill.ca/mvs/mvsteth.htm.

References

1. Greenberger N, Hinthorn D. *History taking and physical examination.* St. Louis, MO: Mosby—Year Book, 1993.
2. Kasper D, Braunwald E, Wilson JD, eds. *Harrison's principals of internal medicine.* New York, NY: McGraw-Hill, 2005.
3. Bonow RO, Carabello B, de Leon AC Jr, et al. ACC/AHA guidelines for the management of patients with valvular heart disease: a report of the American College of Cardiology/American Heart Association Task Force on Practice Guidelines (Committee on Management of Patients With Valvular Heart Disease). *J Am Coll Cardiol* 1998;32:1486–1588.
4. Mangione S, Nieman LZ, Gracely E, et al. The teaching and practice of cardiac auscultation during internal medicine and cardiology training. *Ann Intern Med* 1993;119:47–54.
5. Favrat B, Pecoud A, Jaussi A. Teaching cardiac auscultation to trainees in internal medicine and family practice: does it work? *BMC Med Educ* 2004;4:5.

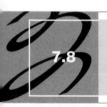

7.8

HYPERTENSION
Raymond D. Heller

Hypertension (HTN) is a leading cause of morbidity and mortality in the United States. Estimates suggest that of all individuals with HTN, 34% are receiving adequate therapy, 25% are receiving inadequate therapy, 11% are receiving no therapy, and 30% of individuals with HTN do not know they have the condition (1).

I. BACKGROUND. According to *The Seventh Report of the Joint National Committee on Prevention, Detection, Evaluation, and Treatment of High Blood Pressure*, the classification of blood pressure in adults age 18 years and older is as follows (see Table 7.8.1):

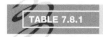

TABLE 7.8.1	Classification of Blood Pressure in US Adults 18 Years of Age and Older	
Blood pressure classification	Systolic blood pressure (mm Hg)	Diastolic blood pressure (mm Hg)
Normal	<120	<80
Prehypertension	120–139	80–89
Stage 1 HTN	140–159	90–99
Stage 2 HTN	≥160	≥100

HTN, hypertension.
Department of Health and Human Service, National Institutes of Health, *The seventh report of the Joint National Committee on prevention, detection, evaluation, and treatment of high blood pressure*. www.nhlbi.nih.gov/guidelines/hypertension

A. A systolic blood pressure of 120 mm Hg or less is considered normal.

B. A new classification, "prehypertension" is a systolic blood pressure of 120 to 139 mm Hg and/or a diastolic blood pressure of 80 to 89 mm Hg. Prehypertension is not a disease category and individuals who fall into this category *are not* candidates for drug therapy. Patients who fall into this category are identified as being considered at high risk of HTN and should be counseled regarding lifestyle modification to reduce their risk of developing HTN in the future.

C. Stage 1 HTN is defined as a systolic blood pressure of 140 to 159 mm Hg and/or a diastolic blood pressure of 90 to 99 mm Hg.

D. Stage 2 HTN is defined as a systolic blood pressure of 160 mm Hg or greater based on the average of 2 or more readings taken at each of 2 or more visits after initial screening (2).

II. PATHOPHYSIOLOGY

A. Etiology. The cause of 90% to 95% of the cases of HTN is not known (1). Patients with no identifiable cause of HTN are said to have primary or essential HTN. Patients with a specific structural organ or gene defect responsible for their HTN are classified as having secondary HTN (3).

B. Epidemiology. Approximately one in three adults in the United States have HTN, and approximately 28% or 59 million of American adults 18 years of age and older have "prehypertension" (1). Approximately 50% of individuals who suffer a first myocardial infarction and two-thirds who undergo a first stroke have a blood pressure higher than 160/95 mm Hg. Compared to normotensive individuals, the relative risk for a stroke is four times greater for individuals with a systolic blood pressure of 160 mm Hg or higher and/or a diastolic blood pressure of 95 mm Hg or higher. Individuals at the lower educational and income levels tend to have higher levels of blood pressure.

III. EVALUATION

A. History. After the documentation of HTN is established, a detailed history should reveal information about target end organ damage, the patient's cardiovascular risk status, and secondary causes of HTN. Questions to assess the extent of target organ damage should include any history of acute episodic or progressive visual change, or occipital headaches upon arising in the morning that fade in several hours. Review any symptoms consistent with angina pectoris, ischemic heart disease, peripheral vascular disease, congestive heart failure, cerebral vascular disease, retinopathy, and nephropathy (3). Symptoms suggestive of a secondary cause of HTN need to be explored. The patients' age and gender should also be considered. A higher percentage of men than women have HTN until 55 years of age. After 55 years of age, a much higher percentage of women have HTN than men (2). Other important medical history includes previous documentation of HTN by a health care provider. Part of the health history must address comorbid health conditions such as diabetes mellitus, dyslipidemia, obesity, and family history.

1. **Medication history.** It is important to review current or past antihypertensive medication use. Patients stop antihypertensive therapy for various reasons, including stated reasons such as they were "feeling better" or they "could not afford the medication." It is also necessary to review the herbal and over-the-counter (OTC) therapies the patient currently uses or previously used. Many OTC cough and cold remedies and weight loss pills contain products that can potentially elevate blood pressure. Unfortunately, some OTC herbal therapies may interact with prescription medications, altering the metabolism, serum level, effectiveness, and side effects of many prescription medications, and potentially complicating treatment. Potencies of herbal medications can vary dramatically between manufacturers. Therefore, health care practitioners should have ready access to a guide for herbal medicines that describes their origin, uses, side effects, metabolism, excretion, toxicities, and known potential prescription drug interactions. In addition, many prescription medications may elevate blood pressure.

2. **Social history.** Factors to review include tobacco, caffeine, alcohol, and illicit drug use. A dietary history may illuminate approximate quantities of saturated fats and sodium intake. Time spent in exercise and type of leisure activities should be determined.

B. **Physical examination**
1. **Blood pressure measurement.** Errors can be minimized by choosing the proper size blood pressure cuff and utilizing a standardized technique. Guidelines for a proper size blood pressure cuff are listed in Table 7.8.2. Patient preparation guidelines to minimize erroneous blood pressure readings are listed in Table 7.8.3. To determine a proper cuff inflation pressure, palpate the radial pulse while inflating the cuff bladder. When the radial pulse is no longer palpable, note this pressure on the manometer and add 30 mm Hg to it. Deflate the cuff and wait approximately 30 seconds before attempting cuff reinflation. Place the stethoscope bell lightly over the brachial artery, inflate the cuff rapidly to the above determined pressure. Deflate it at a rate of about 2 to 3 mm Hg per second. Note the pressure level when at least two consecutive beats are first heard. This level is the systolic pressure. Continue lowering the cuff pressure until the sounds become muffled and disappear, again note the pressure on the manometer. Confirm sound disappearance by listening as the pressure falls an additional 20 mm Hg. If no further sounds occur, deflate the cuff rapidly to zero. The disappearance point represents the diastolic blood pressure. Measure the blood pressure in each arm (4).

2. **Other important features.** The physical examination should include the eye examination looking for retinal changes consistent with HTN. Palpate the thyroid to evaluate for masses, enlargement, or asymmetry. The cardiovascular examination should include palpation and auscultation of the carotid and femoral pulses, noting symmetry of pulse strength or bruits. Palpate distal

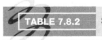

TABLE 7.8.2	**Selecting the Correct Blood Pressure Cuff**

- Width of the inflatable bladder of the cuff should be approximately 40% of the upper arm circumference (approximately 12–14 cm in the average adult)
- Length of inflatable bladder should be approximately 80% of upper arm circumference (almost long enough to encircle the arm)
- If aneroid, recalibrate periodically before use.

Bickley LS, Szilagyi PG. Beginning the physical examination: general survey and vital signs. In: *Guide to physical examination and history taking*, 8th ed. Philadelphia, PA: Lippincott Williams & Wilkins, 2003:75–78.

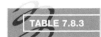

TABLE 7.8.3   **Preparing to Measure Blood Pressure**

- Ideally, ask the patient to avoid smoking or drinking caffeinated beverages for 30 min before the blood pressure is taken and to rest for at least 5 min.
- Check to make sure the examining room is quiet, warm, and comfortable.
- Make sure the arm selected is *free of clothing*. There should be no arteriovenous fistulas for dialysis, scarring from prior brachial artery cutdowns, or signs of lymphedema (seen after axillary node dissection or radiation therapy).
- Palpate the brachial artery to confirm that it has a viable pulse.
- Position the arm so that the brachial artery, at the antecubital crease is *at heart level* — roughly level with the fourth interspace at its junction with the sternum.
- If the patient is seated, rest the arm on a table a little above the patient's waist; if standing, try to support the patient's arm at the midchest level.

Bickley LS, Szilagyi PG. Beginning the physical examination: general survey and vital signs. In: *Guide to physical examination and history taking*, 8th ed. Philadelphia, PA: Lippincott Williams & Wilkins, 2003:75–78.

extremity pulses and perform a complete cardiac examination, noting any cardiac heave, murmurs, gallops, rubs, jugular venous distension, and intensity of S_1 and S_2 heart sounds. Abdominal examination should evaluate for bruits, pulsatile and nonpulsatile masses, or renal enlargement. A complete pulmonary examination should be performed. Examination of extremities should note edema, and changes consistent with peripheral vascular disease. A thorough neurologic and skin examination should be performed.

C. Testing

1. Basic laboratory tests, when evaluating a patient with HTN, include uric acid, urinalysis including screening for microalbuminuria, complete blood count, serum creatinine, potassium, calcium, and blood urea nitrogen. A fasting serum glucose and a complete lipoprotein profile should be obtained. The lipoprotein profile should include a total cholesterol, triglyceride, low-density lipoprotein cholesterol, and high-density lipoprotein cholesterol. The estimated glomerular filtration rate (GFR) or creatinine clearance should be calculated using available formulas (see Table 7.8.4). If a secondary cause of HTN is suspected, the appropriate specific laboratory workup should be included.

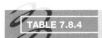

TABLE 7.8.4   **Equations for Estimation of GFR from Plasma Creatinine Concentration (P_{cr})**

1. Equation from the Modification of Diet in Renal Disease Study[a]
   Estimated GFR (mL/min/1.73 m^2) = $1.86 \times (P_{cr})^{-1.154} \times (age)^{-0.203}$
   Multiply by 0.742 for women
   Multiply by 1.21 for African-Americans
2. Cockcroft-Gault equation
   Estimated creatinine clearance (mL/min) = $\dfrac{(140 - Age) \times body\ weight\ (kg)}{72 \times (P_{cr})(mg/dL)}$
   Multiply by 0.85 for women

[a]Kasper DL, Braunwald E, Fauci AS, et al. *Harrison's principles of internal medicine*, 16th ed. Part 8; Chapter 230. McGraw-Hill Companies, 2005.

    2. An electrocardiogram may assist with recognizing a previously damaged myocardium, rhythm disturbances, or changes consistent with left ventricular hypertrophy (LVH).

    3. Imaging studies may be useful. A chest x-ray may be useful when attempting to evaluate the patient for cardiomegaly, but a limited echocardiogram will give more detailed information about cardiac function and LVH.

  D. Genetics. To date, genetic studies have not identified any single gene or combination of genes that appreciably accounts for HTN in the general population.

III. DIAGNOSIS

A. Differential diagnosis

    1. Essential HTN

    2. Secondary HTN

      a. Renovascular HTN

        i. Stenosis of main renal arteries and/or major branches is responsible for 2% to 5% of patients with HTN.

        ii. Initial workup involves Doppler ultrasonography with measurement of the intrarenal resistance index.

        iii. This diagnosis includes the subgroups preeclampsia and eclampsia.

      b. Renal parenchymal HTN. Diseases that injure renal parenchymal tissue result in inflammatory and fibrotic changes of small intrarenal vessels, thereby causing decreased profusion and resultant HTN.

      c. Primary aldosteronism. A tumor or bilateral adrenal hyperplasia should be sought.

      d. Cushing's syndrome

        i. Truncal obesity, fatigability, purplish abdominal striae, amenorrhea, Hirsutism, edema, glucosuria, moon facies, and buffalo hump

        ii. Most common in third or fourth decade of life

        iii. Failure to suppress cortisol level with dexamethasone challenge

      e. Pheochromocytoma

        i. Most common in young to mid adult life

        ii. Headaches, palpitations, excessive sweating, impaired glucose tolerance, hypercalcemia, weight loss, and anxiety

        iii. Twenty-four hour urine collection assayed for vanillylmandelic acid, metanephrine, and "free" catecholamines

      f. Coarctation of the aorta

        i. Cardiac murmur, possibly heard in the back, over spinous processes, and lateral thorax

        ii. Decreased, delayed, or absent femoral pulses

        iii. Chest x-ray reveals "the three sign" at coarctation sight and notched ribs

      g. Hyperparathyroidism

        i. Hypercalcemia

        ii. Renal parenchymal damage due to nephrocalcinosis and renal stones

    3. Oral contraceptive medications

    4. Malignant HTN (3)

      a. Diastolic blood pressure usually greater than 130 mm H

      b. Papilledema, retinal hemorrhages, and exudates

      c. Possibly vomiting, severe headache, transient visual changes or loss, stupor, coma, oliguria, and cardiac decompensation

B. Clinical manifestations. Individuals may have high blood pressure for years and not know it. Sometimes HTN may have subtle symptoms such as epistaxis, hematuria, and episodic weakness, dizziness, palpitations, easy fatigability, and impotence. If HTN is part of a disease process, such as secondary HTN, it may be joined by other symptoms of the influencing disease process.

References

1. American Heart Association Inc. www.americanheart.org, accessed on 11 April, 2006.
2. Department of Health and Human Service, National Institutes of Health, The Seventh Report of the Joint National Committee on Prevention, Detection, Evaluation, and

Treatment of High Blood Pressure. www.nhlbi.nih.gov/guidelines/hypertension, accessed on 11 April, 2006.
3. Kasper DL, Braunwald E, Fauci AS, et al. *Harrison's principles of internal medicine*, 16th ed. Part 8; Chapter 230. New York, NY: McGraw-Hill Companies, 2005.
4. Bickley LS, Szilagyi PG. Beginning the physical examination: general survey and vital signs. In: *Guide to physical examination and history taking*, 8th ed. Philadelphia, PA: Lippincott Williams & Wilkins, 2003:75–78.

PALPITATIONS
John Winters

7.9

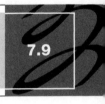

I. BACKGROUND. Palpitations are an unpleasant abnormal awareness of the heartbeat. They are usually described as a pounding or racing of the heart.

II. PATHOPHYSIOLOGY

A. Etiology. Palpitations are a common presenting complaint encountered by the primary care physicians and cardiologists. The list of underlying causes of palpitations is extensive (see Table 7.9.1).

B. Epidemiology. One prospective cohort study of 190 patients showed that 43% had palpitations due to cardiac causes, 31% due to anxiety or panic disorder, and

TABLE 7.9.1	Some Causes of Palpitations
Cardiac	**Medications**
Arrhythmias	Alcohol
Atrial fibrillation/Atrial flutter	Anticholinergics
Multifocal atrial tachycardia	Caffeine
Premature ventricular contractions	Illicit drugs
Sick sinus syndrome	Nicotine
Sinus node dysfunction	Sympathomimetics
Sinus tachycardia	**Endocrine/metabolic**
Supraventricular tachycardia	Hyperthyroidism
Ventricular tachycardia	Hypoglycemia
Wolf-Parkinson-White syndrome	Pheochromocytoma
Other cardiac causes	**Psychiatric**
Cardiac shunts	Anxiety disorder
Cardiomyopathy	Panic attacks
Pacemaker	Somatization disorder
Valvular heart disease	**Others**
	Anemia
	Fever
	Strenuous physical activity

l6% due to an undetermined etiology (1). Remembering that the heart is electrically paced, a good mnemonic to assist in recalling causes of palpitations is E-PACED (**E**lectrolytes, **P**sychiatric, **A**nemia, **C**ardiac, **E**ndocrine and **D**rugs) (2).

III. EVALUATION. Because patients rarely experience an episode while in the physician's office, the history and physical examination are the most crucial elements of the investigation. Moreover, only occasionally does physical examination provide clues or supporting evidence to affirm a diagnosis, thereby making a thorough and descriptive history assume even greater importance.

A. History. The history should focus on information such as the circumstances during occurrence, intermittency, duration, precipitating and resolving factors, a detailed description of the palpitations, and associated signs and symptoms.

1. The circumstances during which palpitations occur may indicate an association with anxiety or panic attacks, although one should also keep in mind excess catecholamine during times of stress. Validated screening tools are readily available to assist in identifying patients with such psychiatric illness (3). Occurrence at night while lying down could result from atrial or ventricular premature contractions. Positional changes might indicate atrioventricular nodal tachycardia.

2. Isolated or skipped beats could be premature contractions or benign ectopy.

3. Palpitations precipitated by exercise may be associated with supraventricular arrhythmias or atrial fibrillation. Palpitations terminated by vagal maneuvers point to paroxysmal supraventricular tachycardia.

4. Palpitations described as rapid and regular may indicate paroxysmal supraventricular tachycardia and ventricular tachycardias. Palpitations described as rapid and irregular could imply atrial fibrillation, multifocal atrial tachycardia, and atrial flutter with variable block. Flip-flopping or stopping–starting sensations may be caused by supraventricular or ventricular premature contractions. Palpitations may be sensed as a pounding in the neck. Notably, atrioventricular nodal reentrant tachycardia is associated with a rapid regular pounding in the neck, whereas such a sensation that is less regular and more intermittent may be premature ventricular contractions.

5. The physician should keep in mind that dizziness, presyncope, or syncope accompanying palpitations are factors that help identify patients at risk for fatal results. These symptoms should prompt an investigation for ventricular tachycardias.

6. Age at onset in childhood may suggest supraventricular tachycardia. Symptoms of hyperthyroidism such as heat intolerance should be elicited. Illicit drugs, caffeine, and nicotine habits as well as anemia and metabolic disorders are all important possible associations that should be considered.

B. Physical examination. The findings of the physical examination may give clues such as a heart murmur, indicating the possibility of valvular disease or cardiomyopathies or the midsystolic click of mitral valve prolapse. A brisk walk down a corridor might reveal a poorly controlled ventricular response and resultant palpitations in a patient with atrial fibrillation and palpitations (1). It is necessary to search for signs of congestive heart failure.

C. Testing. Twelve-lead electrocardiography (ECG) is indicated and should be analyzed for short PR interval and delta waves (ventricular pre-excitation), Q waves indicating left ventricular hypertrophy or prior infarction, premature contractions, long QT intervals, heart blocks, or any other abnormality. Laboratory testing can usually be limited to investigation of anemia, thyroid function, and electrolyte disturbances (potassium and magnesium). Ambulatory ECG can be used for further investigation. Holter monitoring should suffice for patients with daily symptoms; otherwise, a continuous-loop event recorder should provide a better diagnostic yield (4, 5).

IV. DIAGNOSIS. The list of causes of palpitations is extensive (Table 7.9.1). In most cases, the cause is benign. Life-threatening causes are suggested by associated symptoms such as dizziness or syncope. The history is the most important diagnostic tool, and a thorough and descriptive inquiry should he made. The physical examination may provide further clues or supporting evidence. Testing involves 12-lead ECG and a limited laboratory investigation.

References
1. Abbott AV. Diagnostic approach to palpitations. *Am Fam Physician* 2005;71:743–750.
2. Weber BE, Kapoor WN. Evaluation and outcomes of patients with palpitations. *Am J Med* 1996;100:l38–148.
3. Taylor RB, ed. *The 10-minute diagnosis manual*, 1st ed. Philadelphia, PA: JB Lippincott, 1994.
4. Zimetbaum P, Josephson ME. Evaluation of patients with palpitations. *N Engl J Med* 1998;338:1369–1373.
5. Zimetbaum P, Josephson ME. The evolving role of ambulatory monitoring in general clinical practice. *Ann Intern Med* l999;130:848–856.

PERICARDIAL FRICTION RUB
Kamlesh G. Ansingkar

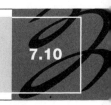

7.10

I. **BACKGROUND.** The pericardium consists of an outer fibrous layer called *parietal pericardium* and an inner serous layer called *visceral pericardium*. The visceral layer folds onto itself to form the parietal layer. In general, there is approximately 50 mL of ultrafiltrate of plasma between these two layers, which primarily drains into the right pleural space through the thoracic duct (1). Pericardial friction rub (caused by the deposition of fibrinous material between the two inflamed layers), associated with chest pain and serial electrocardiographic changes, is the most common finding in acute pericarditis (AP) (1,2).

II. **PATHOPHYSIOLOGY**

A. **Etiology of AP.** Disease may be idiopathic or caused by a bacterial (*Staphylococcus, Haemophilus, Pneumococcus, Salmonella*, tuberculosis, *Meningococcus*, syphilis), viral (coxsackievirus, echovirus, Epstein-Barr virus, influenza virus, human immunodeficiency virus, mumps), fungal (histoplasmosis, blastomycosis, coccidioidomycosis, aspergillosis), or parasitic (echinococcosis, amebiasis, *Rickettsia, Toxoplasma*) infection. Other causes include rheumatoid arthritis, systemic lupus erythematosus, scleroderma, rheumatic fever, sarcoidosis, pericarditis associated with other inflammatory conditions (Sjögren syndrome, mixed connective tissue disease, Reiter's syndrome, ankylosing spondylitis, inflammatory bowel disease, Wegener's granulomatosis, vasculitis such as giant cell arteritis and polyarteritis, polymyositis, Behçet's syndrome, Whipple's disease, familial Mediterranean fever, and serum sickness), renal failure with and without dialysis, hypothyroidism, cholesterol pericarditis, acute myocardial infarction (AMI), Dressler's syndrome, postpericardiotomy syndrome, neoplasms (primary from pericardial mesothelioma and angiosarcoma, and metastatic from breast, lung, lymphoma, melanoma, and leukemia), irradiation, drugs (penicillin, cromolyn sodium, doxorubicin, cyclophosphamide, procainamide, hydralazine, methyldopa, isoniazid, mesalazine, reserpine, methysergide, dantrolene, phenytoin, and minoxidil) and miscellaneous causes, including aortic dissection and penetrating and nonpenetrating cardiac trauma (1,2).

B. **Epidemiology of AP.** The prevalence of AP in hospitalized patients is estimated to be approximately 0.1% and is more common in males and adults than in females and in children, (1,3). Up to 15% of patients may experience recurrence of symptoms in the first few months (2). Before the era of reperfusion therapy, the incidence of infarction-associated pericarditis ranged from 7% to 25%, whereas in one study, after percutaneous transluminal coronary angioplasty (PTCA) in Q wave AMI, the pericardial rub was detected in 8% (4).

III. EVALUATION

A. History

1. Patients with AP usually present with chest pain that is typically a sharp precordial pain but may also present with a dull, aching, burning, or a pressing pain. It may be referred to the trapezius ridge (a symptom characteristic of AP) and is worse with inspiration, lying down, during swallowing, or with body motion and is relieved by sitting upright or leaning forward.

2. Associated symptoms may include dyspnea (especially with tamponade), fever, myalgia, and malaise (with viral or bacterial AP), weight loss (malignancy), and productive cough (with pneumonia and purulent pericarditis) or hemoptysis (tuberculosis). Other nonspecific symptoms include hiccups, cough, hoarseness, palpitations, nausea, and vomiting.

3. Past medical history may be suggestive of an associated illness that may cause AP, examples of which include history of recent pericardiotomy, renal failure with or without dialysis, collagen-vascular diseases, malignancy, or use of medications (1–3,5).

B. Physical examination.
Pericardial friction rub, which is like creaking leather or a scratching sound, is usually auscultated along the lower left sternal border. It is best heard with the diaphragm of a stethoscope in a quiet room. It is usually triphasic (atrial systole rub, ventricular systole rub, and early ventricular diastole rub) but may be biphasic or monophasic, and serial examinations may be necessary because it can be evanescent. Associated physical findings may include fever, tachycardia, and tachypnea. Hypotension, pulsus paradoxus, elevated systemic venous pressure, and muffled heart sounds may occur with cardiac tamponade (1,2).

C. Testing

1. **Laboratory tests.** A complete blood count may show leukocytosis, and erythrocyte sedimentation rate, C-reactive protein, and antistreptolysin titer may be elevated. Blood urea nitrogen and serum creatinine may be useful to evaluate uremia. Cardiac enzymes may be elevated if associated with myocarditis and AMI. Rheumatoid factor, antinuclear antibody test, and anti-DNA values may be helpful in evaluating autoimmune disorders and connective-tissue diseases. Tuberculin testing may aid in ruling out tuberculous pericarditis. Thyroid function tests may be helpful to rule out hypothyroidism. Antibody titers to various infectious agents can be tested as clinically indicated.

2. **Electrocardiogram (ECG).** ECG is most useful in diagnosing AP. ECG changes include diffuse upward ST elevation, except in aVR and V_1. Initially, T waves are upright in the leads with ST elevation, and the PR may be depressed in the epicardial leads. Several days later, the ST segment returns to baseline, and the T wave flattens and then gradually becomes inverted. Low-voltage QRS complexes indicate presence of a pericardial effusion.

3. **Imaging studies.** Chest radiography may show a flask-shaped enlarged heart in the presence of a large effusion. If clinical signs of pericardial tamponade or large effusion are present, then echocardiography is helpful for diagnostic and therapeutic pericardiocentesis (1,2).

IV. DIAGNOSIS.
Differential diagnosis includes aortic dissection, coronary artery vasospasm, esophageal rupture, esophagitis, esophageal spasm, acute gastritis, myocardial infarction, myocardial ischemia, and peptic ulcer disease. Each condition should be evaluated appropriately (1).

References

1. Philip J, Gentlesk PJ, McCabe J, et al. *Acute pericarditis*. March 2005. http://www.emedicine.com.cuhsl.creighton.edu/med/topic1781.htm, accessed on 1 July, 2005.
2. Marinella MA. Electrocardiographic manifestations and differential diagnosis of acute pericarditis. *Am Fam Physician* 1998;57:699–704.

3. Grimm RA, Hesse B. *Pericardial disease: acute pericarditis*, 2003. http://www.clevelandclinicmeded.com/diseasemanagement/cardiology/pericardial/pericardial.htm#table1, accessed on 1 July, 2005.
4. Sugiura T, Takehana K, Abe Y, et al. Frequency of pericardial friction rub ("pericarditis") after direct percutaneous transluminal coronary angioplasty in Q-wave acute myocardial infarction. *Am J Cardiol* 1997;79(3):362–364.
5. Ross AM, Grauer SE. Acute pericarditis. Evaluation and treatment of infectious and other causes. (Review). *Postgrad Med* 2004;115(3):67–70,73–75.

RAYNAUD'S DISEASE
Sandra B. Baumberger

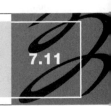

7.11

I. BACKGROUND. Raynaud's disease is a vasospastic disorder that causes episodic ischemia of the digits of the hands, lasting a variable amount of time. It was named after Maurice Raynaud, who first noted the disorder in 1862. Although the disorder mainly affects the hands, it can also affect the tongue, the nose, the nipples, or the toes. There are two classifications of Raynaud's disease: Primary Raynaud's disease (PRD), formerly known as Raynaud's phenomenon, is not associated with an underlying illness. Secondary Raynaud's disease (SRD), formerly known as Raynaud's syndrome, is often associated with an underlying illness (1).

II. PATHOPHYSIOLOGY

    A. Etiology. Emotional stress and cold seem to be the biggest triggers of attacks. The duration of these attacks may be a few minutes or a few hours. Classically, during the attacks there is a three-stage color change. Stage one involves the pallor of the skin, which is sometimes associated with coldness, numbness, and/or paresthesias. The second stage, if present, involves cyanosis and may include some of the symptoms associated with stage one. Finally, the third stage involves erythema, which may be associated with throbbing of the digits (2). PRD carries a low risk of progression to an autoimmune disorder if after 2 years of attacks no other signs or symptoms of autoimmune processes are present. Conversely, Raynaud's can be the presenting sign for scleroderma. It has been proved that those who suffer from PRD or SRD have abnormal blood flow to the digits and abnormal recovery from cold stimulus. In patients with scleroderma, the blood vessels are already narrowed because of proliferation of the intimal area. This exacerbates the ischemia caused by the cold stimulus (3).

    B. Epidemiology. Raynaud's disease affects approximately 3% to 4% of the general population. Although the prevalence varies, it appears to be more common in women than in men. PRD usually begins in the second or third decade of life. SRD may begin with the underlying disorder and/or be the presenting sign of an autoimmune disorder. Raynaud's disease is more common in cold climates and can be associated with certain occupations such as those that require exposure to mechanical vibration on an ongoing basis (4). Other disorders associated with SRD include systemic lupus erythematosus (SLE), rheumatoid arthritis, dermatomyositis, polymyositis, and hyperviscosity syndromes, as well as vasospastic processes such as vascular headaches, atypical angina, and primary pulmonary hypertension (5).

III. EVALUATION

    A. History. When interviewing the patient, it is important to determine when the symptoms normally appear. Exposure to cold temperatures and stress are the most common triggers. Medications used and history of tobacco use are also important topics to be covered in the history (5). Questions about the use of machines or tools that produce vibration or other repetitive activities done with the fingers may help determine if the patient has a variant of Raynaud's disease known as *hand–arm vibration syndrome* (1).

B. Physical examination. The examination should focus on a thorough assessment of the digits. Inspect the digits carefully for sclerodactyly or digital ulcers, and examine the nail fold capillaries for abnormally large capillary loops, alternating with areas without any capillaries. This pattern is suggestive of scleroderma (5). It is also important to inspect for Malar rash, persistent cyanosis, and/or necrotic tissue of the digits.

C. Genetics. There is often a family history of the disorder (5). Currently, however, no genetic marker that can be tested for has been identified.

IV. DIAGNOSIS

A. Differential diagnosis. PRD is the most likely diagnosis in a young woman with less severe symptoms and no underlying disease. SRD should be considered in anyone with a known autoimmune disease such as scleroderma or SLE. Other diagnoses that could be considered include thromboangiitis obliterans in a man who smokes, thoracic outlet syndrome, carpal tunnel syndrome related to repetitive use of the hands, acrocyanosis, and cryoglobulinemia, especially associated with hepatitis B or C. Drugs that may induce SRD include, but are not limited to, β-blockers, antineoplastic drugs, oral contraceptives, ergot alkaloids, cyclosporine, and α-interferon (3).

B. Clinical manifestations. Color change of the digits when exposed to the cold is the classic presentation. Patients may not undergo all the three color changes. Some literature states that pallor followed by cyanosis is the most common pattern, whereas other sources note that in patients who have episodes with cyanosis the severity of the disease is higher (1). The most important thing to keep in mind when diagnosing patients with Raynaud's disease is that patients with SRD almost always have other symptoms of connective-tissue disease in addition to PRD.

References

1. Block JA. Raynaud's phenomenon. *Lancet* 2001;357:2042–2048.
2. National Institute of Arthritis and Musculoskeletal and Skin Diseases. www.niams.nih.gov, accessed on 11 April, 2006.
3. *Raynaud's phenomenon*, 2004. www.imedicine.com.
4. Canada's National Occupational Health and Safety Resource. www.ccohs.ca/oshanswers/diseases/raynaud/html, accessed on 11 April, 2006.
5. *Raynaud's phenomenon*, 2004. www.firstconsult.com.

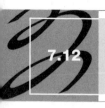

7.12

TACHYCARDIA
Mike Dukelow

I. BACKGROUND. Tachycardia is defined as a condition in which the heart rate greater than 100 beats/minute. It can be categorized into two main types, supraventricular or ventricular, with the former being further categorized into either wide complex tachycardia or narrow complex tachycardia (1).

II. PATHOPHYSIOLOGY. In the evaluation of the patient with tachycardia, one needs to discover the etiology of the tachycardia and then identify the specific dysrhythmia. Symptoms of tachycardia include palpitations, irregular rhythm, lightheadedness or presyncope, syncope, and congestive heart failure (Chapters 2.12, 7.5, and 7.9).

Conditions to look for in the previous medical history may include myocardial infarction, cardiomyopathy, arrhythmias, pulmonary hypertension, cardiac surgery, and valvular heart disease. Medications that can precipitate tachycardia and hence need to be watched out for are class IA and III antiarrhythmic medications, over-the-counter cold remedies, or even some antibiotics combined with some of the nonsedating antihistamines.

III. EVALUATION

A. History. Determine if the patient is hemodynamically stable and if he or she is symptomatic (distressed or unconscious) or asymptomatic (awake and not distressed).

B. Physical examination. Auscultate the heart, listening for murmurs, rubs, and gallops. A respiratory and visual examination of the patient that demonstrates lung crackles, jugular venous distention, and lower extremity edema indicates heart failure.

C. Testing
   1. **Electrocardiogram (ECG).** Obtain a 12-lead ECG and determine the rate, rhythm, and QRS duration on the rhythm strip (most times it is lead II).
   2. **Laboratory tests.** Look for hypomagnesemia, hypokalemia, anemia, hyperthyroidism, hypoxemia, illicit drugs, and digitalis toxicity.

IV. DIAGNOSIS

A. Narrow complex tachycardia (QRS <120 millisecond)
   1. **Sinus tachycardia.** Sinus tachycardia is normal in infants up to children younger than 2 years. There are numerous reasons for tachycardia in adults: pathologic (anemia, thyrotoxicosis, hypoxemia, hypotension, pulmonary embolism), physiologic (anemia, fever), and pharmacologic (β-agonist). Normal P wave and PR interval are seen on the ECG. Therapy consists in treating the underlying cause.
   2. **Atrial fibrillation.** Atrial fibrillation is an irregularly irregular rhythm with a variable rate (normal up to >200 beats/minute) with an absence of P waves on the ECG. If there is an aberrant conduction from the atria to ventricles or prior bundle branch block, it may be difficult to distinguish atrial fibrillation from ventricular tachycardia (VT). Usually, atrial fibrillation has an irregular rhythm, and VT has a regular rhythm.
   3. **Atrial flutter.** In atrial flutter, cardiac monitoring shows the classic "sawtooth" appearance in leads II, III, and aVF with a rate between 280 and 320 beats/minute. The ventricles have a slower rate, demonstrating a block of either 2:1 or 4:1 with a corresponding rate of 150 to 75 beats/minute. By doing a carotid massage or using adenosine if the massage fails to slow the atrial rate, one may be able to show flutter waves.
   4. **Paroxysmal supraventricular tachycardia.** Paroxysmal supraventricular tachycardia is a rhythm that is most commonly caused by the reentry of the atrial impulse at the atrioventricular (AV) node. Morphology of the rhythm shows a sudden onset with a narrow and regular QRS complex without obvious P waves and a rate from 120 to 190 beats/minute. Wolff-Parkinson-White syndrome occurs when there is antegrade conduction via an accessory pathway, producing delta waves (upsloping prior to the QRS complex) and shortened PR intervals.
   5. **Multifocal atrial tachycardia (MAT).** Multifocal atrial tachycardia is an arrhythmia that may occur in cases of metabolic or electrolyte disorders, pulmonary diseases, or digitalis toxicity. The rate of MAT is up to 140 beats/minute with an irregularly irregular rhythm and varying PP, RR, and PR intervals.

B. Wide complex tachycardia (QRS >120 millisecond). There can be much difficulty in distinguishing supraventricular tachycardia with an aberrant conduction from VT. The Brugada criteria can help discern the two patterns (2, 3).
   1. If an RS complex cannot be identified in any precordial leads, VT can be made with 100% specificity.
   2. If there are RS complexes in more than one lead, then the RS interval (the start of the R wave up to the deepest part of the S wave) is measured. If this is >100 milliseconds, then VT can be diagnosed with 98% specificity.

3. If the RS interval is <100 milliseconds, then there maybe either a ventricular or a supraventricular origin site of the tachycardia and AV dissociation must be evaluated. AV dissociation is 100% specific for VT but has a low sensitivity.

4. If the RS interval is <100 milliseconds and there is no demonstrable AV dissociation, then look for a RBBB-like pattern (QRS polarity is positive in leads V_1 and V_2 with an rS complex in V_6) or a LBBB-like pattern (QRS polarity negative in leads V_1 and V_2 and a Q or QS wave in lead V_6). If these are present, then VT is indicated.

C. **Ventricular fibrillation.** This is technically not a tachycardia but rather represents abnormal ventricular depolarizations in several areas that prevent an unified contraction of cardiac muscle. The rhythm on the ECG has the appearance of a "bag of worms", showing varying amplitudes of either coarse waves or fine waves.

References

1. Scheinman M. Tachyarrhythmias in primary cardiology. In: Goldman L, Braunwald E, eds. *Heart disease: a textbook of cardiovascular medicine*. Philadelphia, PA: WB Saunders, 1998:330–352.

2. Wellens HJ. Electrophysiology: ventricular tachycardia: diagnosis of broad QRS complex tachycardia. *Heart* 2001;86:579.

3. Brugada P. A new approach to the differential diagnosis of a regular tachycardia with a wide QRS complex. *Circulation* 1991;83:1649–1659.

Respiratory Problems

Joseph E. Scherger

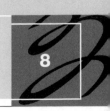

8

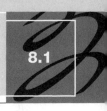

COUGH
Désirée A. Lie

I. **BACKGROUND.** Cough is among the top ten reasons for visits to family physicians in the United States and the fifth most common symptom presenting in outpatient care. It accounts for 200 to 400 million episodes of illness per year.

II. **PATHOPHYSIOLOGY.** Three causal conditions increasing in frequency over the past two decades are asthma, gastroesophageal reflux disease (GERD), and chronic obstructive pulmonary disease (COPD) (1,2). Bronchitis is one of the most common causes of cough in the primary care setting (3). Postnasal drip, asthma, and GERD account for almost 90% of cases of chronic cough (4).

III. **EVALUATION**

    A. **History.** A thorough history is vital to accurate diagnosis.

        1. **Cough characteristics.** In evaluating cough as a symptom (5), a distinction has to be made among the following:

           a. Normal versus pathologic cough

           b. Acute (<3 weeks) versus chronic (>3 weeks) cough

           c. Respiratory versus nonrespiratory causes

           d. Pediatric versus adult conditions.

        2. **Characteristics of the cough.** What is the type of cough (barking, brassy, wheezy, nocturnal, or paroxysmal)? What are the duration, timing, and triggers? Are there associated symptoms of fever, sputum production, dyspnea, hemoptysis, and weight loss? Are there clear relieving factors? Ask specifically about postnasal drip, because patients often do not volunteer this information. A good history is the key to diagnosis.

           a. Upper respiratory causes most commonly relate to postnasal drip. In adults, sinusitis, pharyngitis, and allergic rhinitis should be considered. In children, concomitant otitis media should be excluded.

           b. Lower respiratory causes include lung (bronchitis, asthma, pneumonia, and bronchiectasis, and in children, foreign body aspiration) and cardiac (congestive heart failure [CHF] and mitral stenosis) conditions.

           c. Nonrespiratory causes include GERD, drug effects (e.g., angiotensin-converting enzyme [ACE] inhibitors), and psychogenic conditions.

        3. **Smoking.** Patients who smoke should be identified early, because of the possible risk of bronchitis and lung cancer. Passive smoking is also a risk factor, especially in children. Office visits for cough provide an opportunity for smoking cessation education. Smoking cessation has been shown to reduce respiratory symptoms by 50%. In smokers, bronchogenic cancer should be considered a possible etiology in the presence of a new or recent change in chronic "smoker's cough"—a cough persisting for more than 1 month after smoking cessation and hemoptysis without infection.

        4. **Psychosocial factors.** The psychosocial impact of cough reflects severity and the need for further workup. Has the patient missed school or work? Is the sleeping partner disturbed? Is there avoidance of exercise because it triggers cough? In chronic, episodic cough, a correct diagnosis of asthma can considerably improve quality of life. A psychogenic cause for cough and behavioral problems in children may be unmasked here.

        5. **Other information.** Associated chest pain should direct the history toward pleurisy or rib fracture secondary to chronic cough. Occupational exposures (toxic fumes, chemicals, birds, and animals), systemic diseases (rheumatoid

arthritis, breast and prostate cancer metastases, and human immunodeficiency virus [HIV] disease), and drug exposure (ACE inhibitors, cyclophosphamide, and methotrexate) are important factors to consider. Cough with significant weight loss should trigger a workup for tuberculosis (TB), HIV, or lung cancer in the smoker.

B. Physical examination

1. Focused physical examination. This should include vital signs (temperature, pulse, respiratory rate, and blood pressure), ear, nose, sinuses, throat (ENST), and a full lung examination with the chest uncovered. Normal lung examination often excludes pneumonia but not asthma, bronchitis, COPD, GERD, or lung cancer. It is more effective to examine the lung before the ENST in young children because the ENST examination is more traumatic and can induce crying. In the older patient, especially the postmenopausal woman, rib palpation may be included to isolate fracture secondary to osteoporosis.

2. Additional physical examination. Cardiovascular examination is directed at a diagnosis of CHF. Associated lymphadenopathy suggests infection or neoplasm. Wasting can be ominous (cancer or HIV). Abdominal examination may reveal a tender enlarged liver in CHF or epigastric tenderness in GERD (Chapters 7.5 and 9.6).

C. Testing

1. Clinical laboratory tests. Most acute presentations of cough do not require blood, urine, or other laboratory tests. White blood count with differential count and blood cultures are indicated for pneumonia. Gram's stain and culture of sputum are rarely practical in the office. A purified protein derivative test should be placed early if TB is suspected, unless the patient is known to be anergic or thought to have overwhelming active TB. Systemic causes require testing specific to the disease in question.

2. Radiologic tests. A chest x-ray is not indicated for upper respiratory causes or bronchitis. It is only useful when pneumonia, TB, COPD, CHF, or cancer (primary or metastatic) is being considered. Computed tomography of the sinuses is more sensitive and specific than physical examination to differentiate sinusitis from other causes of cough.

3. Pulmonary function tests. A simple peak flowmeter used with a therapeutic trial of bronchodilators will identify most cases of asthma. This important test should be supervised by the physician or an experienced nurse. Additional testing is suggested for COPD and pulmonary fibrosis.

4. Invasive tests. Bronchoscopy is useful for foreign body aspiration, cancer, or chronic interstitial lung disease. Esophageal pH monitoring most likely confirms suspected GERD.

IV. DIAGNOSIS

A. Differential diagnosis. *Acute cough* is likely to be infectious. A pertinent observation is that physicians overtreat acute bronchitis with antibiotics. The literature suggests that most cases are viral in origin, and antibiotics are ineffective. *Chronic cough* has a longer list of differential diagnoses. Asthma tends to be underdiagnosed in adults and children. Smoking-related causes should prompt educational intervention and workup, especially in older patients. GERD is a diagnosis often missed because it is not considered. Often, more than one office visit is needed to unravel the cause of chronic cough. Up to 80% of cases have multiple causes (6). Making an accurate diagnosis is essential to successful treatment. Of those presenting with cough, 90% can be adequately managed in the family physician's office, although it can take 3 to 5 months to arrive at a correct diagnosis in some cases (2). Referral to a pulmonary specialist is needed only in complicated cases (e.g., cancer, occupational and connective tissue diseases, and failed therapy).

B. Special concerns. Failure to improve with appropriate management over 4 weeks signals a need for more extensive workup to exclude TB, adult-onset asthma, penicillin-resistant *pneumococcus*, lung cancer, and immunosuppression.

References

1. Weiss BD. *20 common problems in primary care.* New York, NY: McGraw-Hill, 1999.
2. Lawler WR. An office approach to the diagnosis of chronic cough. *Am Fam Physician* 1998;58(9):2015–2022.
3. Heath JM. Chronic bronchitis: primary care management. *Am Fam Physician* 1998; 57(10):2365–2372,2376–2378.
4. Mello CJ, Irwin RS, Curley FJ. Predictive values of the character, timing and complications of chronic cough in diagnosing its cause. *Arch Intern Med* 1996;156:997.
5. Irwin RS. Managing cough as a defense mechanism and as a symptom. A consensus report of the American college of chest physicians. *Chest* 1998;114:133S–181S.
6. Irwin RS. Silencing chronic cough. *Hosp Pract* 1999;34:53–60.

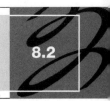

CYANOSIS
Janis F. Neuman

8.2

I. **BACKGROUND.** Cyanosis is a bluish discoloration of the skin and mucous membranes caused by increased amounts of unsaturated hemoglobin in the blood.

II. **PATHOPHYSIOLOGY.** For cyanosis to appear, 5 g/100 mL of reduced blood hemoglobin is required. An O_2 saturation $<75\%$ or a Pao_2 of 40 mm Hg results in cyanosis (1). Oxygen delivery to the tissues depends on an intact respiratory system to provide oxygen for hemoglobin saturation, the concentration of hemoglobin, the cardiac output and regional microvasculature, and an oxyhemoglobin unloading mechanism (2). Cyanosis can be considered central or peripheral, based on the underlying abnormality.

A. Central cyanosis includes conditions that lead to arterial desaturation such as decreased inspired oxygen tension, pulmonary disease, and conditions causing right to left shunts (e.g., congenital heart disease and intrapulmonary shunts). Abnormal hemoglobin levels are also considered central. Decreased blood oxygenation (central cyanosis) is usually caused by one of the following:

1. Obstruction to the intake of oxygen (epiglottitis and acute laryngotracheobronchitis, asthma, chronic bronchitis or emphysema, and foreign body aspiration).

2. Decreased absorption of oxygen, as occurs with an alveolar capillary block (sarcoid, pulmonary fibrosis, pneumonia, pulmonary edema, alveolar proteinosis). Ventilation–perfusion (V̇/Q̇) defects from emphysema, pneumoconioses, and sarcoid also decrease O_2 absorption.

3. Decreased perfusion of the lung with blood (shock, septic, or cardiogenic; pulmonary embolus; pulmonary vascular shunts from pulmonary hemangioma; congenital heart disease).

4. Reduced intake of oxygen from an atmosphere with a decreased oxygen concentration.

5. A defective hemoglobin unable to attach to oxygen (methemoglobinemia, sulfhemoglobinemia, carbon monoxide poisoning, and other hemoglobinopathies).

B. Peripheral cyanosis is caused by reduced cardiac output, cold exposure, and arterial or venous obstruction. Peripheral cyanosis occurs with the following:

1. Reduced cardiac output from acute myocardial infarction or other causes of pump failure

2. Local or regional phenomenon from cold exposure, arterial obstruction from embolus or thrombosis, and venous stasis or obstruction

3. Cold exposure (Raynaud's disease) (Chapter 7.11)

III. EVALUATION
A. History

1. When did the cyanosis appear? Is the cyanosis of recent onset or has it been present since birth? A history of "squatting" episodes in childhood and congenital cyanosis suggest congenital heart disease. Chronic cyanosis caused by methemoglobinemia can be congenital or acquired. Other causes of chronic cyanosis include chronic obstructive pulmonary disease (COPD), pulmonary fibrosis, and pulmonary atrioventricular fistula. Acute and subacute cyanosis are caused by acute myocardial infarct, pneumothorax, pulmonary embolus, pneumonia, or upper airway obstruction.

2. Is the patient symptomatic or asymptomatic? Asymptomatic patients may have methemoglobinemia (congenital or drug-induced), or sulfhemoglobinemia. Exposure to drugs (prescribed and illicit) or environmental factors are important in these patients. Intermittent cyanosis, skin color changes, and pain with cold exposure suggest Raynaud's phenomenon. Symptomatic patients, especially with chest pain and respiratory distress, are more likely to have a cardiac or pulmonary cause of cyanosis.

3. Does the patient have known risk factors for cardiac or pulmonary disease, including smoking, hyperlipidemia, asthma, drug abuse (especially methamphetamines), severe obesity (sleep apnea), neuromuscular disease, or autoimmune disease? Does the patient have chest pain or intermittent cyanosis with exercise, suggesting angina? Chest pain can be present with acute pulmonary emboli or pneumothorax. Is there a cough and fever suggesting pneumonia? Has the patient had any occupational or environmental exposures that might cause pulmonary problems?

4. Is there a family history of abnormal hemoglobins or pulmonary disease? Has the patient suffered an episode of hypotension that could produce adult respiratory distress syndrome (ARDS), such as sepsis or heart failure?

B. Physical examination

1. **Initial assessment.** Vital signs are very important; tachycardia suggests cardiac arrhythmia, shock, volume depletion, anemia, or fever (Chapter 7.12). An increased or decreased respiratory rate and use of accessory musculature suggest hypoxia from any cause. Hypotension can signal vascular collapse from myocardial infarction, septic shock, or pulmonary embolus.

2. **Additional physical examination.** Stridor suggests upper airway obstruction. Examine the pharynx for evidence of obstruction. If epiglottitis or the presence of a foreign body is suspected, be prepared to intubate the patient. Check the neck for evidence of jugular venous distention. Auscultate the chest for rales, suggestive of pulmonary edema; wheezing and rhonchi consistent with reactive airway disease; or absence of breath sounds, suggestive of pneumonia, or pneumothorax. Auscultate the heart for murmurs, arrhythmias, and abnormal heart sounds. Feel the pulses in the extremities to assess for arterial embolus or venous thrombosis, especially if cyanosis is localized to one extremity. Examine the abdomen for evidence of intraabdominal catastrophe or aneurysm. Examine the nails for evidence of clubbing, which is suggestive of chronic pulmonary disease.

C. Testing

1. Pulse oximetry estimates oxygen saturation but does not measure it directly. Direct measurements using arterial blood gases (ABGs) are necessary to assess a patient with cyanosis. Patients with abnormal hemoglobins have a normal PaO_2 but decreased hemoglobin O_2 saturation. Patients with cyanosis have O_2 saturation <75% and PaO_2 <40 mm Hg if they have a normal hemoglobin concentration. A low PaO_2 is caused by respiratory or cardiac problems in most circumstances.

2. A chest radiograph helps assess heart size and lung parenchyma. Infiltrates suggest pneumonia, ARDS, or pulmonary edema. Exclude pneumothorax. Look for evidence of interstitial lung disease. Pleural effusion can represent infection, malignancy, or pulmonary edema (Chapter 8.4).

3. An electrocardiogram may demonstrate acute myocardial infarction, arrhythmia, or pericardial process. P pulmonale, right ventricular hypertrophy, and R axis suggest chronic pulmonary disease.

4. Other tests include ventilation–perfusion scanning, which may demonstrate pulmonary embolus. Pulmonary artery catheterization and pressure measurements help distinguish cardiac causes from pulmonary causes of cyanosis. Pulmonary function testing can help in the diagnosis of various pulmonary diseases.

IV. DIAGNOSIS

A. Focused history, physical examination, and diagnostic testing elucidate the cause of cyanosis in affected patients. Response to supplemental O_2 can also help pinpoint the cause of cyanosis (2). Decreased oxygenation secondary to mild to moderate ventilation–perfusion mismatches caused by pneumonia, pulmonary embolus, and asthma may be reversible with supplemental oxygen. Severe $\dot{V}/\dot{Q}$ mismatch caused by intrapulmonary shunting from severe pulmonary edema or ARDS may be refractory to supplemental O_2. Moderate $\dot{V}/\dot{Q}$ mismatch associated with ventilatory failure COPD may respond to supplemental O_2, but be aware of increasing CO_2 levels. ABGs directly measure PaO_2 and O_2 saturation. Abnormal hemoglobins will also be measured and they help guide therapy. Hypoxia with an elevated CO_2 suggests COPD or asthma, whereas hypoxia with a normal or decreased CO_2 suggests pneumonia, ARDS, pulmonary edema, pulmonary emboli, or interstitial lung disease (1).

B. Once the cause of the cyanosis is determined, the objective is to treat the underlying process. Causes of pseudocyanosis include argyria or bismuth poisoning (slate blue-gray color), hemochromatosis (brownish color), or polycythemia (ruddy red color). For peripheral cyanosis caused by decreased cardiac output, correct the causes of hypovolemia (e.g., dehydration, shock, heart failure from whatever cause). Surgical consultation may be required for acute embolization of an extremity, and anticoagulation for venous thrombosis.

References

1. Khan MG. *Cardiac and pulmonary management.* Philadelphia, PA: Lea & Febiger, 1993:818–825.
2. Woodley M, Whelan A. *Manual of medical therapeutics.* Boston, MA: Little, Brown and Company, 1993:179–181.

Suggested Readings

Hurst JW. *Medicine for the practicing physician.* Boston, MA: Butterworth-Heineman, 1983:973–975.

Collins RD. *Dynamic differential diagnosis.* Philadelphia, PA: J.B. Lippincott, 1981:386–388.

HEMOPTYSIS

Kathryn M. Larsen and Mary D. Knudtson

8.3

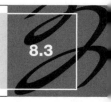

I. BACKGROUND. Hemoptysis is defined as the coughing up or expectoration of blood from the tracheobronchial tree, which can be from the trachea, the major airways, or the lung parenchyma. It is an alarming symptom that usually prompts the patient to seek immediate medical attention.

II. PATHOPHYSIOLOGY. Hemoptysis can range in severity from trivial to life-threatening, and is due to numerous causes. The clinician must determine the anatomic bleeding site and the underlying cause for the bleeding (1). Bleeding originating from the nasopharynx or bleeding from the gastrointestinal tract can mimic hemoptysis (Chapter 9.7). A thorough evaluation is necessary because the amount of blood expectorated does not correlate with the seriousness of the cause. After extensive evaluation, there is no identifiable cause of hemoptysis in up to 30% of affected patients; these patients are classified as having cryptogenic hemoptysis.

  A. Etiology. The pathogenesis of hemoptysis generally results from inflammation or injury to the tracheobronchial mucosa (e.g., bronchitis, bronchiectasis, tuberculosis, sarcoidosis, bronchogenic carcinoma); injury to the pulmonary vasculature (e.g., lung abscess, necrotizing pneumonia, pulmonary infarction secondary to emboliza-tion); or elevation of the pulmonary capillary pressure (e.g., pulmonary edema, Wegener's granulomatosis, Goodpasture's syndrome).

  B. Epidemiology. The most common causes are acute and chronic bronchitis, fol-lowed by bronchogenic carcinoma and pneumonia (2). Lung tumors account for 20% of the cases of hemoptysis; they are usually associated with smokers older than 40 years who have had a change in cough pattern with an ache or pain in the chest. A bleeding diathesis or the use of anticoagulant medicine may present with hemoptysis but underlying pulmonary disease must always be excluded. Chest trauma is a less common cause of hemoptysis.

III. EVALUATION

  A. History

  1. Identification of the bleeding site. What is the source of the bleeding? Is the problem truly hemoptysis or could the bleeding originate in a nonpulmonary location such as the nose and oropharynx or the gastrointestinal tract? Blood that is coughed from the respiratory tract is bright red in color and may be frothy or mixed with sputum. Hemoptysis is more likely associated with a history of underlying pulmonary disease, smoking, or mitral valve disease. Hematemesis is associated with blood that is dark red, brown, or ground coffee in color and may be mixed with food particles. Hematemesis is favored in the presence of a preexisting gastrointestinal condition, especially with a history of liver disease, alcohol use, or peptic ulcer disease. Sputum that is blood-streaked often arises from the nasal mucosa and oropharynx.

  2. Characteristics of the sputum. What are the characteristics of the sputum in terms of color, odor, and consistency? A description of the sputum can assist in defining the disease process causing the hemoptysis: (a) frothy, pink sputum is suggestive of pulmonary edema fluid; (b) putrid or foul-smelling sputum suggests a lung abscess; (c) currant jelly sputum may suggest a necrotizing pneumonia; (d) the sputum of pneumococcal pneumonia is typically rust-colored and can be confused with true hemoptysis; (e) large amounts of blood-streaked sputum often suggest bronchiectasis.

  3. Other information. Does the patient have other associated symptoms? Cough, dyspnea, and sputum production over several years may suggest chronic bron-chitis or bronchiectasis. Weight loss and fatigue may suggest an underlying malignancy, and fever and night sweats might indicate tuberculosis. Does the patient have a history of known pulmonary, cardiac, or hematologic problems? Does the patient have hematuria, which might suggest a pulmonary–renal syn-drome (Chapter 10.2)? Does the patient smoke or have specific environmental exposures? Is the patient taking medications, especially anticoagulants, that might contribute to the bleeding?

  B. Physical examination. A focused physical examination should include vital signs and examinations of the nose, sinuses, oropharynx, neck, lungs, and heart. The neck should be palpated for the presence of lymphadenopathy and inspected for jugular venous distension. The lower extremities should be checked for edema. Examination of the skin may reveal lesions associated with systemic lupus erythe-matosus; Kaposi's sarcoma; clubbing (consistent with neoplasm, bronchiectasis, or lung abscess); or ecchymosis related to a coagulopathy.

  C. Testing

  1. Evaluation should begin with a chest x-ray to look for possible clues to the diag-nosis: a mass lesion, focal or diffuse parenchymal disease, pneumonitis, abscess, infiltrate, hilar adenopathy, enlarged heart, pulmonary edema, coin lesion of aspergilloma, or the peribronchial cuffing suggestive of bronchiectasis. A com-puted tomography scan may be necessary to define a lesion seen on chest x-ray film (3). Additional basic testing should include a complete blood count with differential and a coagulation profile. For patients in whom infection is suspected, skin testing, a Gram's stain, acid-fast stain, or sputum cultures may be appropriate. Cytologic examination of the sputum is indicated in cases of suspected malignancy.

2. Other special tests include fiberoptic bronchoscopy, which is used to localize the bleeding site of specific lesions noted on x-ray film. It is also used in cases of persistent or recurrent bleeding and for smokers older than 40 years with a negative chest x-ray study. Ventilation–perfusion scanning is indicated if pulmonary embolism is suspected.

IV. DIAGNOSIS. Determining the site of bleeding is the first step. If the bleeding is from the nasopharynx or gastrointestinal tract, then it is not classified as hemoptysis. The basic approach depends on the severity of the bleeding. Most cases of blood-tinged sputum are upper respiratory in nature and do not require extensive workup. Bronchitis is the most common cause. However, bronchogenic carcinoma, and bronchiectasis are also common causes that require further evaluation (4). Mild hemoptysis can be evaluated with elective bronchoscopy of the respiratory tract. Massive hemoptysis (definitions in the literature range from 100 mL in 24 hours to 1,000 mL over several days) requires an emergent diagnostic approach, typically with rigid bronchoscopy (5). If hemoptysis persists despite treatment of a presumed infection, bronchial arteriography with embolization or resection of the involved segment may be necessary.

References
1. Colice GL. Hemoptysis: three questions that can direct management. *Postgrad Med* 1996;100(1):227–236.
2. DiLeo MD, Amedee RG, Butcher RB. Hemoptysis and pseudohemoptysis: the patient expectorating blood. *Ear Nose Throat J* 1995;74(12):822–824,826–828.
3. Marshall TJ, Flower CD, Jackson JE. The role of radiology in the investigation and management of patients with hemoptysis. *Clin Radiol* 1996;51(6):391–400.
4. Marwah OS, Sharma OP. Bronchiectasis: how to identify, treat, and prevent. *Postgrad Med* 1995;97(2):149–150,153–156,159.
5. Cahill BC, Ingbar DH. Massive hemoptysis: assessment and management. *Clin Chest Med* 1994;15(1):147–167.

PLEURAL EFFUSION
Mark F. Giglio

8.4

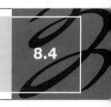

I. BACKGROUND. Pleural effusions occur in a variety of illnesses. The underlying causes range from benign atelectasis to malignancy. Pleural effusions develop in 1 million patients each year in the United States (1). Although effusions occur within the lungs and pleura, the source is often from outside the pulmonary system.

II. PATHOPHYSIOLOGY. Pleural effusions are of two distinct types: transudative and exudative.

A. Transudative effusions result from an elevated net hydrostatic pressure gradient. Common causes include congestive heart failure (CHF), nephrotic syndrome, and cirrhosis. Generally, they require no further workup when identified and respond to treatment of the primary problem.

B. Exudative effusions result from increased permeability of the pleural vessels. The differential diagnosis encompasses a broader range of conditions, including malignancy and infections.

III. EVALUATION

A. History. The patient's history can often suggest that a pleural effusion is present. Small effusions, however, may cause no symptoms. Frequently, an underlying disease causes the patient's initial symptoms.

1. **Pulmonary.** Dyspnea is the most common symptom. Did it develop acutely or gradually? Is there a dry cough present? Does the patient experience chest pain, especially pleuritic pain? Does the pain vary in quality (Chapter 8.5)?

2. **Associated symptoms.** The main goal here is to think about underlying illnesses that might produce a pleural effusion. Orthopnea, paroxysmal nocturnal dyspnea, dyspnea on exertion, and pedal edema suggest CHF. Does the patient have exertional chest pain that may be angina? Hemoptysis, weight loss, and anorexia point to malignancy. Has the patient been acutely ill? Productive cough, fever, chills, and night sweats suggest pneumonia. Does the patient have risk factors for deep venous thrombosis (e.g., recent travel, prolonged immobilization, or fracture)? Symptoms of pulmonary embolism include tachycardia, hemoptysis, and dyspnea.

3. **Past medical history.** Has the patient had prior pulmonary diseases? Are cardiac risk factors present? Is there a history of hepatic or renal disease? Has the patient had cancer?

4. **Family history.** Are there family members with premature coronary artery disease, tuberculosis, or malignancy?

5. **Social history.** Does the patient smoke? Does the patient use alcohol excessively? Where does the patient work? Is there solvent or asbestos exposure at work?

B. Physical examination

1. **Focused physical examination.** Observe the patient's appearance and respiratory effort. Is the patient splinting or showing signs of respiratory distress? Vital signs should include respiratory rate. Is tachycardia present (Chapter 7.12)? Typical findings on pulmonary examination include decreased or absent breath sounds over the affected side, dullness to percussion, decreased tactile fremitus, and possibly splinting of the affected side. Findings can be bilateral (e.g., CHF) or unilateral. Examination can also vary with the severity of the effusion. Findings are usually normal when less than 300 mL of fluid is present. A pleural rub may be noted. With a large effusion (>1,500 mL), the affected hemithorax is often larger with bulging interspaces (2).

2. **Additional physical examination.** It is necessary to think in terms of differential diagnosis when looking for signs of underlying causes. Cardiac examination should look for signs of congestive heart failure, including cardiomegaly, displaced point of maximal impulse, and an S_3 gallop. Is a heart murmur present? Abdominal examination may reveal hepatomegaly, liver tenderness, a fluid wave, and other signs of ascites. Are there signs of malignancy, including generalized or regional lymphadenopathy (Chapters 15.1 and 15.2)?

C. Testing

1. **Radiography.** Initial testing focuses on confirming that a pleural effusion is present. A chest x-ray study is the typical starting point. On the upright anteroposterior view, a small effusion may show up as blunting of the costophrenic angle. Larger effusions show a meniscus sign at the air fluid border. Lateral decubitus views help estimate the size of the effusion.

2. **Ultrasound and other modalities.** Unfortunately, chest x-rays can fail to show small effusions, even with decubitus views. Ultrasound can detect as little as 5 to 50 mL of fluid. It is also helpful in locating pockets of fluid and guiding thoracentesis for small effusions. Computed tomography, which is very sensitive, can differentiate pleural fluid from pleural thickening and focal masses.

3. **Thoracentesis.** Thoracentesis allows evaluation of any undiagnosed pleural effusion. Note that not all effusions require diagnostic thoracentesis. If the cause is apparent from the clinical presentation (e.g., CHF), observation may be appropriate (3). In general, parapneumonic effusions require thoracentesis to confirm diagnosis and assess the need for chest tube placement.

   a. Relative contraindications include bleeding diathesis, systemic anticoagulation, small volume of pleural fluid, mechanical ventilation, inability of the patient to cooperate, and cutaneous disease at the needle entry site.
   b. Transudate or exudate? On the basis of a revision of the "modified" Light's criteria, pleural fluid is an exudate if it meets one or more of the following parameters (4):
      i. Pleural fluid serum lactate dehydrogenase (LDH) level >0.45 the upper limit of normal LDH
      ii. Pleural. Serum LDH >0.6
      iii. Pleural. Serum protein >0.5
   c. Other measures used to test for an exudate include pleural fluid cholesterol, fluid:serum albumin gradient and fluid:serum bilirubin ratio. Cell count, pH, glucose, Gram's stain, and culture help assess for infection.

IV. DIAGNOSIS. In developing a diagnostic assessment for the patient with pleural effusion, it is important to consider that pleural fluid analysis does not establish a specific diagnosis, but supports a clinical impression. Ordering and interpreting tests must be guided by pretest clinical impressions (5). Initially, it may be appropriate to order only pleural fluid LDH and protein levels to determine the presence or absence of an exudate. Additional fluid can be reserved for further testing if an exudate is found.

   A. If the pleural fluid analysis shows a transudate, the most likely diagnosis is CHF. Additional possibilities include cirrhosis with ascites, nephrotic syndrome, hypoalbuminemia, and acute atelectasis. Further diagnostic evaluation of the pleural fluid is not necessary.
   B. If the pleural fluid is exudative, the most likely diagnostic possibilities are malignancy, infection, or tuberculosis, but the differential diagnosis is quite broad. In one study, malignancy accounted for 25% of all pleural effusions seen in the general hospital setting. Cytology is helpful in looking for malignancy. In 54% to 63% of patients with malignant effusions, pleural fluid cytology is positive (5). Glucose level, cell count, and pH help guide management in the setting of parapneumonic effusions and aid in determining the need for chest tube placement. Tuberculous effusions may require pleural biopsy to confirm the diagnosis. Amylase can be elevated in pancreatitis, pancreatic pseudocyst, malignancy, and esophageal rupture. Triglycerides are elevated in the setting of chylothorax.
   C. Studies on pleural fluid yield a definitive or presumptive diagnosis in 74% of cases (5). Those cases that are undiagnosed may require repeat thoracentesis, pleural biopsy, bronchoscopy, or thoracoscopy to ascertain the cause.

References

1. Stagner SW, Campbell GD. Pleural effusion: what can you learn from the results of the a "tap"? *Postgrad Med* 1992;91:439–454.
2. Jay SJ. Diagnostic procedures for pleural disease. *Clin Chest Med* 1985;6:33–48.
3. Burgher LW, Jones FL, Patterson JR, et al. Guidelines for thoracentesis and needle biopsy of the pleura. *Am Rev Respir Dis* 1989;140:257–258.
4. Heffner JE, Brown LK, Barbier C. Diagnostic value of tests that discriminate between exudative and transudative pleural effusions. *Chest* 1997;111:970–980.
5. Bartter T, Santarelli R, Akers S, et al. The evaluation of pleural effusion. *Chest* 1994; 106:1209–1214.

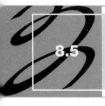

PLEURITIC PAIN
Hal S. Shimazu

I. **BACKGROUND.** Pleuritic pain is the characteristic pain of inflamed pleura (i.e., pleurisy—a term often used synonymously with pleuritic pain). Pleuritic pain arises from parietal pleura and is typically sharp, stabbing, unilateral, and aggravated by deep inspiration and coughing. The visceral pleura is insensitive.

II. **PATHOPHYSIOLOGY**
   A. **Etiology.** It is important to distinguish true pleuritic pain (see Table 8.5.1) from conditions that mimic this pain (see Table 8.5.2). In acute pleuritic pain, urgent exclusion of pulmonary embolism (PE) is paramount; mortality from PE is <10% in treated patients and 30% in untreated patients (1). Because of the low specificity of the presenting signs and symptoms of PE, in the absence of an obvious cause for acute pleuritic pain, suspicion for PE must remain high; further evaluation is required, typically with a ventilation–perfusion ($\dot{V}/\dot{Q}$) lung scan (2, 3).
   B. **Epidemiology.** Pleuritic pain as a clinical manifestation with a multitude of etiologies is not as such a reportable clinical entity. Therefore, specific data on the prevalence and incidence of pleuritic pain are lacking.

III. **EVALUATION**
   A. **History**
      1. **Initial history.** History begins with assessing the characteristics of the pleuritic pain—the acuity, its location, and exacerbating features. Acute onset

TABLE 8.5.1   **Causes of Pleuritic Pain**

Pleuritis/pleurisy: Infectious (viral, especially coxsackievirus B; primary or reactivated tuberculosis, fungal), autoimmune (e.g., systemic lupus, rheumatoid arthritis, Dressler's syndrome—pleuropericarditis), uremic, radiation-induced, drug reaction, and idiopathic

Pulmonary embolism

Pneumonia

Spontaneous pneumothorax

Trauma (hemothorax, pneumothorax)

Neoplasia

Asbestos

TABLE 8.5.2   **Conditions that Mimic Pleuritic Pain**

Chest wall: Costochondritis, rib fracture, muscle strain/spasm, herpes zoster
Abdominal: Pancreatitis, abscess (hepatic, splenic, subphrenic), splenic infarction
Cardiac: Pericarditis

suggests sudden development as viral or idiopathic pleurisy, PE, pneumonia, or pneumothorax. Insidious onset suggests a slower inflammatory or irritative process, usually resulting in a pleural effusion with the pain generally diminishing as fluid accumulates (Chapter 8.4). Pleuritic chest pain localizes above the underlying pleural pathology through intercostal innervation. Shoulder pain through phrenic innervation can indicate ipsilateral diaphragmatic involvement, usually by abdominal pathology (see Table 8.5.2). Substernal pain that decreases by leaning forward, suggests pericarditis (Chapter 7.1). Provocation of pain by shoulder movement indicates a musculoskeletal cause.

2. **Review of symptoms.** A focused review of systems might suggest a respiratory infection, PE, or malignancy as the etiology for the pleuritic pain. Nonproductive cough is nonspecific, and productive cough suggests infection. Hemoptysis suggests malignancy, tuberculosis, or pulmonary embolism. Fever suggests infection but can occur with PE. Recent surgery or lower extremity trauma or swelling increases the risk of PE. Unexplained weight loss suggests malignancy or tuberculosis (TB).

3. **Past medical history.** This can provide clues to the cause including malignancy, recent myocardial infarction, uremia, lupus, and rheumatoid arthritis.

4. **Other inquiries.** Additional history could be helpful with inquiries about oral contraceptives (PE risk), TB, or asbestos exposure.

B. Physical examination

1. A focused examination should include vital signs with attention to temperature, respiratory rate, and examination of the chest. Tenderness to palpation indicates a musculoskeletal cause. Dullness to percussion suggests pleural effusion or parenchymal pathology and hyperresonant percussion indicates pneumothorax. On auscultation, a pleural friction rub is the only sign of pleurisy; crackles suggest pneumonia; and decreased breath sounds indicate pneumothorax or effusion. The result of the examination is frequently normal.

2. Additional physical findings such as abdominal tenderness can suggest a subdiaphragmatic process (Table 8.5.2). Lower extremity edema, tenderness, or Homans' sign can imply deep vein thrombosis (DVT) and PE. Lymphadenopathy can represent lymphoma or metastatic disease.

C. Testing

1. Routine laboratory studies (e.g., complete blood count and metabolic panels) are of limited usefulness; leukocytosis in pneumonia, uremia, or hepatic abnormalities may suggest the cause.

2. Imaging studies

   a. A chest x-ray (CXR) is essential, potentially revealing pneumonia, neoplasm, pneumothorax, or pleural effusion; the decubitus view is sensitive at 100 mL effusion. Nonspecific findings of atelectasis, pulmonary parenchymal abnormalities, or both are seen in 68% of PE; pleural effusion is found in 48% of PE (3). The CXR is generally normal. Notably, PE and viral pleurisy frequently have a normal CXR.

   b. Ultrasound has diagnostic and therapeutic adjunctive roles with pleural effusions.

   c. Computed tomography (CT) scan has a role with both effusions and parenchymal abnormalities.

3. Diagnostic thoracentesis is indicated for pleural effusion if the cause of the effusion and pain is not apparent (diagnostic assessment of pleural effusion is discussed in Chapter 8.4). Effusion associated with pleuritic pain is nearly always an exudate with a notable exception of PE, which can be a transudate (4).

4. Additional studies are indicated for evaluation of a potential PE. The standard or rapid enzyme-linked immunosorbent assay of D-dimer, the degradation product of cross-linked fibrin, is a highly sensitive but nonspecific test for venous thromboembolism that, when coupled with low clinical probability of PE, can safely rule out PE (Chapter 17.5) (5). $\dot{V}/\dot{Q}$ lung scan is typically obtained for any significant suspicion of PE. If the $\dot{V}/\dot{Q}$ scan has low or intermediate probability

for PE, then evaluating for possible DVT with leg impedance plethysmography or ultrasound is useful. If the DVT study is negative, then a pulmonary angiogram can be obtained if there is intermediate or high clinical suspicion for PE (5). Optionally, serial leg venous studies can be obtained if there is only intermediate clinical suspicion (3). The helical CT angiogram has an emerging role in suspected PE evaluation, especially in patients with conditions that would cause a nondiagnostic $\dot{V}/\dot{Q}$ scan. The sensitivity and specificity of the CT angiogram are both 90% in main and lobar pulmonary emboli; however, sensitivity is 71% to 84% in subsegmental pulmonary artery emboli, which can represent from 6% to 30% of patients with pulmonary emboli (5).

D. Genetics. Except for a hereditary hypercoagulable state increasing the risk of PE, genetics has no relevance to the clinical manifestation of pleuritic pain.

IV. DIAGNOSIS

A. Differential diagnosis. After ruling out mimics of pleuritic pain (Table 8.5.2), there are many potential causes of pleuritic pain to consider (Table 8.5.1). Considering the possibility of PE is of paramount importance.

B. Clinical manifestations. The CXR study may reveal an obvious cause (e.g., neoplasm, pneumonia, or pneumothorax) or may nonspecifically reveal a pleural effusion. Commonly, the CXR may be normal. Causes of pleuritic pain in a patient with a normal CXR result are PE, viral or idiopathic pleurisy, and serositis, especially from systemic lupus. Viral pleurisy, usually coxsackievirus B, is characterized by unilateral acute pleuritic pain, variable low-grade fever, and nonproductive cough with typically a normal CXR, which is an indistinguishable presentation from PE— 20% presenting with acute pleuritic pain to the emergency department have PE and approximately 50% have viral or idiopathic pleurisy (1,2). Hence, acute pleuritic pain without an obvious cause on history and physical examination and CXR film requires exclusion of PE. A possible exception to this tenet is the young adult (age <40 years) who is highly unlikely to have a PE if all three of the following clinical features are *absent*: (a) risk factors for or past history of venous thromboembolic disease, (b) physical findings of phlebitis and (c) pleural effusion on CXR (2). In the presence of an effusion without a clear cause of the pleuritic pain and PE either ruled out or clinically highly unlikely, a diagnostic thoracentesis is indicated. The effusion associated with pleuritic pain is nearly always an exudate. The most common causes of exudates in descending order of frequency are malignancy (most commonly lung cancer, breast cancer, lymphoma), pneumonia, PE, and viral infections, which, together constitute 95% of these effusions (4).

References

1. Palevsky HI, Kelley MA, Fishman AP. Pulmonary thromboembolic disease. In: Fishman AP, ed. *Fishman's pulmonary diseases and disorders.* New York, NY: McGraw-Hill, 1997:1297–1329.
2. Hull RD, Raskob GE. Pulmonary embolism in outpatients with pleuritic chest pain. *Arch Intern Med* 1988;148:838–844.
3. Stein PD. Acute pulmonary embolism. *Dis Mon* 1994;40(9):467–515.
4. Light RW. *Pleural diseases,* 3rd ed. Baltimore, MD: William & Wilkins, 1995:75–82, 187–191.
5. Fedullo PF, Tapson VF. The evaluation of suspected pulmonary embolism. *N Engl J Med* 2003;349:1247–1256.

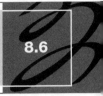

PNEUMOTHORAX
Charles Vega

8.6

I. **BACKGROUND.** Pneumothorax occurs when air enters the pleural space, the area between the visceral and parietal pleura. It is a common problem with a variety of different causes. In all cases, air enters the space because of a disruption or break in either the visceral or parietal pleura.

II. **PATHOPHYSIOLOGY.** Pneumothorax can be classified into two major categories—spontaneous and traumatic.

   A. **Spontaneous pneumothorax**

   1. Primary spontaneous pneumothorax occurs in previously healthy individuals. It can be found more frequently in tall, slender individuals (1). It is most common in individuals in their early twenties and is uncommon in those older than 40 years of age. Primary spontaneous pneumothorax is often caused by a rupture of apical blebs or bullae. Cigarette smoking increases the possibility of primary spontaneous pneumothorax (1). The estimated annual incidence of primary spontaneous pneumothorax is 7.4 to 18 cases per 100,000 men and 1.2 to 6 cases per 100,000 women (2).

   2. Secondary spontaneous pneumothorax occurs as a complication in individuals with underlying pulmonary disease. It is most common in individuals with chronic obstructive pulmonary disease (COPD). Secondary spontaneous pneumothorax is also seen in individuals with interstitial lung disease, with infections, particularly *Pneumocystis carinii* pneumonia and tuberculosis, and with neoplasms, either primary lung or metastatic tumors. The incidence is similar to that of primary spontaneous pneumothorax, with an estimated 10,000 cases per year in the United States (3).

   B. **Traumatic pneumothorax**

   1. Iatrogenic pneumothorax occurs as a complication of medical procedures such as transthoracic needle biopsy, central venous catheter placement, thoracentesis, and bronchoscopy, or as a complication of mechanical ventilation.

   2. **Penetrating and blunt trauma.** Penetrating trauma, such as a stab wound, as the causative factor of pneumothorax is obvious: the wound allows air to enter through the chest wall. Pneumothorax can also be a result of blunt trauma, as sometimes occurs when a rib fracture pierces the visceral pleura. More often, however, decelerating forces of blunt chest trauma can lead to chest compression that can directly cause pneumothorax.

III. **EVALUATION**

   A. **History**

   1. **Spontaneous pneumothorax.** Chest pain, most often pleuritic and localized to the side of the pneumothorax, and dyspnea are the major symptoms. Onset is generally sudden. In primary spontaneous pneumothorax, the symptoms are often mild, onset is usually at rest, and patients often do not immediately seek medical attention (4). Symptoms are generally more severe in patients with underlying lung disease (secondary spontaneous pneumothorax) who have impaired pulmonary reserve (5).

   2. **Traumatic pneumothorax.** The symptoms are the same as in spontaneous pneumothorax; although, in iatrogenic pneumothorax, they may not occur for 24 hours or more after the diagnostic or therapeutic procedure (5). The clinical deterioration of patients on ventilators should raise the suspicion of pneumothorax. This is more likely in patients with acute respiratory distress syndrome, necrotizing or aspiration pneumonia, COPD, or interstitial lung disease (5).

B. Physical examination. Vital signs can be normal, but tachycardia is the most common sign of spontaneous pneumothorax (2). Significant tachypnea can occur in patients with large pneumothoraces, or in patients with underlying pulmonary disease. Hypotension and severe tachycardia can be present in patients with tension pneumothorax or secondary spontaneous pneumothorax. On chest and lung examination may be found unilateral enlargement of the chest cavity, loss of tactile fremitus, hyperresonance to percussion, and decreased, or absent, breath sounds on the affected side. Tracheal deviation may be seen, especially with tension pneumothorax.

C. Testing

1. Arterial blood gas typically shows hypoxia and, occasionally, hypocarbia secondary to hyperventilation.
2. Electrocardiographic changes may be seen, especially with left-sided pneumothorax, including axis deviation, nonspecific ST- and T-wave changes, ST depression, and T-wave inversion (5).
3. Chest x-ray is generally paramount in the diagnosis, with visualization of the visceral pleural line and the absence of lung markings distal to this line. This is best seen on an upright inspiratory film, and the value of adding additional expiratory films has been questioned (3). Lateral decubitus films may be helpful in critically ill patients who cannot sit upright (6).
4. Computed tomography can also be useful when the chest x-ray is not diagnostic.

IV. DIAGNOSIS

A. Differential diagnosis

1. Pneumothorax can be diagnosed by the history and physical examination in slender patients who have had acute onset of chest pain and dyspnea, and confirmed with a chest radiograph visualizing the visceral pleural line. Patients who have had primary spontaneous pneumothorax are at risk of recurrence.
2. Secondary spontaneous pneumothorax can be a bit more difficult to diagnose. Although the symptoms are more prominent, the signs on physical examination are often subtle, especially in patients with COPD who tend to have decreased breath sounds and decreased tactile fremitus, because of their underlying disease. Radiographic evaluation can also be more difficult. Because of the lack of interstitial markings in the emphysematous lung, little difference is seen in the appearance proximal and distal to the visceral line. Also, an emphysematous bleb might be mistaken for a visceral line.

B. Clinical manifestations

1. It is common to obtain a chest x-ray after procedures that might lead to pneumothorax. Pleuritic chest pain and dyspnea, after associated diagnostic or therapeutic procedures, should alert practitioners, even if these symptoms occur many hours after the procedure. All patients with significant blunt trauma to the chest should be evaluated for pneumothorax, including all patients with rib or scapula fractures.
2. Tension pneumothorax occurs when a one-way valve allows air into, but not out of the pleural space. As pressure in the pleural space exceeds the atmospheric pressure, the ipsilateral lung, mediastinum, and contralateral lung are compressed. This is a medical emergency. The diagnosis of tension pneumothorax must be made clinically, because there is not enough time for imaging studies. The diagnosis can be confirmed by treatment: a large bore needle is placed through the second intercostal space approximately 2 to 3 cm from the edge of the sternum. A rush of air and relief of symptoms confirm the diagnosis.

References

1. Baum GL, Wolinsky E. *Textbook of pulmonary diseases*, 5th ed. Vol. II. Boston, MA: Little, Brown and Company, 1994:1871–1875.
2. Sahn SA, Heffner JE. Spontaneous pneumothorax. *N Engl J Med* 2000;342:868–874.

3. Schramel FMNH, Postmus PE, Vanderschueren RGJRA. Current aspects of spontaneous pneumothorax. *Eur Respir J* 1997;10:1372–1379.
4. Light RW. *Pleural diseases*, 3rd ed. Baltimore, MD: Williams & Wilkins, 1995:242–277.
5. Jantz MA, Pierson DJ. Pneumothorax and barotrauma. *Clin Chest Med* 1994;15(1): 75–91.
6. Spillane RM, Shepard JO, Deluca SA. Radiographic aspects of pneumothorax. *Am Fam Physician* 1995;51(2):459–464.

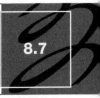

SHORTNESS OF BREATH
Robert M. Theal

8.7

I. **BACKGROUND.** Shortness of breath, or dyspnea, accounts for 3.7% of all visits to medical clinics (1).

II. **PATHOPHYSIOLOGY.** Fortunately, only a handful of disorders cause most of the cases; therefore, the most economical approach is to exclude acute life-threatening problems during the initial clinical examination. These include pneumonia, pulmonary embolus, acute heart failure, toxic exposure or ingestion, myocardial infarction, pneumothorax, life-threatening neuromuscular disease, or airway obstruction. If these are unlikely, the next step is to then systematically evaluate the patient for the most frequent disorders using common tests.

Shortness of breath has a long differential diagnosis, but respiratory and cardiac diseases account for 85% of the cases; in the remaining 15%, only a few illnesses are usually found (2). Of all the final diagnoses in patients with dyspnea, the frequency of asthma is 18% to 33% and chronic obstructive pulmonary disease is 9% to 19% (1–4). Congestive heart failure (CHF) or pulmonary edema represents 11% to 63% of the cases (1–4). Other important diagnoses are deconditioning or obesity in 3% to 5% (1–4). Final diagnoses ranging between 0% and 10% include interstitial lung disease and ischemic heart disease (1–4). Table 8.7.1 lists less common diagnoses.

III. **EVALUATION.** The initial history, physical examination, and chest x-ray (CXR) are diagnostic in 66% to 92% of the patients (1).

   A. **History.** Are historical features helpful? Historical findings are neither sensitive nor specific; however, some symptoms are associated with specific diseases. Regardless of the cause, individuals associate shortness of breath with words that describe a sense of "work" or "effort" to breathe. Asthma is associated with words that denote a sense of "tightness." Patients with interstitial lung disease choose terms emphasizing the sense of "rapid" breathing. Does the patient select terms indicating difficulty with both inhalation and exhalation? This is often reported by patients with CHF (Chapter 7.5). Patients who are deconditioned select rapid, breathing more, or heavy to describe their dyspnea. Patients suffering from neuromuscular disorders select terms denoting rapid breathing or difficulty with inhalation. Is the patient younger than 40 years of age? Are the patient's symptoms episodic? Reactive airway disease and hyperventilation are associated with these terms (3).

   B. **Physical examination.** In the physical examination, focus on signs of respiratory or cardiac disease. For the respiratory system, this means a careful examination starting at the nose. Specifically, on head, eyes, ear, nose, and throat examination look for evidence of obstruction, infection, or postnasal drip. Exclude obstruction, subcutaneous emphysema, or tracheal deviation. On cardiac examination, look for evidence of cardiomegaly, S_3 gallop, or hepatojugular reflux (HJR). In this setting, HJR is very specific for CHF (1). Assess the lungs for abnormal breath sound intensity, rales, wheezing, rhonchi, or tachypnea. Examine the chest for abnormal movements

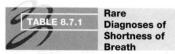

TABLE 8.7.1	Rare Diagnoses of Shortness of Breath

Anemia Acidosis

Thyroid disease

Neuromuscular disease

Pulmonary infection

Pulmonary embolus

Pulmonary hypertension

Pulmonary effusion

Neoplasia

Airway obstruction

Arrhythmia

Acute myocardial infarction

Atrial septal defect

Ventricular septal defect

Mitral stenosis

Pericardial disease

Chest wall deformity

Gastroesophageal reflux disease

Postnasal drip

Sleep apnea

Hyperventilation

[a]Frequencies between 0% and 5%.

or deformities. Exclude abdominal masses, ascites, pregnancy, or abdominal distention. Evaluate the extremities for edema, tenderness, or asymmetry. Perform a complete neurologic examination, and screen for weakness atrophy, sensory loss, and fasciculations.

C. Testing

1. Most patients require a CXR and pulse oximetry to screen for cardiac and pulmonary diseases. Use an arterial blood gas (ABG) analysis to confirm hypoxia, hypercapnia, hypocapnia, and acidosis. Complete blood count (CBC), electrolytes, thyroid-stimulating hormone (TSH), and drug screens are useful for suspected cases of anemia, acidosis, hyperthyroidism, hypothyroidism, or drug ingestions.

2. Pulmonary function tests (PFTs) are important to document the presence of obstructive or restrictive lung diseases. A methacholine challenge test is used if the symptoms are intermittent, if the patient is younger than 40 years of age, or if lung disease is suspected and the PFTs are normal. In this setting, the results will confirm or exclude asthma (2). In patients with dyspnea, a diffusing capacity of lung for carbon monoxide (DLCO) has a high positive predictive value and a high negative predictive value for interstitial lung disease (2). Low maximal inspiratory and expiratory pressures suggest neuromuscular disease.

3. An electrocardiogram (ECG) or exercise stress test (EST) screens for arrhythmias and ischemic heart disease. **Warning:** A negative EST does not exclude ischemia in patients with dyspnea (2) (Chapter 7.1). The cardiac causes of dyspnea are CHF, intracardiac shunts, valvular heart disease, pulmonary hypertension, and pericardial disease. They have abnormal or characteristic findings on echocardiography and Doppler echocardiography.

4. Other tests are used in selected patients. A high-resolution computed tomography (CT) scan of the chest detects early interstitial lung disease in patients with normal CXR films. Electromyogram (EMG) and nerve conduction studies are useful for confirming and differentiating the most common neuromuscular problems: myasthenia gravis and Guillain-Barré syndrome. A therapeutic response to H_2 blockers confirms gastroesophageal reflux disease (GERD) in most patients with dyspnea (3). Screen for acute or chronic pulmonary embolism with a nuclear medicine ventilation and perfusion ($\dot{V}/\dot{Q}$) scan.

IV. **DIAGNOSIS.** The initial assessment usually requires a clinical evaluation, CXR, and pulse oximetry. This identifies about 70% of the underlying diseases (1). For the remainder, a systematic evaluation for the most common diseases correctly identifies the cause. If appropriate, consider obtaining an ECG, CBC, TSH, and electrolytes. If these are nondiagnostic, further testing is then indicated.

  A. Exclude pulmonary diseases if the initial evaluation is nondiagnostic, or if pulmonary diseases are suspected, which account for 75% of the cases (2). Start with PFTs and an ABG. If the PFTs are normal, order a methacholine challenge test to rule out asthma. If interstitial lung disease is suspected or if the PFTs show a restrictive pattern, then order a DLCO. Abnormally low maximal inspiratory and expiratory pressures suggest neuromuscular disease. Confirm the diagnosis with an EMG.

  B. When pulmonary disease has been excluded, or if cardiac disease is suspected, the next step should be a cardiac evaluation. An echocardiogram suggests or identifies most of the cardiac causes. If the echocardiogram is normal, consider exercise stress testing or a Holter monitor. If these are normal, most patients will have either GERD or deconditioning, or psychogenic disorders. Other low frequency causes of shortness of breath that need further evaluation include neuromuscular diseases, pulmonary emboli, postnasal drip, and sleep apnea. With a clinical suspicion of these disorders, obtain an EMG, $\dot{V}/\dot{Q}$ scan, or polysomnogram. Otherwise, they are not indicated.

References

1. Mulrow CD, Lucey CR, Farnett LE. Discriminating causes of dyspnea through clinical examination. *J Gen Intern Med* 1993;8:383–392.
2. Pratter MR, Curley FJ, Dubois J, et al. Cause and evaluation of chronic dyspnea in a pulmonary disease clinic. *Arch Intern Med* 1989;149:2277–2282.
3. DePaso WJ, Winterbauer RH, Lusk JA, et al. Chronic dyspnea unexplained by history, physical examination, chest roentgenogram, and spirometry. *Chest* 1991;100:1293–1299.
4. Schmitt BP, Kushner MS, Wiener SL. The diagnostic usefulness of the history of the patient with dyspnea. *J Gen Intern Med* 1986;1:386–393.

Suggested Readings

Mahler DA, Harver A, Lentine T, et al. Descriptors of breathlessness in cardiorespiratory diseases. *Am J Respir Crit Care Med* 1996;154:1357–1363.

STRIDOR
Alexandra Duke and Tahany Maurice-Habashy

8.8

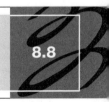

I. **BACKGROUND.** Stridor is a common type of wheezing (Chapter 8.9). It is characterized by a harsh, raspy, medium-pitched sound, produced as air flows through a partially blocked airway. It is usually seen in early childhood.

II. **PATHOPHYSIOLOGY.** Stridor can be inspiratory, indicating an obstruction at or above the larynx; or expiratory, indicating an obstruction below the larynx. Biphasic

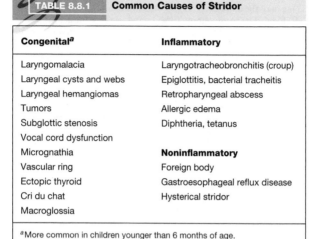

TABLE 8.8.1   Common Causes of Stridor

Congenital[a]	Inflammatory
Laryngomalacia	Laryngotracheobronchitis (croup)
Laryngeal cysts and webs	Epiglottitis, bacterial tracheitis
Laryngeal hemangiomas	Retropharyngeal abscess
Tumors	Allergic edema
Subglottic stenosis	Diphtheria, tetanus
Vocal cord dysfunction	
Micrognathia	**Noninflammatory**
Vascular ring	Foreign body
Ectopic thyroid	Gastroesophageal reflux disease
Cri du chat	Hysterical stridor
Macroglossia	

[a]More common in children younger than 6 months of age.

stridor is an obstruction in the trachea; it is heard with inspiration and expiration. When hoarseness or aphonia accompanies stridor, the vocal cords are involved (see Table 8.8.1) (1–5).

III. EVALUATION

A. History

1. **Characteristics of stridor.** When confronted with stridor, check the age of the patient and the duration of the symptoms. A child younger than 6 months of age with stridor lasting a few weeks to months has a congenital cause of stridor. A patient older than 6 months of age with stridor lasting hours to days usually has an acquired cause of stridor, most commonly viral croup, epiglottitis, or aspiration of a foreign body.

   a. A typical history is a child younger than 6 years of age with a 2- to 3-day history of upper respiratory infection (URI) and gradually worsening cough, especially at night. A barking cough with the inspiratory stridor heralds the diagnosis of croup, which accounts for 90% of all cases of stridor. This condition classically improves with moist air (1, 3).

   b. A history of choking, coughing, or gagging points to aspiration or ingestion of a foreign body.

   c. In older children and adults, a concomitant sore throat and fever may indicate acute supraglottitis, which constitutes an emergency.

2. Other information

   a. It is necessary to learn whether the stridor is acute, recurrent, or chronic.

   b. A personal or family history of atopy suggests spasmodic croup, which presents with stridor at night, not necessarily associated with a URI.

B. Physical examination

1. Focused physical examination

   a. The examination should include vital signs, notably temperature and respiratory rate, and pulse, with an emphasis on general appearance, and examination of the head and neck, including ears, nose, and throat.

   b. Signs of respiratory distress may be present, including dyspnea, tachypnea, chest retractions, nasal flaring, and stridor. If cyanosis is present, this is an ominous sign (2, 4) (Chapter 8.2).

2. Additional physical examination

   a. A toxic-appearing child with high fever has drooling, severe respiratory distress, and a preference for a sitting and forward-leaning position (1, 4).

b. Varying degrees of anxiety, which increase during examination, cause a worsening of stridor (1,4).

C. Testing

1. The best test is a lateral neck x-ray study to assist with a diagnosis that is mostly made on clinical grounds. Films of the larynx and trachea in anteroposterior and lateral neck views may show a narrowing of the trachea or extrinsic pressure on the tracheobronchial airway. Acutely, lateral neck radiographs showing the classic swollen glottis described by some as a thumbprint assist with the diagnosis of acute supraglottitis and eminent respiratory collapse. Chest x-ray studies are of little value. Films showing hyperinflation or bronchial thickening may help to make a diagnosis of asthma, rather than stridor. Additionally, foreign body aspiration or mass is elucidated in x-ray studies (2).

2. Tomograms or a computed tomography (CT) scan of the neck may provide additional information, especially in chronic stridor (2).

3. Blood tests (e.g., complete blood count) can be useful in the acutely ill patient, especially if viral or bacterial infection is suspected.

4. If it is suspected that the stridor is a result of a laryngomalacia or laryngeal lesions such as papilloma, direct laryngoscopy is the test of choice for accurate diagnosis. Direct observation through fiber-optic bronchoscope positioned in the pharynx provides diagnostic views of the larynx (2,4).

IV. DIAGNOSIS.

In making the diagnosis of stridor, two key elements exist: acute onset in a toxic-appearing patient versus chronic stridor in a relatively stable patient.

A. Acute stridor

1. The most likely cause of acute stridor in the febrile child with the additional features of barking cough and antecedent coryza is laryngotracheobronchitis or croup. Acute stridor is a non–life-threatening condition accounting for 90% of stridor cases. Classically, it improves with exposure to moist air. It has a viral cause, usually from one of the following: respiratory syncytial virus, rhinovirus, adenovirus, parainfluenza virus, or influenza virus. Generally, this diagnosis is made on clinical grounds (1). The child is less ill and, although often febrile, not toxic appearing. The entire illness usually abates in 5 days. Hospitalization, unlike with epiglottitis, is rarely needed (2).

2. In the toxic patient with fever, respiratory distress, sore throat, or drooling, especially in the younger age-group, epiglottitis—a medical emergency—should be considered. Use of the *Haemophilus influenzae* vaccine has increased in recent years; therefore, acute epiglottitis is becoming increasingly rare. *H. influenzae* is the most common bacterial cause of stridor, although streptococcus, staphylococcus, and viral agents are also possible causes.

3. The patient with a history of suspected foreign body aspiration has similar symptoms without fever. Foreign body aspiration is common in 1- to 2-year-old children, although it does occur in adults. It can be a cause of chronic stridor (3).

4. Additionally, an acute allergic reaction can cause stridor. The history should herald a possible offending agent and, although respiratory collapse may be eminent, the patient is not toxic, as no infectious agent is involved.

5. Trauma can also cause laryngeal damage; however, the history assists with this diagnosis.

B. Chronic stridor.

For the most part, these causes of stridor occur in early childhood. With the exception of laryngeal papillomas, tumors, and subglottic stenosis after instrumentation, as in intubation (there is a congenital form also), foreign body aspiration with partial obstruction and hysterical stridor can occur at any age. Laryngomalacia and laryngeal lesions are caused by webs, hemangiomas, and cysts; they are usually identified early in life (1–3).

References

1. Pryor MP. Noisy breathing in children. *Postgrad Med* 1997;101:103–112.
2. Behrman RE, Kliegman RM, Arvin AM. *Nelson textbook of pediatrics.* Philadelphia, PA: WB Saunders, 1996:241, 1173, 1198,1238.

3. Behrman RE, Vaughan VC. *Nelson textbook of pediatrics*. Philadelphia, PA: WB Saunders, 1983:1031–1032,1076–1077.
4. Tintinalli JE, Ruiz E, Krome RL. *Emergency medicine: a comprehensive study guide*. New York: McGraw-Hill, 1996:247–251.
5. Campbell AGM, MacIntosh N. *Textbook of pediatrics*. London: Pearson Ltd, 1998: 508–513,563.

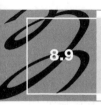

WHEEZING
Thomas C. Bent

I. **BACKGROUND.** Wheezing is one of the most common respiratory complaints to present to primary care physicians.

II. **PATHOPHYSIOLOGY.** Although asthma and chronic obstructive pulmonary disease (COPD) account for most cases of wheezing, there are multiple causes. The National Asthma Education and Prevention Program (NAEPP) recommends an accurate diagnosis be made by medical history, physical, and spirometry (1).

A. **Wheezing in infants, children, and adults.** The reasons why patients wheeze vary dramatically, depending on age. For example, whereas asthma is the most common chronic pediatric disease in industrialized nations, inhalant allergens appear to be unimportant precipitants of wheezing in infancy (2) (see Table 8.9.1). Wheezing that begins in infancy or early childhood is associated with progressive and persistent disease (3).

B. **Wheezing versus stridor.** Stridor, discussed in Chapter 8.8, is characterized as an inspiratory wheeze that implies major obstruction of the upper airway. Wheezing, in contrast, is defined as high-pitched, continuous (or long duration) lung sounds that are superimposed on the normal breath sounds (4). The inspiratory phase of respiration is usually normal, and the expiratory phase is prolonged. Unfortunately, the difference is not always obvious to the clinician. Vocal cord dysfunction, which is a psychosomatic disorder, can be difficult to differentiate from asthma. These episodes can include both inspiratory and expiratory wheezing and an upper airway cause is not clear (5).

TABLE 8.9.1   **Etiology of Wheezing by Age-Group**

Infants
Bronchiolitis, pertussis, recurrent aspiration during feeding, gastroesophageal reflux disease, foreign body inhalation, bronchopulmonary dysplasia, cystic fibrosis, tracheoesophageal fistula, congenital malformations
Children
Asthma, bronchiolitis, tracheomalacia, gastroesophageal reflux, sinusitis, foreign bodies, cystic fibrosis, and pulmonary hemosiderosis
Adults
Asthma, chronic obstructive pulmonary disease, acute infections, foreign body inhalation, intra-airway tumor, extrinsic tumor with airway compression, interstitial lung disease

III. EVALUATION

A. History

1. **Onset.** Is this the first episode? If so, were there problems with wheezing or asthma in childhood?
2. **Exposures.** Triggers to wheezing should be identified and controlled (1).
   a. Cigarette smoke is one of the most potent and ubiquitous avoidable allergens.
   b. Occupational exposures can frequently be identified, especially between agricultural and industrial workers.
   c. Family or household exposure to tuberculosis or pertussis can indicate an infectious cause.
3. **Comorbid conditions.** Has the patient recently suffered an upper respiratory infection or sinusitis? Is there a history of gastroesophageal reflux disease? Congestive heart failure? Aspirin sensitivity? Allergic rhinitis?
4. **Family history.** A history of asthma, allergies, or atopic disease in family members can support the diagnosis of asthma.
5. **Past history.** A childhood history of atopic disease or allergies suggests adult onset asthma. Past history of exercise-induced wheezing also supports this diagnosis.
6. **Psychosocial aspects.** Emotional stress can lead to exacerbation of chronic asthma. Psychogenic wheezing is a conversion disorder, which can coexist with other psychopathology.

B. Physical examination

1. **Vital signs.** A complete set of vital signs is essential to the assessment of the patient with wheezing. The respiratory rate and the pulse are a more objective, and often more accurate, assessment of the severity of wheezing, rather than the auditory volume of the wheezing itself. Fever suggests a concurrent respiratory infection. Hypotension is an ominous sign that points to a decompensating patient.
2. **Lung examination.** During auscultation, note the location, intensity, and the duration of wheezing. Wheezing caused by asthma, COPD, or interstitial disease should be diffuse and symmetric and present during expiration. The expiratory phase is prolonged. Focal obstruction (e.g., tumors and foreign bodies) can give asymmetric findings and inspiratory wheezing. Mucous plugging changes with cough. Rhonchi and crackles suggest a concurrent infectious process. Percussion and egophony can be present with consolidation.

C. Testing

1. **Pulmonary function.** A peak flowmeter is a valuable initial assessment of airway obstruction, and can be done quickly and cheaply in the office. It is also an excellent measurement of progression of disease or success of treatment. Pulse oximetry is another quick, noninvasive office technique to assess the severity of both chronic disease and acute respiratory distress. Full spirometry, although not available in all primary care offices, gives additional diagnostic information that can differentiate among asthma, COPD, and fixed airway obstruction.
2. **Chest x-ray.** Plain chest films identify consolidation, masses, mediastinal shifts, and hyperaeration.
3. **Clinical laboratory tests.** A complete blood count may demonstrate signs of an acute bacterial infection. Polycythemia is a sign of chronic hypoxia (Chapter 16.5). Eosinophilia can indicate asthma or allergic disease (Chapter 16.2). Angiotensin-converting enzyme levels are elevated in sarcoidosis. A tuberculin skin test should be considered in all patients with wheezing or chronic cough.

IV. DIAGNOSIS

A. Differential diagnosis.

The history and physical examination are the key elements to an acute diagnosis. A consistent exposure or reaction history, coupled with an elevated serum immunoglobulin E or eosinophilia, indicates allergic disease. Wheezing in the setting of acute bronchitis or sinusitis is not true asthma, and the patient can be reassured that this is not the beginning of a chronic disease. Inspiratory wheezing, or stridor, indicates upper airway obstruction or psychogenic wheezing. A normal, or nearly normal, peak flow is reassurance that good air exchange is occurring, regardless of the loudness of the wheezing. The pulse oximetry differentiates between severe obstruction and poor cooperation with the peak flow testing. When confusion still exists, spirometry clarifies the diagnosis in most cases.

B. Clinical manifestations. The immediate assessment of the patient with acute wheezing is essential. Regardless of whether the patient presents with an initial episode or a chronic condition, it is necessary to determine the degree of airway obstruction and the potential deterioration of the patient quickly. The reduction in the intensity of wheezing can indicate acute decompensation, as air obstruction becomes too severe to allow the mechanical sounds of wheezing.

References

1. Key clinical activities for quality asthma care: recommendations of the National Asthma Education and Prevention Program. www.guidelines.gov/summary/summary.aspx?doc_id=3734&nbr=2960&string=asthma, accessed on May, 2006.
2. Martinati LC, Boner AL. Clinical diagnosis of wheezing in early childhood. *Allergy* 1995;50:701–710.
3. Castro-Rodríguez JA, et al. A clinical index to define risk of asthma in young children with recurrent wheezing. *Am J Respir Crit Care Med* 2000;162:1403–1406. http://www.aafp.org/afp/20010501/tips/12.html.
4. Meslier N, Charbonneau G, Racineux JL. Wheezes. *Eur Respir J* 1995;8:1942–1948.
5. Goldman J. All that wheezes is not asthma. *Practitioner* 1997;241:35–38.

Gastrointestinal Problems

Michael R. Spieker

9

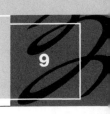

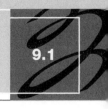

ABDOMINAL PAIN
David R. Congdon

9.1

I. **BACKGROUND.** Abdominal pain is a common complaint and comprises up to 5% of total visits to the emergency department. The etiology may be quite varied and may result from extra-abdominal pathology or intra-abdominal sources.

II. **PATHOPHYSIOLOGY.** The common reasons for abdominal pain that causes concern are presented in Table 9.1.1 (1). Selected causes of severe abdominal pain are listed in Table 9.1.2.

III. **EVALUATION**
   A. **History**
      1. The history should include the following: **P**alliative/alleviating factors, **Q**uality of pain, **R**adiation or referred pain pattern, **S**everity, and **T**ime of onset/temporal

TABLE 9.1.1	Common Causes of Abdominal Pain

Diagnosis	Etiology	Epidemiology
Acute appendicitis	Appendiceal obstruction, inflammation, ischemia	Adolescence to young adulthood
		Higher perforation rate in children, women, and elderly
		Mortality rate of 0.1% (2%–6% with perforation)
Biliary tract disease	Stone in cystic or common duct is the typical cause.	Peak age of 35–60 y
		Rare in patients <20 y of age
		Female-to-male ratio of 3:1
		Risk factors: multiparity, obesity, alcohol intake, birth control pills
Ureteral colic	Family history, dehydration, urinary tract infections, certain medications	Average age of 30–40 y, less common in children
Diverticulitis	Diverticular infection/inflammation or perforation; peritonitis may develop.	Incidence increases with advancing age; occurs in men more than in women
		Recurrences are common.
Peptic ulcer	Sometimes associated with *Helicobacter pylori* infection.	Occurs in all age-groups; peaks at the age of 50 y
	Risk factors include nonsteroidal anti-inflammatory drug use, tobacco and alcohol use.	Men affected twice as much as women. Severe bleeding or perforation is rare.

King KE, Wightman JM. Abdominal pain. In: Marx JA, ed. *Rosen's emergency medicine: concepts and clinical practice*, 5th ed. St. Louis, MO: Mosby, 2002:185–194.

TABLE 9.1.2	Selected Life-threatening Causes of Abdominal Pain	
Ruptured aortic aneurysm	Atherosclerosis, intimal dissection; leakage causes shock.	More frequent in men Risk factors: hypertension, diabetes mellitus, smoking, chronic obstructive pulmonary disease, coronary artery disease
Acute pancreatitis	Obstructive biliary stone, alcohol, hypertriglyceridemia, hypercalcemia.	More frequent in men, rare in childhood
Mesenteric ischemia	Often multifactorial, including transient hypotension in the presence of atherosclerosis. Thrombosis occurs in up to 65% of cases.	Most common in elderly people with cerebrovascular disease, congestive heart failure, diabetes mellitus

relationships. The character of pain is particularly helpful (e.g., colicky, steady, sharp, burning, tearing, gnawing). The associated symptoms should be identified (e.g., dysuria, hematuria, hematochezia, change in bowel habits, persistent vomiting). The exact sequence of symptoms may be especially helpful. For example, in acute appendicitis, pain and anorexia typically precede point tenderness.

2. A thorough gynecologic history should be performed in all women with abdominal pain, and pregnancy (including ectopic pregnancy) should be considered. The last normal menstrual period should be determined.

3. Small bowel obstruction in patients with prior abdominal surgery should be considered. Alarming symptoms generally involve escalating symptoms, fever, profound illness, and extremes of age.

B. Physical examination

1. Analysis of the general appearance is especially helpful. Patients with colicky (hollow viscus obstruction) pain often writhe about, seeking a comfortable position. Peritonitis causes patients to be still and jarring the bed or heel tap may exacerbate the pain. Check complete vital signs, identify fever, tachycardia, or hypotension. The abdomen should be inspected for distension, pulsations, or ecchymosis (Grey Turner's or Cullen's sign). It is necessary to auscultate for the presence of bowel sounds or bruits suggestive of aneurysms. Bowel sounds are sometimes absent in appendicitis.

2. Palpation begins distal to areas of pain and should be gentle. Guarding and rigidity should be noted. Masses and organomegaly should be assessed. Murphy's sign may help identify gallbladder pathology. The iliopsoas and obturator signs may indicate appendicitis. Genital examination is important to exclude hernia and a rectal examination may help identify a retrocecal appendicitis.

C. Testing

1. **Laboratory evaluation.** It is necessary to obtain a serum human chorionic gonadotropin from any patient who could potentially be pregnant. Electrolytes can rule out metabolic abnormalities such as hypercalcemia. A complete blood count should be considered in infectious etiologies and for the purpose of monitoring hematocrit stability and platelet count. Elevated liver tests can identify hepatocellular or obstructive biliary disease. Elevated amylase may be found in pancreatitis, salivary disease, mesenteric ischemia, and fallopian pathology. Lipase is very specific to the pancreas. Urinalysis is useful to exclude urinary tract infections. Hematuria is found in 90% of renal stones. Pyuria can be present when an inflammatory mass (e.g., appendicitis) is close to the urinary tract (2).

TABLE 9.1.3	Types of Abdominal Pain
Visceral pain	Results from stretching nerve fibers surrounding an organ; may be crampy or colicky, often intermittent; many times located in midline. This type of pain is often ill-defined and diffuse. Examples include appendicitis, cholecystitis, bowel obstruction, and renal colic. Foregut structures often refer to the epigastrium (stomach, duodenum, pancreatic-biliary tree), and midgut structures (small bowel, ascending colon) refer to periumbilical area. Hindgut structures (descending colon) often refer to the suprapubic area or the back.
Somatic pain	Arises from pain fibers in parietal peritoneum; usually sharper, localized, and more constant; may develop after visceral pain. Usually it represents peritoneal inflammation from various sources (bleeding, chemical irritation, infectious causes) and most often causes great concern.
Referred pain	Defined as pain felt at a distance from the diseased organ. Diaphragmatic irritation often radiates to shoulders, and ureteral colic often radiates to groin. Referred pain is often localized to the developmental dermatome and can be misleading in localizing the source (4).

   2. Imaging. Plain film acute abdominal series (upright and supine) identify free air and abnormal gas patterns. Plain films may identify calcifications associated with renal stones (85%), biliary lithiasis (15%), and pneumonia as an extra-abdominal cause for pain. Ultrasound is useful to rule out ectopic pregnancy, appendicitis, biliary tract disease, abdominal aortic aneurysm, and hydroureter. Computed tomography (CT) scan is largely replacing other modalities, because it provides a quick accurate imaging modality to detect appendicitis, urolithiasis, cholecystitis, diverticulitis, and pancreatitis. In elderly patients with abdominal pain, CT scan alters the initial diagnosis in 45% of cases and affects admission decisions in 26% of cases (3).

IV. DIAGNOSIS
   A. Differential diagnosis. The differential diagnosis is usually broad and frequently reconsidered. If a chosen treatment modality is unsuccessful, the working diagnosis must be questioned and the differential diagnosis expanded. Serial examination and close follow-up are necessary if the diagnosis is in question.
   B. Clinical manifestations. Patterns associated with the different types of abdominal pain are presented in Table 9.1.3. Multiple causes necessitate a broad differential diagnosis. Numerous diagnostic modalities exist, including physical examination, laboratory studies, and ancillary studies.

References
1. King KE, Wightman JM. Abdominal pain. In: Marx JA, ed. *Rosen's emergency medicine: concepts and clinical practice*, 5th ed. St. Louis, MO: Mosby, 2002:185–194.
2. Kamin RA, Nowicki TA, Courtney DS, et al. Pearls and pitfalls in the emergency department evaluation of abdominal pain. *Emerg Med Clin North Am* 2003;21:61–72.
3. Esses D, Birnbaum A, Bijur P, et al. Ability of CT to alter decision making in elderly patients with acute abdominal pain. *Am J Emerg Med* 2004;22:270–272.
4. Fales WD, Overton DT. Abdominal pain. In: Tintinalli JE, ed. *Emergency medicine*, 4th ed. New York, NY: McGraw-Hill, 1996:217–221.

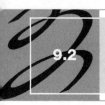

ASCITES
William M. Lucas

I. **BACKGROUND.** Ascites is a fluid collection in the peritoneal cavity. In approximately 85% of the patients in the United States with ascites, hepatic cirrhosis is the etiology (1), and the second most common cause is carcinomatosis. The 5-year survival rate for patients with ascites is 30% to 40% (2). Liver transplant increases the chances of survival by 40% (2).

II. **PATHOPHYSIOLOGY.** The most common cause of ascites—cirrhosis—leads to increased portal pressures followed by development of collateral flow through lower pressure pathways. Portal hypertension triggers the release of nitric oxide, causing vasodilatation and an enlarged intravascular space. The body attempts to correct this perceived hypovolemia by triggering vasoconstrictor and antinatiuretic factors that lead to salt and fluid retention, thereby interrupting the balance among the Starling forces

TABLE 9.2.1   **Paracentesis Fluid Findings and Their Significance**

Characteristic	Specific findings	Significance
Appearance	Clear	Cirrhosis
	Turbid/cloudy	Infection
	Opalescent	Elevated triglyceride concentration
	Milky	Elevated triglyceride concentration
	Pink/bloody	Traumatic tap, malignancy
	Brown	Patient with jaundice, ruptured gallbladder, duodenal ulcer
Cell count and differential	Polymorphonuclear leukocytes count >250	Spontaneous bacterial peritonitis
Serum to ascites albumin gradient (serum albumin − ascites albumin) (g/dL)		
	>1.1	**Portal hypertension**-cirrhosis, alcoholic hepatitis, compression from large liver metastases, portal vein thrombosis, Budd-Chiari Syndrome, cardiac ascites, acute fatty liver of pregnancy, myxedema, mixed ascites
	<1.1	**No portal hypertension**-present, peritoneal carcinomatosis (most common), tuberculosis, pancreatic or biliary ascites, bowel infarction or obstruction, nephritic syndrome

that maintain fluid hemostasis. Then, fluid "sweats" from the surface of the liver and collects in the abdominal cavity. The kidneys eventually lose their ability to clear free water, causing a dilutional hyponatremia and ultimately hepatorenal syndrome.

III. EVALUATION

A. History. The history should focus on alcohol consumption, transfusions, human immunodeficiency virus and hepatitis risk factors, tattoos, family history of liver disease, obesity, diabetes, hyperlipidemia, and tuberculosis risk factors.

B. Physical examination. Detecting ascites by physical examination is variably sensitive and examiner dependent. Approximately 1,500 mL of fluid must be present to identify ascites reliably. Of the specific physical examination techniques described to detect ascites, flank dullness is the most reliable predictor. Fluid wave and puddle signs are of little clinical value. Spider angiomas, palmer erythema, muscle wasting, large abdominal wall collateral veins, and jaundice are suggestive of portal hypertension.

C. Testing. Following confirmation of ascites by ultrasound, all patients with ascites should be evaluated with a diagnostic paracentesis. Other indications of paracentesis include fever, abdominal pain, tenderness, hypotension, ileus, renal failure, mental status changes, and therapeutic relief of excess fluid. Coagulopathy is not a contraindication to this procedure and rarely causes complications except in the setting of disseminated intravascular coagulopathy. Paracentesis findings and their significance are described in Table 9.2.1, while their association is presented in Table 9.2.2. Paracentesis fluid analysis of pH, lactate, cholesterol, and fibronectin are unhelpful in diagnosis (3). When obtaining cultures, 10 to 20 cc of peritoneal fluid should be collected at the bedside for best results.

IV. DIAGNOSIS

A. Differential diagnosis. The differential diagnosis of ascites is listed in Table 9.2.3. Uncommon causes include trauma to lymphatics or ureters, *Chlamydia*, nephrotic syndrome, serositis in connective tissue disease, myxedema, acquired immunodeficiency syndrome, and Fitz-Hugh-Curtis syndrome.

B. Clinical manifestations. The symptoms of ascites are nausea, anorexia, early satiety, heartburn, increased abdominal girth, shortness of breath, abdominal pain, orthopnea, weight gain, and leg swelling. Physical findings include fever, encephalopathy, jaundice, jugular venous distension, gastrointestinal bleeding, bulging flanks, abdominal distension, hepatomegaly, splenomegaly, penile and scrotal edema, or umbilical hernia.

 TABLE 9.2.2 **Clinical Association of Paracentesis Fluid Results**

Characteristic	Association
Amylase	Elevated in small bowel or pancreatic injury
LDH	In uncomplicated ascites, LDH is fewer than half the serum values. Peritonitis > SBP > serum LDH.
Glucose concentration	Mildly depressed in carcinomatosis and SBP. In bowel perforation or late SBP the glucose level may be as low as 0.
Cytology	This is of benefit when carcinomatosis is present. This test requires the release of malignant cells into the ascitic fluid, sensitivity 67% of all malignancy related cases.
Renal panel	Assess for hepatorenal syndrome.

LDH, lactate dehydrogenase; SBP, spontaneous bacterial peritonitis.

TABLE 9.2.3 **Differential Diagnosis of Ascites**

Cause	Comment
Cirrhosis	Etiology in ~80% of ascites (3)
Alcoholic hepatitis	
Carcinomatosis	Two thirds of malignancy-related ascites
Metastases	One third of malignancy-related ascites
Congestive heart failure	History of heart failure or severe lung disease
Tuberculosis	Cause in ~1% of ascites (3)
Hepatitis B and C	Leads to cirrhosis
Pancreatic disease	Ascites amylase is five times the serum values
Wilson's disease	Effects range from liver test abnormalities to hepatic failure
Hemochromatosis	Iron deposition causes cirrhosis
Constrictive pericarditis	Leads to hepatic congestion
Mixed ascites	~5% (cirrhosis + another etiology)

References

1. Runyon BA. Management of adult patients with ascites due to cirrhosis. AASLLD practice guidelines. *Hepatology* 2004;39:1–16.
2. Gines P, Cardenas A, Arroyo V, et al. Current concepts: management of cirrhosis and ascites. *N Engl J Med* 2004;350:1646–1654.
3. Haubrich WS, Schaffner F, Brek J, et al. *Bockus gastroenterology.* 5th ed. Philadelphia, PA: WB Saunders, 1994:2009.

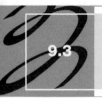

9.3 CONSTIPATION
Joseph T. LaVan

$\mathcal{C}$onstipation is a symptom, and not a diagnosis. Most cases of constipation are "functional" or idiopathic in nature, so evaluation is targeted at identifying the few causes that can be corrected. Once these causes have been ruled out, treatment is symptomatic.

I. **BACKGROUND.** The meaning of "constipation" varies from patient to patient and provider to provider. In 1999, an international panel developed a consensus definition for constipation (1). The Rome-II criteria (see Table 9.3.1) helped standardize research and offer an objective path to clinical diagnosis.

II. **PATHOPHYSIOLOGY.** The colon and rectum are responsible for both digestive and excretive functions, including continued mixing of the output of the ileum, further processing of undigested carbohydrate (including digestion and absorption), absorption of water to create semisolid or solid stool, and ultimately evacuation of stool from the body. These processes are coordinated through a variety of neurotransmitters, a parasympathetic neural plexus and a variety of other voluntary and involuntary mechanisms.

A. **Etiology.** Changes in the texture of the stool, the peristaltic function or internal diameter of the colon or the expulsive function of the rectum and pelvic floor can lead to constipation (2, 3). Table 9.3.2 lists some of the more common causes.

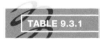

TABLE 9.3.1   **Rome-II Criteria for the Diagnosis of Functional Constipation**

Adults

- Two or more of the following symptoms are present at least 12 wk in 12 mo (not required to be consecutive):
  - Straining during more than one in four bowel movements
  - Lumpy or hard stools during more than one in four bowel movements
  - Sensation of incomplete defecation in more than one in four bowel movements
  - Sensation of blockage or obstruction in anus or rectum during more than one in four bowel movements
  - Use of manual maneuvers (e.g., digital expression of stool, pelvic floor support) with more than one in four bowel movements
  - Fewer than three bowel movements per week
- Absence of diarrhea or loose stools
- Symptoms do not meet the criteria for irritable bowel syndrome

Infants and young children

- Two or more weeks of one of the following symptoms:
  - Hard stools (pebblelike = scybalous) in most bowel movements
  - LESS THAN three FIRM stools per week
- Symptoms not explained by a metabolic, endocrine, or anatomic cause

Adapted with permission from Thompson WG, Longstreth GF, Drossman DA, et al. Functional bowel disorders and functional abdominal pain (Rome II: a multinational consensus document on functional gastrointestinal disorders). *Gut* 1999;45(suppl 2):1143–1147.

TABLE 9.3.2   **Causes of Constipation (Rated by the Likelihood of Being a Cause of Constipation)**

Functional (common)

Low-fiber diet
Sedentary lifestyle
Dehydration
Slow transit time
Outlet delay
Irritable bowel syndrome
Inflammatory bowel disease
Excessive milk intake
Stool withholding

Medications (less common)

Antacids
Anticholinergics
Antidepressants
Calcium channel blockers
Cholestyramine
Nonsteroidal anti-inflammatory drugs
Clonidine
Diuretics
Sinemet
Narcotics
Sympathomimetics
Psychotropics

Structural (less common)

Anal fissures
Hemorrhoids
Colonic strictures
Diverticulitis
Ischemia
Radiation colitis
Adenocarcinoma
Imperforate anus
Pelvic masses

Neurogenic (rare)

Cerebrovascular events
Multiple sclerosis
Parkinson's disease
Hirschsprung's disease
Spinal cord tumors or abnormalities
Cerebral palsy
Chagas disease
Botulism
Down syndrome
Prune-belly syndrome

Endocrine/metabolic (rare)

Diabetes mellitus
Hypercalcemia
Hyperparathyroidism
Hypokalemia
Hypothyroidism
Uremia
Celiac disease
Cystic fibrosis
Pregnancy

Psychogenic (less common)

Anxiety
Depression
Somatization

Connective tissue (rare)

Amyloidosis
Scleroderma

Systemic lupus erythematosus

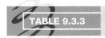

Component	Finding	Condition suggested
	History	
Age at onset	Childhood onset	Congenital causes
Duration	Acute onset	Correctable causes
	Longer duration	Functional cause
The most troubling symptom	Straining	Pelvic floor dysfunction
	Need for manual maneuvers for evacuation	
	Cramping/bloating between bowel movements	Irritable bowel syndrome
Medication history	See the list of common offenders in Table 9.3.2	
	Physical examination	
Digital rectal examination	Tender puborectalis	Puborectalis spasm
	Inability to expel rectal finger	Pelvic floor dysfunction
	Rectal mass, anal stricture	Obstruction
	Anal fissure	Cause or effect?
	Impacted stool	Slow transit constipation
Simulated defecation	Laxity of anal verge	Neurogenic causes
Perineal function during simulated expulsion and retention	Low activity	Pelvic floor dysfunction
Vaginal examination (women)	Observe for rectocele	Pelvic relaxation
Neurologic examination	Other focal neurologic deficits	Neurogenic causes
Abdominal examination	Masses, scars	Causes of obstruction

TABLE 9.3.3 History and Physical Examination Findings

B. Epidemiology. Various studies have found prevalence rates ranging between 2% and 28% (4). Constipation is the reason for 2.5 million physician visits per year. Prevalence is higher in women and the elderly. Risk factors include inactivity, low-calorie diets, higher number of medications (independent of side effect profiles) and lower socioeconomic status (5). Low-fiber diets do not seem to be a risk factor.

III. EVALUATION

A. History and physical examination. The initial focus of the evaluation should be on distinguishing idiopathic constipation from secondary causes. Table 9.3.3 presents significant findings in the history and physical examination that aid in distinguishing idiopathic or functional causes from secondary causes. Most secondary causes can be identified by history, physical examination, and a limited laboratory evaluation.

B. Testing. Initial laboratory tests should include serum chemistries (including calcium and glucose), complete blood count and thyroid function tests. Additional laboratory tests such as serum protein electrophoresis, urine porphyrins, or parathyroid hormone are indicated only if the initial evaluation is abnormal. Flexible sigmoidoscopy, colonoscopy, or barium enema are indicated when obstructive symptoms are present or when the patient is older than 50 years.

C. Genetics. Although some causes of constipation have genetic components, a detailed discussion is outside the scope of this review.

IV. DIAGNOSIS

A. Differential diagnosis. The differential diagnosis of functional constipation is presented in Table 9.3.1.

B. Clinical manifestations. Although physicians seem to focus on a decreased frequency of bowel movements, patients complain of straining, infrequency, hard stools, the need to defecate without being able to, and the persistent urge to defecate immediately after a bowel movement.

References
1. Thompson WG, Longstreth GF, Drossman DA, et al. Functional bowel disorders and functional abdominal pain. (Rome II: a multinational consensus document on functional gastrointestinal disorders). *Gut* 1999;45(suppl 2):1143–1147.
2. Arce DA, Ermocilla CA, Costa H. Evaluation of constipation. *Am Fam Physician* 2002;65:2283–2290.
3. Faigel DO. A clinical approach to constipation. *Clin Cornerstone* 2002;4(4):11–21.
4. Satish-Rao SC. Constipation: evaluation and treatment. *Gastroenterol Clin North Am* 2003;32:659–683.
5. AGA Technical Review: Constipation. Up To Date 2005. http://www.uptodateonline. com/ application/topic.asp?file=gihepgui/26493&type=A &selectedTitle=7~62>.25, accessed on May-2005.

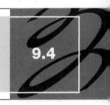

DIARRHEA
David C. Krulak

9.4

I. BACKGROUND. The clinically most useful definition of diarrhea is actually the most vague and patient-centric, namely, frequent, loose stools. These stools are often watery, excessive, and can be uncontrolled. Diarrhea can be associated with fever, abdominal cramping, weight loss, painful defecation, and bloody stools. Additionally, the duration of diarrhea is of significant clinical importance. Diarrhea of <14 days duration is termed *acute*, whereas diarrhea that extends beyond 30 days is termed *chronic*.

II. PATHOPHYSIOLOGY

A. Etiology

    1. Acute diarrhea can be infectious or noninfectious. Infectious organisms affect either the colon (often a febrile, bloody diarrhea) or small intestine (typically large volume, watery stools).

    2. Chronic diarrhea is categorized as one of four types: fatty, inflammatory, secretory, or osmotic.

        a. Fatty diarrhea contains excess stool fat, shown by direct measurement or Sudan staining.

        b. Inflammatory diarrhea demonstrates mucus, blood, and fecal leukocytes in the stool.

        c. Secretory diarrhea is watery and does not have a significant osmotic gap (<50 mOsm/kg).

        d. Osmotic diarrhea is also liquid in nature but is characterized by an osmotic gap (>125 mOsm/kg).

B. Epidemiology

    1. The epidemiology of diarrhea in the United States has not been well studied. It is well established that acute diarrhea is the leading cause of childhood death worldwide. In the US population, viruses are likely the most common cause, with bacterial infection producing most of the severe cases. In the United States, acute diarrhea rarely requires a significant diagnostic evaluation and usually no more than symptomatic oral rehydration and reassurance. However, in selected clinical settings (e.g., impoverished or immunocompromised patients), this ailment can be life threatening.

2. Chronic diarrhea is a worldwide childhood problem, with infection being the most common cause. In developed countries, chronic diarrhea is most frequently because of irritable bowel syndrome, inflammatory bowel disease, and malabsorption syndromes.

III. EVALUATION. Most patients with acute diarrhea experience a mild, self-limited illness and no laboratory testing is necessary. The challenge of the initial evaluation is to distinguish these patients from those with more serious disorders. "Red flags" associated with severe illness include hypovolemia; bloody diarrhea; fever; more than five unformed stools in 24 hours; severe abdominal pain; recent antibiotic use or hospitalization; or diarrhea in an infant, geriatric, or immunocompromised patient (1).

A. History. Evaluation of acute diarrhea begins with a history regarding occupation, travel, sexual practices, pets, and hobbies that could signal exposure to potential pathogens. Other key points include inquiries about recent fevers, medication use, a dietary history, and a complete past medical history (to determine risk of nosocomial infection or immunocompromised status). A complaint of chronic diarrhea requires a detailed history that should thoroughly explore the onset, duration, pattern, and characteristics of the stools. Major findings include significant weight loss, diarrhea for longer than one year, nocturnal diarrhea, and straining with stool. Other questions should focus on social and epidemiologic history (travel, foods, sexual practices, living conditions, water sources), family history, associated symptoms (fever, fecal incontinence, abdominal pain), and aggravating or palliative

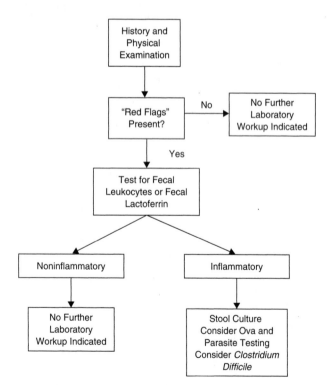

Figure 9.4.1. Laboratory evaluation of acute diarrhea. (Adapted from Thielman NM, Guerrant RL. Clinical practice. Acute infectious diarrhea. *N Engl J Med* 2004;350:38.)

factors (diet, stress, medication). A detailed medical history evaluates for iatrogenic causes (medication, surgery), immunocompromised states, and possible psychiatric pathology. A thorough review of systems provides evidence of systemic processes that can cause diarrhea such as diabetes mellitus, hyperthyroidism, rheumatologic disease, and tumors. (The physical examination in these cases is usually normal; however, an evaluation of volume and nutritional status is essential.)

B. Physical examination. Examination should focus on signs of hypovolemia (e.g., dry mucous membranes, orthostatic hypotension). Observation for fever or peritoneal signs can indicate an invasive source (2). Abdominal (masses, ascites, liver changes) and anorectal findings (loss of tone, presence of disease), lymphadenopathy, mouth ulcers, skin changes, or thyroid masses can provide diagnostic clues (3).

C. Testing. See Figures 9.4.1 and 9.4.2 for evaluation of acute and chronic diarrhea.

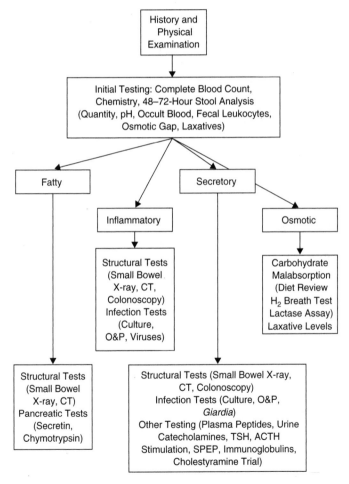

Figure 9.4.2. Laboratory evaluation of chronic diarrhea. ACTH, adrenocorticotropic hormone; CT, computed tomography; O&P, ova and parasites; SPEP, serum protein electrophoresis; TSH, thyroid-stimulating hormone. (Adapted from Fine KD, Schiller LR. AGA technical review on the evaluation and management of chronic diarrhea. *Gastroenterology* 1999;116:1464.)

IV. DIAGNOSIS

A. Differential diagnosis. See Table 9.4.1 for a differential diagnosis of diarrhea.

B. Clinical manifestations

1. Acute diarrhea features a few well-described patterns. Traveler's diarrhea commonly begins 3 to 10 days after arrival in a foreign location where the patient is exposed to foods or water contaminated with diarrheagenic *Escherichia coli*, *Salmonella*, or *Campylobacter*, among others. Diarrhea that develops within 6 hours of food ingestion is likely because of a preformed bacterial toxin. Symptoms that begin after more than 8 hours suggest a bacterial or viral infection. A febrile diarrhea is suggestive of invasive bacteria, enteric viruses, or a cytotoxic organism. If diarrhea occurs in the setting of a recent course of antibiotic therapy, *Clostridium difficile* toxin should be considered.

2. Chronic diarrhea has fewer recognizable patterns simply because of the myriad possible underlying etiologies. However, crampy abdominal pain with

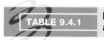

| TABLE 9.4.1 | Differential Diagnosis of Acute and Chronic Diarrhea |

Acute diarrhea

Infectious

Bacteria (*Salmonella, Campylobacter, Shigella, Escherichia coli*)

Virus (rotavirus, norovirus)

Protozoa (*Cryptosporidium, Giardia, Entamoeba histolytica*)

Noninfectious

Food intolerance

Medications

Inflammatory bowel disease

Carcinoid

Thyroid disease

Chronic diarrhea

Fatty

Intestinal malabsorption

Maldigestion

Inflammatory

Inflammatory bowel disease

Infection

Ischemia

Neoplasia

Secretory

Medications

Motility disorder

Neoplasia

Inflammatory bowel disease

Toxin

Osmotic

Carbohydrate malabsorption

Ingestion of magnesium, sulfates, or phosphates

bowel habits varying between diarrhea and constipation is common in irritable bowel syndrome. Diarrhea with abdominal pain, weight loss, and fever are hallmarks of inflammatory bowel disease. Finally, malabsorption classically presents with weight loss and voluminous, fatty, malodorous stools.

References

1. Thielman NM, Guerrant RL. Clinical practice. Acute infectious diarrhea. *N Engl J Med* 2004;350:38.
2. DuPont HL. Guidelines on acute infectious diarrhea in adults. The practice parameters committee of the American college of gastroenterology. *Am J Gastroenterol* 1997;92:1962.
3. Schiller LR. Chronic diarrhea. *Gastroenterology* 2004;127:287.

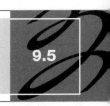

DYSPHAGIA
Michael R. Spieker

9.5

I. **BACKGROUND.** Dysphagia (difficulty in swallowing) is a common complaint in primary care practices, especially in aging persons. Up to 10% of adults older than 60 years, 25% of hospitalized patients, and 30% to 40% of nursing home patients experience swallowing problems.

II. **PATHOPHYSIOLOGY.** Organic swallowing problems occur at two primary sites: at the initiation of the swallow reflex in the oropharynx or with propulsion of food through the esophagus. Dysfunctional transfer of the food past the upper esophageal sphincter into the esophagus causes oropharyngeal dysphagia symptoms, and disordered peristalsis or conditions that obstruct the flow of a food bolus through the esophagus cause esophageal dysphagia symptoms. Mechanical obstruction or neuromuscular motility disorders occur in both the oropharynx and the esophagus. Common causes of oropharyngeal and esophageal dysphagia are listed in Table 9.5.1 (1).

III. **EVALUATION.** Choosing the best study depends on many factors including age, acuity of onset, comorbidities, and availability of testing modalities in the community. The Agency for Health Care Policy and Research (AHCPR) has published a limited review that evaluates diagnostic and therapeutic modalities, primarily focusing on stroke patients with dysphagia (2).

A. **History.** A careful history identifies 80% to 85% of causes by differentiating whether the dysphagia is oropharyngeal or esophageal in location and whether it is obstructive or neuromuscular in nature. The onset, severity, and duration of dysphagia combined with questions about associated symptoms can help narrow the differential diagnosis (see Table 9.5.2) (3). Alcohol and tobacco consumption histories provide important information. Medications can cause direct esophageal injury, dysmotility, decreased lower esophageal sphincter tone with reflux, or xerostomia with subsequent dysphagia (see Table 9.5.3) (4).

B. **Physical examination.** Examination, including gag reflex testing, typically provides limited information unless the patient has experienced an obvious cerebrovascular accident. Gag reflexes are absent in up to 13% of nondysphagic, "normal" patients. However, two clinical items combined (cough on swallowing and positive "three-ounce water test") provide a useful and potentially cost-effective screening tool in aspiration risk evaluation. Patients subjectively localize esophageal strictures within 4 cm approximately 75% of the time.

TABLE 9.5.1	Differential Diagnosis of Dysphagia

Oropharyngeal dysphagia

Neuromuscular disease (diseases of the central nervous system)

Cerebrovascular accident

Parkinson's disease

Brain stem tumors

Degenerative diseases

Amyotrophic lateral sclerosis

Multiple sclerosis

Huntington's disease

Postinfectious

Poliomyelitis

Syphilis

Peripheral nervous system

Peripheral neuropathy

Motor end-plate dysfunction

Myasthenia gravis

Skeletal muscle disease (myopathies)

Polymyositis

Dermatomyositis

Muscular dystrophy (myotonic dystrophy, oculopharyngeal dystrophy)

Cricopharyngeal (upper esophageal sphincter), achalasia

Obstructive lesions

Tumors

Inflammatory masses

Trauma/surgical resection

Zenker's diverticulum

Esophageal webs

Extrinsic structural lesions

Anterior mediastinal masses

Cervical spondylosis

Esophageal dysphagia

Neuromuscular disorders

Achalasia

Spastic motor disorders

Diffuse esophageal spasm

Hypertensive lower esophageal sphincter

Nutcracker esophagus

Scleroderma

(continued)

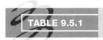

TABLE 9.5.1	Differential Diagnosis of Dysphagia (Continued)

Obstructive lesions

Intrinsic structural lesions

   Tumors

   Strictures

   Peptic

   Radiation-induced

   Chemical-induced

   Medication-induced

   Lower esophageal rings (Schatzki's ring)

   Esophageal webs

   Foreign bodies

Extrinsic structural lesions

   Vascular compression

   Enlarged aorta or left atrium

   Aberrant vessels

   Mediastinal masses

   Lymphadenopathy

   Substernal thyroid

From Castell DO. Approach to the patient with dysphagia. In: Yamada T, ed. *Textbook of gastroenterology*, 2nd ed. Philadelphia, PA: Lippincott Williams & Wilkins, 1995.

C. Testing. Few screening laboratory tests are indicated in the evaluation of dysphagia unless history or clinical examination findings dictate otherwise. However, special studies, including barium swallow for suspected intrinsic and extrinsic obstructive lesions, esophagogastroscopy for assessing esophageal mucosa or masses identified by barium swallow, and videoradiography in stroke patients with suspected swallowing disorders, are typically required for definitive diagnosis. In patients with acute onset dysphagia while eating, upper endoscopy can directly remove an impacted food bolus and dilate strictures. For all dysphagia diagnoses, endoscopy is more sensitive (92% vs. 54%) and more specific (100% vs. 91%) than double-contrast upper gastrointestinal radiography.

IV. DIAGNOSIS

A. Differential diagnosis. The diagnosis of dysphagia centers on the answers to two questions: is the dysphagia oropharyngeal or esophageal in location? Is it neuromuscular or obstructive in nature? (Table 9.5.1) Patients with oropharyngeal dysphagia present with difficulty in initiating swallowing and have associated coughing, choking or nasal regurgitation. Speech quality may have a nasal tone. Oropharyngeal dysphagia is associated with stroke, Parkinson's disease, or other long-term neuromuscular disorders. Local structural lesions are less common. Esophageal dysphagia often causes the sensation of food sticking in the throat or chest. Motility disorders and mechanical obstructions are common. Several medications have been associated with direct esophageal mucosal injury, whereas others can decrease lower esophageal sphincter pressures and cause reflux (Table 9.5.3) (4, 5).

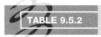

TABLE 9.5.2	Associated Symptoms and Possible Causes of Dysphagia

Condition	Diagnoses to consider
Progressive dysphagia	Neuromuscular dysphagia
Sudden dysphagia	Obstructive dysphagia, esophagitis
Difficulty in initiating swallow	Oropharyngeal dysphagia
Food "sticks" after swallow	Esophageal dysphagia
Cough	
Early in swallow	Neuromuscular dysphagia
Late in swallow	Obstructive dysphagia
Weight loss	
In the elderly	Carcinoma
With regurgitation	Achalasia
Progressive symptoms	
Heartburn	Peptic stricture, scleroderma
Intermittent symptoms	Rings and webs, diffuse esophageal spasm, nutcracker esophagus
Pain with dysphagia	Esophagitis
	Postradiation
	Infectious: herpes simplex virus, monilia
	Pill-induced
Pain made worse by	
Solid food only	Obstructive dysphagia
Solids and liquids	Neuromuscular dysphagia
Regurgitation of old food	Zenker's diverticulum
Weakness and dysphagia	Cerebrovascular accidents, muscular dystrophies, myasthenia gravis, multiple sclerosis
Halitosis	Zenker's diverticulum
Dysphagia relieved with repeated swallows	Achalasia
Dysphagia made worse with cold foods	Neuromuscular motility disorders

From Johnson A. Deglutition. In: Scott-Brown WG, Kerr AG, eds. *Scott-Brown's otolaryngology*, 6th ed. Boston, MA: Butterworth-Heinemann, 1997.

B. Clinical manifestations. Patients with neuromuscular dysphagia experience gradually progressive difficulty in swallowing solid food and liquids. Cold foods often aggravate the problem. Patients may succeed in passing the food bolus by repeated swallowing, by performing the Valsalva maneuver, or by making a positional change. They are more likely to experience pain when swallowing than patients with simple obstruction. Achalasia, scleroderma, and diffuse esophageal spasm are the most common causes of neuromuscular motility disorders. Obstructive pathology is typically associated with dysphagia of solid food but not liquids. Patients may be able to force food through the esophagus by performing a Valsalva maneuver, or they may regurgitate undigested food. Rapidly progressing dysphagia of a few months' duration suggests esophageal carcinoma. Weight loss is more predictive of a mechanical obstructive lesion. Peptic stricture, carcinoma, and Schatzki's ring are the predominant obstructive lesions.

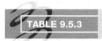 **TABLE 9.5.3** | **Medications Associated with Dysphagia**

Medications that can cause direct esophageal mucosal injury

Antibiotics

Doxycycline (Vibramycin)

Tetracycline

Clindamycin (Cleocin)

Trimethoprim-sulfamethoxazole (Bactrim, Septra)

Nonsteroidal anti-inflammatory drugs

Alendronate (Fosamax)

Zidovudine (Retrovir)

Ascorbic acid

Potassium chloride tablets (Slow-K)[a]

Theophylline

Quinidine gluconate

Ferrous sulfate

Medications, hormones, and foods associated with reduced lower esophageal sphincter tone and reflux

Butylscopolamine

Theophylline

Nitrates

Calcium antagonists

Alcohol, fat, chocolate

Medications associated with xerostomia

Anticholinergics: atropine, scopolamine (Transderm Scop)

α-Adrenergic blockers

Angiotensin-converting enzyme inhibitors

Angiotensin II–receptor blockers

Antiarrhythmics

Disopyramide (Norpace)

Mexiletine (Mexitil)

Ipratropium bromide (Atrovent)

Antihistamines

Diuretics

Opiates

Antipsychotics

[a]Especially the slow-release formulation.
From Boyce HW. Drug-induced esophageal damage: diseases of medical progress. [Editorial] *Gastrointest Endosc* 1998;47:547–550; Stoschus B, Allescher HD. Drug-induced dysphagia. *Dysphagia* 1993;8:154–159.

References
1. Castell DO. Approach to the patient with dysphagia. In: Yamada T, ed. *Textbook of gastroenterology*, 2nd ed. Philadelphia, PA: Lippincott Williams & Wilkins, 1995.
2. Agency for Health Care Policy and Research. *Diagnosis and treatment of swallowing disorders (dysphagia) in acute-care stroke patients*. Evidence Report/Technology Assessment: Number 8. AHCPR Publication No. 99-E024. Rockville, MD: AHCPR, July 1999:9.
3. Johnson A. Deglutition. In: Scott-Brown WG, Kerr AG, eds. *Scott-Brown's otolaryngology*, 6th ed. Boston, MA: Butterworth-Heineman, 1997.
4. Boyce HW. Drug-induced esophageal damage: diseases of medical progress [Editorial]. *Gastrointest Endosc* 1998;47:547–550.
5. Stoschus B, Allescher HD. Drug-induced dysphagia. *Dysphagia* 1993;8:154–159.

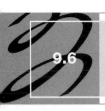

EPIGASTRIC DISTRESS
Pamela L. Pentin

9.6

I. **BACKGROUND.** Epigastric discomfort is caused by a variety of conditions occurring in multiple organs across the gastrointestinal, cardiovascular, and pulmonary systems. Serious causes, such as gastric, esophageal, bowel, and pancreatic cancers are rare but must also be considered. Overlapping symptoms make initial diagnosis difficult, and in many patients a definite cause is never established. Pulmonary, cardiac, and vascular causes of epigastric discomfort are reviewed in other chapters.

II. **PATHOPHYSIOLOGY**
   A. **Etiology.** Gastroesophageal reflux disease (GERD) is caused by weakness of the lower esophageal sphincter, allowing stomach contents to move in a retrograde direction, irritating the esophagus. Esophagitis can be related to GERD but also can be caused by hypersecretory conditions. Esophagitis and gastritis can also be primarily inflammatory conditions, related to medications such as nonsteroidal anti-inflammatory drugs (NSAIDs) and toxins such as alcohol. Most peptic ulcer diseases (PUDs) are related to *Helicobacter pylori* infection. Gallstones, formed by supersaturation of bile, cause pain by obstructing the cystic duct. Obstruction of the cystic duct by gallstones can cause cholecystitis, an acute inflammatory and often condition process.
   B. **Epidemiology.** Epigastric discomfort and dyspepsia occur in 25% of the population each year, but most affected persons do not seek medical care (1). Patients at increased risk for gallstones include the elderly, the obese (especially with rapid weight loss), the pregnant, and those on medications such as fibrates, estrogens, and contraceptives. Also at increased risk for gallstones are certain ethnicities, those with maternal family history, the female gender, and those with metabolic diseases such as diabetes, cirrhosis, and hypertriglyceridemia.

III. **EVALUATION**
   A. **Clinical approach.** Typical **history, physical examination**, and **laboratory findings** associated with common causes of epigastric distress are listed in Table 9.6.1.
   B. **Genetics.** Most causes of epigastric discomfort result from environmental factors, but some, such as cholelithiasis, exhibit hereditary components. Colonic and esophageal malignancies arise in certain inherited disorders. Hereditary pancreatitis is caused by a mutation in the cationic trypsinogen gene.

IV. **DIAGNOSIS**
   A. **Differential diagnosis.** The differential diagnosis of gastrointestinal causes of epigastric discomfort is presented in Table 9.6.2.

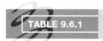

TABLE 9.6.1	Typical Historical, Physical Examination, and Laboratory Findings for Gastrointestinal Etiologies of Epigastric Discomfort		
	History	**Physical examination**	**Laboratory tests**
GERD	Heartburn, regurgitation, sour belches, pain radiating to throat, pain worsened by lying supine, chronic cough, hoarseness, beneficial trial of treatment with proton-pump inhibitors	Dental erosions, examination often normal	Usually normal
PUD	Personal or family history PUD, smoking history, nonsteroidal anti-inflammatory drug use, pain reduced by the intake of meals	Hypotension or tachycardia (GI bleeding), melena	Positive *Helicobacter pylori* antibody testing, positive urea breath test, stool *H. pylori* testing, heme positive stools
GI malignancy	Dysphagia, weight loss, continuous pain, anorexia, protracted vomiting, age >50 y, smoking or alcohol history, family history	Weight loss, palpable mass, Virchow's nodes, hypotension or tachycardia (GI bleeding), melena, acanthosis nigricans, brittle nails, cheilosis, conjunctival pallor	Anemia, heme positive stools
Pancreatitis	Abrupt onset pain, stabbing, severe, and radiating to back; history of alcohol use	Diffuse, severe pain	Elevated amylase, lipase
Cholelithiasis	Rapid onset pain, increasing intensity, <3-h duration, radiation to scapula or right shoulder, sweating, vomiting, pain brought on by meals, more common at night, genetic component	No palpable mass	Usually normal
Cholecystitis	>3-h duration of pain, shifts from epigastrium to right upper quadrant, acholic stools, dark urine	Palpable mass (30%–40%), fever, jaundice (15%), positive Murphy's sign	Leukocytosis (with left shift), elevated sedimentation rate, elevated bilirubin, elevated aminotransferases, elevated alkaline phosphatase, elevated amylase
Irritable bowel	Constipation and/or diarrhea, pain relieved by defecation	Normal	Normal

GERD, gastroesophageal reflux disease; GI, gastrointestinal; PUD, peptic ulcer disease
From Bazaldua OV, Schneider FD. Evaluation and management of dyspepsia. *Am Fam Physician* 1999;60:1773–1788; Dyspepsia and GERD Practice Guideline. Institute for Clinical Systems Improvement (ICSI); 2004 Jul; Marshall BJ. Gastritis and peptic ulcer disease. In: Rakel RE, ed. *Conn's current therapy*, 57th ed. Elsevier, 2005:600–603; Ahmad M, et al. Differential diagnosis of gallstone induced complications. *South Med J* 2000;93:261–264.

B. Clinical manifestations

1. A very useful diagnostic test for GERD is a simple trial of treatment with a double-dosed proton-pump inhibitor, such as omeprazole. If symptoms remit, further workup may not be necessary. If symptoms do not remit, then an upper endoscopy is warranted. Dysphagia (difficulty in swallowing) suggests an early symptom of esophageal cancer or can be an acid-induced stricture. The biliary colic of gallstones causes epigastric or right upper quadrant pain of rapid onset that increases in intensity over a 15-minute interval and lasts as long as 3 hours,

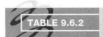

TABLE 9.6.2	Differential Diagnosis of Gastrointestinal Causes of Epigastric Discomfort

Esophagus

Esophagitis
Gastroesophageal reflux disease
Medications

Lung
Pneumonia
Pulmonary embolism
Pneumothorax

Pancreas
Pancreatitis

Heart
Cardiac ischemia
Pericarditis

Stomach
Gastritis
Peptic ulcer disease
Bleeding
Gastroparesis
Medications

Gallbladder
Cholelithiasis
Cholecystitis

Bowel
Irritable bowel syndrome
Bleeding

usually without any palpable mass. Pain may radiate to the interscapular region or to the right shoulder. Associated sweating and vomiting are common. Attacks of biliary colic are often brought on by eating, especially a fatty meal, and are more common at night, possibly because the gallbladder shifts to a horizontal position, facilitating entry of stones into the cystic duct. (2).

2. Acute cholecystitis causes epigastric or right upper quadrant tenderness or mass and fever. The pain typically lasts longer than 3 hours, and over time, shifts from the epigastrium to the right upper quadrant. In the elderly, localized tenderness may be the only presenting sign. The gallbladder is palpable 30% to 40% of the time, and jaundice is seen in about 15% of patients with acute cholecystitis. Patients with cholecystitis may also have acholic stools.

3. Malignancies that cause epigastric discomfort are rare. However, symptoms of gastric and esophageal cancers are similar to those of other causes of epigastric distress. Dysphagia, unexplained weight loss, history of gastrointestinal bleeding, or clinical signs of anemia can differentiate patients with a more serious disease. Numerous medications (see Table 9.6.3) induce nonulcer dyspepsia. By identifying medication-associated dyspepsia, costly diagnostic studies can be avoided. Irritable bowel syndrome is generally associated with abnormal bowel habits.

TABLE 9.6.3	Medications Associated with Epigastric Discomfort
Acarbose	
Bisphosphonates	
Iron supplements	
Nonsteroidal anti-inflammatory drugs	
Oral antibiotics	
Potassium supplements	
Systemic corticosteroids	

4. Though discussed in Chapter 7.5, it must be mentioned here that the pain of ischemic heart disease may originate in the epigastrium and must be ruled out. Metabolic disorders are a rare cause of epigastric discomfort, but a complete differential should include malabsorption syndromes, collagen vascular disorders, Zollinger-Ellison syndrome and Crohn's disease.

References
1. Bazaldua OV, Schneider FD. Evaluation and management of dyspepsia. *Am Fam Physician* 1999;60:1773–1788.
2. Ahmed A, Cheung RC, Keeffe EB. Management of gallstones and their complications. *Am Fam Physician* 2000;61:1673–1680, 1687–1688.

UPPER GASTROINTESTINAL BLEEDING

Charles S. Blackadar

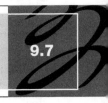

9.7

I. **BACKGROUND.** Upper gastrointestinal (GI) bleeding, defined as bleeding proximal to the ligament of Treitz, is responsible for 350,000 hospital admissions in the United States, with a mortality of 10% (1). Bleeding can be either acute or chronic, and the source can be overt or occult. The patient may be either hemodynamically stable or unstable on presentation.

II. **PATHOPHYSIOLOGY.** Bleeding from the upper GI tract usually results when disruption occurs between the protective barriers to the vasculature and the harsh environment of the digestive tract. The most common causes (as percentages) are listed in Table 9.7.1.

III. **EVALUATION.** The key to successful evaluation and diagnosis is a systematic approach with emphasis on the overall hemodynamic status of the patient (see Figure 9.7.1).

   A. **History.** Clinical history accurately points to the source of bleeding in only 40% of cases (2). Hematemesis and melena are the most common presentations of acute upper GI bleeding. The examiner must get answers to several important questions: Is there a prior history of bleeding (60% rebled from the same site) (2). Does the patient have any comorbid diseases (peptic ulcer disease, pancreatitis, cirrhosis, cancer)? Particular attention must be given to the patient's cardiopulmonary status because this affects urgency and degree of resuscitative efforts. Table 9.7.1 lists other diagnostic clues to common causes, and Table 9.7.2 lists the less common causes.

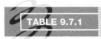

TABLE 9.7.1	Common Causes of Gastrointestinal Bleeding and Diagnostic Clues

Cause	Diagnostic clue
Peptic ulcer (55%)	Nonsteroidal anti-inflammatory drug use, *Helicobacter pylori* infection, stress
Esophagogastric varices (14%)	Ethanol use, umbilical or rectal varices, palmar erythema, ascites, spider hemangiomas
Arteriovenous malformations (6%)	History of previous episodes
Mallory-Weiss tears (5%)	Vomiting prior to hematemesis, ethanol use, occurs in young men
Tumors (4%)	Ethanol use, smoking, smoked foods, gastroesophageal reflux disease, Barrett's esophagus, weight loss

From Jutabha RJ, Jensen DM. Approach to the patient with upper gastrointestinal bleeding. UpToDate June 2005.

B. Physical examination
   1. Vital signs. The single most important aspect of the initial physical examination is determining the patient's hemodynamic stability. Unstable patients should be managed as trauma patients. Placement of a nasogastric (NG) tube is considered the "fifth vital sign" in patients with acute upper GI bleeding (3). After ensuring hemodynamic stability, the initial physical examination should eliminate a nasal or oropharyngeal source of bleeding.
   2. Skin examination. Ecchymoses, petechiae, and varices should be noted. Conjunctival pallor is a sign of chronic anemia. Numerous mucosal telangiectasias can point to an underlying vascular abnormality.
   3. Abdominal examination. Look for stigmata of chronic liver disease (hepatosplenomegaly, spider angiomata, ascites, palmar erythema, caput medusae, gynecomastia, and testicular atrophy).
   4. Rectal examination. Rectal varices, hemorrhoids, and fissures should be noted.
C. Testing. Basic laboratory studies should include a complete blood count (CBC) with particular attention to the hematocrit, coagulation studies (prothrombin time [PT]) and partial thromboplastin time [PTT]), liver function tests (LFTs), serum chemistries (blood urea nitrogen is elevated disproportionate to creatinine in patients with GI blood loss), electrocardiogram (ECG), and NG aspirate analysis. Initially, the hematocrit is a poor indicator of blood loss; however, serial hematocrits can be useful in assessing ongoing blood loss. The CBC indices, particularly an elevated red cell distribution width and low mean corpuscular volume, point toward a chronic bleed. A prolonged PT or PTT suggests an underlying coagulopathy. Elevated LFTs suggest underlying liver disease. An ECG is important, especially in elderly patients, to search for evidence of cardiac ischemia. If the aspirate is bright red, or "coffee grounds" in appearance, an upper GI source of bleeding is likely. Additionally, NG lavage removes blood and helps with the performance of endoscopy. In cases in which no source can be identified, lower endoscopy should be considered in the search for a lower GI bleed.
IV. DIAGNOSIS. The differential diagnosis of an upper GI bleed should include bleeding from the upper airways or pharynx that is swallowed and regurgitated and lower GI bleeding that may be manifested as melanic stools due to delay in transit through the colon. In most cases, diagnosis can be confirmed with lavage and the source localized and treated with upper endoscopy. In rare cases in which endoscopy is unable to adequately identify the source of GI bleeding, specialized nuclear medicine and angiographic studies can be used.

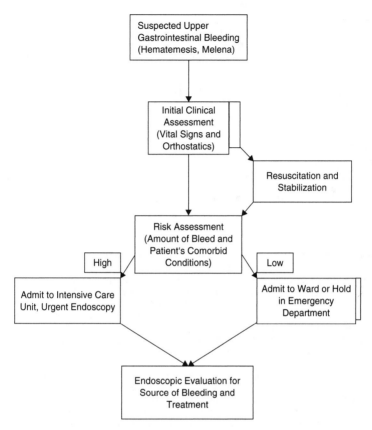

Figure 9.7.1. Approach to upper gastrointestinal bleeding. (Modified from Eisen GM, Dominitz JA, Faigel DO. An annotated algorithmic approach to upper gastrointestinal bleeding. *Gastrointest Endosc* 2001;53:853–858.)

TABLE 9.7.2   **Uncommon Causes of Upper Gastrointestinal Bleeding**

Cause	Diagnostic clue
Dieulafoy's lesion	Congenital lesion usually diagnosed during endoscopy
Gastric antral vascular ectasia	Associated with cirrhosis and elderly women
Hemobilia	Usually associated with recent biliary tree injury
Aortoenteric fistulas	Primary cases associated with AAA, secondary cases with fistulas from AAA repairs; may present with back pain and fever

AAA, abdominal aortic aneurysm.
From Jutabha RJ, Jensen DM. Approach to the patient with upper gastrointestinal bleeding. UpToDate June 2005.

References

1. Eisen GM, Dominitz JA, Faigel DO. An annotated algorithmic approach to upper gastrointestinal bleeding. *Gastrointest Endosc* 2001;53:853–858.
2. McGuirk TD, Coyle WJ. Upper gastrointestinal tract bleeding. *Emerg Med Clin North Am* 1996;14:523–545.
3. Laine L. Acute and chronic gastrointestinal bleeding. In: Feldman M, Sleisinger MH, Scharschmidt BF, eds. *Gastrointestinal and liver disease: pathophysiology, diagnosis, and management.* Philadelphia, PA: WB Saunders, 1998:198–218.

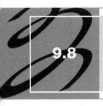

HEPATITIS
9.8
Brian A. Smoley

I. **BACKGROUND.** Hepatitis is an inflammation of the liver that is usually caused by a viral infection but can result from a number of different etiologies.
II. **PATHOPHYSIOLOGY.** The inflammation due to hepatitis produces cellular injury and necrosis. Even with fulminant acute hepatitis, recovery is possible. Fibrosis distorts the liver's architecture in chronic hepatitis and can cause cirrhosis and portal hypertension. Whether acute or chronic, liver failure ensues when enough necrosis has occurred to compromise hepatic function.
   A. **Etiology.** Viral hepatitis has multiple causes. The highly contagious hepatitis A and E viruses (HAV, HEV) are spread by the fecal-oral route and typically produce an acute, self-limited, "infectious hepatitis." Hepatitis B, C, and D viruses (HBV, HCV, HDV) are spread parenterally, vertically, or by intimate contact and cause acute and chronic "serum hepatitis." HDV requires the presence of HBV, causing coinfection when they are transmitted together and superinfection when HDV follows HBV.
   1. Toxin- or drug-induced hepatitis can be difficult to diagnose and is probably underreported. An offending drug may have been started months earlier and exposure to toxins may not be known. Acetaminophen is the best known and most common drug culprit, but other known offenders include nonsteroidal anti-inflammatory drugs, anticonvulsants, and various antimicrobials. Hepatotoxins include organic solvents, mushroom amatoxin, rat poisons, and yellow phosphorus (found in fire works). Alcohol is also an important agent, either as a toxin or through its effect on the metabolism of other toxins.
   2. Fatty liver disease starts with an accumulation of lipids within hepatocytes (steatosis) and can progress to frank steatohepatitis and even cirrhosis. Alcohol consumption is a common cause, but many drugs and metabolic disorders (especially insulin-resistant syndromes) are associated with nonalcoholic steatosis and steatohepatitis.
   3. As with most autoimmune diseases, autoimmune hepatitis occurs more commonly in women. It presents in a number of ways but is progressive and ultimately leads to end-stage liver disease if not treated. α_1-Antitrypsin (A1AT) is a hepatically produced proteinase inhibitor. A1AT-deficient individuals who produce a particular abnormal form of the enzyme and lack the ability to degrade it develop hepatitis because of its accumulation within hepatocytes. Iron overload leads to iron deposition in the liver and other tissues. Hepatic iron overload usually takes at least 40 years to become symptomatic. Hereditary hemochromatosis, ineffective erythropoiesis, multiple blood transfusions, and excessive dietary intake iron are known causes. A deficient copper-transporting enzyme causes Wilson's disease. Copper first accumulates within hepatocytes and later in other tissues as it spills into the serum. Ischemia can also cause hepatitis (1,2).

B. Epidemiology. Acute hepatitis affects up to 1% of Americans each year. HAV, HBV, and HCV are the causes in 97% of cases (48%, 34%, and 15%, respectively). There were an estimated average of 92,000 new cases of hepatitis A, 78,000 of hepatitis B, and 30,000 of hepatitis C each year in the United States from 2000 to 2003. The estimated prevalence of chronic hepatitis is 2%. Approximately, 5% of HBV infections and 75% of HCV infections result in chronic disease, yielding an estimated 1.25 million cases of chronic hepatitis B and 2.7 million cases of chronic hepatitis C in the United States (1,3). Asymptomatic elevations of aminotransferases occur in 1% to 4% of individuals, but at least half likely represent the 2.5% whose values are expected to fall above the "normal range." Fatty liver disease is believed to be the most common cause of mild (less than five times the upper limit of normal) liver enzyme elevations (2).

III. EVALUATION

A. History. Initial history should focus on identifying risk factors for viral and alcoholic hepatitis. History of contact with a person with jaundice or hepatitis, travel to endemic areas, ingestion of shellfish or other suspect foods, work in a health care or other high-risk setting, day-care attendance, institutionalization, history of blood transfusion, sexual promiscuity, or any use of injected illicit drugs all suggest viral hepatitis. Screening for alcohol abuse is done with questionnaires (e.g., CAGE) or by looking for "red flags" (e.g., social or occupational difficulties, depression or anxiety, poorly explained trauma, convictions for driving while being intoxicated). Review of all medications (prescribed, over the counter, traditional, and complementary) and occupational exposures can identify potential hepatotoxins. Family history can yield evidence of inherited disorders such as A1AT deficiency, hereditary hemochromatosis, and Wilson's disease (1,4).

B. Physical examination. Examination serves to confirm or refute initial suspicions and reveal other clues to the cause and severity of disease. Icterus, jaundice, and liver tenderness are expected findings in acute hepatitis; hepatosplenomegaly can occur in severe cases. Patients with chronic hepatitis can have only mild liver tenderness. The liver can be small or enlarged; and smooth, nodular, or hard. Patients with advanced disease present with signs of chronic disease (e.g., muscle wasting), altered hormone metabolism (e.g., alopecia, gynecomastia, palmar erythema, testicular atrophy), and portal hypertension (e.g., ascites, caput medusa, splenomegaly) (1).

C. Testing

1. The likelihood and severity of disease must be considered when ordering or interpreting laboratory tests. Commonly used tests (see Table 9.8.1) include serum alanine and aspartate aminotransferases (ALT and AST), alkaline phosphatase, and γ-glutamyl transpeptidase (GGT); serum albumin and bilirubin levels; and prothrombin time (PT). Specific antigens, nucleic acids, or antibodies used to diagnose viral hepatitis and laboratory tests for rare causes of hepatitis are listed in Table 9.8.2.

2. Imaging studies are not generally indicated in the initial evaluation except to exclude biliary tract obstruction or screen for fatty liver disease. Liver biopsy is sometimes necessary for both diagnosis and estimation of prognosis. A review (2) and algorithm (5) for the evaluation of abnormal liver chemistries are available on the Internet.

D. Genetics. Genetic studies are not used in the initial evaluation of hepatitis but can be used if an inherited condition is suspected (e.g., hereditary hemochromatosis).

IV. DIAGNOSIS

A. Differential diagnosis. A differential diagnosis of hepatitis is given in Table 9.8.3.

B. Clinical manifestations

1. **Acute hepatitis.** The clinical presentation can be quite variable. Some patients experience no symptoms, whereas others (1%–2%) suffer fulminant disease with life-threatening liver failure (1). Table 9.8.4 outlines a classic presentation.

2. **Chronic hepatitis.** Any hepatitis that persists beyond 6 months is considered to be chronic. Symptoms tend to be less severe or absent. When present, they are nonspecific, intermittent, and mild and include fatigue, malaise, poor

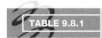

TABLE 9.8.1	Common Laboratory Tests for Evaluating Liver Disease

Test	Implication	Notes
ALT and AST	Hepatocellular injury or necrosis	Do not correlate with disease severity; AST/ALT ≥ 2 in alcoholic liver disease
Direct bilirubin	Hepatobiliary disease	Bilirubinuria occurs with conjugated (direct) hyperbilirubinemia and is always pathologic
GGT	Hepatobiliary disease	Increased by alcohol ingestion; used to confirm hepatic origin of alkaline phosphatase
Alkaline phosphatase	Cholestatic disease	Not liver-specific; used to rule out cholestasis
Prothrombin time and albumin	Hepatic function	Short-term and long-term indicators; not specific

ALT, alanine aminotransferase; AST, aspartate aminotransferase; GGT, γ-glutamyl transpeptidase.
From Goldman L, Ausiello D, eds. *Cecil textbook of medicine,* 22nd ed. Philadelphia, PA: Saunders, 2003; Green RM, Flamm S. AGA technical review on the evaluation of liver chemistry tests. *Gastroenterology* 2002;123:1367–1384. http://www2.us.elsevierhealth.com/inst/serve?action= searchDB&searchDBfor=art&artType=abs&id=agast1231367&nav=abs&special=hilite&query= [all_fields](liver+chemistry+tests,).

concentration, sleeping difficulties, and right upper quadrant pain. More severe anorexia, nausea, weakness, weight loss, pruritus, icterus, and jaundice can occur in the setting of advanced disease or an acute exacerbation. Although typically less severe in presentation, the inflammation of chronic hepatitis can lead to cirrhosis and end-stage liver disease. Such patients suffer abdominal swelling, edema, easy bruising, gastrointestinal bleeding, and mental confusion (with the onset of hepatic encephalopathy). Serum aminotransferase levels are

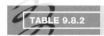

TABLE 9.8.2	Diagnostic Tests for Suspected Hepatitis

Hepatitis A	Anti-HAV IgM
Hepatitis B	Hepatitis B surface antigen, antihepatitis B core IgM
Hepatitis C	Anti-HCV antibody (ELISA or RIBA), HCV RNA
Uncommon	
A1AT deficiency	Serum A1AT activity, A1AT phenotyping
Autoimmune hepatitis	Antinuclear, antismooth muscle, liver–kidney microsomal antibodies
Iron overload	Serum ferritin and transferrin saturation
Wilson's disease	Serum ceruloplasmin, 24-h urine copper

A1AT, α_1-antitrypsin; ELISA, enzyme-linked immunosorbent assay; HAV, hepatitis A virus; HCV, hepatitis C virus; RIBA, recombinant immunoblot assay.
From Goldman L, Ausiello D, eds. *Cecil textbook of medicine,* 22nd ed. Philadelphia, PA: Saunders, 2003; Green RM, Flamm S. AGA technical review on the evaluation of liver chemistry tests. *Gastroenterology* 2002;123:1367–1384. http://www2.us.elsevierhealth. com/inst/serve?action=searchDB&searchDBfor=art&artType=abs&id=agast1231367&nav= abs&special=hilite&query=[all_fields](liver+chemistry+tests,).

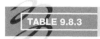

TABLE 9.8.3	Differential Diagnosis of Hepatitis

Biliary tract obstruction	Conditions such as choledocholithiasis, neoplasm, pancreatitis, primary sclerosis cholangitis
	SURGICAL CAUSES MUST BE EXCLUDED EARLY
Liver infiltration	Granulomatous liver disease: immunologic and hypersensitivity disorders; fungal, mycobacterial, parasitic, other infections; inflammatory bowel disease; lymphoma; primary biliary cirrhosis; drug, foreign body, toxic reactions; rheumatic diseases; sarcoidosis
	Infiltrating malignancy
Other infections	Bacterial: ehrlichiosis, gonococcal perihepatitis, Legionnaires' disease, leptospirosis, listeriosis, Lyme disease, pyogenic abscess, Q-fever, Rocky Mountain spotted fever, salmonellosis, secondary syphilis, tularemia
	Fungal: candidiasis
	Parasitic: amebic abscess, babesiasis, malaria, toxoplasmosis
	Viral: adenovirus, cytomegalovirus, Epstein-Barr virus, herpes simplex virus
Pregnancy	Acute fatty liver of pregnancy, HELLP syndrome, hyperemesis gravidarum

HELLP syndrome, hemolysis, elevated liver enzymes, and low platelet count.
From Goldman L, Ausiello D, eds. *Cecil textbook of medicine,* 22nd ed. Philadelphia, PA: Saunders, 2003; Green RM, Flamm S. AGA technical review on the evaluation of liver chemistry tests. *Gastroenterology* 2002;123:1367–1384. http://www2.us.elsevierhealth.com/inst/serve?action= searchDB&searchDBfor=art&artType=abs&id=agast1231367&nav=abs&special=hilite&query= [all_fields](liver+chemistry+tests,).

usually less than five times the upper limit of normal but are highly variable. Because of the varying severity of inflammation and the gradual decrease in liver function that occurs in the course of chronic hepatitis, serial examination of laboratory tests is probably more important than the absolute values at any given time (1).

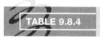

TABLE 9.8.4	Phases of "Classic" Acute Hepatitis

Phase	Symptoms	Findings	Duration
Preicteric	Anorexia, nausea, fatigue, malaise, vague right upper quadrant pain	Greater than tenfold elevation of ALT and AST	3–10 d
Icteric	Worsening of preicteric symptoms, dark urine, jaundice	Jaundice, liver tenderness, hyperbilirubinemia	1–3 wk
Convalescent	Gradual resolution	Gradual resolution	≤ 5 mo

ALT, alanine aminotransferase; AST, aspartate aminotransferase.
From Goldman L, Ausiello D, eds. *Cecil textbook of medicine,* 22nd ed. Philadelphia, PA: Saunders, 2003.

References
1. Goldman L, Ausiello D, eds. *Cecil textbook of medicine*, 22nd ed. Philadelphia, PA: Saunders, 2003.
2. Green RM, Flamm S. AGA technical review on the evaluation of liver chemistry tests. *Gastroenterology* 2002;123:1367–1384. http://www2.us.elsevierhealth.com/inst/serve? action=searchDB&searchDBfor=art&artType=abs&id=agast1231367&nav=abs& special=hilite&query=[all_fields](liver+chemistry+tests,).
3. National Center for Infectious Diseases. Burden from hepatitis A, B, and C in the United States. 2005. http://www.cdc.gov/ncidod/diseases/hepatitis/resource/dz_burden02.htm.
4. Mersy DJ. Recognition of alcohol and substance abuse. *Am Fam Physician* 2003;67: 1529–1532. http://www.aafp.org/afp/20030401/1529.html.
5. American Gastroenterological Association medical position statement: evaluation of liver chemistry tests. *Gastroenterology* 2002;123:1364–1366. http://www2.us.elsevierhealth. com/inst/serve?action=searchDB&searchDBfor=art&artType=abs&id=agast1231364 &nav=abs&special=hilite&query=[all_fields](liver+chemistry+tests,).

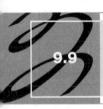

HEPATOMEGALY
9.9
Darryl G. White

I. **BACKGROUND.** Hepatomegaly is a physical finding associated with hepatobiliary disease. It is not specific or sensitive to one cause and defining it can be enigmatic because of the highly variable liver size that makes establishment of what constitutes normal somewhat difficult. The normal adult liver has a midclavicular range of 8 to 12 cm for men and 6 to 10 cm for women, with most studies defining hepatomegaly as a liver span greater than 15 cm in the midclavicular line (1).

II. **PATHOPHYSIOLOGY**
   A. **Etiology.** Liver enlargement can have multiple pathophysiologic pathways. Enlargement occurs in the early hepatic inflammatory response to viral pathogens, toxic substances, and other stimulants and is then followed by scarring and shrinking in chronic conditions. Fatty infiltration causes enlargement in obesity and metabolic syndrome. Vascular congestion results in swelling in acute and chronic heart diseases as well as in conditions of decreased vascular out flow. Focally enlarging lesions such as vascular cysts, infectious cysts, and cancerous growths also occur. Abnormal deposition of amyloid, lipids, or iron can also result in liver enlargement.
   B. **Epidemiology.** The incidence of hepatomegaly has not been studied in any large population group. However, a recent summary article of multiple studies found that a palpable liver margin had a likelihood ratio of 2.5 (confidence interval [CI], 2.2–2.8) for hepatomegaly and a nonpalpable liver margin had a negative likelihood ratio of 0.45 (CI, 0.38–0.52). (2).

III. **EVALUATION**
   A. **History.** Initial evaluation of hepatomegaly centers on two questions: Does the patient have known risk factors for liver disease (see Table 9.9.1)? Does the patient have symptoms associated with liver disease (see Table 9.9.2)?
   B. **Physical examination.** Examination of the liver is difficult given its irregular shape and its location within the abdomen.
      1. It is typical to use one of the two directions for palpation of the right upper quadrant: palpate from below using the fingertips to palpate superiorly or from above with the fingertips hooked over the lower rib. Either method is facilitated by the patient's deep inspiration. Palpation must include the midline to identify an enlarged left lobe of the liver. On palpation, note the liver position, the extent of its palpation below the costal margin, and its texture and consistency. Palpate

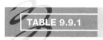

TABLE 9.9.1	Risk Factors for Liver Disease	
Acupuncture	Alcoholism	Bisexuality
Blood product transfusion	Dietary supplements	Family history liver disease
Gallstones	Gastrointestinal bleeding	Irritable bowel disease
Sexually transmitted disease	Male homosexuality	International travel
Tattoos		

for the lower edge and percuss for the upper margin. These two points give the highest accuracy in estimating liver size. (3) If the margin is not palpated but hepatomegaly is suspected, attempt direct percussion of both margins. The "scratch method" (gently stoking or scratching the skin surface in a parallel plane while listening with the stethoscope for change in sound and intensity of frequency) has been used to identify margins: however, a recent study comparing ultrasound to the results of the scratch test found that this test was unreliable and inaccurate. (4)

2. Auscultation of the right upper quadrant has poor clinical utility. Other physical examination findings consistent with liver disease include jaundice, vascular spiders, palmar erythema, gynecomastia, ascites, splenomegaly, testicular atrophy, peripheral edema, Dupuytren's contracture, parotid enlargement, and encephalopathy. Although none of these physical examination signs are pathognomonic for hepatobiliary disease, their presence prompts further diagnostic tests for hepatic disease.

C. **Testing.** Diagnostic tests should include computed tomography (CT) scan of the right upper quadrant and initial laboratory tests (complete blood count, serum blood tests [CHEM-7]), liver enzyme tests (aspartate aminotransferase, alanine aminotransferase, γ-glutamyl transpeptidase, alkaline phosphatase), and true liver function tests (albumin, prothrombin time, partial thromboplastin time, and bilirubin). If liver enzymes are elevated, proceed with hepatitis serology. Ultrasound can be used when CT scan is contraindicated or not available. Further testing used to elucidate the differential diagnosis is listed in Table 9.9.3.

IV. DIAGNOSIS

A. **Differential diagnosis.** This can be approached on the basis of the findings of physical examination.

1. Smooth nontender liver. Suspect fatty infiltration, congestive heart failure (CHF), portal cirrhosis, lymphoma, portal obstruction, hepatic venous thrombosis, hepatic vein thrombosis, lymphocystic leukemia, amyloidosis, schistosomiasis, or kala-azar.

2. Smooth tender liver. Suspect early CHF, acute hepatitis, amoebic abscess, or hepatic abscess.

3. Nodular liver. Suspect late portal cirrhosis, tertiary syphilis, hydatid cyst, or metastatic carcinoma.

4. Very hard nodular liver. This nearly always indicates metastatic carcinoma.

TABLE 9.9.2	Symptoms of Liver Disease		
Abdominal pain	Pruritus	Nausea	Loss of appetite
Confusion	Arthralgias	Rashes	Night sweats
Fatigue	Diarrhea	Chills	Sleep disturbance
Gastric bleeding	Fever	Easy bruisability	Vomiting
Myalgia	Heavy menses	Frequent epistaxis	

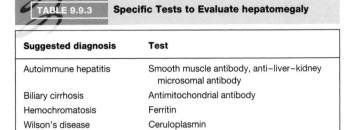

Suggested diagnosis	Test
Autoimmune hepatitis	Smooth muscle antibody, anti–liver–kidney microsomal antibody
Biliary cirrhosis	Antimitochondrial antibody
Hemochromatosis	Ferritin
Wilson's disease	Ceruloplasmin
Hepatocellular cancer	α-Fetoprotein
α_1-Antitrypsin deficiency	Enzyme assay of the same

TABLE 9.9.3   Specific Tests to Evaluate hepatomegaly

    B. Clinical manifestations. The clinical manifestations of hepatomegaly, although somewhat ill defined, should prompt a thorough evaluation and workup. Appropriate diagnostic tests generally provide a quick and accurate diagnosis. New therapies for chronic liver diseases make early diagnosis critical for obtaining good results.

References

1. Unal B, Bilgili Y, Kocacikli E, et al. Simple evaluation of liver size on erect abdominal plain radiography. *Clin Radiol* 2004;59:1132–1135.
2. Seupaul RA, Collins R. Physical examination of the liver. *Ann Emerg Med* 2005;45:553–555.
3. Naylor CD. Physical examination of the liver. *JAMA* 1994;27:1859–1865.
4. Tucker WN, Saab S, Leland SR, et al. The scratch test is unreliable for determining the liver edge. *J Clin Gastroenterol* 1997;25:410–414.

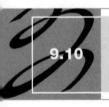

9.10 JAUNDICE

Ronald F. Dommermuth

  I. BACKGROUND. Jaundice refers to a yellowish discoloration of the skin, sclerae, and mucous membranes caused by the deposition of bile pigments. Typically, physical examination is unable to detect elevations of bilirubin until the serum level exceeds 2.0 to 3.0 mg/dL.

  II. PATHOPHYSIOLOGY

    A. Etiology. Bilirubin is formed primarily through the metabolic breakdown of heme rings, predominantly from the catabolism of red blood cells. Dysfunction of any of the phases of bilirubin metabolism (prehepatic, intrahepatic, or posthepatic) can lead to jaundice. Normally, 96% of plasma bilirubin is unconjugated (indirect). When the plasma elevation is caused predominantly by unconjugated bilirubin, the defect is likely to be the result of overproduction, impaired hepatic uptake, or abnormalities in conjugation. When the plasma elevation includes a substantial contribution from conjugated (direct) bilirubin, then hepatocellular disease, defective canalicular excretion, and biliary obstruction are the more likely causes.

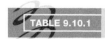

TABLE 9.10.1	Medications Associated with the Development of Jaundice

Alcohol

Diuretics

Acetaminophen

Cholesterol-lowering agents

Anticonvulsants

Sex hormones

Psychotropic medications

Antibiotics

Diuretics

Oral hypoglycemics

Inhaled anesthetics

Chemotherapy agents

Nonsteroidal anti-inflammatory drugs

Herbal compounds

B. Epidemiology. Among adults presenting with jaundice, serious underlying disease is common. In one study, 20% of patients with jaundice had pancreatic or biliary carcinoma, 13% experienced gallstone disease and 10% suffered from alcoholic cirrhosis (1). Jaundice rarely represents a medical emergency but can present as massive hemolysis, kernicterus, ascending cholangitis, and fulminant hepatic failure.

III. EVALUATION

A. History

1. Sudden onset is consistent with viral hepatitis, acute biliary obstruction, trauma, or toxin-mediated fulminant liver failure. More gradual onset is indicative of chronic liver disease (including alcoholic cirrhosis) or malignancy. A lifelong history suggests an inherited metabolic or hemolytic cause. Acholic stools, dark urine, and right upper quadrant (RUQ) pain, especially following a fatty meal, should suggest cholestasis or cholelithiasis. A history of fever or prior biliary surgery, especially if RUQ pain is present, points to cholangitis. Charcot's triad of cholangitis includes fever, RUQ pain, and jaundice. In the presence of a history of anorexia, malaise, or myalgias, a viral etiology should be considered. Typically, pruritus or weight loss is associated with noninfectious etiologies such as primary biliary cirrhosis in which pruritus is commonly the initial symptom (2). Numerous medications can induce hepatocellular injury or cholestasis (see Table 9.10.1).

2. Blood transfusions, intravenous drug use, sexual contacts, travel to endemic regions, or ingestion of contaminated foods can also expose patients to viral-related hepatocellular injury. Past medical history and surgical history, prior episodes of jaundice, and a history of a rheumatologic disease or inflammatory bowel disease should be examined. Family history may reveal an inherited defect in bilirubin conjugation or transport, Wilson's disease, α_1-antitrypsin deficiency, or hemochromatoses.

B. Physical examination. In addition to icterus, examination findings of ascites, splenomegaly, spider angiomas, caput medusa, gynecomastia, testicular atrophy, palmar erythema, or Dupuytren's contracture suggest chronic liver disease and portal hypertension. Altered consciousness and asterixis point toward liver. Kayser-Fleischer rings are seen in Wilson's disease, and Courvoisier's sign (a painless palpable gall bladder) is suggestive of pancreatic cancer.

C. Testing
1. Initial laboratory testing for a jaundiced patient includes a complete blood count and peripheral smear, a fractionated serum bilirubin (total and direct), and a urinalysis. Additional testing should include aspartate aminotransferase/alanine aminotransferase (AST/ALT), γ-glutamyl transpeptidase, and alkaline phosphatase. Pure liver function should be evaluated by obtaining an albumin and a prothrombin time.
2. Further laboratory testing and imaging are predicated on obtaining the initial results and may include serologic testing for viral hepatitis, autoimmune markers (antimitochondrial antibodies: primary biliary cirrhosis, or anti–smooth muscle antibodies and antimicrosomal antibodies: autoimmune hepatitis), serum iron, transferring and ferritin (hemochromatosis), ceruloplasmin (Wilson's disease), and α_1-antitrypsin activity (α_1-antitrypsin deficiency). Ultrasound and computed tomography can help distinguish obstructive disease from hepatocellular disease.

IV. DIAGNOSIS.
Historical features corroborated by physical examination and laboratory studies should distinguish obstructive causes from nonobstructive causes, differentiate acutely presenting conditions from more chronic diseases, and discriminate unconjugated and conjugated sources of bilirubin (see Table 9.10.2). Dubin-Johnson and Rotor's syndrome are inherited disorders that affect transportation of conjugated bilirubin.

Results of the patient's aminotransferases further refine the differential diagnosis. Hepatocellular injury is distinguished from cholestasis by substantial elevations in the aminotransferases (AST/ALT). A ratio of AST/ALT of >2.0 suggests alcoholic liver disease. Normal aminotransferases argue against hepatocellular injury and increase the

---

TABLE 9.10.2   Differential Diagnosis of Jaundice

Disorders of unconjugated hyperbilirubinemia		
Overproduction	**Impaired uptake**	**Impaired conjugation**
Intravascular hemolysis	Congestive heart failure	Crigler-Najjar syndrome, types I and II
Extravascular hemolysis	Cirrhosis	Advanced cirrhosis
Dyserythropoiesis	Gilbert's disease	Wilson's disease
	Medication	Antibiotics
Disorders of conjugated hyperbilirubinemia		
Extrahepatic cholestasis	**Intrahepatic cholestasis**	**Hepatocellular injury**
Sclerosing cholangitis	Viral hepatitis	See Table 9.10.1
Choledocholithiasis	Alcoholic hepatitis	
Pancreatitis	Nonalcoholic steatohepatitis	
Tumors	Biliary cirrhosis	
AIDS cholangiopathy	Toxins	
Strictures	Infiltrating diseases	
Parasitic infections	Total parenteral nutrition	
	Pregnancy	
	End-stage hepatic disease	

AIDS, acquired immunodeficiency syndrome.

likelihood that hemolysis or a disorder of bilirubin processing exists. However, this can be misleading in chronic liver disease when there is little liver parenchyma left for being injured.

References
1. Reisman Y, Gips GH, Lavelle SM, et al. Clinical presentation of (subclinical) jaundice. *Hepatogastroenterology* 1996;43:1190.
2. Leuschner U. Primary biliary cirrhosis-presentation and diagnosis. *Clinics in Liver Disease* 2003;7:741.

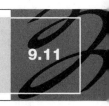

RECTAL BLEEDING
Christine Romascan

9.11

I. **BACKGROUND.** Primary care physicians are frequently faced with the clinical quandary of rectal bleeding in the outpatient or emergency department setting. The spectrum of rectal bleeding can range from just a few drops of blood on the toilet paper to more ominous symptoms of hematochezia or melena. Many patients with rectal bleeding do not seek health care for this problem (1).

II. **PATHOPHYSIOLOGY. Rectal bleeding is typically a sign of local mucosal or vascular disease, but it can also signify proximal intestinal disease in the small or large bowel.** Scant or minimal rectal bleeding is a common problem present in up to 15% of the population. Hard, compacted stools associated with poor diet and bowel habits traumatize local venous and mucosal tissues. Physiologic states such as pregnancy can inhibit venous blood flow in the pelvis and lead to hemorrhoid formation. Bleeding from sources proximal to the duodenum tend to produce stools that are black and tarry because of metabolism of heme.

III. **EVALUATION.** The initial evaluation should determine the acuity and hemodynamic stability of the patient and establish the origins of the bleeding as upper or lower gastrointestinal tract in nature. Characteristics of anorectal versus other gastrointestinal sources of bleeding are compared in Table 9.11.1 (2–4).

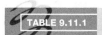 **Factors Associated with Anorectal versus Other Sources of Gastrointestinal Bleeding**
Suspected anorectal disease (hemorrhoids, anal fissure, proctitis, malignancy)
Age <50 y
Amount of bleeding minimal (bright red drops: on toilet paper, stool or in toilet bowl only)
Constipation or diarrhea
Pain while defecating
Anal symptoms (pain, pruritus, prolapse, protrusions)
From Bounds B, Friedman L. Lower gastrointestinal bleeding. *Gastroenterol Clin* 2003;32:1107–1125; Gopal D. Diseases of the rectum and anus: a clinical approach to common disorders. *Clin Cornerstone* 2002;4:34–48; Peter D, Dougherty J. Evaluation of the patient with gastrointestinal bleeding: an evidence-based approach. *Emerg Med Clin North Am* 1999;17:239–261.

A. History. Investigate about any comorbid illness such as liver disease, kidney disease, ulcers, or cancer. What are the dietary influences, such as fiber content or food ingestion (toxins or infections), that could be occurring? Is the patient taking any medications known to increase the risk of gastrointestinal bleed such as nonsteroidal anti-inflammatory drugs, aspirin, warfarin, tobacco, or alcohol? Has the patient engaged in anoreceptive intercourse or been exposed to sexually transmitted diseases? Are genitourinary symptoms such as urinary pain or prostatitis present (3,4)?

B. Physical examination
   1. It is important to check the following:
      a. Vital signs, orthostatic assessment "tilts"
      b. Skin pallor, jaundice, or turgor
      c. Abdominal tenderness, masses
      d. Ascites and/or hepatosplenomegaly
      e. Genitourinary examination
      f. Rectal examination: external visual inspection, digital rectal examination, stool assessment
   2. Potential hemodynamic compromise warrants volume resuscitation with two large-bore intravenous lines, preferably in an intensive care setting.

C. Testing
   1. Initial laboratory tests assess hemodynamic stability and clotting ability. Consider performing the following tests: complete blood count to assess for anemia, type and screen, stool Hemoccult test, serum blood urea nitrogen and creatinine, and coagulation panel.
   2. Imaging studies can be directed at the most likely source of bleeding. Younger patients with intermittent mild rectal bleeding can be evaluated with anoscopy or flexible sigmoidoscopy. Persons older than 50 years of age with painless bleeding are assumed to have colon cancer until proved otherwise by colonoscopy, even if the rectal examination is abnormal.

D. Genetics. A family history of gastrointestinal illness such as inflammatory bowel disease (Crohn's or ulcerative colitis), polyposis, or cancer significantly increases the likelihood of inherited rectal disease (4).

IV. DIAGNOSIS
   A. Differential diagnosis. Differential diagnosis includes any upper or lower gastrointestinal tract bleeding source from inflammatory bowel disease, diverticular bleeding, polyposis, malignancy, infection, trauma, or coagulopathy.
   B. Clinical manifestations. Clinical assessment of the patient should always begin with evaluation of hemodynamic status. If rectal bleeding is minimal or has stopped, and the patient is stable, evaluation can occur in the outpatient setting. By far, the most common anorectal bleeding source is hemorrhoidal disease. Risks of hemorrhoids increase with advancing age, pregnancy, prolonged sitting or standing, chronic diarrhea or constipation. Associated complaints from hemorrhoids include anal pruritus, pain and prolapse. Other anorectal sources of minimal bleeding include anal fissures, polyps, proctitis, rectal ulcers, and cancer (3).

References
1. Talley NJ, Jones M. Self-reported rectal bleeding in a United States community: prevalence, risk factors, and health care seeking. *Am J Gastroenterol* 1998;93:2179–2183.
2. Bounds B, Friedman L. Lower gastrointestinal bleeding. *Gastroenterol Clin* 2003;32: 1107–1125.
3. Gopal D. Diseases of the rectum and anus: a clinical approach to common disorders. *Clin Cornerstone* 2002;4:34–48.
4. Peter D, Dougherty J. Evaluation of the patient with gastrointestinal bleeding: an evidence based approach. *Emerg Med Clin North Am* 1999;17:239–261.

STEATORRHEA
Charles L. Bryner, Jr.

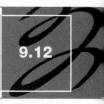

9.12

I. BACKGROUND. Steatorrhea, the third most common cause of chronic diarrhea, arises from the malabsorption of fat. By definition, it is the excretion of more than 7 g of fat in the stool during a 24-hour period while the patient is on a diet containing no more than 100 g of fat per day. It manifests as a history of greasy, foul-smelling stools that leave an oily residue in the toilet bowl, increased flatulence, and weight loss.

II. PATHOPHYSIOLOGY

  A. Etiology. The problem of fat malabsorption may stem from an intraluminal digestive disorder, a mucosal blockage of absorption at the enterocyte level, or a postmucosal blockage. The postmucosal blockages (e.g., intestinal lymphangiectasis or acanthocytosis) are quite uncommon and are beyond the scope of this brief discussion.

   1. Acute or chronic liver disease may cause steatorrhea. Impaired synthesis or impaired excretion of conjugated bile salts results in a bile salt deficiency and maldigestion of fats. Hepatitis, primary biliary cirrhosis, alcohol-induced liver diseases, or extrahepatic biliary obstruction (including cancer of the head of the pancreas) may be the causes. Prolonged, severe cardiac failure or hemochromatosis can cause cirrhosis, which can produce steatorrhea.

   2. The short bowel syndrome is a well-known cause of steatorrhea (1) and can follow actual resection of the ileum or arise from conditions that render large portions of the small bowel nonfunctional, such as Crohn's disease, chemotherapy, or radiation enteritis. Loss of a functional ileum leads to inadequate reabsorption of bile acid salts and causes a faulty digestion of fats. Pancreatic enzymes may be inactivated by exposure to excess gastric acids such as would occur in the Zollinger-Ellison syndrome. Segmental stasis of intestinal contents can also occur with the dysmotility of diabetes or scleroderma. Stasis permits bacterial overgrowth of the affected segment. The bacteria subsequently deconjugate and metabolize the bile acids in the small bowel rather than the colon.

   3. Ingestion of certain foods has been shown to cause steatorrhea. Ingestion of a large amount of peanuts or the use of liquid paraffin to treat constipation may result in significant steatorrhea. In patients attempting to lose weight, ingestion of the fat substitute Olestra can cause steatorrhea (2).

   4. Laxative abuse hastens gastrointestinal (GI) transit and may preclude adequate absorption of fats. Other drugs that can cause steatorrhea through a variety of mechanisms include bile acid sequestering resins (cholestyramine and colestipol), colchicine, para-aminosalicylic acid, paromycin sulfate (Humatin), and antibiotics such as tetracycline and neomycin. Thyrotoxicosis can cause a secondary steatorrhea due to the rapid transit of intestinal contents, which precludes proper digestion and absorption of fats. Infection with *Giardia lamblia* can lead to fat malabsorption. Travel within the tropics (excluding Africa) suggests tropical sprue, a chronic diarrheal disease, possibly of infectious origin.

   5. Even seemingly unrelated events have been shown to trigger steatorrhea; 3% of patients develop steatorrhea as a complication of bone marrow transplantation. The mechanism is believed to be graft versus host disease that affects the exocrine pancreatic function (3).

  B. Epidemiology. The incidence and prevalence of steatorrhea are difficult to estimate because this condition arises from an array of diverse underlying conditions that are difficult to amass into an overall figure. These other conditions are nonreportable illnesses or surgical procedures performed for other reasons and so are not readily tabulated in the literature.

III. EVALUATION

A. History. A careful history often provides clues to probable diagnoses and guides the astute clinician to tests most likely to provide a definitive diagnosis. The frequency of stools and duration of the complaint are important, as well as whether there has been an actual loss of weight. Recent travel to the tropics or a history of pancreatitis can be important clues. A family history of similar problems can help pinpoint a cause. Does the patient exhibit any signs or symptoms of hyperthyroidism?

B. Physical examination. Physical findings associated with steatorrhea are limited. A thorough examination of the abdomen to exclude palpable masses should be undertaken along with a search for signs of alcoholic liver disease.

C. Testing

1. The gold standard for diagnosis remains the quantitative determination of fecal fat from stool samples collected over 72 hours while the patient ingests a diet with a limited fat content. Collecting the stool is cumbersome and difficult for the patient and the test requires strict adherence to the prescribed diet. Spot tests of a single stool sample with Sudan III or the newer fecal elastase determination are simpler tests to administer. The validity of the fecal elastase test is still controversial but most agree that it has a very strong negative predictive value (4). Once true steatorrhea is demonstrated, further testing helps determine the underlying disorder.

2. Liver function testing and appropriate use of ultrasound or computed tomography (CT) scan of the liver and pancreas may demonstrate the source. Serum antibody testing can now identify gluten enteropathy (5). Sweat chloride testing is indicated in young children; cystic fibrosis is the leading cause of steatorrhea in this age group.

3. The D-xylose test measures the absorptive capacity of the proximal small bowel mucosa. D-xylose does not require pancreatic exocrine function to be absorbed. Disorders of the intestinal mucosa that impede absorption lead to low levels of the sugar in both serum and urine samples. Inadequate renal function, dehydration, or hypothyroidism can also depress urine levels, so determinations of serum thyroid-stimulating hormone, blood urea nitrogen, and creatinine are warranted. Bacterial overgrowth of the small intestine can also produce an abnormal D-xylose test.

   a. An abnormal D-xylose test should prompt referral for small intestine biopsy to search for evidence of mucosal diseases including gluten enteropathy, Whipple's disease, giardiasis, tropical sprue, or intestinal lymphoma. Some of these entities may also be diagnosed by their characteristic appearance on an upper GI series.

   b. A normal D-xylose test indicates proper mucosal function and so the problem is usually the digestion of fats within the intestinal lumen. The most frequent etiology is pancreatic insufficiency (see Table 9.12.1). A secretin test may be required to measure pancreatic function. A therapeutic trial of pancreatic enzymes with improvement in symptoms is considered presumptive proof of the diagnosis. Abdominal ultrasonography, CT scan, or endoscopic retrograde cholangiopancreatography may also be useful in the evaluation of suspected pancreatic disease.

4. The bile salt breath test, a nuclear medicine study, measures bile acid absorption. Because the terminal ileum is also the site of vitamin B_{12} absorption, the Schilling test may also be utilized to search for disorders of absorption. Disorders of the terminal ileum (Crohn's disease, granulomatous ileitis, prior ileal resection) result in poor absorption of bile salts, which then pass into the colon where bacteria deconjugate them. Poor reabsorption depletes the supply of bile salts, resulting in maldigestion of fats.

5. Noninvasive testing for small bowel bacterial overgrowth (SBBO) is available by the C-xylose breath test, the bile acid breath test, or the breath hydrogen test. A therapeutic trial of oral tetracycline with resolution of steatorrhea is presumptive confirmation of bacterial overgrowth, avoiding a more costly testing. The upper small intestine is normally bacteriologically sterile except for contaminants from

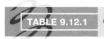

TABLE 9.12.1	Causes of Pancreatic Exocrine Insufficiency
Alcohol-induced liver diseases	Cystic fibrosis
Chronic pancreatitis	Zollinger-Ellison syndrome
Hypertriglyceridemia	Gastrectomy
Cancer of the pancreas	Vagotomy
Resection of the pancreas	Hemochromatosis
Blockage of the pancreatic duct	Shwachman-Diamond syndrome
Traumatic pancreatitis	Trypsinogen deficiency
Hereditary pancreatitis	α_1-Antitrypsin deficiency
Enterokinase deficiency	Somatostatinoma
Graft vs. host disease	

the mouth and upper respiratory tract. Aspiration of fluid through an endoscope or a small-intestine tube placed under fluoroscopic guidance that yields a bacterial colony count greater than 100,000/mL is diagnostic of SBBO.

    D. Genetics. Genetics plays little role in this disorder with the exception of those conditions with familial tendencies such as cystic fibrosis, gluten enteropathy, and acanthocytosis. In approximately 25% of cases, Zollinger-Ellison syndrome occurs in association with a genetic syndrome, multiple endocrine neoplasia type 1.

IV. DIAGNOSIS

    A. Differential diagnosis. As indicated in the preceding text, the differential diagnosis of steatorrhea is extensive. The degree of steatorrhea can lend clues to the source. Mild steatorrhea can occur with any disorder that causes rapid transit of intestinal contents, because the shortened exposure of the fats prevents proper absorption. The explosive urgent diarrhea of irritable bowel syndrome can mimic steatorrhea, but the fecal fat content does not usually meet the criteria for true steatorrhea. The proper workup of this symptom frequently requires specialized testing and procedures, necessitating consultation with a gastroenterologist if initial history and the more readily available tests fail to reveal its source.

    B. Clinical manifestations. The clinical expression as foul, greasy loose stools that are difficult to flush accompanied by weight loss is unchanged no matter what the underlying etiology of the steatorrhea is. The urgency and occasional incontinence may lead the patient to avoid social gatherings, cease physical exercise, or at times withdraw from even friends and family rather than experience the shame of an accident. Aggressively seeking the underlying condition and treating the diarrhea until the cause is found helps avoid this situation.

References

1. Gruy-Kapral C, Little KH, Fordtran JS, et al. Conjugated bile acid replacement therapy for short-bowel syndrome. *Gastroenterology* 1999;116:15.
2. Balasekaran R, Porter JL. Positive results on tests for steatorrhea in persons consuming olestra potato chips. *Ann Intern Med* 2000;132(4):279–282.
3. Grigg AP, Angus PW, Hoyt R, et al. The incidence, pathogenesis and natural history of steatorrhea after bone marrow transplantation. *Bone Marrow Transplant* 2003;31(8):701–703.
4. Beharry S, Ellis L, Corey M, et al. How useful is fecal pancreatic elastase 1 as a marker of exocrine pancreatic disease? *J Pediatr* 2002;141(1):84–90.
5. Murray JA. Serodiagnosis of celiac disease. *Clin Lab Res* 1997;17:445–464.

Renal and Urologic Problems

R. Whitney Curry, Jr.

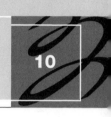

10

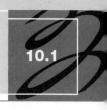

I. BACKGROUND. Dysuria is defined as "painful urination." Acute dysuria is a frequent problem seen in ambulatory practices, accounting for >3 million office visits a year. The most common diagnosis given for patients with dysuria is a urinary tract infection (UTI). The estimated cost of traditional management of acute UTIs approaches $1 billion per year in the United States. Although a UTI is the most common cause of dysuria symptoms, many other causes need to be accurately diagnosed. The differential diagnosis for patients with dysuria can be separated into broad categories. With a few notable exceptions, the differential diagnoses for men and women are similar, although the incidences are greatly different and change with age (1).

II. PATHOPHYSIOLOGY

    A. Causes of dysuria—female (2)

        1. Infectious

            a. Cystitis, lower UTI, with or without pyelonephritis

            b. Urethritis caused by a sexually transmitted disease (STD): *Chlamydia, Neisseria gonorrhoeae*, herpes simplex virus (HSV)

            c. Vulvovaginitis—bacterial vaginosis, trichomoniasis, yeast, genital HSV

        2. Noninfectious—trauma, irritant, allergy, sexual abuse

    B. Causes of dysuria—male (3)

        1. Infectious

            a. Urethritis caused by *Chlamydia, N. gonorrhoeae*, yeast (uncircumcised → balanitis), HSV

            b. Cystitis (if culture positive, possible anatomic abnormality, further workup indicated)

            c. Prostatitis, acute more common than chronic (4)

        2. Noninfectious

            a. Penile lesions, trauma, sexual abuse

            b. Benign prostatic hypertrophy (BPH) particularly in older men (5). Infection can be evident but is primarily an obstructive process.

III. EVALUATION

    A. History. A good general history is critical and can help direct further questions. Careful questioning about other associated symptoms and risk factors is the key to sorting out the diagnosis.

        1. Internal dysuria versus external dysuria. Internal dysuria is where the discomfort seems to be centered inside the body and begins before or with the initiation of voiding.

            a. Inflammation of the bladder or urethra
            External dysuria is when the discomfort appears after voiding has initiated

            b. Vaginitis, vulvar inflammation, or external penile lesions.

        2. Other important history items

            a. New sex partner → STD cause

            b. Diaphragm usage → bladder infection

            c. Gradual onset → urethritis and external causes

            d. Suprapubic pain, costovertebral angle tenderness, fever, and flank pain → pyelonephritis

            e. Older men → questioning about BPH

    B. Physical examination. The examination is essential in narrowing the diagnosis.

        1. Rule out pyelonephritis

            a. Fever

     b. Flank tenderness

     c. Suprapubic tenderness

  2. Genital examination

     a. Speculum examination in women

     b. Foreskin retraction in uncircumcised men

     c. Prostate examination

  3. Collection of samples for testing

     a. HSV lesions

     b. Discharge—yeast, bacterial vaginosis, gonorrhea, and trichomoniasis

     c. Trauma

C. Testing

  1. Urine analysis dipstick test—nitrates and leukoesterase (urea-fixing bacteria and leukocytes)

  2. Direct microscopic examination of the urine can detect the following:

     a. Leukocytes, bacteria, and blood

     b. Pyuria (defined as white blood cell count $>10/mm^3$ of urine)

  3. Urine culture: takes up to 48 hours

IV. DIAGNOSIS. Given the many causes of dysuria, an accurate diagnosis can be difficult without a thorough approach to each patient. Because most causes have other associated symptoms and findings, a diagnosis can usually be made with a carefully taken history, a focused physical examination, and appropriate laboratory tests. Separating an uncomplicated UTI or STD from the more serious pyelonephritis and other possible diagnoses is the challenge in these patients.

References

1. Johnson JR, Stamm WE. Diagnosis and treatment of acute urinary tract infections. *Infect Dis Clin North Am* 1987;4(1):773–791.
2. Kurowiski K. The woman with dysuria. *Am Fam Physician* 1998;57(9):2155–2164, 2169–2170.
3. Ainsworth JG, Weaver T, Murphy S, et al. General practitioners' immediate management of men presenting with urethral symptoms. *Genitourin Med* 1996;72(6):427–430.
4. Roberts RO, Lieber MM, Rhodes R, et al. Prevalence of a physician-assigned diagnosis of prostatitis: the Olmsted County study of urinary symptoms and health status among men. *Urology* 1998;51(4):578–584.
5. Bremnor JD, Sadovsky R. Evaluation of dysuria in adults. *Am Fam Physician* 2002;65(8):1589–1596.

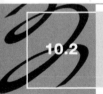

HEMATURIA
Siegfried O. F. Schmidt and Ku-Lang Chang

10.2

I. BACKGROUND. Hematuria, defined as "blood in the urine," is frequently encountered in family practice. It can be manifested as gross (macroscopic) hematuria with obvious reddish discoloration, or it can occur as microscopic hematuria detected with a dipstick followed by a microscopic examination. Although there is existing controversy pertaining to what constitutes microhematuria, most clinicians consider three or more red blood cells per high-power field (400×) as abnormal.

II. PATHOPHYSIOLOGY

  A. Etiology. The list of the potential causes of hematuria is lengthy and includes diseases of the urinary tract, as well as nonurologic causes. Some of these are life threatening (e.g., renal and bladder cancer), whereas others are insignificant (e.g., exercise-induced hematuria, bladder polyps, renal cysts). It is important to note that hematuria in an adult is more often urologic than renal in origin. The extent of the workup should be determined by considering factors such as the likelihood of coexisting illnesses, potential complications from procedures, and the cost to the patient. Benign causes such as menstruation, infection, and trauma should always be excluded before further evaluation and referral to urology or nephrology is initiated.

B. Epidemiology. Overall prevalence varies greatly (0.1%–13%) and depends on many variables (e.g., the number of screening tests performed, the type of population studied). However, screening of the general population for microscopic hematuria is not recommended. The decision to check for hematuria should depend on various risk factors for significant underlying disease, and remains a physician's judgment call. Risk factors for significant urologic disease include age >40 years, cigarette smoking (past or present, including second-hand smoke), history of urinary tract infections, history of hematuria, exposure to various drugs (analgesic, anti-inflammatory drugs, cyclophosphamide, human immunodeficiency virus therapy), exposure to occupational hazards (benzenes, 2-naphthylamine, aromatic amines, and aniline dyes), and pelvic radiation. In many cases of microhematuria, no cause can be found despite a complete evaluation.

III. EVALUATION

A. History. A thorough history is of utmost importance.

1. General questions should cover the type of hematuria (macroscopic/gross/microscopic), and the relationship between urination and the timing of hematuria. The three-container method assists in separating the micturition into three portions—initial, middle, and final portions. Anatomically, initial hematuria usually originates from anterior urethral disease, and final hematuria results from disease of the bladder neck, posterior urethra, or prostate. Hematuria throughout the micturition suggests pathology more proximal. Wormlike clots suggest a location above the bladder neck. Urine color should be questioned, which can be affected by the following: phenazopyridine (orange), nitrofurantoin (brown), rifampin (yellow-orange), L-dopa, methyldopa, and metronidazole (reddish brown), phenolphthalein in laxatives, red beet and rhubarb consumption, food coloring, and vegetable dyes (red).

2. Associated symptoms can hint at various particular problems; for example, a recent sore throat, fever, chills, and flulike symptoms may be the first signs of immunoglobulin A nephropathy or postinfectious glomerulonephritis. Urinary frequency, urgency, dysuria, fever, and chills point to an infectious process. Diminished urine flow and abdominal or flank pain radiating into the groin can indicate the presence of urinary tract obstruction. Vaginal discharge or bowel movement changes may hint at a nonurinary tract cause such as a foreign body (especially in children). A rash, joint pain, photosensitivity, flulike symptoms, and Raynaud's phenomenon point to a collagen vascular disease.

3. Past medical history should also include travel history. If the patient has traveled to areas where bilharzia (*Schistosoma haematobium*) is endemic, parasitic infestation is highly probable. Furthermore, if the history includes the use of analgesics, especially anti-inflammatory drugs, renal papillary necrosis should be considered. Past exposure to cyclophosphamide may cause chemical cystitis, because past exposure to antibiotics (e.g., penicillin, cephalosporins) may cause interstitial nephritis. Of special note is that the mere use of oral anticoagulants does not cause hematuria. To the contrary, these patients may in fact present earlier in their disease process and should be evaluated promptly (1).

4. Family history may lead to the suspicion of polycystic kidney disease, sickle cell trait and disease, nephrolithiasis, various glomerular diseases, tuberculosis, and benign familial hematuria. The combination of renal failure, deafness, and hematuria suggests Alport's hereditary nephritis.

B. Physical examination. Examination should focus on signs of systemic disease (e.g., fever, rash, lymphadenopathy, joint swelling, and abdominal or pelvic mass) and underlying medical or renal disease (e.g., hypertension, peripheral and generalized edema). Multiple telangiectasias and mucous membrane lesions indicate hereditary hemorrhagic telangiectasia (Rendu-Osler-Weber disease). The finding of an abdominal mass may indicate a Wilms' tumor in children or abdominal cancer and aneurysm in adults. On rectal and genitourinary examination, one can find signs of prostatitis, prostate hypertrophy, prostate cancer, vaginal and urethral changes, and pelvic masses.

C. Testing

1. Laboratory testing initially begins with examining a freshly voided, clean catch urine sample by a dipstick. It is important to confirm hematuria by a microscopic examination of the urine sediment. This sediment is obtained by centrifugation of a fixed volume of urine (5 mL) for 5 minutes at 3,000 rotations/minute. Afterward, the supernatant is poured off, and the remaining sediment is re-suspended in the centrifuge tube by gently tapping the bottom of the tube. A pipette is used to sample the residual fluid and transfer it to a glass slide, and a coverslip is applied to the slide for microscopic evaluation (2). The specimen is examined under high magnification (400×) to determine the cell type and distinct morphologic features. Results are recorded as the number of red blood cells per high-power field. If a patient is asymptomatic and has no particular risk factors, two additional urine analyses should be obtained. If one of them is abnormal, it is not necessary to perform other studies. If at least two out of three urine analyses are abnormal, further workup is necessary (3). When the dipstick testing is positive for blood, but urine microscopy reveals no red blood cells, hemoglobinuria or myoglobinuria should be considered. The use of a benzidine dipstick allows the differentiation of these discolorations from those of hematuria and myoglobinuria. As a next step, a urine culture can be obtained to rule out an infection.

2. Blood tests include a renal panel and a complete blood count with differential, sedimentation rate, prothrombin time, and partial thromboplastin time.

3. Any further evaluation is highly dependent on the suspected cause. Further blood tests may include serum complement titer (significant if low), antistreptolysin-O titer (significant if high), antinuclear antibody and extended panels with antideoxyribonuclease B titer (significant if high), and hemoglobin electrophoresis. The urine can also be sent for cytology. A tuberculin skin test or chest x-ray can be performed to detect tuberculosis. Intravenous pyelogram, abdominal and pelvic ultrasound, computer tomography, or magnetic resonance imaging may detect benign conditions such as urolithiasis, obstructive uropathy, renal cysts, parenchymal abnormalities, and nonurinary tract lesions, as well as malignancies of various anatomical areas. One should then proceed with a cystoscopy, looking for abnormalities of the urethra and bladder. Biopsies of various areas, as well as invasive vascular studies, may be necessary.

4. Recently developed urinary tumor markers (e.g., BTA TRAK and telomerase) have been used in tumor surveillance, but their role in screening of patients with hematuria is unclear at this time (1). At any time during an evaluation, it remains within the physician's judgment to refer the patient to a subspecialist.

IV. DIAGNOSIS.

The keys to the diagnosis of hematuria are found in the clinical history and the physical examination. Laboratory and imaging studies only help confirm or rule out initial suspicions. The goal is to diagnose a variety of serious illnesses, including malignancies and renal parenchymal diseases. In general, the degree of hematuria is of little diagnostic or prognostic value (2). As little as 1 mL of blood can cause a visible color change. In addition, a variety of drugs, foods, and food coloring can discolor the urine. Also, it is necessary to remember that transient hematuria, especially in a young individual, is quite common and rarely indicative of significant pathology (4). When present in patients older than 40 years of age, however, transient hematuria warrants a comprehensive evaluation to rule out malignancy. Similarly, a diagnostic workup should be performed when persistent hematuria is found in patients of any age. A summary of the best practice policy recommendations by the American Urologic Association is contained in the article, "Asymptomatic Microscopic Hematuria in Adults," available at the website http://www.aafp.org/afp/20010315/1145.html. It contains an excellent flow chart of the workup of asymptomatic microscopic hematuria, plus a strategy to identify patients with significant disease, while minimizing cost and morbidity associated with unnecessary tests.

Repeat evaluations are indicated for those patients with a negative evaluation, and in whom a malignancy is suspected (mainly older adults). A reasonable time frame appears to be 3 to 6 months for less invasive tests and 1 year for more invasive tests (5).

A. Clinical manifestations. Other important clinical manifestations should also be considered. Until otherwise proven, painless gross hematuria in the absence of infection in elderly men is caused by malignancy, just as hematuria associated with "sterile" pyuria is caused by genitourinary tuberculosis or interstitial nephritis. Finally, other medical problems such as prostate hypertrophy, diabetes mellitus (nephrosclerosis), nephrolithiasis, trauma (including vigorous masturbation), previous urinary tract malignancies with recurrence, and sickle cell disease (papillary necrosis) may cause hematuria.

References
1. Yun EJ, Meng MV, Carroll PR. Evaluation of the patient with hematuria. *Med Clin North Am* 2004;88:329–343.
2. Thaller TR, Wang LP. Evaluation of asymptomatic microscopic hematuria in adults. *Am Fam Physician* 1999;60:1143–1154.
3. Grossfeld GD, Wolf JS, Litwin MS, et al. Asymptomatic microscopic hematuria in adults: summary of the AUA best practice policy recommendations. *Am Fam Physician* 2001;63(6):1145–1154.
4. Murakami S, Igarashi T, Hara S, et al. Strategies for asymptomatic microscopic hematuria: a prospective study of 1034 patients. *J Urol* 1990;144:99–106.
5. Messing EM, Young TB, Hunt VB, et al. Hematuria home screening: repeat testing results. *J Urol* 1995;154(1):57–61.

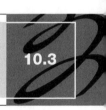

IMPOTENCE
Louis Kuritzky

10.3

I. **BACKGROUND.** Impotence, defined as the consistent inability to get or maintain an erection sufficient for intercourse, is, in essence, a patient-defined diagnosis (1, 2). The role of the clinician is to confirm impotence, rule out correctable secondary causes, and expeditiously restore sexual function. To encourage hopefulness, clinicians would do well to explain at the outset that essentially 100% of men can have restoration of sexual function using currently available treatments.

II. **PATHOPHYSIOLOGY.** The most recent large epidemiologic survey of American men found some degree of impotence in 52% of men older than 40 years of age. Most organic impotence is on a vascular basis. Because integrity of the endothelium is necessary to provide adequate penile engorgement, disorders that cause endothelial dysfunction are predictably associated with erectile dysfunction (ED). Diabetes, smoking, hypertension, dyslipidemia, and peripheral vascular disease are all associated with impaired endothelial function, and may hence induce or contribute to ED. Whether the correction of vasculopathic factors improves erectile function in men with ED remains to be determined.

III. **EVALUATION**
   A. **History**
      1. Although written questionnaires may elicit sexual dysfunction, most patients prefer to communicate such issues in the privacy of verbal communication with their primary care provider. Initial inquiry can simply be "Are you sexually

active?" For sexual dysfunction evaluation, gender orientation is not relevant to diagnosis or therapy, so that whether the patient is homosexual, heterosexual, or bisexual has no distinct bearing on the diagnostic or therapeutic direction. For individuals who are not sexually active, the next inquiry should be to determine whether this is a matter of choice, or an obstacle that prevents sexual activity (e.g., lack of partner, impotence, physical disorder).

2. For individuals who are sexually active, a series of follow-up questions uncovers most relevant psychosexual pathology. You could begin with "How would you rate your sex life on a scale of 1 to 10?" If the response is 10, sexual dysfunction is decidedly unlikely. However, most individuals respond "Oh, about a 7." You can follow with, "What would have to be different to change your sex life from a 7 to a 10?" This forced-choice inquiry often produces responses that directly indicate problematic underlying issues such as "Well, if I could just get a good erection" or "If my erection could last >30 seconds." Inquiry about libido is a crucial diagnostic point for testosterone deficiency. Men who present with good libido only have a remote possibility of having testosterone deficiency.

3. A medication history should be taken. Most medication-induced impotence is evident by the temporal relationship between the onset of impotence and medication initiation. On the other hand, agents such as thiazides may produce impotence after months of use. Similarly, some antidepressants may produce sexual dysfunction early, or after weeks of therapy. Relationship of medications to impotence can often be clarified by a drug holiday.

B. **Physical examination.** Although physical examination is usually not enlightening, there is general agreement that the genitals should be examined for evidence of overt testicular atrophy and the penis for Peyronie's disease. Peyronie's disease produces palpable plaques in the corpora cavernosa that can lead to angulation upon erection, pain, or both. Treatment is surgical. A rectal examination to document rectal sensation as well as tone can be complemented by the bulbocavernosus reflex. This reflex is elicited by briskly squeezing the glans penis in one hand while a single digit from the other is in the rectum. A normal examination, indicating an intact reflex arc, is manifest as a rectal contraction in response to the glans squeeze. Prostate examination is pertinent at this point, in the event testosterone therapy is required.

C. **Testing.** Reasonable screening tests for impotence include plasma glucose, lipid profile (seeking vasculopathic risk factors), total morning testosterone, and a urinalysis. If total morning testosterone is low, luteinizing and follicle-stimulating hormone levels should be measured, because an increase in these indicates gonadal failure, for which testosterone replacement is indicated; a decrease indicates potential hypothalamic or pituitary insufficiency, necessitating central nervous system (CNS) imaging to rule out a mass lesion. Similarly, testosterone may be suppressed by an elevated prolactin, whether induced by a CNS lesion, hypothyroidism, medications, or other factors. A low (or low–normal) total testosterone should be repeated and confirmed by means of measuring the free testosterone, which is more sensitive, but substantially more expansive than total testosterone.

IV. **DIAGNOSIS**

A. **Differential diagnosis.** Impotence is broadly divided into psychogenic and organic categories, although there is often a substantial degree of overlap. Men who report sudden, complete loss of sexual function, or "circumstantial" impotence: (i) good function with one partner, but not another; (ii) good erections with masturbation but not with a partner; (iii) good morning erections, but not with a partner, are much more likely to have psychogenic impotence. Because organic impotence generally leads to psychological consequences, many patients suffer a combination of psychogenic and organic impotence.

B. **Clinical manifestations**

1. Psychogenic impotence may reflect depression, relationship conflict, performance anxiety, or partner-directed hostility. The history is definitive in most cases. Sudden complete loss of function, situation or partner variability, along with maintenance of morning or masturbatory erections, is typical. Occasionally,

patients with dysfunctions other than impotence seek advice; for instance, believing that premature ejaculation is impotence. In such cases, corrective education combined with appropriate attention to the alternate diagnosis is the logical next step.

2. Organic sexual dysfunction is characterized by incremental loss of erectile function. In middle age, men with organic ED note reduced erectile turgidity, increasing requirement for tactile stimulation to produce an erection, and a lengthening refractory period (i.e., the amount of time required after ejaculation before the male is receptive to restimulation and erection). Such stepwise loss of sexual function corroborates organicity.

3. In primary care, as many as 98% of patients have no correctable cause of impotence discerned after appropriate history and physical examination. That need not delay the immediate provision of highly effective oral agents (PDES inhibitor [phosphodiesterase type 5 inhibitors]), vacuum constriction devices, or intracorporeal injection, any of which may be provided in the primary care setting. Patients who fail to respond to the standard treatment tools should be referred.

References
1. Kuritzky L. Primary care issues in the management of erectile dysfunction. In: Seftel AD, ed. *Male and female sexual dysfunction*. Edinburgh: Mosby, 2004.
2. Kuritzky L, Ahmed O, Kosch S. Management of impotence in primary care. *Comp Ther* 1998;24(3):137–146.

URINARY INCONTINENCE IN ADULTS
Richard Rathe

10.4

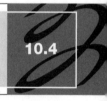

I. BACKGROUND. Urinary incontinence (UI) is the involuntary loss of urine at times and in amounts that interfere with hygiene and activities of daily living. UI is one of the most prevalent and underdiagnosed afflictions in the United States. It is a major cause of social withdrawal and loss of independent living. Victims are often too embarrassed to discuss this problem, even with their physician. Some even view it as a natural part of aging, but this is not the case. UI is a symptom, not a disease. Understanding the types of disorders that cause incontinence is the key to correct diagnosis and effective treatment.

II. PATHOPHYSIOLOGY

   A. Etiology. (See Tables 10.4.1 and 10.4.2). The DRIP mnemonic is often cited to remember the reversible (and curable) causes of UI:

      1. D—delirium and drugs

      2. R—restricted mobility and retention

      3. I—infection, inflammation, and impaction

      4. P—polyuria from uncontrolled diabetes and other conditions

   B. Epidemiology

      1. Thirteen million Americans are incontinent; 11 million are women.

      2. One in four women ages 30 to 59 have experienced an episode of UI.

      3. More than 50% of elderly individuals are incontinent.

      4. Every year $16.4 billion is spent on incontinence-related care.

      5. Every year $1.1 billion is spent on disposable products for adults (1).

III. EVALUATION

   A. History

      1. Voiding history. It is important to fully characterize the patient's problem by taking a detailed history, including the duration of the symptoms, timing of

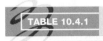

TABLE 10.4.1   Classification of Urinary Incontinence

Type	Definition	Mechanism	Disorders
Urge	Inability to delay voiding once the urge occurs	Detrusor hyperactivity	Idiopathic (common in the elderly) Genitourinary conditions (cystitis, stones)
Stress	Loss of urine with increased abdominal pressure	Sphincter failure	Weak or injured pelvic muscles Sphincter weakness
Overflow	Partial retention of urine behind an obstruction	Outlet obstruction Loss of innervation	Obstruction (prostate, cystocele) Neuropathic (diabetes, nerve injury)
Functional	Inability to get to the toilet in time	Physical or cognitive impairment	Dementia or delirium Physical limitations (lack of mobility) Psychological/behavioral
Mixed	Any combination of the above	Any combination of the above	Any combination of the above

voluntary/involuntary voiding, amounts voided involuntarily, and the relationship to voluntary voiding. Focus on the following areas:

   a. Need for pads or diapers (measure of severity)
   b. Loss of urine with coughing or laughing (suggests stress type)
   c. Inability to hold urine after having the urge to urinate (suggests urge type)
   d. Pain or discomfort (suggests infection or inflammation)
   e. Inability to fully empty bladder (suggests obstruction)
   f. Decreased urinary stream (suggests obstruction)
   g. Impact of UI on the patient's life
   h. What the patient thinks is going on
2. **Voiding journal.** A voiding journal is a good way to get additional information about the patient's problem. Have the patient record the time and approximate amount of each voiding, and whether they were wet or dry.

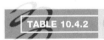

TABLE 10.4.2   Major Causes of Urinary Incontinence

Acute	Chronic
Primary disorders	Local processes
Infection, medications, delirium	Pelvic floor weakness following childbirth, bladder tumor or deformity, tumors, obstruction by an enlarged prostate, cystocele or fecal impaction
	Postsurgical
Exacerbations of systemic diseases	Systemic processes
Diabetes mellitus, diabetes insipidus, congestive heart failure, stroke	Menopause, neuropathy (diabetes, alcoholism), dementia, depression, stroke, tumor, Parkinson's disease

3. **Major medical problems.** Does the patient have any known condition that is associated with UI? These include diabetes, heart failure, menopause, and neurologic problems. Does the patient have other genitourinary symptoms? In female patients, be sure to take a detailed obstetrical history.

4. **Medication history.** Because medications are a major cause of incontinence, be sure to take a thorough medication history. Offending agents include diuretics, older antidepressants, antihypertensives, narcotics, and alcohol.

5. **Diabetes insipidus.** Central or nephrogenic diabetes insipidus can present with UI due to increased urine output (many liters per day). These patients frequently have a concomitant polydipsia that closely matches their water loss. You should consider this diagnosis when the patient gives a history of voiding large volumes of urine.

B. **Physical examination.** The examination is often normal in cases of UI. You should focus your efforts in an attempt to uncover the underlying cause(s):

1. General (is the patient physically capable of getting to the toilet?)
2. Mental status (can the patient understand and act on their urge to void?)
3. Neurologic including the anal reflex (focal signs suggest a neurologic cause)
4. Abdominal (is the bladder distended?)
5. Rectal/prostate (impaction or enlarged prostate present?)
6. Pelvic (atrophic vaginitis, prolapse, or mass present?)

C. **Testing**

1. **Urinalysis.** Be cautious interpreting the urinalysis; in the absence of other symptoms, bacteriuria is seldom the primary cause of UI. Treat cystitis or urethritis when they are confirmed by the rest of the clinical picture. A urologist should investigate unexplained, persistent microhematuria.

2. **Postvoiding urine volume.** The patient should be straight catheterized immediately after voiding. In general, the postvoid urine volume should be <50 mL. Volumes in the range of 100 to 200 mL may suggest impaired bladder contractility or obstruction. Volumes >200 mL strongly suggest obstruction.

3. **Blood urea nitrogen, creatinine, and glucose.** These simple blood tests help rule out underlying renal disease and diabetes.

4. **Special tests.** Certain tests are available through urologic consultation to further delineate the cause of UI. These include cystoscopy, cystometry, and other voiding studies. Up to two-thirds of patients can be successfully treated without urologic referral (2).

D. **Genetics.** Recent research indicates that there may be a genetic predisposition for UI in women. For a woman with a history of incontinence in her mother or older sisters the relative risk was 1.3. This increased to 1.9 if the symptoms were reported as "severe." These results were consistent, regardless of the type(s) of incontinence present (3).

IV. **DIAGNOSIS.** Clinical history is the most important factor leading to the correct diagnosis and successful treatment of UI. However, it is an imperfect tool at best. In one review, clinical history had a sensitivity and specificity for stress incontinence of 0.90 and 0.50 respectively. For detrusor instability the figures were 0.74 and 0.55 (4). The task becomes even more problematic when one considers the reluctance of patients to talk about their symptoms, and the tendency for UI to be of a mixed type. Response to therapy (or lack thereof) often drives the practical management of this condition. Lack of response to multiple trials of therapy is a good indication for consulting an urologist. Remember that your initial assessment is often incorrect, so keep an open mind and do not discount any possible diagnosis. Finally, remember that there are often multiple simultaneous factors leading to UI. For example, many otherwise healthy elderly individuals have physical limitations that can contribute a functional component to their problem.

References

1. *Overview: urinary incontinence in adults, clinical practice guideline update.* (March 1996) http://www.ahrq.gov/clinic/uiovervw.htm, accessed on July 2005.

2. Weiss BD. Diagnostic evaluation of urinary incontinence in geriatric patients. *Am Fam Physician* 1998;57(11):2665–2687. http://www.aafp.org/afp/980600ap/weiss.html, accessed on July 2005.
3. Hannestad YS. Familial risk of urinary incontinence in women: population based cross sectional study. *BMJ* 2004;329:889–891. http://bmj.bmjjournals.com/cgi/content/full/329/7471/889/, accessed on July 2005.
4. Jensen JK, Nielsen FR, Ostergard DR. The role of patient history in the diagnosis of urinary incontinence. *Obstet Gynecol* 1994;83(5):904–910.

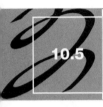

10.5 NOCTURIA
Vincent H. Ober

I. BACKGROUND. Nocturia is urination during the time that a patient is usually sleeping. Nocturia is a unique clinical syndrome but may be associated with many different medical problems (1).

II. PATHOPHYSIOLOGY

A. Etiology. The causes of nocturia are usually divided into three groups: conditions that increase urine volume, conditions associated with disordered sleep, and disturbances of the lower urinary tract (2). However, a patient may have multiple contributing etiologies.

1. Volume-related conditions
   a. Excessive intake of fluids
   b. Dietary substances and medications that increase urine output, including alcohol, caffeine, diuretics, lithium, and theophylline
   c. Diseases associated with increased solute excretion such as diabetes mellitus and hypercalcemia
   d. Diabetes insipidus (central and nephrogenic)
   e. Peripheral edema from excessive sodium ingestion, congestive heart failure, hepatic disease, sleep apnea, renal insufficiency, hypoalbuminemia, and medications (e.g., dihydropyridine calcium channel blockers and thiazolidinediones)
   f. Increased nighttime urine secretion (nocturnal polyuria) due to age-related decreased renal concentrating ability, decreased renal sodium conservation, decreased nocturnal antidiuretic hormone secretion, and increased atrial natriuretic hormone secretion (3)

2. Sleep-related conditions
   a. Insomnia
   b. Restless leg syndrome
   c. Chronic pain syndromes
   d. Shortness of breath associated with pulmonary or cardiac disease
   e. Dietary substances such as caffeine or drugs (e.g., very short acting hypnotics)
   f. Neurologic disorders such as dementia and Parkinson's disease

3. Lower urinary tract conditions
   a. Urinary tract infection, including cystitis and prostatitis
   b. Chronic interstitial cystitis
   c. Small bladder capacity because of pelvic mass, adhesions, or surgery
   d. Detrusor hyperactivity (both neurogenic and non-neurogenic)
   e. Urinary retention due to bladder outlet obstruction or detrusor weakness
   f. Decreased bladder compliance due to aging, tumor, or radiation

B. Epidemiology. The incidence of nocturia is reported in 4% of children 7 to 15 years (4) and in up to 91% of men older than 80 years of age. Overall, the incidence is higher in men (1,5). There are many causes for the increased incidence with age, but increased nocturia is mainly related to a decrease in bladder capacity and an increase in nocturnal urine secretion (with no change in 24-hour urine production).

III. EVALUATION

A. History. The history should include the following: (i) a voiding diary (for 24–72 hours), with measurement of urine volumes to establish bladder capacity (average voiding volume), total urine output, and diurnal voiding patterns; (ii) the volume of fluid intake; (iii) the medical history; (iv) the surgical history; (v) the medications used; (vi) dietary habits; (vii) sleep history; and (viii) response to self treatments such as fluid, caffeine, and alcohol restriction.

B. Physical examination. The examination should include pulmonary, cardiac, abdominal, female pelvic, rectal, and neurologic evaluations.

C. Testing

1. Laboratory tests should include routine dipstick urinalysis and blood chemistries (to include blood urea nitrogen [BUN], creatinine, glucose, calcium, albumin). Postvoid residual urine should be measured (<50 mL is normal). Urine culture may be useful if the patient has symptoms of frequency and dysuria and a normal urinalysis.

2. Specialized testing such as cystoscopy, urodynamic testing, and sleep studies are rarely needed.

IV. DIAGNOSIS

A. Volume-related causes for nocturia are indicated by a total daily urine output >40 mL/kg/day. Excessive fluid, caffeine, and alcohol intake are detected by the patient history. Serum glucose is elevated in diabetes mellitus. Serum calcium is elevated in hypercalcemia. Urine specific gravity is <1.010 in diabetes insipidus. The history and physical examination should detect medical or surgical problems and medications associated with increased nocturnal urine production. Renal insufficiency is diagnosed by an elevated serum creatinine and BUN. Nocturnal polyuria is indicated by nocturnal urine volume >33% of the total 24-hour urine volume.

B. Sleep-related causes are suggested by a patient history of insomnia, acute or chronic pain, or breathlessness. Dietary substances or drugs that disrupt sleep, as well as dementia and neurologic diseases, should be detected by the history and physical. Sleep studies are usually not required. Nighttime voided volume with each micturition less than average daytime voided volume (bladder capacity) suggests disordered sleep or urinary tract abnormalities.

C. Lower urinary tract causes are identified by the history, urinalysis, and measurement of postvoid residual urine. Pyuria usually indicates urinary tract infection. Lower urinary tract irritative symptoms (frequency and dysuria) and a normal urinalysis and urine culture suggest interstitial cystitis (and is confirmed by cystoscopy). Small voided volume throughout the day and night indicates small bladder capacity, decreased bladder compliance, or detrusor hyperactivity. Postvoid residual urine >50 mL indicates urinary retention that may be caused by prostatic obstruction or inadequate detrusor contractions. Urodynamic studies can be helpful in complex cases.

References

1. Van Kerrebroeck P, Abrams P, Chaikin D, et al. The standardization of terminology in nocturia: report from the standardization subcommittee of the international continence society. *BJU Int* 2002;90(S3):11–15.
2. Resnick NM. Urinary incontinence. In: Cassel CK, Cohen HJ, Larson EB, et al., eds. *Geriatric Medicine*, 3rd ed. New York, NY: Springer-Verlag, 1997:562–566.
3. Miller M. Nocturnal polyuria in older people: pathophysiology and clinical implications. *J Am Geriatr Soc* 2000;48(10):1321–1329.
4. Mattsson S. Urinary incontinence and nocturia in health schoolchildren. *Acta Paediatr* 1994;83:950–954.
5. Malmsten UGH, Milson I, Molander U, et al. Urinary incontinence and lower urinary tract symptoms: an epidemiological study of men aged 45 to 99 years. *J Urol* 1997; 158(5):1733–1737.

OLIGURIA AND ANURIA
Marcia W. Funderburk

10.6

I. BACKGROUND. Oliguria and anuria should be recognized promptly so that the cause can be identified and treatment initiated to preserve renal function and prevent life-threatening complications. Oliguria is defined as urine volume <500 mL/24 hour or <20 mL/hour (in small children, <0.8 mL/kg/hour). Anuria is strictly defined as the total absence of urine; in the clinical setting, however, a urine output of <50 to 100 mL/24 hour is often considered anuria (1). The amount of urine output must be reliably established (most reliably measured using an indwelling catheter).

II. PATHOPHYSIOLOGY

  A. Etiology

    1. Oliguria. It is helpful to think of oliguria as prerenal, renal, or postrenal.

      a. Prerenal disorders are characterized by decreased renal perfusion, leading to decreased glomerular filtration rate such that the daily endogenous load of nitrogenous wastes cannot be excreted, therefore the term prerenal azotemia.

      b. Renal disorders are characterized by pathology within the kidney parenchyma itself, which can be the end result of prolonged decreased renal perfusion.

      c. Postrenal disorders causing oliguria are characterized by the partial obstruction of the urinary tract at an anatomic position distal to the kidney. This can be confusing, because these disorders can also cause polyuria.

    2. Anuria results from the total obstruction of the urinary tract, or as an end result of the prerenal and renal causes of oliguria. A sudden cause of anuria, especially in the elderly, is bilateral renal artery occlusion (or unilateral occlusion in a single kidney) typically caused by embolism. Early recognition of this entity is imperative to restore blood flow to the ischemic kidney(s).

III. EVALUATION

  A. History

    1. Pertinent present history. A patient may complain of decreased urine output in some clinical situations. More often, however, the clinical situation and pertinent history should lead to an evaluation of the presence of oliguria or anuria.

      a. Are there symptoms of illness or trauma leading to hypotension?

        i. Hypovolemia (e.g., hemorrhage, diuretic overuse, gastrointestinal fluid loss, skin fluid loss owing to burns or heat exposure, third spacing secondary to burns, peritonitis, pancreatitis, or trauma)?

        ii. Decreased cardiac output (e.g., congestive heart failure, myocardial infarction, pericardial tamponade, or acute pulmonary embolus)?

        iii. Peripheral vasodilatation (e.g., septic shock, anaphylactic shock)?

      b. Are there symptoms of vascular disease? Consider bilateral renal vascular obstruction due to severe renal artery stenosis, thrombosis, or embolism.

      c. Is there any history consistent with renal parenchymal injury (e.g., recent radiocontrast agent, nephrotoxin exposure such as ethylene glycol, nonsteroidal anti-inflammatory drug overdose, acute nephritis, acute vasculitis, pyelonephritis [in the elderly], papillary necrosis [in patients with diabetes], or prolonged hypotension with hypoperfusion of the kidney)?

      d. Is there any history consistent with urinary tract obstruction?

        i. Bladder neck obstruction (e.g., benign prostatic hypertrophy, prostate cancer, bladder cancer, or functional obstruction due to drug side effects)?

        ii. Obstruction of the urethra or bilateral ureters—internally (secondary blood clots, stones, sulfonamide or uric acid crystals, pyogenic debris, necrotizing papillitis or edema), or externally (secondary tumors, periureteral fibrosis, accidental ureteral ligation during pelvic surgery, ascites, pregnancy, pelvic abscess, or hematoma).

   e. Medication use must be considered—diuretics, antihypertensives, anticholinergics, aminoglycosides, amphotericin B, or chemotherapeutic drugs.
   2. Pertinent past history. Is there a history of cancer, recent surgery, kidney stones, neurologic disorder, vascular disease, chronic liver disease (hepatorenal syndrome), or kidney transplant?
B. Physical examination
   1. Focused physical examination. This should include vital signs (notably blood pressure, pulse, and temperature). Orthostatic blood pressure and pulse may be necessary. Signs of hypovolemia, hypotension, and dehydration—skin turgor and color, mucous membranes, capillary refill, warmth of extremities—should be noted.
   2. Additional physical examination. Depending on the history (e.g., skin rash, cardiac examination, bruits over kidneys), palpate for a distended bladder; if a cancer or outlet obstruction is suspected, perform a rectal or pelvic examination.
C. Testing
   1. An indwelling urinary catheter serves as a diagnostic tool (if obstruction has occurred at the bladder neck or urethra) and for accurate urine volume measurement. Urine output and blood pressure monitoring can often lead to expedient correction of prerenal causes, thereby avoiding further complications.
   2. Urinalysis is often normal in prerenal causes of oliguria or anuria, except being highly concentrated with possible qualitative proteinuria because of the high concentration. Microscopic analysis is usually unremarkable (or reveals few hyaline or granular casts) in prerenal causes; whereas proteinuria, casts, and hematuria can point to renal causes.
   3. Urine osmolality is typically high in prerenal causes (>500 mOsm/kg H_2O) versus impaired in renal causes (<350 mOsm/kg H_2O) (2).
   4. Urine sodium is typically <20 mEq/L in prerenal causes (unless diuretics have been used) versus >40 mEq/L in renal causes (1).
   5. Blood urea nitrogen and creatinine levels are elevated. The ratio must be interpreted considering the entire clinical situation. Urine:plasma creatinine ratio (U:P Cr) is calculated to help differentiate between prerenal (U:P Cr >40) and renal (U:P Cr <20) causes (1).
   6. Diagnostic imaging, which may be necessary in some cases, is guided by the history and physical examination findings (e.g., ultrasound, computed tomography [CT], retrograde pyelogram, renal biopsy).
IV. DIAGNOSIS. The key to a diagnosis of oliguria or anuria is to actively anticipate when it is likely to manifest and accurately measure using an indwelling catheter. Once recognized and a cause is suggested, (i) prerenal causes can be further assessed by measuring hemodynamic status and administering fluids; (ii) renal causes can be further assessed with urinalysis (qualitative and quantitative), renal ultrasound, or renal biopsy; and (iii) postrenal causes can be further assessed using ultrasound, CT scan, or retrograde pyelography.

References

1. Molitoris BA. Oliguria and anuria. In: Massry SG, Glassock RJ, eds. *Massry and Glassock's textbook of nephrology*, 4th ed. Philadelphia, PA: Lippincott, Williams & Wilkins, 2001:489–491.
2. Glassock RJ, Massry SG, Humes HD. Acute renal failure including cortical necrosis, Part 2 diagnosis, clinical presentation, and management. In: Massry SG, Glassock RJ, eds. *Massry and Glassock's textbook of nephrology*, 4th ed. Philadelphia, PA: Lippincott, Williams & Wilkins, 2001:971.

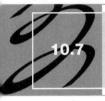

10.7 PRIAPISM
David B. Feller

I. **BACKGROUND.** Priapism is defined as a persistent, often painful, penile erection not associated with sexual stimulation. No time course is specifically defined, but priapism is usually diagnosed when the erection lasts >4 hours. Although relatively uncommon (incidence 1.5/100,000 person-years and 2.9/100,000 person-years for men 40 years of age and older) (1), priapism represents a urologic emergency (2).

II. **PATHOPHYSIOLOGY**

A. **Etiology.** Two types of priapism (low-flow or veno-occlusive and high-flow or arterial) have been described based on the underlying precipitating event (3). Arterial priapism usually occurs after injury to the cavernous artery from perineal or direct penile trauma. This injury then leads to uncontrolled high arterial inflow within the corpora cavernosa. Veno-occlusive priapism is characterized by inadequate outflow and is far and away the most common. Distinction between the two is imperative because ultimate treatment varies significantly.

B. **Epidemiology.** A history of penile or perineal trauma almost always precedes arterial priapism, and is the most important historical information that distinguishes between the two types of priapism. Studies have suggested that up to 41% of patients who present with priapism (veno-occlusive) have taken some type of psychotropic medication, usually neuroleptics, or trazodone, and even with the α-blocker prazosin (4). Priapism has been commonly reported (1%–17%) after intracavernous injection with prostaglandins for the treatment of erectile dysfunction. Subsequently, therapeutically induced prolonged erection has become the primary and most common cause of priapism. Patients with any history of malignancy, especially genitourinary or pelvic carcinoma and new-onset priapism, should be evaluated for penile metastasis. In one review, 20% to 53% of cases with penile metastases presented initially with priapism (5).

The most common cause of priapism in children is sickle cell disease. It has been reported that over 60% of all children with this disease eventually develop priapism.

III. **EVALUATION**

A. **History.** Specific questions may help identify the type of priapism, cause, and urgency of treatment. Always inquire how long the priapism has been present. How much pain does the patient experience? Moderate to severe, persistent pain is characteristic of veno-occlusive priapism and results from tissue ischemia. Pain is generally much more mild or transient with arterial priapism. Is there a history of penile or perineal trauma? Trauma more commonly precedes arterial priapism. Does the patient take any medications that may predispose to priapism? Is there any history of malignancy? Is there any history of sickle cell disease?

B. **Physical examination.** The examination should include a thorough genitourinary examination to look for trauma or malignancy. The corpora cavernosa but not the corpora spongiosum is involved with priapism and, therefore, the glans remains flaccid while the shaft is erect and tender. The examination should also include palpation for inguinal lymphadenopathy (genitourinary malignancy), and an abdominal examination (abdominal or genitourinary malignancy and trauma).

C. **Testing**

1. In most instances, the history and physical examination determine the cause of priapism. A complete blood count and sickle cell screen may be useful, looking for malignancy and sickle cell disease respectively. Coagulation studies are also recommended (in case aspiration is contemplated for treatment). Blood gas measurement from a cavernosal sample may be useful if differentiation between low-flow versus high-flow priapism is difficult (2).

2. In most cases, further diagnostic testing is not needed. If objective studies are needed, color flow Doppler cavernosonography is the method of choice followed by technetium-99m penile scanning and magnetic resonance imaging. If pelvic malignancy is suspected, computed tomography is generally the next step. If trauma preceded priapism, arteriography may be indicated.

D. Genetics. Sickle cell anemia, an autosomal recessive disorder is associated with a high incidence of priapism (>40% of affected adults and >60% of affected children).

IV. DIAGNOSIS

A. Differential diagnosis. The key to determining the cause of priapism is the clinical history. Examination reveals an erect, usually tender penis, with flaccid glans. Early distinction between arterial and veno-occlusive priapism should be made; the former is often associated with trauma and less painful or painless erections. Evaluation of priapism is aimed at determining how long it has been present, because permanent damage may occur within as little as 4 hours, and at determining the cause. The most common causes are due to psychotropic medications or medications for erectile dysfunction. Less common causes include trauma, sickle cell disease, and pelvic malignancy.

B. Clinical manifestations. Priapism is considered a urologic emergency and should be managed aggressively. Without prompt recognition and treatment, priapism may result in urinary retention, cavernosa fibrosis, impotence, or even gangrene. Treatment within 4 to 6 hours of onset has been shown to decrease morbidity, the need for invasive procedures, and decrease impotence (4).

References

1. Eland IA, van der Lei J, Strickler BH, et al. Incidence of priapism in the general population. *Urology* 2001;57:970–972.
2. Vilke GM, Harrigan RA, Ufberg JW, et al. Emergency evaluation and treatment of priapism. *J Emerg Med* 2003;26(3):325–329.
3. Montague DK, Jarow J, Broderick GA, et al. American Urological Association guideline on the management of priapism. *J Urol* 2003;170:1318–1324.
4. Thompson JW Jr, Ware MR, Blashfield RK. Psychotropic medication and priapism: a comprehensive review. *J Clin Psychol* 1990;51:430–433.
5. Chan PT, Begin LR, Arnold D, et al. Priapism secondary to penile metastasis: a report of two cases and a review of the literature. *J Surg Oncol* 1998;68:51–59.

SCROTAL MASS
Kendall M. Campbell and Robert L. Hatch

10.8

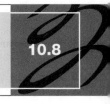

I. BACKGROUND. Scrotal masses are common, occurring in all age-groups, from infants to elderly men. In fact, up to 20% of adult males have a varicocele. Many scrotal masses are benign and require no treatment, whereas others require immediate recognition and emergent treatment.

II. PATHOPHYSIOLOGY. Testicular torsion is a true emergency, because the best results occur if patients are in the operating room within 6 hours of onset of symptoms. Strangulated inguinal hernias and testicular ruptures also present urgent situations, whereas testicular cancers and incarcerated hernias require prompt but less urgent treatment. Hydroceles in children and certain varicoceles in adolescents may require surgery to preserve future fertility. When evaluating scrotal masses, the primary objective is to rapidly identify and refer patients who require immediate intervention.

III. EVALUATION

A. History

1. **Pain.** Is the mass painful? How painful? Testicular torsion usually presents with severe pain, although several other conditions are also quite painful. These include strangulated hernias, epididymitis, orchitis, and torsion of a testicular or epididymal appendage. Varicocele, hydrocele, spermatocele, epididymal cysts, and testicular tumors are typically painless but may present with a dull ache or heaviness of the scrotum.

2. **Inciting event.** Did the mass first appear after vigorous activity or testicular trauma? Torsion is often precipitated by one of these factors. Another surgical emergency, testicular rupture, can result from high force injuries such as athletic injuries or car accidents. A new swelling following minor trauma, on the other hand, suggests bleeding associated with a tumor. Tumors can also be associated with metastases or gynecomastia.

3. **Patient age.** In a review of 238 testicular masses in children, torsion of an appendage was the most common cause of acute masses in children aged up to 13 years. In men older than 13 years, epididymitis and testicular torsion become more common (1). Testicular torsion peaks in men between the ages of 13 and 15 years (1) but occurs from infancy to middle age. Indeed, torsion accounts for 83% of acute scrotal masses in children aged <1 year (1). Epididymitis is the most common cause of acute scrotum in adolescents and adults. In men younger than 35 years of age, *Chlamydia* and gonorrhea are the most common pathogens. In infants and men older than 35 years of age, epididymitis usually results from an underlying urinary tract infection, and *Escherichia coli* and *Proteus mirabilis* predominate (2). The average age for patients with testicular cancer is 32 years. Hydrocele, epididymitis, varicocele, and hernias are more common in adults, but they too occur over a wide range of ages.

4. **Duration.** How long has the mass been present? Torsion typically presents with sudden onset of symptoms, leading patients to seek care soon after onset. Other acute conditions can also have an abrupt onset. Many benign scrotal masses have been noted for some time by the patient. Abrupt appearance of a varicocele in an older man can signal venous obstruction (spermatic vein if on the left, vena cava if on the right).

5. **Symptoms of infection.** Is there a history of fever, penile discharge, mumps, or any other recent infection? Infection is the most common cause of acute testicular pain. Epididymitis often presents with discharge and mild fever. A high fever often accompanies orchitis. Mumps orchitis, the most common cause of orchitis without epididymitis (2), typically occurs 3 to 4 days after the parotitis. It is bilateral in 14% to 35% of cases (2). Scrotal wall cellulitis is common in patients who are immunocompromised, obese, or diabetic (2). Many other infections, including tuberculosis and syphilis, can produce epididymitis or orchitis.

6. **Previous history.** Have the symptoms previously appeared? Patients with torsion may have had similar, milder symptoms in the past (torsion that spontaneously resolved). Patients with chronic epididymitis generally describe an initial severe bout that has been followed by milder recurrences.

7. **Other associated symptoms.** Are there any other symptoms? Nausea often accompanies torsion and orchitis.

B. Physical examination

1. **Palpate the scrotum and contents**

   a. **Determine the orientation of the testicle.** A torsed testicle is usually retracted upward and rotated to an abnormal position. This may be indicated by an epididymis that appears to lie in an abnormal location (normally, the head of the epididymis lies at the superior pole of the testicle and its body extends posterolateral along the testicle). Comparison with the other testicle may help with this determination. Normal position does not rule out torsion, however, because the testicle may have rotated a full 360°. In epididymitis and orchitis, testicular lie can be difficult to determine due to swelling (3).

    b. Assess for swelling and tenderness. Torsion, orchitis, and epididymitis all develop swelling and tenderness soon after onset.

    c. Determine location of mass. Consider whether the mass is intratesticular or extratesticular. The most common extratesticular scrotal masses include inguinal hernias, epididymal cysts, and varicoceles. The most concerning intratesticular lesions are malignant germ cell tumors, which make up 90% to 95% of intratesticular primary tumors. Appendices of the epididymis and testicle can extend from the superior pole of either structure. Spermatocele is most commonly found superior and posterior to the testicle. Varicocele occurs in a similar location, usually on the left side. In epididymitis, the swollen epididymis is often difficult to distinguish from the testicle.

    d. Assess the consistency of the mass. A varicocele typically has the consistency of a bag of worms. Hydrocele and spermatocele usually have a cystic consistency. Hydrocele can become more tense as the day progresses (because of the dependent position).

  2. Assess the cremasteric reflex. When the inner thigh is lightly stroked, the testicle on that side should rise noticeably. Absence of this reflex suggests testicular torsion.

  3. Elevate the testicle above the symphysis pubis. This usually relieves the pain of epididymitis but not of torsion (Prehn's sign) (2).

  4. Transilluminate the mass. Hydroceles and spermatoceles transilluminate.

  5. Examine the patient in both the supine and standing positions. Hernias and varicoceles usually become more prominent on standing, especially with Valsalva.

C. Testing. Reliance on clinical findings alone produces false-positive rates for testicular torsion of approximately 50% (2). Doppler ultrasound has replaced radioisotope scans as the imaging modality of choice (3). It avoids false-positive results from skin hyperemia and is far superior for detecting other causes of testicular pain or masses (3). In the presence of acute or stuttering symptoms that suggest torsion, a Doppler ultrasound should be obtained as soon as possible (comparing the affected testicle to the unaffected one). Parenteral narcotics may be administered if it is necessary to alleviate pain and allow a better examination. Specificity of 97% is reported for detecting torsion (1). False-negative results may occur even with ultrasound, producing lower sensitivity (86%) (1). In this series, most false-negative results occurred either in prolonged torsion in which the testicles were no longer salvageable, or in cases of intermittent torsion. An ultrasound can be helpful in differentiating many other masses, but showed a disappointing ability to differentiate malignant from benign masses in children (4). Aspiration of a spermatocele usually reveals dead sperm (1). Pyuria is almost always present in epididymitis, but it has also been found in up to 27% of patients with torsion (>5 white blood cells/high-power field) (5). Similarly, leukocytosis suggests an infectious cause but it has also been found in 33% of patients with torsion (5).

IV. DIAGNOSIS. Due to considerable overlap in the presentation, laboratory findings, and imaging studies of these conditions, establishing a diagnosis is challenging in some cases. If the diagnosis of testicular torsion cannot be rapidly and confidently excluded, emergent referral or ultrasound is strongly recommended. Less urgent consultation is recommended if the diagnosis is unclear but torsion is not suspected.

References

1. Lewis AG, Bukowski TP, Jarvis PD. Evaluation of acute scrotum in the emergency department. *J Pediatr Surg* 1995;30:277–282.
2. Dogra V, Bhatt S. Acute painful scrotum. *Radiol Clin North Am* 2004;42:349–363.
3. Blaivas M, Brannam L. Testicular ultrasound. *Emerg Med Clin North Am* 2004;22: 723–748.
4. Aragona F, Pescatori E, Talenti E. Painless scrotal masses in the pediatric population: prevalence and age distribution of different pathological conditions—a 10-year retrospective multicenter study. *J Urol* 1996;155:1424–1426.
5. Kattan S. Spermatic cord torsion in adults. *Scand J Urol Nephrol* 1994;28:277–279.

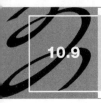

SCROTAL PAIN
George R. Wilson

I. BACKGROUND
A. Scrotal pain can result from pathology within the scrotum, trauma to the scrotum, pathology of the scrotal sac, extrascrotal pathology, and referred pain from intra-abdominal pathology. It can be acute, chronic, or intermittent.

B. Scrotal pain is a common problem in adults, most often due to epididymitis or varicocele. With the exception of trauma, scrotal pain in an adult rarely requires emergent surgical intervention. On the other hand, scrotal pain in children and adolescents, although less common than in adults, is often due to causes that require urgent intervention. The most common cause of scrotal pain in a child or adolescent that requires timely diagnosis and surgical intervention is testicular torsion (1). The highest probability for saving a torsed testicle occurs within the first 6 hours. After 6 hours, the probability of success declines, reaching zero at approximately 48 hours. Choice of diagnostic modality in this early period can play an important role in determining what intervention is appropriate.

II. PATHOPHYSIOLOGY
A. Etiology
1. Intrascrotal pathology—testicular torsion, torsion of testicular appendage, epididymitis, orchitis, varicocele, spermatocele, primary or metastatic testicular tumor

2. Pathology of the scrotal sac—usually confined to blunt trauma or infection

3. Extrascrotal pathology—direct/indirect hernia, incarcerated hernia, hydrocele, urinary tract infection (UTI), prostatitis, sexually transmitted disease (STD)

4. Scrotal trauma—falls, animal bites, sexual abuse

5. Pain referred from intra-abdominal pathology or systemic disease—renal colic, Henoch-Schönlein purpura, mononucleosis, Buerger's disease, coxsackie B virus, polyarteritis nodosa (2).

B. Epidemiology
1. Intrascrotal pathology
a. Testicular torsion is highest in incidence at 12 to 18 years of age (1,3). It is the most common cause of scrotal pain in the first year of life (often misdiagnosed as colic or intra-abdominal disorder), (1) and is uncommon in adults.

b. Torsion of testicular appendage is common at 10 to 15 years of age. It is rare in neonates and adults (3).

c. Epididymitis is the most common cause of acute scrotal pain in adults (1). It is rare in prepubertal children (3). If it occurs in prepuberty, urogenital anomaly or dysfunction should be suspected.

d. Orchitis is usually due to extension of epididymitis. Mumps orchitis, which occurs only postpuberty in approximately 20% of mumps cases, is unilateral in 70% of cases. It is less common since the mumps vaccine.

e. Varicocele occurs primarily in adults and adolescents. It is rare but can occur in prepubertal children; in such cases, an intra-abdominal lesion obstructing venous drainage should be considered.

f. Spermatocele is common postvasectomy. Not seen in prepuberty, it is very rare in adolescents.

g. Primary or metastatic testicular tumor is highest in incidence at 18 to 30 years of age. Metastatic tumor is rare but does occur.

2. Pathology of the scrotal sac
a. Bacterial infection secondary to fungal disease or contact dermatitis

b. Inclusion/sebaceous cysts

3. **Extrascrotal pathology**
   a. Direct/indirect hernia or incarcerated hernia is equally prevalent in adults and children.
   b. Hydrocele occurs primarily in neonates. Although it occurs in adults, it is not common. The condition often resolves spontaneously.
   c. UTI must be considered in small children, especially infants. It is often associated with congenital anomaly and/or urine reflux.
   d. Prostatitis is postpubertal. Not seen in prepuberty, it is rare in adolescents.
   e. STDs are generally postpubertal. They are rarely prepubertal; sexual abuse should be suspected.
4. **Scrotal trauma.** Significant damage to a testicle from trauma, in any age-group, is rare. Scrotal pain due to trauma is generally self-evident or self-reported. Traumatic damage in prepuberty is rare due to the small size of the testicle. When it does occur, self-experimentation or sexual abuse is often the cause. Scrotal pain due to trauma usually resolves in <1 hour (2). Pain persisting longer than 1 hour suggests testicular rupture. Testicular rupture from minor trauma is consistent with occult testicular neoplasm.

III. EVALUATION

A. **History.** The primary piece of historical information to be obtained is the time of the onset of pain (4). This is critical in testicular torsion, because it determines how rapidly diagnostic tests need to be accomplished and may dictate the order of tests that need to be performed. Other historical information includes whether the pain is severe or mild; acute or chronic; or constant or intermittent. History of trauma needs to be elicited. Fever, nausea and/or vomiting, dysuria, and other medical conditions need to be determined. When appropriate, the options of sexual experimentation and/or unusual sexual practices should be explored.
   1. Testicular torsion usually presents with an abrupt onset of pain. Nausea and vomiting are common. History of previous ipsilateral pain is associated with a 44% incidence of testicular torsion (1). Early fever is not part of the history.
   2. Torsion of the testicular appendage has less intense pain than testicular torsion. Pain may persist for days, beginning in the lower abdomen before moving into the scrotum. Malaise is common. Fever is not usually part of the history.
   3. Epididymitis can be abrupt or insidious in onset. Fever is common. Voiding symptoms may occur.

B. **Physical examination**
   1. Infants and small children should be observed prior to examining the scrotum. Testicular torsion generally causes restlessness, irritability, and crying. All neonates and small children with a history of abdominal pain require an examination of the scrotum.
   2. Scrotum is examined for evidence of trauma, changes is color, discoloration, unilateral or bilateral swelling, infection, and masses. If pain is present longer than 24 hours without scrotal changes, torsion is unlikely (2). Discoloration is usually due to trauma but can be seen with torsion and epididymitis. The cremasteric reflex should be checked. If present on the painful side, testicular torsion is ruled out. For the absence of a cremasteric reflex to be a reliable indicator, its presence must be demonstrated on the non–painful side. Unilateral swelling without skin changes indicate hernia or hydrocele. Elevating the scrotum increases pain with testicular torsion, and decreases pain with epididymitis (Prehn's sign) (3).
   3. The testes are examined for presence or absence of torsion. High transverse lie suggests torsion. Testicular torsion causes early swelling. Appendiceal torsion and epididymitis are palpable as a mass or swelling along the margin of the testis. Transillumination of the scrotum may reveal a "blue dot sign" in appendiceal torsion (2,3).

C. **Testing.** Very few laboratory tests are indicated in the evaluation of scrotal pain.
   1. Urinalysis is usually negative. If it is positive, the diagnosis is more likely to be epididymitis, rather than testicular or appendiceal torsion.

2. White blood cell count may indicate nonspecific leukocytosis. It is more commonly elevated in epididymitis and may be elevated with testicular or appendiceal torsion after 24 hours.

3. Serology and erythrocyte sedimentation rate are not helpful, and they may unnecessarily delay diagnosis.

4. **Imaging studies**

   a. Color Doppler is the first-line modality for diagnosis. This provides a definitive diagnosis of testicular torsion in 91.7% of cases. A negative test is 96.2% reliable—testicular torsion is not present (5).

   b. Gray-scale Doppler is not reliable in diagnosing testicular torsion. It may give false-negative results early. Once changes become evident, the testicle may no longer be salvageable (3).

   c. Nuclear scanning has been shown to be an effective method for evaluating acute scrotum. However, the process is often too slow to be universally used in determining the need for surgical intervention in a narrow therapeutic window. The primary uses are evaluation in trauma, with asymptomatic masses, and when elective surgical exploration is contraindicated and Doppler studies are equivocal.

   d. Magnetic resonance imaging provides good anatomical data but is not useful to evaluate for blood flow in the acute setting.

D. Genetics. This plays a very small role in scrotal pain.

IV. DIAGNOSIS

A. Differential diagnosis. Most critical is testicular torsion due to the finite survival of the testis. Other etiologies (appendiceal torsion, epididymitis, trauma, hernia/hydrocele, tumor) have a larger window of opportunity. All tests should be directed toward initially excluding testicular torsion—and as rapidly as possible.

B. Clinical manifestations. The two primary pieces of clinical history are (1) the age of the patient and (2) the time lapsed since the onset of pain. Severe unilateral pain of <6 hours, worsened by the elevation of the scrotum, in an adolescent, is testicular torsion until proven otherwise. Every neonate with abdominal symptoms must have a scrotal examination as a part of the workup. Color Doppler ultrasonography is the diagnostic modality of choice for the evaluation of acute scrotal pain. Surgical exploration must always be considered whenever the history and/or physical examination is consistent with testicular torsion, or when the data does not *completely* rule it out. The opportunity to salvage the testis is in the first 6 hours.

References

1. Espy PG, Koo HP. Torsion of the testicle. In: Graham SD, Glenn JF, Keane TE, eds. *Glenn's urologic surgery*, 6th ed. Philadelphia, PA: Lippincott Williams and Wilkins, 2004:513–517.

2. Kass EJ, Lundak B. The acute scrotum. *Pediatr Clin North Am* 1997;44(5):1251–1266.

3. Sandock DS, Herbener TE, Resnick MI. Disorders of the scrotum and its contents. In: Resnick MI, Older RA, eds. *Diagnosis of genitourinary disease*, 2nd ed. New York: Thieme-Stratton Inc., 1997:465–483.

4. Galejs LE. Diagnosis and treatment of the acute scrotum. *Am Fam Physician* 1999;59(4): 817–824.

5. Karmazyn B, Steinberg R, Kornreich L, et al. Clinical and sonographic criteria of acute scrotum in children: a retrospective study of 172 boys. *Pediatr Radiol* 2005;35(3): 302–310.

URETHRAL DISCHARGE
George PN Samraj

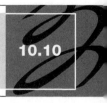

10.10

I. BACKGROUND. Urethral discharge (UD) is a common symptom, with etiology varying from sexually transmitted infection to cancer. UD may be profuse or scanty; clear, yellowish or white, brown or green; mucopurulent or serous; or bloody, watery, or frank pus. UD may be an acute or chronic condition, and patients may or may not have symptoms.

II. PATHOPHYSIOLOGY. UD is the presenting sign of many disorders and can be classified as noted below.

A. Sexually transmitted diseases (STDs)

    1. Gonococcal (GC) infection. GC infection is more common in men than women. The Centers for Disease Control and Prevention reports that in 2004, 330,132 cases of (113.5 cases per 100, 000 population in 2004) gonorrhea were reported in the United States. It is 20 times more common in young patients from large cities and in African-American individuals (1).

    2. Nongonococcal (NGC) infection. This is the most common STD in the United States, with 2.8 million new cases occurring annually (1). As many as 85% of women with chlamydial infections and 40% of infected men are asymptomatic.

      a. *Chlamydia trachomatis,* (20%–40% of NGC)

      b. *Ureaplasma urealyticum,* (10%–20% of NGC)

      c. *Mycoplasma genitalium*

      d. Other organisms linked to UD:

        i. Bacteria. *Gardnerella vaginalis, Escherichia coli,* tuberculosis, *Corynebacterium genitalium, Bacteroides,* mycoplasmas

        ii. Viruses. Herpes simplex virus, adenoviruses, cytomegalovirus, human papilloma virus, and others

        iii. Protozoal. *Trichomonas vaginalis* (about 5 million cases occur annually in the United States)

        iv. Fungal. *Candida* species

B. Nonsexually transmitted diseases

    1. Infections. Cystitis, prostatitis

    2. Anatomic and congenital abnormalities. Urethral stricture, phimosis

    3. Iatrogenic. Catheterization, instrumentation, and other procedures

    4. Chemical irritation from douches, lubricants, and other chemicals

    5. Tumors. Malignant lesions and new growths

    6. Foreign bodies. Common in children and teenagers

    7. Substance abuse. Chronic use of amphetamines or other stimulants produces a serous discharge. Caffeine and alcohol are also implicated in UD.

    8. Miscellaneous factors linked to UD. Sexual practices, masturbation, oral sex

    9. Unknown. No organisms may be found in up to one-third of patients.

III. EVALUATION

A. History. A comprehensive medical history is essential for the evaluation of UD. It should include (a) dysuria, (b) UD, (c) itching at the urethra, (d) hematuria, (e) rectal symptoms, (f) contact with infectious agents, (g) testicular pain, (h) low back pain and constitutional symptoms. The characteristic of UD is characterized in relation to color (purulent, mucoid, or bloody); quantity, odor, consistency, frequency, past history, or any previous treatment and relationship to urination. Profuse, thick yellow to grayish UD 3 to 7 days after sexual exposure is characteristic of GC infection. Clear to white scanty, or mucopurulent UD (23%–55%) that develops gradually at least a week after exposure and waxes and wanes in intensity is suggestive of chlamydial infection. Mucoid, scant watery discharge that develops over a period of 2 to 3 weeks is common with NGC UD. A bloody discharge is suggestive of urethral carcinoma. Sexual history should include sexual orientation, past sexual history, sexual behaviors, condom usage, and number of sexual partners, recent sexual contacts, and the orifices used for sexual contacts. Consistent usage of condoms prevents sexually transmitted urethritis. Oral sex increases UD due to infections from oral flora.

B. Physical examination

1. A focused physical examination includes vital signs and urologic and rectal examination. In men, this should include examination of the penis, perimeatal region for the evidence of erythema, urethral meatus, scrotum, testicles, epididymis, prostate, perianal, and the inguinal region for lymph nodes. Stains present on the patient's underwear may indicate the characteristics of the discharge, particularly in a patient who has urinated shortly before examination. Recent micturition can eliminate much inflammatory discharge. Sometimes it may be necessary to examine the patient in the morning before voiding to enhance the diagnosis. In women, a complete urogynecologic examination should be performed.

2. A complete examination of the abdomen may be indicated to rule out intra-abdominal pathology such as masses, inflammation, obstruction, and distention of organs. Additional physical examination should include an examination of the skin and other systems as needed. If a GC infection is suspected, it may be necessary to check the patient's joints, skin, throat, eyes, and other organs.

C. Testing

1. UD sample collection. Proper collection and handling of UD specimens is essential for diagnosis. When the discharge is not spontaneous, the urethra should be gently stripped. This is best accomplished by grasping the penis firmly between the thumb and forefinger with the thumb pressing on the ventral surface. The examiner's hand is then moved distally, compressing the urethra. This maneuver may express a small amount of discharge. UD for testing should preferably be collected without contamination by the various bacteria present in the urethral meatus. The urethral meatus can be gently spread and UD collected by gently inserting (2–4 cm into the urethra) a calcium alginate urogenital swab (cotton swabs are uncomfortable due to the large size and may interfere with the culture) by rotating for 3 to 6 seconds. UD should be collected 1 to 4 hours (preferably 4 hours) after urination. Pharyngeal swabs may be collected when clinically indicated. The specimen should be directly placed into the culture medium. The same swab may be used for a Gram stain (2, 3).

2. Gram's stain and culture. The presence of polymorphs with intracellular diplococci is diagnostic of GC disease. Polymorphs without the intracellular diplococci are suggestive of NGC disease. Few or no polymorphs are suggestive of other etiologies. The Gram stain is quite accurate for men but it is not very sensitive for women (50%), where cultures of the throat, rectum, and sometimes conjunctivae are required to establish the diagnosis.

3. Wet preparation of UD. This test is performed to establish the diagnosis of trichomonas, candidiasis, and some viral and bacterial infections (e.g., bacterial vaginosis; clue cells, viral inclusions).

4. Urethritis confirmation. This is confirmed with one of the three clinical findings.

a. Presence of purulent or mucopurulent discharge

b. More than five white blood cells (WBCs) per field in the oil immersion (1000×) microscopy of the Gram stain of the discharge

c. Presence of leukocyte esterase in the first voided urine or the presence of >10 WBCs per high-power field (400×) in the sediment of the spun urine

5. Urinalysis and urine cultures are essential for the diagnosis of urinary infections. Collection of a urine specimen as described by Stamey (4) with four sterile containers (before and after prostatic massage) is sometimes useful to identify the site of infection in men. Urinary leukocyte esterase is a useful screening test for chlamydial and GC infections in asymptomatic men.

6. Nucleic acid–based tests (nucleic acid amplification assay, nucleic acid hybridization test, nucleic acid genetic transformation test) are now used by many centers because of their simplicity, high sensitivity, and specificity when compared with the difficulties encountered with the traditional culture test (low sensitivity and storage problems). Nucleic acid amplification assays are more popular and use various techniques (polymerase chain reaction, ligase chain reaction, or strand displacement amplification of deoxyribonucleic acid) to identify an infection. These tests can be performed from UD or 20 to 40 mL (more volume can interfere with the test) of first voided, first catch initial stream of urine. Female patients should not cleanse the labial and urethral region before the collection of the first stream of urine. Some centers prefer a urine specimen for its simplicity and increased detection rate, especially with scanty UD (5).

7. **Blood studies.** A complete blood count, chemistry profile, rapid plasma reagin, human immunodeficiency virus, and immunologic studies may be required.

8. **Diagnostic imaging.** A urethrogram and pelvic, vaginal, and rectal ultrasound studies may be indicated in some clinical conditions.

9. **Other procedures.** Examination under anesthesia for children and elderly patients is sometimes necessary in the evaluation of UD. Anoscopy is appropriate for patients who have anal intercourse or for those with anal and rectal symptoms. Cystourethroscopy and laparoscopy may also be useful in certain conditions.

IV. **DIAGNOSIS AND SPECIAL CONCERNS.** *Neisseria gonorrhoeae* and *Chlamydia trachomatis* infections are reportable to State Health Departments, and a specific diagnosis is essential. UD secondary to STD involves many psychosocial and medicolegal implications for the patient, their partners, their families, and society. Sexual partners should be traced, tested, and treated. In children with UD, sexual abuse should be suspected. Pregnant women with GC infection or chlamydia may infect the infant at birth (ophthalmia neonatorum).

References

1. *Sexually transmitted diseases surveillance and statistics*, 2004, Reports 2004 National Report CDC, http://www.cdc.gov/std/stats/gonorrhea.htm.
2. Berger RE, Lee JC. Sexually transmitted disease: the classic disease. *Campbell's urology*, 8th ed. Philadelphia, PA: WB Saunders, 2002:671–678.
3. Lyon CJ. Urethritis. *Clin Fam Pract* 2005;l7(1):31–41.
4. Meares EM, Stamey TA. Bacteriologic localization patterns in bacterial prostatitis and urethritis. *Invest Urol* 1968;5:492–518.
5. http://www.cdc.gov/STD/LabGuidelines/1-LG.htm. Screening Tests To Detect *Chlamydia trachomatis* and *Neisseria gonorrhoeae* Infections CDC- 2002.

Problems Related to the Female Reproductive System

Kathryn M. Andolsek

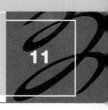

11

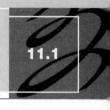

I. BACKGROUND. Amenorrhea is the absence or abnormal cessation of menses.

II. PATHOPHYSIOLOGY. Excluding pregnancy, amenorrhea is caused by dysfunction somewhere along the female reproductive pathway.

A. Etiology of primary amenorrhea

1. **Hypothalamic/pituitary dysfunction.** Physiologic delay of puberty or absence of gonadotropin-releasing hormone (GnRH) secretion from the hypothalamus (e.g., Kallmann's syndrome—primary amenorrhea with impaired sense of smell)

2. **Ovarian dysfunction.** Ovarian failure due to chromosomal abnormality (i.e., Turner's syndrome)

3. **Outflow tract dysfunction.** Müllerian dysgenesis (missing upper two-thirds of vagina, uterus, and fallopian tubes), imperforate hymen, transverse vaginal septum, and testicular feminization (genotypically male but phenotypically female except for the absence of a normal female genital tract)

B. Etiology of secondary amenorrhea (1, 2)

1. **Hypothalamic dysfunction.** Low GnRH secretion due to stresses, such as intense exercise, weight loss/low body mass index (BMI) and/or malnutrition (consider eating disorder and/or the female athlete); chronic disease; autoimmune disorders (e.g., hyperthyroidism, hypothyroidism, diabetes mellitus, hypoparathyroidism, systemic lupus erythematosus); depression or other psychiatric disorders; psychotropic medication use; or recreational drug abuse

2. **Pituitary dysfunction.** Pituitary tumors (prolactinoma, adrenocorticotropic hormone–secreting adenoma (Cushing's syndrome) or growth hormone–secreting adenoma (acromegaly), Sheehan's syndrome (postpartum pituitary necrosis), panhypopituitarism, empty sella syndrome, infiltrative disease of pituitary (sarcoidosis, tuberculosis), head irradiation, or trauma

3. **Ovarian dysfunction**

   a. **No evidence of androgen excess**—premature ovarian failure (women younger than 40 years of age), radiation/chemotherapy treatment

   b. **Evidence of androgen excess (hirsutism, virilization)**—polycystic ovary disease, androgen-secreting adrenal or ovarian tumors

4. **Uterine dysfunction.** Asherman's syndrome (uterine adhesions), endometrial hyperplasia, or cancer

C. Epidemiology. The prevalence of secondary amenorrhea is 5% (3).

III. EVALUATION (3, 4)

A. History

1. **Menstrual and reproductive history**

   a. Menarche

   b. Last menstrual period

   c. Frequency of menses and duration

   d. History of prior pregnancies

   e. History of pregnancy or delivery

   f. History of spontaneous or therapeutic abortions or dilatation and curettage

   g. History of uterine surgeries

2. **Systemic processes**

   a. Weight loss or gain

   b. Frequency and level of intensity of exercise

   c. Psychosocial or medical stressors/crises

    d. Nipple discharge
    e. Headaches or decreased peripheral vision
    f. Hot flashes
    g. Painful intercourse
    h. Mood swings
    i. Detailed medical and psychiatric history, including diagnoses and medications
    j. Detailed social history, particularly illicit drug use
B. Physical examination
  1. Vital signs
  2. General. Assess for general health, affect, Tanner staging, and measure BMI.
  3. Skin. Inspect for virilization/hirsutism (acne, male pattern baldness, excessive hair on face or chest, increased muscle mass) versus sparse axillary or pubic hair growth. Look for acanthosis nigricans or buffalo hump, thin skin, and/or purple striae.
  4. Neck. Palpate for thyromegaly or thyroid nodules.
  5. Breast. Inspect for galactorrhea.
  6. Pelvic. Inspect for anatomic abnormalities, clitoromegaly, or signs of vaginal atrophy.
C. Testing
  1. Laboratory tests
    a. *Obtain a pregnancy test in all women of reproductive age.*
    b. In any woman with amenorrhea who is not pregnant, obtain the following:
      i. Serum prolactin
      ii. Thyroid-stimulating hormone
      iii. Follicle-stimulating hormone
      iv. Estradiol
    c. If the patient has amenorrhea with hirsutism and virilization, obtain the following:
      i. Serum total testosterone
      ii. 17-Hydroxyprogesterone levels
      iii. Dehydroepiandrosterone (DHEA-S)
    d. If the woman has been anovulatory for more than a year, consider endometrial biopsy. Consider hysteroscopy in patients at risk for uterine adhesions.
  2. Progestin challenge test (5). This test is used to demonstrate estrogen effect at the level of the endometrium. Medroxyprogesterone acetate 10 mg is given daily for 5 to 10 days, and if menses starts within 10 days of completing therapy, the test is positive and the patient is able to produce enough estrogen to cause endometrial proliferation. The disadvantage is a delay in diagnosis.
  3. Diagnostic imaging. Obtain a magnetic resonance imaging (MRI) scan of the pituitary and hypothalamus in patients with associated headaches, visual field defects, or hyperprolactinemia. Consider a dual-energy x-ray absorptiometry scan in patients at risk of osteoporosis. In patients with suspected androgen-secreting tumors, obtain a pelvic ultrasound and consider adrenal computed tomography scan or MRI. In patients with primary amenorrhea and abnormalities of pelvic anatomy, obtain a pelvic ultrasound.
D. Genetics. In patients with clinical signs of Turner's syndrome, obtain karyotyping. Also consider a karyotype in women who are younger than 30 years of age with premature ovarian failure.
IV. DIAGNOSIS
  A. Differential diagnosis. Always exclude pregnancy first.
  B. Clinical manifestations
    1. Primary amenorrhea. This is defined as follows:
      a. Failure to reach menarche and pubertal milestones by 14 years of age
      b. Failure to reach menarche by 16 years of age in a girl who has developed secondary sexual characteristics
    2. Secondary amenorrhea. This is defined as the disruption of regular menses for the equivalent of more than three cycles or 6 months once they have begun.

3. Complications. The low estrogen levels of prolonged amenorrhea are associated with increased risk of osteopenia and osteoporosis (5).

References
1. Larsen PR. *Williams textbook of endocrinology*, 10th ed. Philadelphia, PA: Elsevier, 2003.
2. Stenchever MD. *Comprehensive Gynecology*, 4th ed. St. Louis, MO: Mosby Inc., 2001.
3. *E-medicine: amenorrhea.* http://www.emedicine.com/med/topic117.htm, 2006.
4. *Up to date: etiology, diagnosis, and treatment of secondary amenorrhea.* http://www.utdol.com, 2006.
5. Apgar B. Diagnosis and management of amenorrhea. *Clin Fam Pract* 2002;4(3):643.

BREAST MASS
Joyce A. Copeland

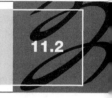

11.2

I. BACKGROUND. A breast mass is a collection of tissue that is not part of the normal physiologic architecture of the mammary gland. The palpable mass is the subject of this chapter.

II. PATHOPHYSIOLOGY

    A. Etiology. The etiology of the breast mass may be malignant or benign. Malignancy is the major concern, especially in older women. Benign changes such as adenomas or cysts are extremely common.

    B. Epidemiology. One of the three most common presentations for breast complaints is a palpable breast mass. Most of these are benign, but this must be tempered with the fact that breast cancer is the most common cancer in women and the second most common cause of cancer death (1). Most cancers are present in women older than 50 years of age, but one-third of them are in younger women (2).

III. EVALUATION

    A. History

        1. Current medical history and chief complaint

            a. When and how was the mass discovered? Does the patient perform regular breast self-examinations? What, if any, changes have occurred since the discovery?

            b. Age and menstrual status. Cancer is more prominent in the age-groups over 50 years of age, although 3% may be seen in the 20- to 29-year age-group. Approximately 85% of masses in the postmenopausal age-group prove to be cancerous (3).

            c. Is the mass painful? If so, is there any cyclic variation in the pain? Has there been any nipple discharge? Has the patient noticed any warmth or redness?

        2. Past medical history

            a. Reproductive history. What is the reproductive history and current menstrual status? Has the patient ever breast-fed an infant? Is she on estrogen replacement therapy (ERT)? A woman who breast-feeds for ≥ 2 years may have a decreased risk of breast cancer. ERT has a controversial role in etiology or advancement of breast cancer. What was her age at the birth of her first child?

            b. Breast history. The patient should be questioned about any previous experience of a breast mass, breast biopsy or surgery, and the clinical outcome. Has she had a personal history of breast cancer or atypical hyperplasia on a previous biopsy? A prior history of breast cancer or atypical hyperplasia on a biopsy increases the risk of malignancy. Does the patient have a history of radiation exposure or chemotherapy? Has there been any recent breast trauma? What is her current lactation status?

3. **Family history.** Is there a family history of breast cancer? If yes, what is the relationship of the family member and at what age was the cancer diagnosed and what was the relative's menstrual status? A mother or sister with premenopausal breast cancer indicates the highest level of risk.

4. **Lifestyle.** Inquire about the patient's alcohol intake and dietary habits. There is a possible link between breast cancer and alcohol consumption, a high-fat diet, and obesity. Ask about smoking history as well.

B. **Physical examination**
1. **Inspection.** Inspect the breasts for symmetry, contour, skin retraction, rashes, *peau d'orange*, nipple discharge, and erythema or edema. Disruptions of symmetry and contour may accompany a breast mass.
2. **Palpation and compression.** Palpate both breasts, including the nipple and areolar region. Palpate the supraclavicular, infraclavicular, and axillary regions for adenopathy. Evaluate the consistency, regularity, location, and mobility of the mass, as well as the presence of tenderness.

C. **Testing**
1. **Imaging studies.** The mammogram is used to characterize the nature of the mass and to provide an assessment of the remainder of the breast tissue and the contralateral breast. It is not a diagnostic procedure. Ultrasound is used to characterize a mass as solid or cystic or identify masses that may not be identified by mammography. It is helpful in evaluating mass in a patient younger than 35 years of age and may be used as an adjunct in the performance of aspiration or biopsy for the indeterminate lesion.
2. **Fine needle aspiration (FNA) (4).** FNA can be used to obtain tissue or fluid in a palpable mass. Fluid aspiration plus resolution of the mass suggests a cystic origin. Grossly bloody fluid demands a further evaluation of the mass. A cystic mass in a postmenopausal woman not receiving ERT requires a more thorough evaluation.

   Reexamine the breast in 4 to 6 weeks if the cyst resolves. If the fluid reaccumulates, reaspirate. Residual mass or asymmetry after aspiration requires mammography and biopsy. If no aspirate is obtained, proceed with excisional biopsy.
3. **Fine needle aspiration biopsy (FNAB) (4).** FNAB has a sensitivity of 0.65 to 0.98 and a specificity of 0.34 to 1.0. The procedure provides material for a cytologic examination. Correlation with imaging studies must be concordant in conclusion or excisional biopsy is indicated. Imaging guidance is indicated for a nonpalpable mass. Atypia of any degree warrants excisional biopsy.
4. **Core needle biopsy.** This technique involves the use of a larger gauge needle and provides histologic material for assessment. It is usually performed in conjunction with stereotactic mammography or ultrasound guidance. There is a 50% concordance with surgical biopsy at 50% of the cost (5).
5. **Triple test for solid mass (6).** The triple test includes physical examination, imaging findings, and cytology through FNAB. This technique has a sensitivity of 97% to 100% and a specificity of 98% to 100%. Concordance for benign findings allows the clinician to stop testing. Malignant cytopathology requires excisional biopsy. Inconclusive results without concordance require open excisional biopsy.
6. **Open excisional biopsy.** A lesion that is highly suspicious on clinical examination and/or mammography is best evaluated with open biopsy and excision. Atypical cells on biopsy also require a more definitive tissue diagnosis.
7. **Emerging technology.** Magnetic resonance imaging with gadolinium has a high sensitivity but its specificity is 47.67%. It is less sensitive than mammography for *in situ* lesions. It may have a role in the evaluation of women with silicone

breast implants, those who have had breast-conserving surgery, and those who have a genetic predisposition for cancer (7).

D. Genetics. A family history of breast cancer, ovarian cancer, colon cancer, or prostate cancer should be elicited. A multigenerational history is particularly useful. Recommendations for genetic testing, although not a part of the acute work up of a breast mass, may be considered if a number of relatives, especially first-degree or multigenerational, have these cancers.

IV. DIAGNOSIS

A. Differential diagnosis. The differential diagnosis of a breast mass includes cyst, fibroadenoma, fibrocystic breast changes, galactoceles, hematoma, abscess, and cancer.

B. Clinical manifestations

1. Age of presentation is a critical feature in the clinical presentation of a breast mass. Women older than 40 years of age have a higher risk of breast cancer. This is particularly true in postmenopausal women with a new mass.

2. Cyclic pain suggests a cystic origin. Persistent pain may represent breast cancer or an inflammatory process. Pregnancy expands the list of possible causes of a mass to include mastitis, galactocele, or a breast abscess.

3. Hard, immobile, irregular masses raise the suspicion of breast cancer. Smooth, cystic, or rubbery masses suggest a cyst or fibroadenoma. These characteristics do not guarantee the benign nature of the mass (8). Fibrocystic changes are often nondiscrete and irregular but are also mobile and relatively soft. Compression of the nipple may express a discharge (Chapter 11.6).

4. Retraction suggests either chronic inflammation or breast cancer due to the adherence of skin to the mass. *Peau d'orange* is a puckering or indentation of the skin over a mass. This feature raises the suspicion of malignancy.

5. A rash may be related to Paget's disease with a related ductal carcinoma.

References

1. American Cancer Society. Cancer facts and figures 2003. Available at: http://www. cancer.org/downloads/STT/CAFF2003PWSecured.pdf, accessed online August 7, 2005.
2. National Cancer Institute. SEER 1973–2001 public-use data. Available at: http://seer. cancer.gov/publicdata/, accessed online August 7, 2005.
3. White G, Griffith C, Nenstiel R, et al. Breast cancer: reducing mortality through early detection. *Clin Rev* 1996;6(9):77–79,83–84,100–106.
4. http://www.medscape.com/viewarticle/443381, accessed on 2006.
5. Liberman L, Fahs MC, Deshaw DD, et al. Impact of stereotaxic core breast biopsy on cost of diagnosis. *Radiology* 1995;195:633.
6. The uniform approach to breast fine-needle aspiration biopsy. [Editorial Opinion]. National Cancer Institute Conference. *Am J Surg* 1997;174(4):371–385.
7. Klein S. Evaluation of palpable breast masses. *Am Fam Physician* 2005;71:1731–1738.
8. Venet L, Strax P, Vent W, et al. Adequacies and inadequacies of breast examinations by physicians in mass screening. *Cancer* 1971;28:1546.

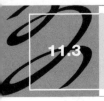

CHRONIC PELVIC PAIN
Paul V. Aitken, Jr. and Albert A. Meyer

I. **BACKGROUND.** Chronic pelvic pain is defined as an episodic or continuous pain that persists for 6 months or longer and is sufficiently severe to have a significant impact on a woman's lifestyle and day-to-day function or relationships. A woman has an approximate 5% chance of having chronic pelvic pain in her lifetime (1).

II. **PATHOPHYSIOLOGY.** Chronic pelvic pain is less likely to be associated with an identifiable pathophysiologic disorder than that lasting <3 months. Every anatomic structure in the abdomen or pelvis could have a role in the etiology of chronic pelvic pain. It is helpful to attempt to categorize the pain as either gynecologic or nongynecologic as the evaluation proceeds toward the more specific diagnosis. Good and consistent scientific evidence shows that gynecologic conditions that cause chronic pelvic pain are endometriosis, gynecologic malignancies, and pelvic inflammatory disease. It also shows that nongynecologic conditions that cause chronic pelvic pain are cystitis, inflammatory bowel disease, pelvic floor myalgia, and somatization disorder (2). Therefore, a comprehensive and detailed multisystem evaluation is warranted.

III. **EVALUATION**

A. **History**

1. Components of an appropriate medical history are as follows (3):
   a. Onset, duration, and pattern of the pain
   b. Location, intensity, character, and radiation of the pain
   c. Aggravating or relieving factors
   d. Review of urinary, musculoskeletal, and gastrointestinal systems
   e. Relationship of the pain to sexual activity or menstruation
   f. Fatigue and anorexia
   g. Medication history (e.g., use of birth control pills or over-the-counter medications)
   h. Past obstetric, gynecologic, and general surgical histories

2. It should be noted that women with a history of pelvic inflammatory disease are four times more likely to develop chronic pelvic pain. An individual with intestinal, sexual, urinary, musculoskeletal, and systemic symptoms may be suffering from a psychiatric disorder (e.g., depression). Specific questions should explore the possibility of a current or remote history of sexual abuse. Often it is possible to obtain this information only when the provider creates an atmosphere of mutual respect and trust.

3. Dyspareunia is often a feature of chronic pelvic pain. Superficial dyspareunia may indicate a urethritis, whereas deep dyspareunia may signify adhesions. Cyclic pain that is related to menstruation usually points to a gynecologic problem. Pain referred to the anterior thigh, or associated with irregular uterine bleeding, or new onset dysmenorrhea may have a uterine or ovarian cause. Urethral tenderness, dysuria, or bladder pain suggests interstitial cystitis or a urethral problem (Chapter 10.1). Pain on defecation, melana, bloody stools, or abdominal pain with alternating diarrhea and constipation can point toward pelvic floor problems, irritable bowel syndrome, or inflammatory bowel diseases.

B. **Physical examination**

1. The general condition of the patient should be noted. Does the patient look chronically ill, which may suggest a pelvic lesion or an inflammatory bowel disorder? Does the patient appear anxious, stressed, or inappropriate?
   a. Can the patient point to the pain with one finger? If so, this can indicate that the pain may have a discrete source.

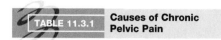

TABLE 11.3.1	Causes of Chronic Pelvic Pain

Endometriosis

Pelvic inflammatory disease

Gynecologic malignancies

Cystitis

Inflammatory bowel disease

Pelvic floor myalgia

Somatization disorders

Depression

Herniated lumbar disc

Lumbar lordosis

Spondylolisthesis

  b. An examination of the lower back, sacral area, and coccyx, including a neurologic examination of the lower extremities, is necessary. A herniated disc,
exaggerated lumbar lordosis, and spondylolisthesis can all cause pelvic pain.
  c. Examine the abdomen, looking for surgical scars, distention, and palpable
tenderness, particularly in the epigastrium, flank, back, or bladder.
  2. A thorough pelvic examination is the most important part of the evaluation.
C. Testing (4). If no obvious cause is apparent, it is reasonable to obtain a complete
blood count, urinalysis, sedimentation rate, and serum chemistry profile. A pelvic
ultrasound may be helpful if pelvic examination is inconclusive. Laparoscopy is
best used to diagnose a definite pelvic mass. Laparoscopy has been used in the
past but various studies have shown a 66% negative laparoscopy rate for patients
with chronic pelvic pain. A multidisciplinary approach using medical, psychologic,
environmental, and nutritional disciplines showed a decrease in pain after 1 year.
IV. DIAGNOSIS. Chronic pelvic pain has an extensive differential diagnosis (1) (see
Table 11.3.1). These complex problems can be assessed using a multisystem approach.
Whereas gastrointestinal, gynecologic, musculoskeletal, and psychiatric conditions can
cause chronic pelvic pain, a thorough gynecologic history and pelvic examination are
the cornerstones of the diagnostic assessment. A few laboratory tests are helpful. A
pelvic ultrasound is useful when the pelvic organs cannot be adequately assessed during
the physical examination. A team approach, coordinated by a trusted family physician,
can bring much relief to patients who have this frustrating clinical problem.

References
1. Ryder RM. Chronic pelvic pain. *Am Fam Physician* 1996;54(7):2225–2232.
2. American College of Obstetricians and Gynecologists. Chronic pelvic pain. ACOG
practice bulletin No. 51 *Obstet Gynecol* 2004;103(3):589–605.
3. Gunter J. Chronic pelvic pain: an integrated approach to diagnosis and treatment.
Obstet Gynecol Surv 2003;58(9):615–623.
4. Chan PD, Winkle CR, eds. *Gynecology and obstetrics, 1999–2000.* Laguna Hills, CA:
Current Clinical Strategies Publishers, 1999:23–25.

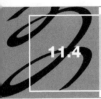

DYSMENORRHEA

Paul V. Aitken, Jr. and Albert A. Meyer

I. **BACKGROUND.** Dysmenorrhea can be defined as a complaint of pain experienced during or immediately before menstruation.

II. **PATHOPHYSIOLOGY.** Dysmenorrhea is the most common gynecologic problem in menstruating women, with up to 90% of women experiencing this symptom at some point in their lives (1). Risk factors include younger age at menarche; cigarette smoking; and the concomitant presence of prolonged, heavy, and irregular periods. Pregnancy history and dietary factors do not seem to correlate with this symptom (2).

III. **EVALUATION**

   A. **History**

   1. A detailed menstrual and gynecologic history is critical to the diagnosis. Given the history, it is extremely important to distinguish primary from secondary dysmenorrhea.

      a. Primary dysmenorrhea starts at the onset of menarche and is thought to be the result of prostaglandin-2α, which produces uterine ischemia. It can be treated with antiprostaglandins and oral contraceptives.

      b. Secondary dysmenorrhea starts later in a woman's ovulatory life and may be caused by endometriosis or pelvic pathology.

         i. If abnormal bleeding is associated with either type of dysmenorrhea, it is important to elicit symptoms of pregnancy, such as missed or late menses, breast tenderness, nausea, or urinary frequency (Chapter 11.1).

         ii. If severe pain develops during the first part of the menstrual cycle, ascertain the history of sexual partners, abnormal vaginal discharge, or dyspareunia. These symptoms could point toward pelvic inflammatory disease (PID) (Chapter 11.3).

         iii. Pain that develops during menses, but not related to pregnancy or infection, can also be caused by tumor. In younger women, secondary dysmenorrhea that is sufficiently severe to affect daily functioning or relationships suggests endometriosis. This condition affects as many as 19% of women (3). Deep dyspareunia and sacral backache with menses are common symptoms. Premenstrual tenesmus or diarrhea correlates with endometriosis of the rectosigmoid area, whereas cyclic hematuria or dysuria may indicate bladder endometriosis.

         iv. Infertility is often a consequence of endometriosis.

   B. **Physical examination**

   1. As with all menstrual complaints, a thorough physical examination is an essential part of making a diagnosis. The general condition of the patient needs to be assessed. Are the vital signs stable or is the patient showing signs of systemic illness such as fever, which can indicate pelvic infection? Hypotension and pallor can indicate a ruptured ectopic pregnancy.

   2. A general physical assessment with attention to the back, sacrum, spine, abdomen, and bladder is important.

   3. A thorough pelvic examination is the key to excluding other possible diagnoses. The external genitalia may show signs of cyanosis, as is seen with pregnancy, or abnormal discharge, as is seen with infection. Palpate the vaginal area for nodules that may present on the anterior *cul-de-sac* or on the posterior vaginal fornix on bimanual examination; they could indicate endometriosis. Cervical motion tenderness and cervical leukorrhea may be present in PID. Uterine tenderness is often present and uterine displacement and fixation may be noted. Ovarian enlargement or adnexa fixation may correlate with endometriosis. An adnexal

mass from a neoplastic or infectious cause may be found. Nodules may also be palpated along the uterosacral ligaments on rectovaginal examination.

C. Testing (4)
   1. A complete blood count looking for anemia or leukocytosis is helpful.
   2. If abnormal bleeding is associated with the dysmenorrhea, thyroid testing and a qualitative serum pregnancy test are indicated.
   3. Urinalysis should be obtained to test for hematuria. With an indication of infection, a urine culture is often helpful.
   4. A pelvic ultrasound may be helpful if any masses seem apparent on pelvic examination.
   5. The definitive diagnosis of endometriosis can only be made with laparoscopy.

IV. DIAGNOSIS (1). Difficult menstrual periods occur at some point for most women during their reproductive years. If it is recurrent and significantly interferes with daily activity or relationships, it warrants treatment. Primary dysmenorrhea not associated with abnormal bleeding can often be treated successfully with nonsteroidal agents or oral contraceptives. If it does not respond to these agents or if it is associated with abnormal bleeding, further diagnostic testing is indicated. Secondary dysmenorrhea, either with or without abnormal bleeding, may point to a pelvic tumor, infection, or pregnancy. Further testing is essential in this case.

References

1. Jamieson DJ, Steege JF. The prevalence of dysmenorrhea, dyspareunia, pelvic pain and irritable syndrome in primary care practices. *Obstet Gynecol* 1996;87:55–58.
2. Proctor ML, Farquhar CM. Dysmenorrhoea. Clinical Evidence Concise 2005;14:573–576.
3. Apgar BS. Dysmenorrhea and dysfunctional uterine bleeding. *Prim Care* 1997;24(1):161–179.
4. Chan PD, Winkle CR. *Gynecology and obstetrics 1999–2000.* Laguna Hills, CA: Current Clinical Strategies Publishers, 1999:25–26.

MENORRHAGIA
Kathryn M. Andolsek

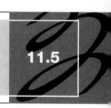

11.5

I. BACKGROUND. Menorrhagia, defined as heavy (≥ 80 mL) bleeding from the uterus occurring at regular (≥ 21–35 days) or lasting ≥ 7 days in duration, is common. Assessing the volume of blood loss has limited utility. It fails to differentiate among etiologies, predict iron status, direct a diagnostic strategy, or indicate prognosis (1). Practically, it is difficult to quantify the amount of blood loss. Diagnose when a woman subjectively reports that menstrual bleeding is heavier or longer than is typical for her.

II. PATHOPHYSIOLOGY
   A. Etiology. The etiology varies considerably with the patient's age, history, and physical findings. Pregnancy and its complications (e.g., spontaneous abortion, ectopic, missed abortion, trophoblastic disease) among women in their reproductive years must always be excluded; if "missed," it may be life threatening. Bleeding as a side effect of hormonal contraceptives, intrauterine devices, and other medications is common. Other frequent causes are anovulation, uterine fibroids, polyps, endometriosis, adenomyosis, coagulation disorders, endocrinopathies, malignancy, pelvic inflammatory disease (PID), and liver or kidney disease (2).
   B. Epidemiology. Menorrhagia is common. In women 30 to 49 years of age, it represents 5% of gynecologic visits. Work loss from increased blood flow is estimated annually to be $1,692 per woman. Once referred, women have an increased risk

of hysterectomy. Menorrhagia accounts for two-thirds of all hysterectomies; no pathology is identified in at least 50% of removed uteri.

III. EVALUATION

A. History

1. **A menstrual and reproductive history is necessary.** Ask about previous patterns of the menstrual cycle; the first day of the last menstrual period and the first day of the previous menstrual period; and the regularity, duration, and frequency of all bleeding, including any intermenstrual flow. Determine if pain is present and attempt to quantify the number of pads or tampons per period.

2. **Pregnancy should always be considered and excluded.** All contraceptive methods, even permanent ones such as tubal sterilization, are subject to failure; women may not reveal sexual activity.

3. **Weight change, excessive patterns, anxiety or stress disorders, as well as symptoms of systemic disease** (e.g., coagulopathy; thyroid, renal, and hepatic diseases) should be evaluated.

4. **Medication history** should include the use of contraceptives (3), anticoagulants, selective serotonin reuptake inhibitors, corticosteroids, antipsychotics, tamoxifen, and herbal modalities such as ginseng, gingko, and soy.

5. **Presence of easy bruising or any abnormal bleeding** such as with teeth brushing or minimal trauma may indicate a bleeding disorder.

6. **The presence of molimenal symptoms** (e.g., edema, abdominal bloating, pelvic cramping, and breast fullness) is more likely with ovulatory cycles; however, these symptoms are not reliable enough to be truly diagnostic.

7. **Psychosocial factors should be considered.** One-third of women with menorrhagia have menstrual blood loss within a normal range. Anxiety, unemployment, and abdominal pain are more common in these women, and these factors may have influenced their decision to seek health care.

8. **Probable etiologies can be classified by age (4)**

   a. **Neonatal period.** Although not "menorrhagia" in this age-group, vaginal bleeding may occur during the first few days of life as the infant experiences a rapid decrease in maternal-derived estrogen levels. This is generally treated with reassurance if no other signs or symptoms are present.

   b. **Neonatal period to menarche.** Similarly, prepubertal bleeding is not "menorrhagia" but should be carefully evaluated to exclude sexual abuse and assault, malignancy, sexually transmitted infections, and trauma.

   c. **Early menarche.** With no molimenal symptoms and irregular menses, anovulatory cycles are likely. Almost all normal adolescents experience some degree of menstrual irregularity; "heavy periods" should be evaluated. Pregnancy should be excluded if there is any question of sexual activity. Abnormal bleeding may also occur as a side effect for contraceptive hormonal methods taken correctly or incorrectly. Fever and pelvic pain can indicate PID. Easy bruising or bleeding may indicate a bleeding disorder. With neurologic symptoms such as blurred vision, visual field defects, headache, or the presence of galactorrhea, a pituitary lesion should be considered.

   d. **Late menarche to late thirties.** Exclude pregnancy and contraceptive-related causes. Anovulation is less common. Polycystic ovarian syndrome, the female athlete triad, and stress-induced conditions, such as eating disorders, may be present. Other gynecologic conditions include endometriosis, endometrial hyperplasia, endometrial polyps, PID, and endocrinopathies (both hypo- and hyperthyroidism, as well as pituitary and hypothalamic conditions).

   e. **Late thirties and older.** Exclude pregnancy. If the patient is not pregnant, abnormal bleeding in this age-group should arouse suspicion of cancer until proved otherwise. Women are increasingly anovulatory as they approach the perimenopause. Inquire about menopausal symptoms, exogenous use of estrogens, and personal or family history of gynecologic malignancy or genetically linked cancers, such as colon and breast. Other causes include adenomyosis.

   f. **Postmenopausal period.** See Chapter 11.8.

9. **In >50% of women with menorrhagia, no etiology is found**; the diagnosis is then dysfunctional uterine bleeding.

B. Physical examination

1. **Assess vital signs and the patient's general appearance, blood pressure, and pulse..** If orthostatic changes are present, evaluate for symptoms of shock. If present, these are usually related to pregnancy and may indicate a ruptured ectopic pregnancy; alternatively, trauma, sepsis, or cancer may be present.

2. **Pallor** with normal vital signs may be present if chronic blood loss has resulted in anemia. Anemia, if present, may be due to the blood loss itself, blood dyscrasia, systemic conditions, or malignancy.

3. **Fever and pelvic tenderness** are suggestive of acute PID.

4. **Physical examination includes the vulva, cervix uterus, and adnexa..** A pelvic mass may indicate abscess, fibroid, ectopic pregnancy, or malignancy. Exclude genital trauma.

5. **Signs of thyroid disease** (e.g., rapid or slow pulse, reflex changes, hair changes, and thyromegaly) can be associated with menstrual abnormalities.

6. **Excessive bruising** can indicate nutritional deficiency, eating disorder, trauma, abuse, medication overuse, or a bleeding disorder.

7. **Jaundice and hepatomegaly** may signify an underlying bleeding disorder.

8. **Obesity, hirsutism, acne, and acanthosis nigricans** suggest polycystic ovary disease.

9. **Galactorrhea** may indicate pituitary pathology.

10. **Edema** may signify renal disease.

C. Testing

1. **Laboratory tests**

   a. **A baseline complete blood count and serum pregnancy test** should be obtained in most women.

   b. A platelet count, bleeding time, and other tests for bleeding disorders should be performed as indicated to exclude a bleeding disorder if no other etiology is readily apparent. Inherited bleeding disorders occur in as many as 11% of patients with menorrhagia compared with 3% of control women; most of them have von Willebrand's disease, which is more common in white women. Establishing this diagnosis is important, because many of the diagnostic and therapeutic options are surgical and may present added risk if an underlying bleeding disorder is present. The available data do not support routinely screening all women with menorrhagia (5).

   c. Screening for sexually transmitted diseases and thyroid dysfunction should be considered.

   d. A Papanicolaou smear should be performed if indicated, although cervical dysplasia rarely causes significant degrees of vaginal bleeding.

   e. Renal and liver function tests are useful if these etiologies are suspected.

2. **Diagnostic imaging**

   a. Any nonpregnant woman with irregular bleeding and a pelvic mass requires complete evaluation with ultrasound, computed tomography (CT) scan, or laparoscopy.

   b. Transvaginal ultrasound detects leiomyoma, endometrial thickening, and focal masses but may miss endometrial polyps and submucous fibroids. Although highly sensitive for endometrial carcinoma, it may miss 4% more cancers than a dilation and curettage (D & C). An endometrial stripe of <5 mm is reassuring but does not conclusively exclude cancer.

   c. Saline-infused sonography (sonohysterography) (5–10 mL sterile saline infused into the endometrial cavity) with ultrasound imaging can be done. The utility of this procedure is comparable to diagnostic hysteroscopy and is more accurate than transvaginal ultrasound alone. The sensitivity is 95% to 97% and the specificity is 70% to 98% when combined with endometrial biopsy. A decision analysis recommends it as the procedure of first choice (6).

   d. Magnetic resonance imaging (MRI) may be useful for adenomyosis.

3. **Endometrial sampling** is recommended in women ≥35 years of age or those at increased risk of endometrial carcinoma. This procedure is best performed on the first day of menses to avoid unexpected pregnancy.

4. **Hysteroscopy**

5. **D & C**

IV. **DIAGNOSIS (7).** Menorrhagia presents most frequently at the extremes of the reproductive years, during menarche and in perimenopause. Pregnancy must be excluded. Any pelvic mass must be evaluated with ultrasound, CT scan, or MRI. If no diagnosis can be made, laparoscopy or hysteroscopy with saline infusion may be indicated.

References

1. Warner PE, Critchley HO, Lumsden MA, et al. Menorrhagia II: is the 80 mL blood loss criterion useful in management of complaint of menorrhagia? *Am J Obstet Gynecol* 2004;190(5):1224–1229.

2. Albers JR, Hull SK, Wesley RM. Abnormal uterine bleeding. *Am Fam Physician* 2004;69:1915–1926.

3. Schrager S. Abnormal Uterine Bleeding Associated with hormonal contraception. *Am Fam Physician* 2002;65(1):2073–2080.

4. Finley B, Harnisch DR, Comer B, et al. *Women's genitourinary conditions: FP essentials*, Monograph No, 314 AAFP Home Study, Leawood, Kan: American Academy of Family Physicians, 2005:28–41 July.

5. James A, Matchar DB, Myers ER. Testing for von Willebrand disease in women with menorrhagia: a systematic review. *Obstet Gynecol* 2004;104(2):381–388.

6. Dijkhuizen FPHLJ, Mol BWJ, Bongers MY, et al. Cost effectiveness of transvaginal sonography and saline infused sonography in the evaluation of menorrhagia. *Int J Gynecol Obstet* 2003;83(1):45–52.

7. Roy SN, Bhattacharya S. Benefits and risks of pharmacological agents used for the treatment of menorrhagia. *Drug Saf* 2004;27(2):75–90.

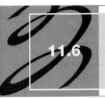

NIPPLE DISCHARGE IN THE NONPREGNANT FEMALE

Joyce A. Copeland

I. **BACKGROUND.** Nipple discharge in the nonpregnant female may be of either physiologic or pathologic origin. Galactorrhea is milk production unrelated to pregnancy. Abnormal discharges other than milk may occur owing to a pathologic etiology.

II. **PATHOPHYSIOLOGY**

A. **Etiology.** Galactorrhea is the result of the stimulation of the pituitary gland resulting in the release of prolactin. Prolactin initiates the production of milk in the lobular and ductal epithelium of the breast.

1. Medications that inhibit dopamine function or the metabolism of other neurotransmitters are often associated with nipple discharge on the basis of the impact of the substances on prolactin production. These physiologically based agents are most often associated with bilateral, multiductal discharge. Common offenders include the following:

a. Phenothiazines, haloperidol, and other antipsychotics

b. Tricyclic antidepressants, benzodiazepines, selective serotonin reuptake inhibitors

c. Metoclopramide, cimetidine

d. Reserpine, methyldopa, digitalis, verapamil

e. Steroid hormones such as oral contraceptives, estrogens, progestins

f. Isoniazid, danazol

2. Significant stress may induce nipple discharge by the same mechanism as medication.
3. Neurologic symptoms in association with bilateral discharge and amenorrhea require investigation for pituitary abnormalities such as pituitary adenoma.
4. Nonphysiologic causes of nipple discharge involve inflammation or friction as well as malignancy.

B. Epidemiology. Between 50% and 80% of women will present with a nipple discharge at some point in their reproductive years. This finding is associated with breast cancer in approximately 5% of these women (1). Risks of malignant etiology increase with age, unilateral and uniductal bloody discharges. The risk of cancer increases after 40 years of age.

III. EVALUATION

A. History (2). Initial history should begin with queries regarding the nature of the discharge and the characteristics of the patient. How old is the patient? What was the circumstance of discovery of the discharge including spontaneity, and the presence of palpable mass? How does the patient describe the characteristics of the discharge? A thorough history should include past breast history, chest trauma, infection, and medication and substance use. Family history of breast cancer is also critical to risk assessment. Is there a history of friction of the nipple? Does the patient smoke?

1. **Reproductive history.** What is the patient's menstrual status? Has there been a recent pregnancy or abortion? This information helps identify normal lactation. Is the patient using hormonal contraception?
2. **Review of systems.** The review of systems should include queries about thyroid function, renal and hepatic disease as well as adrenal or pituitary symptoms. Does the patient have a history of headaches, visual disturbance, and associated amenorrhea or menstrual disturbance?

B. Physical examination
1. **Clinical breast examination**
   a. **Inspection.** Observe the skin of the breast for erythema, crusting, or a rash on the nipple or areolar region. Document the color of any discharge. Look for evidence of nipple retraction. Identify the location of the discharge. Magnification and adequate lighting may assist in the process of localization. Look for chest wall scars, evidence of viral infections (e.g., herpes zoster or simplex), and signs of eczema or inflammation.
   b. **Palpation.** Feel the skin for warmth. Palpate both breasts for a mass or tenderness. Palpate regional lymph nodes for evidence of adenopathy. Document the size, location, consistency, and mobility of any mass.
   c. **Compression.** Compress the base or the areolar region of the breast with the thumb and index finger to attempt expression of the discharge in question. A warm compress prior to the examination may assist in the identification of the discharge. Note the location of any discharge as well as the color of the discharge and the number of ducts involved.
2. **Other examination components.** Palpate the thyroid and liver if history indicates risks of pathology in these organs. A neurologic examination, including visual fields, should accompany any history of visual disturbance or headaches.

C. Testing. Clinical history suggestive of endocrine, renal, or hepatic disease should trigger the evaluation of associated laboratory assessment. Serum prolactin level is indicated for a history of headache, visual disturbance, and menstrual irregularity in the presence of a nipple discharge. Pregnancy testing is also a consideration in the women of reproductive age with menstrual disturbance.

1. **The discharge.** Guaiac testing of the discharge should be performed if from the visual examination the discharge is not obviously bloody or serosanguineous in the unilateral, uniductal presentation. The role of cytology is controversial, but the presence of blood increases the positive predictive value of this modality. A positive cytology is highly predictive of cancer.
2. **Imaging.** Mammography is indicated in all women older than 35 years of age with a spontaneous nipple discharge. The purpose of mammography is to identify occult disease and help in the characterization of any palpable mass. The

role of ductoscopy, ductography, ductal lavage, and magnetic resonance imaging is under investigation. Mammography in younger women is less sensitive. Ultrasound is more useful in women who are younger than 35 years of age.

3. **Possible surgery.** Surgical referral for ductal exploration or further evaluation is indicated for a patient with a unilateral, uniductal nipple discharge or a nipple discharge in the presence of a mass, and for any patient with positive cytology.

D. Genetics. A family history of a parent or sibling with breast cancer or abnormal BRCA1/BRCA2 genes increases the chance that a discharge may be malignant. Genetic testing is not indicated in the evaluation of a nipple discharge.

IV. DIAGNOSIS

A. Differential diagnosis. The chief consideration in the differential diagnosis is the distinction between physiologically and pathologically based etiologies. The differential diagnosis includes pregnancy, "pseudodischarge," friction or manipulation, systemic disease, pituitary disease or stimulation, cancer, ductal ectasia, intraductal papilloma, Paget's disease, eczema, and local inflammation secondary to trauma or infection.

B. Clinical manifestations. Physiologic discharges are multiductal, bilateral, painless, and associated with stimulation or medication. This discharge is usually white, clear, yellow, or green in color. The consistency is usually milky, because this is the physiologic response to the stimulation of the pituitary, resulting in galactorrhea.

Pathologic discharges are usually unilateral, uniductal, and spontaneous. The color is variable and blood or purulence may be apparent. Cancer is present in one-third of bloody discharges. This is even more likely if the woman is older than 40 years of age and/or a mass is present. Benign tumors, infections, and systemic disease are also pathologic causes for this type.

1. "Pseudodischarge" may be indicated by the presence of a stain on the bra or blouse, which may be interpreted as a discharge. Considerations in this circumstance include eczema, infection, trauma, or Paget's disease.

2. Manipulation of the nipple or friction may be responsible for a discharge. Runners or joggers are candidates for friction-related nipple discharge.

3. Discharge associated with thyroid disease, chronic renal failure, and hepatic failure is suggested by a positive review of the systems in these areas.

4. Headache and visual disturbance with a discharge suggests the possibility of pituitary disease.

Intraductal papilloma is the most common cause of benign pathologic discharges. It is associated with a straw-colored or clear transparent discharge.

5. Ductal ectasia is the result of a progression of ductal stagnation and resultant inflammatory process. The incidence of this disorder is higher in smokers and is most prominent in women in the 40- to 60-year-old age-group. Induration and noncyclic burning pain is characteristic of this disorder.

6. Paget's disease involves the skin of the nipple and areola. It is usually associated with ductal carcinoma. Any areolar lesion that does not respond to antibiotics or topical treatment must be biopsied to exclude this disorder.

References

1. Shirley R. Nipple Discharge. Up to Date 2005; Version 13.1; www.uptodate.com.
2. Andolsek K, Copeland J. In: Taylor B, ed. *Conditions of the breast in family medicine: principles and practice*, 5th ed. New York: Springer-Verlag, 1998.

PAP SMEAR ABNORMALITY
Fidel A. Valea

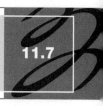

11.7

I. BACKGROUND. The incidence of cervical cancer, once the leading cause of cancer deaths in women, has steadily decreased in the United States since the inception of mass screening with cervical cytology (the Papanicolaou [Pap] smear). Approximately 50 million Pap smears are performed in the United States annually, and approximately 5% reveal abnormalities. Although most of the abnormalities are low grade and will likely regress, a few can progress to cancer; therefore even low-grade abnormalities should be evaluated.

II. PATHOPHYSIOLOGY

A. Etiology

1. The cervix, because of its location in the vagina, is very susceptible to exposure to environmental factors. The squamocolumnar junction, or transformation zone, is the part of the cervix with the greatest likelihood for neoplastic change because it is the junction where the cervical glandular (columnar) epithelium meets the native squamous epithelium of the ectocervix. The exposed columnar epithelium undergoes metaplastic change and is replaced by squamous epithelium in the transformation zone. Because of the constant inflammation, damage, and repair that occur in areas of metaplasia, it is particularly susceptible to the incorporation of viruses and the effects of other carcinogens.

2. The human papilloma virus (HPV) is a double-stranded deoxyribonucleic acid (DNA) virus that replicates within epithelial cells at specific sites and has been linked to cervical intraepithelial neoplasia, or dysplasia, as well as cervical cancer. Epithelial cells become infected with HPV at the basal and parabasal layers. Trauma from intercourse, for example, can abrade the surface epithelium and expose the basal cells. The koilocytes (cells infected with HPV) that develop are present in the superficial layers of the epithelium and further trauma increases shedding of these cells and promotes transmission. After exposure, the incubation period can be anywhere from 1 to 8 months. The first line of host response is to slow viral replication and induce a cell-mediated response to contain the virus. In most healthy individuals with normal immune response, the viral infection is transient with an average duration of viral shedding after a new HPV infection of 8 months (1, 2). Conversely, HPV can evade the host immune response because it is an intracellular infection and is not readily identified as an antigen. The phenotypic expression of an HPV infection also depends on the viral type. Of the >100 types of HPV, >30 infect the lower genital tract. These sexually transmitted types of HPV have generally been divided into two groups: low oncogenic potential and high oncogenic potential. Table 11.7.1 shows the

TABLE 11.7.1	Human Papilloma Virus Types According to the Oncogenic Potential
Oncogenic potential	**Virus type**
Low risk	6, 11, 40, 42–44, 53, 54, 61, 72, 73, 81
High risk	16, 18, 31, 33, 35, 39, 45, 51, 52, 56, 58, 59, 68, 82

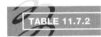

TABLE 11.7.2	Natural History of Cervical Dysplasia			
	Regression (%)	Persistence (%)	Progression to severe dysplasia (%)	Progression to cancer (%)
Mild dysplasia	57	32	11	1
Moderate dysplasia	43	35	22	5
Severe dysplasia	32	~56	—	12

breakdown of the various types. The low oncogenic potential viral types are associated with condyloma and low-grade cervical abnormalities, whereas the high oncogenic potential viral types are associated high-grade cervical dysplasia and cancer. HPV is a necessary but insufficient precursor of squamous cell carcinoma of the cervix. Host factors such as age, nutritional status, immune function, smoking, and possibly silent genetic polymorphisms modulate the incorporation of viral DNA into host cervical cells.

B. Epidemiology

1. HPV is one of the most common sexually transmitted infections in the United States, with an estimated prevalence of 15%, leading to approximately 2 to 5 million abnormal Pap smears in the United States annually. Using modern HPV detection methods, approximately 95% to 100% of squamous cell cervical cancers and 75% to 95% of high-grade cervical intraepithelial neoplasia lesions have detectable HPV DNA. In the United States, peak incidence and prevalence of HPV infection occur among women younger than 25 years of age, but most infections in younger women are transient. In one study, 25% of college freshmen were already exposed to HPV. Of the freshmen who were negative when they enrolled, 42% had evidence of exposure over the next 3 years, leading a prevalence of >60% (2). Infections with HPV in older women are much less prevalent but carry a higher risk of progressing to cervical neoplasia. Although the prevalence of HPV infection is higher among immuno-compromised women such as those with human immunodeficiency virus, the speed of progression to cervical cancer is not increased. Natural history studies confirm that, in most cases, the course of infection and cervical abnormalities that progress do so in an orderly fashion from less severe to more severe lesions, making it an ideal condition for screening (3). This is demonstrated in Table 11.7.2.

2. Risk factors for cervical neoplasia include not only HPV but also early onset of intercourse, multiple sexual partners, young age, male factors (high-risk partner), low socioeconomic status, race, history of other sexually transmitted diseases, compromised immunity, cigarette smoking, oral contraceptive use, and even history of diethylstilbestrol exposure.

3. The American Cancer Society estimates that there will be approximately 10,370 new cases of invasive cervical cancer and 3,710 deaths in the United States in 2005 (4). It is now the 13th most common cancer in women in the United States. Pap smears continue to be one of the few interventions awarded an "A" recommendation from the U.S. Preventive Services Task Force (5).

III. EVALUATION

A. History. Most patients with cervical dysplasia are asymptomatic. They can also present with evidence of external condyloma, vaginal discharge, or even vaginal bleeding. For most, the initial discovery of cervical neoplasia is usually as an abnormality in the Pap smear. The gynecologic history, which is essential in determining a patient's risk, should be shared with the cytopathologist.

B. Physical examination

1. On physical examination, the cervix usually appears normal to the naked eye. Gross cervical lesions should not be evaluated with a Pap smear; instead, they should be biopsied to confirm the diagnosis.

2. There are two general techniques to obtain a cytologic specimen from the cervix. The traditional method uses a spatula to gently scrape the ectocervix and the transformation zone and a cytobrush, or a similar apparatus, to sample the endocervix. Both these specimens are "smeared" evenly on a glass slide and fixed immediately. It is important to not allow the slides to dry before fixation. A more contemporary method is to use a liquid-based system. The cervix and endocervix are sampled with a plastic "broom" or a similar apparatus and the specimen is suspended in a bottle containing the fixative and transported as a suspension. Both are acceptable, although the latter allows for additional HPV DNA testing.

3. The Bethesda System was developed in 1988 and revised in 1991 and again in 2001 by the National Cancer Institute to provide uniform terminology for cervical cytopathology reporting (see Table 11.7.3). In all reports, specific mention should be made about the specimen type, adequacy of the specimen, a general categorization of the results, how the specimen was evaluated, if any other ancillary testing was performed, as well as a final interpretation of findings and recommendations. The evaluation of each abnormality should be individualized on the basis of many factors including age, medical history, reproductive plans, and the presence of risk factors.

4. The American Cancer Society guidelines for cervical cancer screening were last updated in 2002 (6). They reflect the current understanding of the pathophysiology and epidemiology of cervical neoplasia. They recommend that cervical cancer screening should commence approximately 3 years after the onset of vaginal intercourse, but no later than 21 years of age. Screening should be performed annually until 30 years of age, with conventional cytologic smears or every 2 years using liquid-based cytology. After 30 years of age, women who have had three consecutive, technically satisfactory normal results may undergo screening every 2 to 3 years using either technology or can undergo testing for high-risk HPV DNA, in addition to cytology, every 3 years. The American Cancer Society did not recommend screening women older than 70 years of age with three consecutive normal smears and no history of abnormal Pap smears or women who have had total hysterectomies.

C. Testing.
The evaluation of a patient with an abnormal Pap smear begins with the understanding that a Pap smear is a screening test, not a diagnostic test. The correlation between Pap smear and histologic diagnosis is variable. In one series, the most common Pap smear report prior to a histologic diagnosis of severe dysplasia was atypical squamous cells of undetermined significance (ASCUS) (7). Similarly, in a large national trial, <30% of patients with an ASCUS Pap smear were found to have pathology (8). These examples reveal the importance of establishing a histologic diagnosis. However, the evaluation of an abnormal Pap smear may commence with simply repeating the test, depending on the degree of abnormality and the patient's age.

1. Very minimal abnormalities such as ASCUS in younger patients (younger than 30 years of age) can be followed simply by repeating (or confirming) the Pap smear before further testing. HPV DNA testing may be used to help triage these patients; unfortunately, because of the high prevalence of HPV infections in this young age-group, the usefulness of HPV DNA typing in this setting is limited. However, in older patients (older than 30 years of age), it is a very helpful test to help triage patients according to the presence or absence of high-risk HPV DNA (8). In a landmark trial, the ASCUS/low-grade squamous intraepithelial lesion (LGSIL) Triage Study demonstrated that HPV DNA typing for the high-risk strains was useful in the triage of patients older than 30 years of age with an ASCUS Pap smear. Patients older than 30 years of age with high-risk HPV DNA should proceed with diagnostic tests, whereas the similar patient with no high-risk HPV

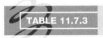

TABLE 11.7.3	Bethesda 2001 Terminology for the Reporting of Cervical Cytopathology

Specimen type

Indicate conventional smear (Pap smear) vs. liquid based vs. other

Specimen adequacy

- Satisfactory for evaluation (*describe presence or absence of endocervical/transformation zone component and any other quality indicators, e.g., partially obscuring blood, inflammation, etc.*)
- Unsatisfactory for evaluation ... (*specify reason*)
  - Specimen rejected/not processed (*specify reason*)
  - Specimen processed and examined, but unsatisfactory for evaluation of epithelial abnormality because of (*specify reason*)

General categorization *(optional)*

- Negative for intraepithelial lesion or malignancy
- Epithelial cell abnormality: see interpretation/result (*specify "squamous" or "glandular" as appropriate*)
- Other: see interpretation/result (*e.g., endometrial cells in a woman over 40 y of age*)

Automated review

If case examined by automated device, specify device and result

Ancillary testing

Provide a brief description of the test methods and report the result so that it is easily understood by the clinician

Interpretation/result

Negative for intraepithelial lesion or malignancy

(*when there is no cellular evidence of neoplasia, record in the General Categorization section and/or in the Interpretation/Result section of the report, whether there are organisms or other non-neoplastic findings*)

Organisms

- *Trichomonas vaginalis*
- Fungal organisms morphologically consistent with *Candida* species
- Shift in flora suggestive of bacterial vaginosis
- Bacteria morphologically consistent with *Actinomyces* species
- Cellular changes consistent with herpes simplex virus

Other non-neoplastic findings *(optional to report; list not inclusive)*

- Reactive cellular changes associated with radiation, intrauterine contraceptive device
- Glandular cells status posthysterectomy
- Atrophy

Other

- Endometrial cells (*in a woman over 40 y of age*) (*Specify if "negative for squamous intraepithelial lesion"*)

Epithelial cell abnormalities

Squamous cell

- Atypical squamous cells of undetermined significance cannot exclude HGSIL (ASC-H)
- Low-grade squamous intraepithelial lesion encompassing: HPV/mild dysplasia/CIN 1
- HGSIL encompassing: moderate and severe dysplasia, carcinoma *in situ*/CIN 2 and CIN 3 with features suspicious for invasion (*if invasion is suspected*)
- Squamous cell carcinoma

(continued)

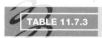

TABLE 11.7.3	Bethesda 2001 Terminology for the Reporting of Cervical Cytopathology *(Continued)*

Glandular cell
- Atypical
  - Endocervical cells (NOS *or specify in comments*)
  - Endometrial cells (NOS *or specify in comments*)
  - Glandular cells (NOS *or specify in comments*)
- Atypical
  - Endocervical cells, favor neoplastic
  - Glandular cells, favor neoplastic
- Endocervical adenocarcinoma *in situ*
- Adenocarcinoma
  - Endocervical
  - Endometrial
  - Extrauterine
  - NOS

Other malignant neoplasms *(specify)*

Educational notes and suggestions *(optional)*

Suggestions should be concise and consistent with clinical follow-up guidelines published by professional organizations (references to relevant publications may be included)

HGSIL, high-grade squamous intraepithelial lesion; CIN, cervical intraepithelial neoplasia; NOS, not otherwise specified, ASC-H, atypical squamous cells-cannot exclude high grade lesion.

DNA can simply be observed and rescreened at a later date. Screening for the low-risk strains of HPV has no usefulness in this setting. In addition, patients with Pap smears showing low-grade changes (LGSILs) or worse did not benefit at all from HPV typing and should proceed with diagnostic tests.

   2. Although postmenopausal patients with ASCUS Pap smears were not specifically evaluated, they may be treated with estrogen vaginal cream if the changes are believed to be caused by atrophy. After a short course of treatment, the Pap smear should be repeated and any subsequent abnormality, even if minimal, should be evaluated further with diagnostic tests.

   3. There is no current role for testing for low-risk HPV DNA, regardless of the patient's age.

V. DIAGNOSIS. The diagnosis of cervical dysplasia, or cancer, should be made only histologically. Colposcopy uses magnification to identify the abnormal areas of the cervix. After excess mucus has been gently wiped away and a Pap smear performed, the cervix, particularly the transformation zone, is moistened with a solution of 3% to 5% acetic acid, allowing for easier visualization of the abnormal areas (punctation, white epithelium, mosaicism, and atypical vessels) and directing the clinician to the specific areas that should be biopsied. The examination is considered satisfactory only if the entire transformation zone can be visualized colposcopically and the most abnormal areas can be biopsied. An endocervical curettage is frequently performed in a blind fashion to evaluate the cells in the endocervical canal that cannot be seen readily. If colposcopy is inadequate, there is an abnormality in the endocervical canal, or there is a suspicion of microinvasive cancer, further diagnostic testing should include either a conization of the cervix or a loop electrosurgical excision procedure (LEEP) to complete the workup. Because of the less-than-perfect correlation between Pap test results and histologic diagnosis, it is imperative that a diagnosis be established histologically and not merely by the Pap test. The differential diagnosis includes the following:

A. ASCUS. Although this may be the lowest grade of abnormality, approximately 30% of patients with an ASCUS Pap smear have dysplasia or significant pathology. The patient younger than 30 years of age can simply be followed with a repeat Pap smear in 4 to 6 months or proceed to diagnostic colposcopy and biopsies, depending on the clinical situation. The patient older than 30 years of age can be triaged according to the high-risk HPV DNA status. If present, she should undergo colposcopy. If high-risk HPV DNA is not present, she can be followed with a repeat Pap test in 1 year.

B. Atypical squamous cells (cannot exclude high-grade squamous intraepithelial lesion [ASC-H]).

This is a new category in the Bethesda reporting system of 2001. Because 30% to 40% of patients with ASC-H have high-grade dysplasia and a very high prevalence of high-risk HPV DNA (approaching 85%), more screening tests are not recommended. They should all have colposcopic evaluation and biopsies.

C. Atypical glandular cells (AGC) (previously called atypical glandular cells of uncertain significance [AGUS]).

This result requires further evaluation on the basis of the impression of the cytopathologist. In the current Bethesda system, the report should include a comment regarding the probable etiology of the AGC. Because the most common abnormality in a patient with an AGC Pap smear is still squamous dysplasia, a colposcopy, including an endocervical curettage, should be performed. Depending on the cell's origin, symptoms, and patient age, the workup may include a conization of the cervix and/or endometrial biopsy, hysteroscopy, or dilation and curettage. An AGC Pap smear should never be "followed" or repeated, because there is a 30% to 60% yield of significant pathology in this patient population. It should never be confused with ASCUS, and HPV typing is not recommended.

D. LGSIL. Depending on the patient's age, this can be managed conservatively with repeat Pap testing or more thoroughly with colposcopy and biopsies. There is no role for HPV DNA testing, because the yield for high-risk HPV DNA is so great that it is not a useful screening tool in this setting. Between 15% and 30% of patients with LGSIL actually have a high-grade lesion.

E. High-grade squamous epithelial lesion (HGSIL). Patients with HGSILs should always be worked up further with very rare exceptions. Colposcopy and biopsies are appropriate, but several patients undergo either diagnostic or therapeutic conization of the cervix or LEEP. HPV typing is not appropriate, because the risk of high-grade dysplasia approaches 75%.

F. Suspicion for invasion. Although this abnormality is frequently evaluated by colposcopy and biopsy, many patients undergo a cervical cone biopsy to confirm the diagnosis. If a gross lesion is present, it should be biopsied to confirm the diagnosis, and a conization is not recommended. On the other hand, the diagnosis of microinvasive cervical cancer can be made only on the basis of a conization specimen, because biopsies are just not sufficient. Patients should be managed by clinicians who are thoroughly familiar with the treatment and management of cervical cancer.

References

1. Tyring SK. Human papilloma infections: epidemiology, pathogenesis, and host immune response. *J Am Acad Dermatol* 2000;43:S18–S26.
2. Ho GY, Bierman R, Beardsley L, et al. Natural history of cervicovaginal papillomavirus infection in young women. *N Engl J Med* 1998;338:423–428.
3. Östor AJ. *Int J Gynecol Pathol* 1993;12:186.
4. Jemal A, Murray T, Ward E, et al. Cancer statistics, 2005. *CA Cancer J Clin* 2005;55:10–30.
5. U.S. Preventive Services Task Force. *Screening for cervical cancer: recommendations and rationale.* http://www.ahrq.gov/clinic/uspstf/uspscerv.htm, accessed on January 2003.
6. Saslow D, Runowicz CD, Solomon D, et al. American Cancer Society guidelines for the early detection of cervical neoplasia and cancer. *CA Cancer J Clin* 2002;52:342–362.
7. Kinney WK, Manos MM, Hurley LB, et al. Where's the high-grade cervical neoplasia? the importance of minimally abnormal Papanicolaou diagnoses. *Obstet Gynecol* 1998;91:973–976.
8. Solomon D, Schiffman M, Tarone R. Comparison of three management strategies for patients with atypical squamous cells of undetermined significance: baseline results from a randomized trial. *J Natl Cancer Inst* 2001;93:293–299.

POSTMENOPAUSAL BLEEDING
Victoria S. Kaprielian

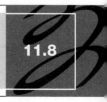

11.8

I. **BACKGROUND.** Postmenopausal bleeding is defined as vaginal bleeding that occurs in a woman who has had no menses for a year or more.

II. **PATHOPHYSIOLOGY**

   A. **Etiology.** Any vaginal bleeding in a postmenopausal woman not on hormone replacement therapy (HRT) requires a diagnosis, because malignant causes are found in 10% to 20% of cases. Women on cyclic HRT are expected to have uterine bleeding; bleeding at unexpected times or in excessive amounts requires investigation.

   B. **Epidemiology.** Abnormal vaginal bleeding is a common outpatient problem, occurring in 10% of women older than 55 years of age (1) and accounting for 70% of gynecologic visits during the perimenopausal and postmenopausal years (2).

III. **EVALUATION**

   A. **History**

      1. **Pattern of bleeding.** Although the amount of bleeding is not helpful in identifying malignancy, it should be assessed to determine the likelihood of significant anemia or hypovolemia that may require intervention. Timing of the bleeding may suggest its cause. Specific relationship to medication courses or cycles suggests drug-induced bleeding. Postcoital bleeding suggests an atrophic cause or cervical polyp. Association with bowel movements or urination suggests a nongenital source.

      2. **Current medications.** Any hormonal therapy, including estrogen, progesterone, tamoxifen, thyroid replacement, or corticosteroids, should be quantified and recorded.

         a. Acyclic bleeding is common in the first 3 to 4 months on continuous estrogen–progestin therapy and usually does not indicate pathology. Bleeding that is excessive, persists after months of therapy, or occurs after amenorrhea has been established on these regimens should be evaluated.

         b. The rate of endometrial cancer in women taking tamoxifen or unopposed estrogen is six to seven times the rate for untreated women. The frequency of endometrial polyps is also increased.

         c. Exogenous corticosteroids and incorrect dosage of thyroid replacement can lead to menstrual irregularities and postmenopausal bleeding.

      3. **Past medical history.** Nulliparity, early menarche, late menopause, and history of chronic anovulation are risk factors for endometrial hyperplasia and carcinoma. Obesity, hypertension, diabetes, and liver disease are commonly associated with estrogen excess and can also increase risk. Past use of oral contraceptives is associated with decreased risk.

      4. **Family history.** A strong family history of endometrial, breast, or colon cancer is a risk factor for endometrial cancer.

   B. **Physical examination**

      1. **Vital signs.** Blood pressure and pulse can indicate the degree and acuity of blood loss; orthostatic changes can be evidence of significant volume depletion. Fever suggests infection as a potential cause (Chapter 2.6).

      2. **Abdomen.** Tenderness or guarding suggests an infectious or inflammatory cause. Palpation for suprapubic masses is necessary as part of the evaluation for malignant causes.

      3. **Pelvis.** It is necessary to examine the external genitalia, vagina, and cervix for lesions or lacerations that could be the source of bleeding. The uterus and ovaries must be palpated to assess for enlargement, masses, and tenderness.

4. **Rectum.** Rectal examination and anoscopy may be warranted to rule out hemorrhoids or other intestinal sources of bleeding (Chapter 9.11).

C. **Testing**

1. **Office laboratory testing.** Urinalysis, stool guaiac testing, or both can be useful to look for nongenital sources of blood. A complete blood count may be helpful in assessing the degree of blood loss and likelihood of infection. Testing for gonorrhea and chlamydia may be warranted when tenderness or fever is present.

2. **Papanicolaou (Pap) smear.** Many sources recommend a Pap smear as part of the evaluation, although its diagnostic yield in these cases is low. Cervical lesions or friability raise the possibility of a cervical bleeding source. Endometrial cells found on the Pap smear of a postmenopausal woman not receiving HRT warrants further evaluation of the endometrium.

3. **Biopsy**
   a. Visible lesions of the vulva, vagina, or cervix should be sent for biopsy.
   b. In the absence of a clear nonuterine source of bleeding, endometrial biopsy is usually recommended. Office-based endometrial biopsy is less invasive and more cost-effective than dilation and curettage (D & C), with comparable sensitivity and specificity (3). There is excellent correlation between the histopathology of specimens taken by office biopsy and D & C (4). Blind sampling of either type is most effective when pathology is global, rather than focal.
   c. If bleeding continues after normal biopsy, further assessment is necessary. This may be done by repeat biopsy, D & C, and/or imaging.

4. **Diagnostic imaging.** Several methods are available; agreement is lacking with regard to the specifics of when each method should be used (1, 5).
   a. Transvaginal ultrasound (TVUS) is gaining popularity as an alternative or adjunct to endometrial biopsy. A clearly identifiable endometrial stripe <4 or 5 mm in thickness is highly unlikely to contain hyperplasia or carcinoma, and biopsy may not be necessary (3). TVUS is better tolerated than endometrial biopsy, with similar detection rates for endometrial abnormalities (1, 4). Fluid in the endometrial cavity has been associated with carcinoma, and its presence warrants further investigation. TVUS should not be used in place of biopsy in women taking tamoxifen, because the drug is known to cause misleading ultrasound findings.
   b. Saline infusion sonohysterography (SIS; ultrasound evaluation after the instillation of fluid into the endometrial cavity) allows the architectural evaluation of the uterine cavity to detect small lesions that may be missed by endometrial biopsy or TVUS. The disadvantage of this method is that no tissue is obtained, so if a lesion is found, hysteroscopy is then necessary for directed biopsy.
   c. Hysteroscopy is becoming the "gold standard" against which other methods of endometrial assessment are compared. This provides direct visualization of the endometrial cavity, allowing targeted biopsy or excision of lesions. However, it is more costly and requires more special expertise than most other modalities. Because lesions are occasionally missed even with this method, some recommend performing D & C along with hysteroscopy (4).
   d. Magnetic resonance imaging is occasionally helpful in determining the presence of fibroids when sonography is not definitive.
   e. Palpable adnexal abnormalities should be evaluated by ultrasound or other imaging as appropriate.

D. **Genetics.** Genetic testing is not helpful in the evaluation of postmenopausal bleeding. Women with a family history of gynecologic malignancy are at high risk and should be evaluated thoroughly. Consideration of the possibility of inherited coagulation deficiency may be warranted in cases of unusually heavy bleeding.

IV. **DIAGNOSIS**

A. **Differential diagnosis.** Causes of postmenopausal bleeding have been reported as atrophy (59%), polyp (12%), endometrial cancer (10%), endometrial hyperplasia (9.8%), hormonal effect (7%), cervical cancer (<1%), and other (2%) (3).

B. Clinical manifestations. Initial clinical evaluation may identify a nonuterine source. Postcoital spotting in conjunction with vaginal atrophy or cervical friability suggests cervical or vaginal mucosal bleeding. If no other source is identified, the key to diagnosis is imaging and tissue sampling of the endometrium. A thin endometrial stripe in a woman in a low-risk category suggests endometrial atrophy. If neither biopsy nor TVUS provides sufficient information, SIS, and/or hysteroscopy with directed biopsy may be used. D & C should be reserved for cases in which other methods are unsuccessful or unavailable.

References

1. Goldstein RB, Bree RL, Benson CB, et al. Evaluation of the woman with postmenopausal bleeding: society of radiologists in ultrasound-sponsored consensus conference statement. *J Ultrasound Med* 2001;20:1025–1036.
2. Clark TJ, Mann CH, Shah N, et al. Accuracy of outpatient endometrial biopsy in the diagnosis of endometrial cancer: a systematic quantitative review. *BJOG* 2002;109:313–321.
3. Goodman A. *Evaluation and management of uterine bleeding in postmenopausal women.* UpToDate online (www.uptodate.com), accessed July 2005, last update October 2004.
4. Feldman S. *Diagnostic evaluation of the endometrium in women with abnormal uterine bleeding.* UpToDate online (www.uptodate.com), accessed July 2005, last update January 2005.
5. Clark TJ, Voit D, Gupta JK, et al. Accuracy of hysteroscopy in the diagnosis of endometrial cancer and hyperplasia: a systematic quantitative review. *JAMA* 2002;288(13): 1610–1621.

VAGINAL DISCHARGE
Sandra M. Carr-Johnson

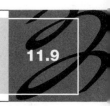

11.9

I. **BACKGROUND.** Vaginal discharge can be physiologic or pathologic. When pathologic, multiple sources (1–3) report that 90% of affected women have bacterial vaginosis (BV), vulvovaginal candidiasis (VVC), or trichomoniasis.

II. **PATHOPHYSIOLOGY.** BV is typically caused by numerous anaerobic organisms found in normal vaginal flora such as *Gardnerella vaginalis*, *Mobiluncus* species, *Prevotella*, and *Mycoplasma hominis* (4) and can occur in up to 33% of women. In nonresistant cases, VVC is caused by *Candida albicans* and accounts for 40% of infections. *Trichomonas vaginalis*, a protozoan parasite, is found in women and men at genitourinary sites. It is responsible for trichomoniasis, which causes 10% to 25% of vaginal infections (4). Although most patients have BV, VVC, or *T. vaginalis*, the other 10% may have pelvic inflammatory disease, sexually transmitted disease, noninfectious causes such as atrophy and allergies, chemical irritation (2), neoplasia, and foreign materials such as retained tampons (5) and intrauterine devices.

III. **EVALUATION**
   A. **History.** In preparation for the clinical encounter, the clinician should consider the following:
      1. **Key points**
         a. Age of the patient
         b. Medical, sexual, and surgical history
         c. Concern for pregnancy
         d. Marital status

      e. Recent treatments

      f. Current health and smoking status

  2. Considerations

      a. The younger patient is more likely to have physiologic discharge that she is not familiar with yet because she is learning about her body and her menstrual cycle.

      b. The adolescent and young adult may be at increased risk of sexually transmitted infections (STIs).

      c. The more mature patient may have vaginal atrophy. Neoplasia may be a concern if a symptom, particularly pruritus, is recurrent.

      d. Patients who have had recent gynecologic surgery or instrumentation are at increased risk of infection that can be evidenced by vaginal discharge.

      e. Marital status and sexual history are helpful in the assessment of STI risk.

      f. Recent treatment provides a direction regarding the treatment of recurrent or resistant infection.

      g. Smoking increases the risk of trichomoniasis (1) and BV (5).

      h. The patient's health status is significant because frequent discharge may suggest chronic illness such as diabetes or human immunodeficiency virus (HIV) or be due to frequent antibiotics and long-term steroids and other conditions.

  3. Discharge characteristics. It is important to know the characteristics of physiologic and pathologic discharge.

      a. Physiologic discharge is often clear and thin and changes with the menstrual cycle.

      b. Pathologic discharge is often diffuse, has color, and may have an odor.

         i. The discharge of BV a homogenous white, noninflammatory discharge that smoothly coats the vaginal walls. The discharge can be fishy or musty before or after the addition of KOH (a positive "whiff" test); see section **III.C** (3).

         ii. The discharge of VVC is often thick, white, and odor free, and it can be associated with vaginal pruritus and erythema.

         iii. The discharge of trichomoniasis may be diffuse, malodorous, and yellow-green, with vulvar irritation (3).

  4. Menses

      a. The last menstrual period assesses menstrual hormonal fluctuations, pregnancy, and menopausal states.

      b. The cause of vaginal discharge in pregnancy is important to know, because BV, VVC, and trichomoniasis can be associated with adverse pregnancy outcomes (1, 3).

  5. Associated symptoms. These can include itching, soreness, dysuria, or post-coital bleeding, lower abdominal pain, pelvic pain, and dyspareunia.

  6. Risk factors for STIs. These can include age <25 years, multiple and frequent partners, previous STIs, unprotected intercourse, and partners with high-risk sexual behavior (5).

B. Physical examination. While examining the female patient, care must be given to her comfort, privacy, and the sensitive nature of the lithotomy position. The entire physical examination should be considered if the patient appears acutely ill, has signs of systemic illness, including abdominal pain, rash, fever, or other complaints. Attention should be given to associated symptoms elicited during the history as well as the highlighted complaint of vaginal discharge and its characteristics. A systematic genitourinary examination with detailed documentation is the standard of care.

C. Testing. Refer to Table 11.9.1.

IV. DIAGNOSIS. Commonly, symptoms resolve after treatment for most patients who present with the complaint of vaginal discharge. However, recurrent vaginitis, particularly with BV and VVC, is not uncommon. Recurrent BV can be due to treatment failure, persistent or reintroduction of foreign bodies, or reintroduction of infection. Recurrent VVC can be caused by non–*C. albicans* infection, which is increasing with

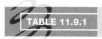

TABLE 11.9.1 **Differential Diagnosis and Clinical Manifestations in Vaginal Discharge**

	Bacterial vaginosis	Vulvovaginal candidiasis	Trichomoniasis
Discharge characteristics	Homogenous, white, noninflammatory	Thick, white, cottage cheese–like	Yellow-green copious, watery, pooling, frothy (4)
Odor	Fishy before and after KOH + "whiff" test	Not typical	Malodorous (10%)
Physical examination	Discharge coats vaginal wall	Excoriation edema, erythema	Strawberry cervix (2% of patients) (4)
Precipitating factors	Changes to vaginal flora, pregnancy, condoms, douching, new or frequent partners (1)	Antibiotics, systemic illness, medication, immunocompromise	Sexually transmitted infection
pH	>4.5	Normally <4.5	>4.5 in 90%
Microscopy/Gram stain	Amsel's diagnostic criteria[a]	Budding yeast or hyphae after 10% KOH	60%–70% sensitive
			Culture most sensitive (3)
	Presence of clue cells highly suggestive (1)		
			Moving flagellae (2)
Associated symptoms	May be asymptomatic	Pruritus, vaginal irritation, dysuria (1)	Vulvar irritation and dysuria, lower abdominal pain; may be asymptomatic (4)

[a]Thin homogeneous discharge, positive "whiff test," clue cells, vaginal pH >4.5 — three out of four is highly suggestive of BV (1).

the frequent use of over-the-counter antifungal medications. Recurrent trichomoniasis is likely the result of treatment failure or reintroduction of infection. Also, it is helpful to consider that noninfectious etiologies as well as less common infectious etiologies may be present.

References

1. Egan ME, Lipsky MS, Diagnosis of vaginitis. *Am Fam Physician* 2000;62(5):1095–1104.
2. Miller KE, Ruiz DE, Graves JC. Update on the prevention and treatment of sexually transmitted diseases. *Am Fam Physician* 2003;67(9):1915–1922.
3. http://www.cdc.gov/mmwr/preview/mmwrhtml/rr5106a1.htm, May 2006.
4. www.infopoems.com, May 2006.
5. Mitchell H. Vaginal discharge-causes, diagnosis and treatment. *BMJ* 2004;328: 1306–1308.

Musculoskeletal Problems

Laeth Nasir

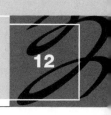

ARTHRALGIA
Iman S. Al-Jabi

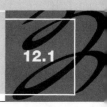

12.1

I. **BACKGROUND.** Arthralgia means joint pain. Joint pain may arise from the joints or periarticular structures such as bones, muscles, ligaments, or nerves.

II. **PATHOPHYSIOLOGY.** The most common cause of arthralgia is mechanical joint dysfunction—often related to trauma—rather than inflammatory or referred pain. Twenty percent of all primary care consultations worldwide are for aches and pains that seem related to muscles and joints. These are most common in the adult population. In the elderly, the most common problem is osteoarthritis; in middle age, inflammatory conditions predominate; and in the young, systemic conditions are more likely (1).

III. **EVALUATION.** Although the causes of arthralgia are numerous, a detailed medical history, thorough physical examination, and judicious use of laboratory testing and radiologic imaging usually allow a diagnosis to be made (2). The history helps determine whether the problem is mechanical or inflammatory, the examination helps define whether the pain is articular, periarticular, or referred.

A. **History.** Factors to consider include the following:
   1. Patient age: diagnostic probabilities differ with each age-group. Infectious causes tend to be less age dependent (3)
   2. History of trauma
   3. Location of the pain and joint swelling
   4. Past medical history
   5. Family history (systemic lupus erythematosus [SLE], rheumatoid arthritis [RA], ankylosing spondylosis, osteoarthritis)
   6. Number of joints involved (if three or more, consider RA)
   7. Limitation of the movement of the joint
   8. Stiffness, weakness, diurnal variation, or effect of exercise
   9. Chronology of symptoms: duration, acuity of onset, pain continuous (inflammatory) or intermittent (mechanical)
   10. Systemic symptoms such as fever, fatigue, rash, or weight loss
   11. Immunization or recent travel
   12. Medication
   13. Review of systems
      a. Skin: malar rash (SLE), Gottron's papules (dermatomyositis), psoriatic rash or nails, mouth ulcers (Behçet's disease)
      b. Cardiovascular: infectious endocarditis, rheumatic fever
      c. Gastrointestinal: inflammatory bowel disease, Henoch-Schönlein purpura
      d. Genitourinary: dysuria, discharge
      e. Hematologic: hemoglobinopathies
      f. Neurologic/psychiatric

B. **Physical examination**
   1. General appearance: conjunctivitis, skin lesions
   2. Vital signs: weight loss, fever
   3. Other signs, such as lymphadenopathy or heart murmur
   4. Joint examination: swelling, warmth, tenderness, deformity, range of movement, muscle wasting

C. **Testing.** Laboratory testing is helpful in diagnosing inflammatory processes. However, it is most often useful in confirming or refuting a diagnosis made on clinical grounds.

| TABLE 12.1.1 | Differential Diagnosis of Arthralgia (4) | | |

Childhood	Adolescence	Middle age	Elderly
Nonaccidental injury	Sports-related pain	Osteoarthritis	Osteoarthritis
Growing pains	Rheumatoid arthritis	Rheumatoid arthritis or other connective tissue disease (e.g., systemic lupus erythematosus, systemic sclerosis, spondyloarthropathies)	Polymyalgia rheumatica
Acute rheumatic fever	Viral (e.g., rubella)	Reactive arthritis (e.g., enteropathic arthritis)	Paraneoplastic syndrome
Juvenile rheumatoid arthritis	Sarcoidosis	Hypothyroidism	Paget's disease
Henoch-Schönlein purpura		Gout	Metabolic bone disease
Viral arthritis		Syphilis, gonococcal infection, human immunodeficiency viral infection	
Leukemia		Brucellosis	
Medication side effects		Depression	

1. **Laboratory tests (5, 6)**
    a. Complete blood count, erythrocyte sedimentation rate, and C-reactive protein are frequently abnormal in inflammatory conditions.
    b. Antinuclear antibody is positive in 90% of SLE cases.
    c. Rheumatoid factor is positive in most cases of rheumatoid arthritis as well as in many autoimmune diseases and chronic infections.
    d. HLA-B27 has a high prevalence in spondyloarthritides (ankylosing spondylosis, Reiter's disease, enteropathic arthritis).
    e. Urinalysis may show proteinuria or hematuria if there is renal involvement in connective tissue disease.
    f. Lyme serology
    g. Liver function testing
2. **Imaging (7)**
    a. Plain radiograph may help in monoarticular joint pain.
    b. Computed tomography and magnetic resonance imaging may be useful for joint derangements.
    c. Synovial fluid aspiration helps distinguish inflammatory from infective and crystal arthropathies. A bloody joint aspirate without elevated white blood count most likely indicates trauma.

IV. DIAGNOSIS. The differential diagnosis is presented in Table 12.1.1.

References
1. Morris D. Osteoarthritis. *Prim care Update.* 2005;3(1):20–26.
2. Ham RJ, Sloane PD, Warshaw GA, eds. *Primary care geriatrics, a case-based approach*, 4th ed. Missouri, MO: Harcourt Health Sciences, 2002.
3. Wilking AP. *An approach to the child with joint pain.* 22 March 2005. http://www.utdol.com/application/topic/topicOutline.asp?file=pedirheu/12386&type=P&

4. Dieppe PA, Klippel JH, eds. *Practical rheumatology*. London: Times Mirror International, 1995.
5. Britten N, Culpepper L, Gass D, et al., eds. *Volume 2: clinical management from Oxford textbook of primary medical care*, 3rd ed. New York, NY: Oxford University Press, 2005.
6. Khot A, Polmear A, eds. *Practical general practice, guidelines for effective clinical management*, 4th ed. Edinburgh: Elsevier Science, 2003.
7. Coumas JM, Howard BA, Jacobson EW. Diagnostic imaging of rheumatologic disorders. In: Noble J, ed. *Textbook of primary care medicine*, 3rd ed. Missouri, MO: Harcourt Health Sciences, 2001.

CALF PAIN

Stephen J. Hartsock and Rebecca L. Spaulding

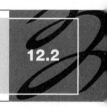

12.2

I. **BACKGROUND.** Calf pain is caused by an array of causes that range from benign to life threatening. The physician must be able to determine quickly which patients require a detailed workup. Deep venous thrombosis (DVT), compartment syndrome, and cellulitis are the most serious conditions requiring prompt recognition and management.

II. **PATHOPHYSIOLOGY.** A number of conditions can result in calf pain (see Table 12.2.1). Musculoskeletal causes account for 40% of calf pain (1). Pain can be referred from the back, hips, or other areas in the lower limb. DVT is one of the most serious causes of calf pain. Risk factors for DVT include elements of Virchow's triad (venous wall damage, stasis, hypercoagulability); therefore immobilization, pregnancy, and recent surgery are classic antecedents. Compartment syndrome usually results from swelling, typically from trauma, and can affect any of the four fascial compartments of the ankle, resulting in increased intracompartmental pressure, ischemia, and irreversible loss of neuromuscular function if not promptly recognized and treated. Rhabdomyolysis can be triggered by trauma, ischemia, drugs, or infection. Peripheral neuropathy can be caused by nerve entrapment or medical causes such as diabetes, vitamin B_{12} and folate deficiencies, thyroid disease, alcoholism, human immunodeficiency virus, or syphilis.

III. **EVALUATION**

A. **History.** The history is critical in narrowing the differential diagnosis. Pertinent information includes the exact location of the pain, as well as quality, severity, duration, and aggravating or alleviating factors. Other symptoms include swelling, color changes, warmth, numbness, weakness, and fever or chills. Related trauma or exercise must be noted, as well as a recent history of immobilization. Current medications, including hormones, statins, or drugs that affect electrolytes such as diuretics, bisphosphonates, and alcohol should be recorded.

B. **Physical examination.** The examination begins by assessing vital signs, specifically blood pressure, temperature, and heart rate. The lower extremities should be examined for swelling, color changes, wounds, hair and nail patterns, and symmetry. The calf circumferences may be measured. Palpation evaluates warmth, tenderness, edema, and bone or muscle defects. Range of motion of the knees, ankles, and toes is noted. Suspicion that the pain is referred should result in evaluation of the back and hips. Vascular examination includes evaluation for venous insufficiency, tender varicosities, or venous cords, arterial pulses, and capillary refill. Neurologic examination includes lower extremity evaluation of motor and sensory function, as well as reflexes. Ability to bear weight and gait is observed. Special tests for DVT exist, including Homan's sign (pain on passive dorsiflexion of the foot). However, the positive predictive value of physical examination findings is only 55%. Therefore, suspicion of the presence of DVT should lead to radiologic evaluation to confirm

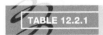

TABLE 12.2.1	Differential Diagnosis of Calf Pain

Vascular
    Venous
        Deep venous thrombosis
        Superficial thrombophlebitis
        Varicose vein
    Arterial
        Claudication
        Ischemia/embolus
Neurologic
    Referred pain
        Hip
        Back
    Peripheral neuropathy or nerve entrapment
    Restless leg syndrome
Musculoskeletal
    Calf muscle strain
    Calf tendon rupture
    Baker's cyst
    Delayed onset muscle soreness
    Compartment syndrome
    Muscle cramps/myalgia
        Electrolyte imbalance
        Rhabdomyolysis
    Trauma
        Fracture
        Bruise/hematoma
Infectious

the presence or absence of thrombosis. Thompson's test (squeezing of the proximal gastrocnemius and soleus tendons, observing for ankle plantar flexion) evaluates possible rupture of the Achilles tendon.

C. Testing. Duplex ultrasound is used to diagnose superficial thrombosis and DVT (sensitivity 89% and specificity 94%) (2). Contrast venography is the gold standard (sensitivity 95% and specificity 97%) but is more invasive (2). The ankle-brachial index (sensitivity 95%, specificity 99%) (3) with duplex ultrasound is used to diagnose peripheral arterial disease (PAD). Angiography is considered the gold standard. Plain radiographs are unnecessary unless there is suspicion of fracture, foreign body, or malignancy. Magnetic resonance imaging can be used for the diagnosis of muscle and soft tissue injuries. Ultrasound can evaluate muscle tears and tendinopathy. Compartment pressure testing is performed to confirm the diagnosis of compartment syndrome. Elevated levels of creatine phosphokinase and transaminases may be seen in patients with muscle injury.

IV. DIAGNOSIS. Pertinent examination findings for DVT include swelling, warmth, tenderness, and discoloration. PAD typically presents with intermittent claudication that resolves rapidly upon rest. Restless leg syndrome presents with an uncomfortable sensation, associated with an uncontrollable urge to move the legs, usually at night. Sudden calf pain in an active patient often represents a muscle strain or tendon rupture. The gastrocnemius is the most commonly injured muscle. Rupture of the Achilles tendon leads to inability to actively plantar flex the ankle and a positive Thompson's test. A ruptured Baker's cyst may cause swelling and discoloration that advances distally into the calf. Exertional, or chronic, compartment syndrome usually occurs with exercise. The patient has pain or numbness that resolves after cessation of exercise. The anterior compartment is involved 70% of the time (4). In acute compartment syndrome, increased pain on passive stretching of the long muscles passing through a compartment is an important sign. Severe pain, pallor, and paralysis are signs of advanced ischemic compartment syndrome. Delayed onset muscle soreness (DOMS) starts approximately 12 hours after exercise and lasts 2 to 3 days. Muscle cramps and soreness may also result from dehydration or rhabdomyolysis. Cellulitis causing redness, pain, warmth, and swelling is usually due to an obvious local area of skin disruption on calf or foot, but occasionally the infection originates in an area such as the interdigital web space and may be missed unless specifically sought for.

References

1. Kahn SR. The clinical diagnosis of deep vein thrombosis: integrating incidence, risk factors, and symptoms and signs. *Arch Intern Med* 1998;158(21):2315–2323.
2. Line BR. Pathophysiology and diagnosis of deep vein thrombosis. *Semin Nucl Med* 2001;31(2):90–101.
3. Comerota AJ. The case for early detection and integrated intervention in patients with peripheral artery disease and intermittent claudication. *J Endovasc Ther* 2003;10:601–613.
4. Korkola M. Avandola A. Exercise induced leg pain. *Phys Sportsmed* 2001;29(6):35–50.

HIP PAIN
Samuel B. Adkins, III

12.3

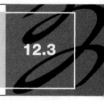

I. **BACKGROUND.** The hip joint is the most inaccessible joint in the any of the limbs. It is located deep within the large muscles of the hip, pelvis, and thigh. It also has more bony support than any other joint.

II. **PATHOPHYSIOLOGY.** The differential diagnosis for the patient with hip pathology (see Table 12.3.1) is significantly influenced by age. The vascular supply to the hip is subject to disruption that can lead to avascular necrosis of the femoral head. This is particularly important in children and adolescents, in whom the presence of active growth centers results in diagnoses specific to people in those age-groups. Both genetic and environmental factors can also lead to degenerative changes in the hip.

III. **EVALUATION**

   A. **History.** Patients may present with a complaint of pain, snapping (lateral snapping suggests iliotibial band tightness, medial snapping suggests iliopsoas tightness), or limp. The history should include specifics about the onset, location, duration, and severity of symptoms. Questioning the patient about associated gastrointestinal symptoms (change in stool frequency, rectal bleeding, abdominal pain), genitourinary symptoms (dysuria, hematuria, menstrual irregularities), or systemic symptoms (night sweats, weight loss, fever) may alert the physician to alternative diagnoses. Steroid use, sickle cell disease, and human immunodeficiency virus infection are all risk factors for avascular necrosis of the femoral head. The menstrual history and possibly the dietary history in young women may indicate an increased likelihood of osteopenia or stress fracture. A careful account of the patient's current and past occupational, domestic, and recreational activities is helpful both diagnostically and in planning for treatment, rehabilitation, and return to normal activities.

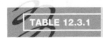

TABLE 12.3.1 Differential Diagnosis of Hip Pain

Diagnosis	Patient age	Suggestive findings
Septic arthritis	Infants and toddlers	Pseudoparalysis, irritability, limp
Transient synovitis	Child, preadolescent	Pain, limp, limited ROM
Legg-Calvé-Perthes disease	Preadolescent	Limp and limited ROM
Slipped capital femoral epiphysis	Adolescent	Obesity, males, pain, limited internal rotation
Avulsion fracture	Young adult	Sudden onset, "pop" heard or felt with injury, pain at insertion site
Femoral neck stress fracture	Young adult	Insidious onset, associated with increased activity or disordered eating, menstrual irregularities, painful ROM
Osteoid osteoma	Young adult	Vague pain, nocturnal pain, decreased ROM
Iliotibial band syndrome	Young adult	Lateral thigh/leg pain/snapping, positive Ober's test
Trochanteric bursitis	Adult	Lateral thigh pain localized over greater trochanter
Avascular necrosis of the femoral head	Adult	Dull pain with weight bearing, decreased ROM
Iliopsoas bursitis	Adult	Medial thigh pain/snapping, pain with standing
Meralgia paresthetica	Adult	Anterior/lateral thigh numbness, obesity, compressive clothing, no weakness
Degenerative joint disease	Adult	Progressive pain, decreased internal rotation early in the disease, pain with weight bearing

ROM, range of motion.

B. **Physical examination.** Although the hip joint is obscured by bone and soft tissues, physical examination of the hip is not difficult. The examination should be carried out in a methodical fashion, and the patient should be appropriately undressed to obtain maximal information.

1. With the patient sitting on the examination table (hips flexed at 90°), test the internal and external rotation of the hip. Also check for hip flexor strength.

2. With the patient lying supine, test abduction. In this position, palpation of the groin may localize the anterior hip pain. Extension is tested with the patient lying on the contralateral side. Ober's test for iliotibial band flexibility and palpation of the greater trochanter area is also performed with the patient in this position (1).

3. Have the patient stand from a sitting position, if able. Observe for signs of discomfort or dysfunction. Inspect the patient's stance. Is the patient able to bear weight without pain? How stable is the stance? Are the lower extremities symmetrical (muscles and alignment)? Next watch the patient walk (slowly first then briskly if able). Is the gait symmetrical? Is the gait phase shortened? This may indicate joint pathology. Is there a lurching (the patient limiting time spent

on the affected hip and the limited range of motion suggest hip joint pathology) or a Trendelenburg (weak abductors causing the pelvis to tilt) gait? Does the patient circumduct the hip (seen with restricted motion)?

4. Examination of the knee (especially in children), lumbar spine, and sacroiliac joints should also be considered.

C. Testing

1. Plain x-rays (anteroposterior pelvis, anteroposterior and frog-leg or lateral views) are indicated for patients with groin or anterior thigh pain, who are more likely to have hip joint pathology, as well as for cases in which there is suspicion of significant pathology, inability to bear weight, unclear diagnosis, or lack of response to therapy.

2. Magnetic resonance imaging (MRI) or computed tomography is helpful if the diagnosis is unclear or a fracture is still suspected after plain radiographs, if a loose body or labral injury is suspected, and in the evaluation of cystic or lytic lesions.

3. Ultrasound can be helpful in detecting small joint effusions when the suspicion of transient synovitis or septic arthritis is high. Bone scanning can also be useful in diagnosing early Legg-Calvé-Perthes disease or aseptic necrosis, although gadolinium-contrast MRI may be preferable if practical and available.

4. Complete blood count, erythrocyte sedimentation rate, and C-reactive protein levels can be helpful in evaluating patients with suspected inflammatory disorders.

5. Occasionally, joint aspiration is needed to make a diagnosis. Fluid should be sent for cell count, gram stain, culture, crystals, and other studies as appropriate.

IV. DIAGNOSIS. Table 12.3.1 lists the differential diagnosis for common hip conditions.

Reference

1. Hoppenfeld Stanley. *Physical examination of the spine and extremities.* New York, NY: Appleton-Century-Crofts, 1976:133–169.

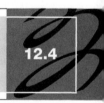

KNEE PAIN
Chris Madden

12.4

I. BACKGROUND. Knee pain is one of the most frequent musculoskeletal complaints in primary care. A careful history, focused physical examination, and occasional diagnostic studies allow for accurate diagnosis of most knee problems.

II. PATHOPHYSIOLOGY

A. Etiology.
Causes of knee pain may include overuse and traumatic injuries, degenerative and inflammatory arthritis, infection, osteonecrosis and osteochondritis, referred pain from the hip and back, and other miscellaneous disorders (1,2).

B. Epidemiology

1. Knee pain in childhood, especially early, is usually caused by minor trauma. Major trauma may result in growth plate or other fractures, whereas inflammatory arthritis (e.g., juvenile rheumatoid arthritis) and infection are less frequent causes. Active children, especially as they mature into preadolescence and become more involved in demanding sports, may experience overuse injuries. Apophysitises such as tibial apophysitis (Osgood-Schlatter disease) are stress injuries to growth plates that are often mistaken for inflammatory injuries and treated with anti-inflammatory medications instead of appropriate rest.

2. Overuse and traumatic injuries to ligaments, tendons, and cartilage may occur in people of any age and are common in active adolescents and adults. It is

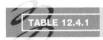

TABLE 12.4.1	Differential Diagnosis of Knee Pain
Overuse	Patellofemoral pain, patellar tendopathy, quadriceps tendinopathy, iliotibial band syndrome, apophysitis (Osgood-Schlatter most common), pes anserine bursitis, synovial plica, bipartite patella
Traumatic	Anterior cruciate ligament rupture, collateral ligament sprain (medial and lateral collateral), fracture (bony and/or chondral), meniscal tear, patellar subluxation or dislocation, prepatellar bursitis, posterior cruciate ligament rupture, quadriceps tendon rupture, patellar tendon rupture
Arthritic	Osteoarthritis, inflammatory (rheumatoid, gout, pseudogout, other)
Infectious	Septic joint
Referred	Back or hip
Miscellaneous	Osteonecrosis, osteochondritis desiccans, Baker (popliteal) cyst, tumor, deep venous thrombosis (presenting as popliteal pain), benign or malignant tumor, pigmented villonodular synovitis
	Other systemic cause (complex regional pain syndrome, fibromyalgia)

a common misconception that maturing youngsters almost always sustain an avulsion fracture of bone or a growth plate rather than rupture a ligament because the ligament is "stronger." Young athletes can rupture ligaments in part because the maturing growth plate is vulnerable to injury, though rupture is less common in them than in adults.

3. Adults and seniors frequently experience pain from knee osteoarthritis. Less frequently, the cause may be other degenerative intra-articular pathology such as meniscal tears or chondral lesions. Inflammatory arthritis, including gout and pseudogout, are more common in adults than in younger patients.

4. A variety of other miscellaneous conditions may cause knee pain in people of all ages (see Table 12.4.1), and these should be considered if pain pattern is atypical, diffuse, occurs at night, or persists despite treatment.

III. **EVALUATION.** Attention to patient age, injury specifics, and pain characteristics and pattern help guide a detailed and careful knee pain history (3).

A. **History**

1. If there is a history of injury, determining the mechanism of injury is the first task in obtaining a history. Identification of knee position and forces involved helps focus the history and physical examination. If a patient does not recall the mechanism, or there was no obvious injury, this is also valuable information that narrows the differential diagnosis.

2. Most knee conditions become apparent after taking a history that focuses on pain characteristics. The mnemonic ChLORIDE may help elicit a comprehensive history.

a. Ch: pain **character** that is described as burning or aching frequently represents patellofemoral pain or osteoarthritis. Traumatic ligamentous pain may be sharp initially and with stress but aching at rest. Dramatic or intense pain and night pain may represent a systemic process. Stiffness, especially after rest, occurs with patellofemoral pain and osteoarthritis.

b. L: pain **location** may be demonstrated by having the patient point to the "most painful area." Relatively localized pain immediately narrows the differential diagnosis to include regional structures. Generalized pain may present a challenge, but having the patient trace the "pain pattern" using his or her fingers may narrow considerations. Circular motions at the anterior knee often represents patellofemoral problems, whereas horizontal motions along the medial or lateral joint lines are common with meniscal tears and osteoarthritis. Sweeps over specific ligament or tendon areas may indicate pathology involving these structures.

c. O: pain **onset**. Determine if the pain began acutely or insidiously. Acute onset implies tissue tearing, bruising, or fracture. Insidious onset implies tissue inflammation or stress injury, often from overuse.

d. R: pain **radiation** can give clues to involved structures. Patellofemoral pain may radiate along medial or lateral patellar retinaculum or retropatellar area. Hamstring tendonitis may radiate into distal posterior thigh. Meniscal pathology can radiate pain almost anywhere in the knee, but frequently radiates posteriorly or to the joint line. Distal or proximal pain should raise the suspicion for nonknee pathology such as referred pain from the back or hip.

e. I: pain **intensity** may provide clues to diagnosis. Severe pain occurs with ligament or tendon rupture, fractures, and gout. Low to moderate intensity pain may be associated with an overuse injury.

f. D: pain **duration** is assessed alongside pain onset. Shorter duration pain correlates most frequently with recent traumatic or inflammatory injury, whereas medium and long duration pain is observed with overuse injuries such as tendinopathy. Prolonged pain, particularly if it is not responding to treatment, should prompt an aggressive search for less common serious causes of knee pain (Table 12.4.1).

g. E: pain **exacerbations** and remitting features are important. Anterior knee pain and/or stiffness after sitting with knees flexed is frequent with patellofemoral pain and is referred to as the "movie goers" sign. Squatting and knee flexion may exacerbate patellofemoral pain but can also cause medial or lateral joint line pain that may represent meniscal or other intra-articular pathology. Cutting, twisting, and pivoting worsens collateral ligament pain and may cause a sense of instability or "sliding" with cruciate ligament injury. Jumping and running worsens pain with patellofemoral, patellar tendon, pes anserine bursa, and other tendon or overuse injuries. Stairs and uneven surfaces or hills can worsen iliotibial band and patellofemoral pain, which frequently occur together. Pain with osteoarthritis may worsen after periods of rest and at the end of the day but can either improve or worsen with activity, depending on the severity. Night pain may indicate tumor or complex regional pain syndrome. If pain and stiffness are most severe upon rising in the morning, inflammatory arthritis should be considered.

3. Associated symptoms. An important feature of knee pain is the presence of mechanical symptoms, which include catching and locking. Mechanical symptoms often represent an unstable structural lesion such as displaced meniscal tears or intra-articular, chondral, or bony fractures and loose bodies that may mandate early orthopaedic referral. A sensation of "giving way" is most frequently a result of reflex inhibition due to patellofemoral pain. However, giving way may also represent underlying knee instability such as that occurring with an anterior, or less frequently, a posterior cruciate ligament tear. Note other pertinent distal or proximal extremity or back symptoms and other systemic or constitutional symptoms.

4. Past medical and family history. Inquire about prior injury, instability, and nontraumatic knee pain. Is the patient on any medications that may modify knee pain? Any prior knee operations? Explore a family history of knee pain, which may represent patellofemoral pain or osteoarthritis.

B. Physical examination

1. Observe the gait. Examine both the affected and nonaffected knees to establish a normal baseline. Focus on structures highlighted in the history. Inspect for asymmetry, extra-articular swelling, intra-articular swelling (effusion), and antalgic gait. Most acute effusions are hemarthroses and represent anterior cruciate ligament (ACL) tears. Palpate injured structures and note the tenderness, thickening, and defects to localize diagnostic considerations. Assess the passive and active ranges of motion and muscle strength. Significant loss of motion occurs

with intra-articular structural lesions, and refusal to move the knee may be due to severe pain associated with a septic joint.

2. Specific testing is helpful with a variety of injuries and dysfunctions. The patellofemoral compression and shrug tests involve compressing the patella into the trochlear groove of the femur. This maneuver elicits pain with patellofemoral problems. The Lachman test involves an anteriorly directed force applied to the proximal tibia while stabilizing the femur at $20°$ of knee flexion, and it reveals increased anterior translation of the tibia on the femur and a soft or absent end point with ACL tears. The McMurray test involves a circumduction maneuver of the flexed knee. A positive test elicits joint line pain and/or popping with meniscal and sometimes with articular cartilage pathology. The varus and valgus stress tests at $30°$ cause joint line opening with lateral and medial collateral ligament injuries, respectively. These tests performed at $0°$ may indicate damage to the posterior cruciate ligament. The posterior drawer test is performed by applying a posterior force to the proximal tibia with the knee flexed at $90°$ and the hip flexed at $45°$, and it reveals increased posterior tibial translation with posterior cruciate ligament injuries.

C. Testing

1. The application of clinical decision rules may help prevent the overuse of plain radiography to detect fractures. The Pittsburgh Knee Rule may be used in adults and children older than 6 years of age, whereas the Ottawa Rule is discouraged in pediatric populations (4). The Pittsburgh Rule recommends a radiograph for anyone with a fall or blunt trauma, anyone younger than 12 years of age or older than 50 years of age, and anyone unable to take four weight-bearing steps in the emergency department after injury (with acute evaluation). One study claims that the rule is 99% sensitive and 60% specific (5). Aside from the decision rules, plain radiography should always be considered with an acute knee effusion to assess for intra-articular fracture.

2. Magnetic resonance imaging (MRI) is the best imaging modality for assessing major ligament and tendon injuries and is most frequently used to confirm ACL rupture. It is usually indicated with an acute knee effusion and for mechanical symptoms not adequately explained by plain radiography. Chronic pain and chronic effusion are less frequent indications for MRI. Other potentially helpful diagnostics that may be applied on an individualized basis include computed tomography, arthrography, bone scan, ultrasound, and arthrocentesis.

IV. DIAGNOSIS.

Accurate diagnosis of knee pathology relies on the ability of the examiner to localize the injury using the history of the injury mechanism and pain characteristics that guide a focused knee examination to address the affected structures using specific testing. Anterior knee pain is usually patellofemoral, which is by far the most common knee complaint in the primary care physician's office. An acute traumatic effusion is an ACL injury until proved otherwise; joint line pain often represents meniscal pathology; and pain of insidious onset occurring along tendons implies tendinopathy. Prolonged or atypical pain warrants immediate and aggressive evaluation to rule out serious pathology.

References

1. Walsh W, Vanicek J. Knee injuries. In: Mellion M, Walsh W, Madden C, et al., eds. *The team physician's handbook*, 3rd ed. Philadelphia, PA: Elsevier Science, 2002:490–509.
2. Calmbach W, Hutchens M. Evaluation of patients presenting with knee pain: Part I. history, physical examination, radiographs, and laboratory tests. *Am Fam Physician* 2003;68:907–912.
3. Calmbach M, Hutchens M. Evaluation of patients presenting with knee pain: Part II. differential diagnosis. *Am Fam Physician* 2003;68:917–922.
4. Ebell M. A tool for evaluating patients with knee injury. *Am Fam Physician* 2005;12: 1169–1172.
5. Seaberg D, Yealy D, Lukens T, et al. Multicenter comparison of two clinical decision rules for the use of radiography in acute, high-risk injuries. *Ann Emerg Med* 1998;32:8–13.

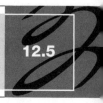

LOW BACK PAIN
Ronald McCoy

12.5

I. BACKGROUND. Low back pain is common in developed countries, affecting approximately 70% of the adult population (1) at some stage during their life.

II. PATHOPHYSIOLOGY. The cause of pain is nonspecific in approximately 95% of people presenting with acute low back pain; serious conditions are rare. The condition is generally self-limited (2) but diagnosis must exclude rarer but potentially serious, life-threatening causes (see Table 12.5.1).

III. EVALUATION

    A. History. The clinician needs to be alert to the presence of indications of potentially serious low back conditions, often called "red flags" (see Table 12.5.2).

        1. Pain characteristics. Assess the nature of the pain, along with the position, onset, and duration of the symptom. Is there any radiating pain, leg weakness, or paresthesia? Does the pain limit the patient physically or socially? Is there a history of previous back problems or back surgery?

        2. Review of systems. Look for any red flag indicators of serious disease (Table 12.5.2). Gastrointestinal and genitourinary symptoms are particularly important, especially incontinence.

TABLE 12.5.1   **Causes of Low Back Pain**

Common causes
Muscle and soft tissue strain
Degenerative disease, including osteoarthritis and spondylosis
Vertebral dysfunction, including facet joint and lumbar disc involvement
Lumbar or sacral nerve root compression: disc herniation, cauda equina syndrome, sciatica, spinal stenosis
Vertebral fracture or subluxation
Inflammatory conditions
Rheumatologic conditions (e.g., rheumatoid arthritis, ankylosing spondylitis)
Sacroiliac joint sprain or degenerative disease
Other less common causes that may also be life threatening
Infection: osteomyelitis, discitis, epidural abscess
Hematologic
Multiple myeloma, myelodysplasia
Cancer (primary or metastatic)
Benign tumors
Aortic aneurysm
Retroperitoneal pathology
Pyelonephritis, renal calculus, cancer
Abdominal pathology
Perforated viscus, pancreatitis

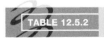

TABLE 12.5.2	"Red Flags" That Indicate Potentially Serious Lower Back Conditions

Age >50 y

History of malignancy

Temperature >37.8°C

Constant pain

Weight loss

History of trauma (may be minor in patients with osteoporosis)

Features of spondyloarthropathy

Neurologic signs

Alcohol or drug disorder

Recent invasive urologic procedures

Sudden onset of sharp back pain with uneven pulses (abdominal aneurysm)

History of anticoagulant use

History of corticosteroid use

Pain not improved after 1 mo

Signs of cauda equina syndrome

- saddle anaesthesia
- recent onset of bladder dysfunction
- severe or progressive neurologic deficit

Adapted from Murtagh J. *General practice*. Australia: McGraw-Hill, 2003.

3. **Psychosocial information.** Look for any "red flag" indicators of serious disease (Table 12.5.2). Have there been any recent events or activities that may be associated with the pain? If work related, assess workplace activities. Assess urinary and sexual function, which can be affected by neurologic compromise. Psychiatric and psychosocial assessment may suggest the presence of psychogenic back pain, but depression may also occur as a consequence of chronic back pain. Disrupted sleep patterns are common in both depression and back pain. Patients seeking drugs of dependence may present with back pain, and addiction may have resulted from previous back pain treatment. A legal history may complicate the diagnosis and management of back pain, and the physician should ask whether there are any legal or insurance issues under consideration.

B. **Physical examination.** Examination aims to identify the location, level, and cause of discomfort, in part by reproducing the pain. For this reason, the most painful parts of the examination are left to the end of the assessment.

1. **General.** Initial impressions of how the patient moves may give important diagnostic clues. Patients with disc lesions may prefer to stand. Gait can be observed as the patient moves about the consulting room, and level of functionality and disability can be observed when the patient sits in chairs and climbs onto the examination table. The patient's clothes should be removed to a minimum to allow close examination of the back and inspection of the gait. Abdominal examination should focus on possible causes of back pain (Table 12.5.1). Systemic examination, especially neurologic examination, is also important to exclude other serious causes of back pain.

2. **Musculoskeletal**

a. **Inspection.** Inspect the contour and shape of the back, looking for scoliosis, lordosis, spasm, and muscle wasting. Assess the range of motion of the spine and lower extremities through extension, lateral flexion, and flexion. Perform the straight leg raising (SLR) test passively with the patient supine. Note the

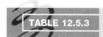

TABLE 12.5.3   Neurologic Findings Seen with Disc Herniation

Disc pain/numbness	Motor weakness	Functional maneuver	Reflex
L3-4/anteromedial thigh and knee	Quadriceps	Deep knee bends	↓ Patellar
L4-5/lateral leg, first three toes	Dorsiflexion of foot or great toe	Heel walking	↓ Achilles
L5-S1/posterior leg, lateral heel	Plantar flexion of foot or great toe	Toe walking	

From Davis S. Low back pain. In: Taylor RB, ed. *Musculoskeletal problems. The 10 minute diagnosis manual.* Philadelphia, PA: Lippincott Williams & Wilkins, 2000.

angle of leg elevation precipitating pain. A positive test for sciatica is buttock pain radiating to the posterior thigh and perhaps to the lower leg and foot. The SLR test is usually negative in spinal stenosis (3).

  b. Palpation. Palpation and percussion of the spine and upper pelvis help identify areas of localized tenderness, as seen in myofascial conditions, fracture, metastatic disease, and some inflammatory conditions. Include an examination of the hip and sacroiliac joint.

 3. Neurologic. Neurologic examination is especially important in the presence of paresthesia, weakness, and radiating pain. Assess strength by having the patient walk on his or her heels (L5), walk on his or her toes (S1), and testing for specific nerve root motor, sensory, and reflex function for each lumbar level. The lower extremity examination includes motor strength, deep tendon reflexes, sensation, proprioception, and certain functional maneuvers (see Table 12.5.3). Romberg and Babinski reflexes should also be assessed. Rectal examination should assess sphincter tone, which can be compromised in sacral root dysfunction. In the primary care setting, most clinically significant disc herniations are detected by the following limited examination: dorsiflexion of the great toe and ankle, Achilles reflex, light touch sensation of the medial (L4), dorsal (L5), and lateral (S1) aspect of the foot, and the SLR test (1, 3).

C. Testing

 1. Clinical laboratory tests

  a. Testing is influenced by the differential diagnosis after the history and physical examination. In the presence of "red flag" indicators, tests may include urinary examination, complete blood count, erythrocyte sedimentation rate, electrolytes, including serum calcium, serum alkaline phosphatase, or prostate-specific antigen. Pain suspected to be caused by a "red flag" condition may require other urgent tests.

  b. Specific tests for inflammatory conditions (such as rheumatoid arthritis or ankylosing spondylitis) or infections may also be needed if indicated from history and examination.

 2. Diagnostic imaging. In low-risk patients, diagnostic imaging is unlikely to be helpful. A posteroanterior and lateral radiograph of the lumbosacral spine may be used to delineate bony structure and alignment but does not provide diagnostic information regarding many serious causes of back pain. Patients with a potential "red flag" condition, such as spinal trauma, or suspected cauda equina syndrome may require computed tomography (CT) scanning and/or magnetic resonance imaging (MRI). MRI is usually the preferred modality if available and the patient is stable. A bone scan may be used when tumor, infection, or occult fracture is suspected. Electromyography may be useful to assess for nerve root dysfunction when symptoms are questionable. Myelography with or without CT scan may be obtained in preoperative planning (1). Persistent, chronic pain may require further diagnostic imaging.

IV. DIAGNOSIS

A. The most common cause of low back pain in primary care is myofascial dysfunction with subsequent muscle spasm. The physical examination reveals limitation of motion of the affected area, with tenderness and increased tone in the affected muscle groups. Spondylolisthesis typically presents in adolescence, particularly in athletes. Low back pain, loss of lumbar lordosis, and a palpable "step off" are classic findings. Lumbar degenerative disc disease may present in older age-groups, with localized or radicular pain due to nerve root compression. Pain radiating below the knee is more likely to be a true radiculopathy.

B. Aching, throbbing pain of insidious onset that is worse in the morning and is unrelieved by rest and worse at night suggests an inflammatory origin of the pain. A deep, dull pain, with intermittent stiffness relieved by rest and worse after activity or the end of the day associated with a precipitating event or a previous history of back pain suggests mechanical origin. Increased pain from standing or walking suggests spinal stenosis, whereas pain on sitting is often due to disc disease. Pain and stiffness in the morning suggests inflammatory disease, whereas continuous pain is more suggestive of neoplasm or infection. A more complicated mixed pattern is seen in the common situation in which mechanical disease coexists with inflammatory disease.

References

1. Deyo RA, Rainville J, Kent DL. What can the history and physical examination tell us about low back pain? *JAMA* 1992;268:760–765.
2. Australian Acute Musculoskeletal Pain Guidelines Group. *Evidence-based management of acute musculoskeletal pain.* Brisbane: Australian Academic Press, 2003.
3. Davis S. Low back pain. In: Taylor RB, ed. *Musculoskeletal problems. The 10 minute diagnosis manual.* Philadelphia, PA: Lippincott Williams & Wilkins, 2000.

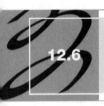

12.6 MONOARTICULAR JOINT PAIN
Trish Palmer

I. **BACKGROUND.** Pain in a single joint is a common presenting complaint.

II. **PATHOPHYSIOLOGY**

A. **Etiology.** Monoarticular joint pain is a sign that can have many causes, including, traumatic, infectious, crystal-induced, degenerative, malignant, and rheumatic conditions. These processes may also involve cartilage, bony structures, surrounding bursae, or ligaments or tendons, resulting in pain.

B. **Epidemiology.** Each year, there are more than 315 million office visits for musculoskeletal complaints (1). This accounts for >10% of all outpatient visits in general medical practice (2). In 2001, a telephone survey revealed arthritis and chronic joint symptoms in one third of all adults (3).

III. **EVALUATION**

A. **History.** A key point is whether the pain stems from trauma. A history of high impact or an inability to bear weight indicates the possibility of a fracture, dislocation, or soft tissue damage. Unusual or exceptional physical demand may indicate a stress fracture (4). Atraumatic joint pain should prompt consideration of diagnoses such as rheumatic disease, degenerative disease, crystal-induced arthropathy, infection, and malignancy. Information about family history of joint disease and rheumatic conditions should be assessed (5). Weight loss, fevers, chills, night sweats,

Condition	Appearance	White blood cells/mm	Polymorpho- nuclear neutrophils (%)	Glucose (% serum level)	Crystals under polarized light
Normal	Clear	<200	<25	95–100	None
Noninflammatory (e.g., degenerative joint disease)	Clear	<400	<25	95–100	None
Acute gout	Turbid	2,000–5,000	>75	80–100	Negative birefringence; needlelike crystals
Pseudogout	Turbid	5,000–50,000	>75	80–1,000	Positive birefringence; rhomboid crystals
Septic arthritis	Purulent/turbid	>50,000	>75	<50	None
Inflammatory (e.g., rheumatoid arthritis)	Turbid	5,000–50,000	50–75	~75	None

Adapted from Roberts JR, Hedges JR, eds. *Clinical procedures in emergency medicine*, 3rd ed. Philadelphia, PA: WB Saunders, 1998.

unrelenting or nocturnal pain, and significant disability may indicate infection or malignancy.

B. Physical examination

1. Examination of the entire patient is imperative. Distribution of pain or swelling can give additional clues regarding the diagnosis. Rheumatoid arthritis (RA) often involves the proximal interphalangeal, metacarpophalangeal, and metatarsophalangeal joints, whereas involvement of the hip, knee, distal interphalangeal joints, or carpometacarpal joint of the thumb suggests osteoarthritis. Elements of physical examination should include inspection, palpation, range of motion (ROM), and special tests.

2. Marked swelling or ecchymosis, laxity, gross deformity, and tendon or muscle dysfunction may indicate fracture or soft tissue injury. Crepitus indicates a derangement of bone, cartilage, or menisci (6). Sensory changes indicate possible neurologic or vascular pathology. Increased ROM may indicate an unstable joint, whereas decreased ROM may represent effusion, capsule fibrosis, or bony abnormality.

3. Bruises inconsistent with the patient's explanation may indicate undetected abuse.

C. Testing. Blood testing (e.g., sedimentation rate, C-reactive protein, rheumatoid factor, antinuclear antibody, uric acid) is useful only if there is a high suspicion of a specific diagnosis. These tests have a high sensitivity but low specificity (7, 8). For example, rheumatoid factor is negative in as many as 30% of cases of RA but may be positive in normal aging individuals as well as in certain disease states (9).

1. Arthrocentesis is urgently indicated when there is a warm, red joint with effusion, especially when there is no history of trauma (10). Absence of fever does not reliably exclude the presence of a septic joint and should not influence this decision (11). Synovial fluid should be sent for the "3 Cs": cell count, culture (Gram's stain), and crystals. Table 12.6.1 reviews the diagnoses consistent with findings on synovial fluid analysis.

2. X-rays should be obtained when there is chronic pain, suspected arthritis, bony tenderness, inability to bear weight, gross deformity, and skeletal immaturity. Magnetic resonance imaging (MRI) is also a choice to further evaluate the

problem and limit exposure to radiation. For clinical questions dealing primarily with soft tissue problems, MRI is the modality of choice except in patients with indwelling metallic devices. Computed tomography (CT) scan is the modality of choice in patients who have indwelling metal for whom plain radiographs are not diagnostic.

3. Injection of iodinated contrast can be performed in conjunction with CT (CT arthrography) to provide information about hyaline cartilage, ligaments, and the joint capsule. MRI with gadolinium injection (MRI arthrography) can visualize intra-articular structures. This modality may also detect early inflammatory arthritis (12).

D. Genetics. Premature development of OA is related to a defect in the type II procollagen gene [COL2A1] and is of dominant inheritance. Genetic studies support a significant genetic contribution to OA (13).

1. RA is genetically complex. Patients with RA have an increased incidence of HLA-DR4 and HLA-DR1 antigens compared to the general population.

TABLE 12.6.2	Differential Diagnosis of Joint Pain

Trauma	Infection	Other
Sprain	Gonococcal	Reflex sympathetic dystrophy
Strain	Nongonococcal: viral, mycobacterial, or fungal	Sjögren's syndrome
Fracture	Lyme disease	Polymyositis
Dislocation	Subacute bacterial endocarditis	Scleroderma
Tear of ligament, tendon, or meniscus	Secondary to enteric and urogenital infections	Sarcoidosis
Tendinitis		Fibromyalgia
		Erythema nodosum
		Sickle cell disease
		Aseptic necrosis
		Charcot's disease
		Drug reaction
		Hypothyroidism
		Irritable bowel syndrome
		Osteochondritis dissecans
Crystal-induced arthropathy	**Degenerative joint disease**	**Malignant**
Gout	Osteoarthritis	Tumor
Pseudogout		Metastases
		Leukemia
	Rheumatic	
	Rheumatoid arthritis	
	Reiter's syndrome	
	Psoriatic arthritis	
	Lupus erythematosus	
	Ankylosing spondylitis	

   2. Classic familial gout may be a monomeric dominantly inherited disorder. Calcium pyrophosphate dehydrate deposition disease occurs in a hereditary form.

IV. DIAGNOSIS

A. Differential diagnosis. Table 12.6.2 shows the differential diagnosis for monoarticular joint pain.

B. Clinical manifestations

   1. Osteoarthritis is usually seen in older patients, presenting symmetrically in large weight-bearing joints. It may manifest initially or during flares as monoarticular joint pain, usually worse at the end of the day or after prolonged weight-bearing. There may be some swelling, usually without erythema or much warmth.

   2. RA often begins with systemic symptoms. Initially, it may affect only one joint but commonly presents as swelling, redness, and warmth of the small joints in the hand and wrist. Morning stiffness is common.

   3. Gouty arthritis occurs suddenly, often during the night. The pain is typically described as excruciating, with the patient unable to even have a sheet touching the affected joint. Commonly, the great toe is warm, swollen, and red.

   4. A septic joint may have an entry point for the bacteria that is obvious, like an abrasion, and is swollen, warm and red. Low-grade fever may accompany joint pain, but lack of fever should not preclude joint aspiration. Children may present with nonspecific symptoms such as irritability, fever, crying with movement of the hip (as with diaper changes), or refusal to bear weight.

References

1. Fauci A, Braunwald E, Isselbacher K, et al., eds. *Harrison's principles of internal medicine.* 14th ed. New York: McGraw-Hill, 1998.
2. Isselbacher K, Martin J, Braunwald E, et al., eds. *Harrison's principles of internal medicine.* 13th ed. New York: McGraw-Hill, 1994.
3. Centers for Disease Control and Prevention. Prevalence of self-reported arthritis or chronic joint symptoms among adults—United States, 2001. *Morb Mortal Wkly Rep* 2002;51:948–950.
4. Reeder MT, Dick BH, Atkins JK, et al. Stress fractures. Current concepts of diagnosis and treatment. *Sports Med* 1996;22(3):198–212.
5. Littman K. A rational approach to the diagnosis of arthritis. *Am Fam Physician* 1996;53(4):1295–1310.
6. Richie AM, Francis ML. Diagnostic approach to polyarticular joint pain. *Am Fam Physician* 2003;68(6):1151–1160.
7. Barth WF. Office evaluation of the patient with musculoskeletal complaints. *Am J Med*;1997(102 1A):3S–10S.
8. Freed JF, Nies KM, Boyer RS, et al. Acute monoarticular arthritis: a diagnostic approach. *JAMA* 1980;243(22):2314–2316.
9. Klippel J, Weyand C, Wortmann R, et al., eds. *Primer on the rheumatic diseases.* 11th ed. Atlanta, GA: Arthritis Foundation, 1997.
10. Till SH, Snaith ML. Assessment, investigation, and management of acute monoarthritis. *J Accid Emerg Med* 1999;16(5):355–361.
11. Learch TJ. Imaging of infectious arthritis. *Semin Musculoskelet Radiol* 2003;7(2):137–142.
12. McGonagle D, Conaghan PG, Wakefield R, et al. Imaging the joints in early rheumatoid arthritis. *Best Pract Res Clin Rheumatol* 2001;15(1):91–104.
13. Felson DT, Couropmitree NN, Chaisson CE, et al. Evidence for a Mendelian gene in a segregation analysis of generalized radiographic osteoarthritis: the Framingham Study. *Arthritis Rheum* 1998;41(6):1064–1071.

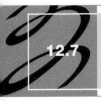

NECK PAIN
James R. Barrett and Brian Coleman

I. **BACKGROUND.** Neck pain is defined as pain occurring anywhere between the base of the skull and thorax. This pain can occur anteriorly, posteriorly, or laterally. The cervical spine is one of the most mobile and complex joints in the body. Considering that, on average, the neck moves over 600 times an hour (1), it is no wonder that it is a common source of pain. Most episodes of neck pain are short lived and resolve spontaneously.

II. **PATHOPHYSIOLOGY**

A. **Etiology**

1. Trauma, job-related causes (e.g., manual labor, driving for long periods, head forward positioning while typing), smoking, and a previous history of low back pain are considered risk factors for neck pain. Often, no specific cause can be elicited.

2. Symptoms due to cervical pathology can be referred to other areas of the body, most commonly the upper back, chest, and arms. Likewise, pain from shoulder or chest pathology can be referred to the neck.

B. **Epidemiology.** Neck pain is extremely common in the general population with a 40% to 70% lifetime prevalence. Cervical arthritis is seen in 80% of individuals over 50 years of age and cervical radiculopathy, in 83.2/100,000 of the general population with most of them in the C6-7 distribution (2).

TABLE 12.7.1 Special Physical Examination Tests of Cervical Spine

Test	Evaluation for	How performed	Positive test
Spurling's test	Nerve root compression (disc herniation)	Head in mild extension and flexion toward side of radicular symptoms	Pain in dermatomal pattern on affected side
Distraction test	Nerve root compression (disc herniation)	Head lifted axially with one hand under chin and other hand around occiput	Pain relief with lifting head
Adson's maneuvers	Thoracic outlet syndrome	Extend patient's symptomatic shoulder while patient rotates neck toward affected side. Pulse is checked during deep inspiration	Loss of pulse in affected extremity
Lhermitte's sign	Spinal canal narrowing (spinal stenosis), multiple sclerosis	Patient sitting with legs extended; ask patient to flex neck forward	Shock like sensation into lower back and/or extremities

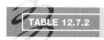

TABLE 12.7.2	Differential Diagnosis of Neck Pain			
Musculoskeletal	**Neurologic**	**Infectious**	**Neoplastic**	**Referred**
Cervical strain or sprain	Thoracic outlet syndrome	Diskitis	Spinal cord tumor	Rotator cuff tendinopathy
Disc herniation	Peripheral neuropathy	Osteomyelitis	Primary neck neoplasm	Myocardial ischemia
Degenerative disc disease	Myelopathy	Meningitis	Malignant neoplasm	Pneumonia
Inflammatory arthritis (rheumatoid, ankylosing spondylitis)	Radiculopathy	Cervical lymphadenitis		
Cervical fracture				
Cervical instability				
Cervical stenosis				
Fibromyalgia				
Whiplash				
Diffuse idiopathic skeletal hyperostosis				
Torticollis				

III. EVALUATION

A. History. Characterizing the location, quality, intensity, radiation, duration, and associated symptoms helps determine the likely cause of neck pain.

1. Key associated neck complaints are radicular symptoms, such as paresthesias, sensory loss, muscle weakness, which can indicate nerve root compression; lower extremity symptoms, such as lower extremity paresthesias, bowel/bladder dysfunction, which can indicate cauda equina syndrome; and fever, weight loss, and other joint involvement that can indicate inflammatory arthritis, infection, or neoplasm.

2. Unusual symptoms can be related to neck pathology and should not be discounted. Sympathetic nervous system activation can cause eye pain, increased tearing, and blurry vision. Irritation of the C3-5 nerve root (due to phrenic nerve involvement) can cause respiratory symptoms such as shortness of breath (3).

B. Physical examination. Examination should include inspection, palpation for tenderness in both midline and paraspinous areas, range of motion, neurovascular examination, and special tests. Inspection of the neck should evaluate for loss of normal lordosis, rash, or other abnormalities. Active range of motion is observed. Reduction of active range of motion may be associated with underlying bony pathology such as arthritis or be due to muscle spasm. Loss of passive range of motion is usually due to underlying bony pathology. Neurovascular examination includes the evaluation of motor strength, sensation, and deep tendon reflexes. Special tests for cervical pathology are reviewed in Table 12.7.1.

C. Testing. Laboratory tests are rarely needed in patients with neck pain. Suspicion of a malignancy or inflammatory arthritis, such as rheumatoid arthritis or ankylosing spondylitis may prompt tests such as rheumatoid factor, sedimentation rate, complete blood count, and/or HLA B27.

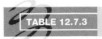

TABLE 12.7.3   **Most Common Causes of Neck Pain**

Etiology	Typical history	Key physical examination findings	Key lab findings
Spondylosis	Dull neck ache	Tender to palpation midline	Radiograph (x-ray) shows degenerative changes that can include narrowing of disc space, sclerosis of posterior elements, and osteophytes
	Older age-group	Decreased active and passive ROMs	
	Occipital headache		
	± radicular symptoms		
Cervical disc herniation	Sharp neck pain	Decreased active ROM	MRI shows disc protrusion or extrusion into spinal canal
	Burning or tingling in upper extremities	Reduced deep tendon reflexes	
	Pain with neck motion	Decreased strength in upper extremities	
	Upper extremity weakness	Positive Spurling's test	
Cervical strain/sprain	Intermittent dull neck pain	Normal ROM	X-ray is normal or shows loss of lordosis
	± Occupational related (postural)	Loss of lordosis	Consider computed tomography to rule out bony injury in trauma
	± Trauma history (motor vehicle accident, fall)	Palpable tightness, ropiness	
	Muscle spasm	Occasional acute edema	
		Muscle spasms	
Fibromyalgia	Diffuse axial skeletal pain	Normal passive ROM	No laboratory test to confirm
	Sleep disturbance	Trigger points	
	Fatigue		
Inflammatory arthritis such as RA or AS	Dull ache	Decreased active and passive ROMs	RA: increased rheumatoid factor and erythrocyte sedimentation rate
	Morning stiffness >1 h	Other joint inflammation	AS: positive HLA B27
	Other joint involvement		

(continued)

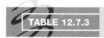

TABLE 12.7.3   **Most Common Causes of Neck Pain (Continued)**

Etiology	Typical history	Key physical examination findings	Key lab findings
Referred pain	Symptoms from other sites (e.g., chest pain, shoulder pain)	Normal ROM of neck	X-ray of other sites electrocardiogram, MRI potentially helpful
		Physical examination findings at other sites (e.g., shoulder strength loss, chest rales)	

ROM, range of motion; MRI, magnetic resonance imaging; RA, rheumatoid arthritis; AS, ankylosing spondylitis.

1. Radiographs are frequently helpful in cases of trauma, radicular symptoms, or prolonged (3–6 weeks) symptoms. Typical views include anteroposterior, odontoid (open-mouth view), and lateral radiographs of the cervical spine. All seven cervical vertebrae should be visualized in the lateral radiograph. Oblique views assist in the evaluation of the neural foramina and posterior elements. Flexion and extension views are obtained when instability of the cervical spine is suspected. It is important to remember that radiographic abnormalities are common in the general population and may not be the cause of the symptoms.
2. Computerized tomography is best used for identifying bony pathology such as subtle fractures, whereas magnetic resonance imaging is ideal for soft tissue pathology, such as disc disease and spinal stenosis. The use of discography to localize the exact disc causing pain is controversial (1). Nerve conduction velocity and electromyogram may be helpful in differentiating the nerve root from peripheral nerve pathology.

D. Genetics. Cervical degenerative disc disease may have a genetic component (4). Genetic predisposition to inflammatory disorders such as rheumatoid arthritis, ankylosing spondylitis, and osteoarthritis is well established (1).

IV. DIAGNOSIS
   A. Differential diagnosis. See Table 12.7.2.
   B. Clinical manifestations. See Table 12.7.3.

References
1. Nankano KK. Neck pain. In: Harris E, Budd R, Firestein G, et al., eds. *Kelley's textbook of rheumatology*, 7th ed. Philadelphia, PA: Elsevier Saunders, 2005:537–554.
2. Devereaux MW. Neck pain. *Prim Care Clin Office Pract* 2004;31:19–31.
3. Bland JH. Disorders of the cervical spine. In: Noble J, ed. *Textbook of primary care medicine*, 3rd ed. St Louis, MO: Mosby, 2001:1125–1137.
4. MacGregor AJ, Andrew T, Sambrook PN, et al. Structural, psychological, and genetic influences on low back and neck pain: a study of adult female twins. *Arthritis Rheum* 2004;51:160–167.

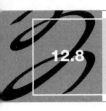

POLYMYALGIA
Martina Kelly and Joseph A. Moran

I. **BACKGROUND.** Multiple (*poly*) muscle aches (*myalgia*) are a common presentation in primary care with a broad differential diagnosis. The challenge for the physician lies in distinguishing benign and self-limiting causes, such as a benign viral infection, from more serious illnesses. In most cases, diagnosis remains primarily a clinical one.

II. **PATHOPHYSIOLOGY.** The most common causes are polymyalgia rheumatica and inflammatory conditions (e.g., polymyositis/dermatomyositis and fibromyalgia). Table 12.8.1 gives a summary of how these may be distinguished. The etiology and epidemiology are dependent on the cause. In many cases, the precise etiology is not known.

III. **EVALUATION.** The key to the evaluation of this condition lies in a careful history and examination (1). Frequently, laboratory investigations are inconclusive, and there is a danger that patients may be overinvestigated.

TABLE 12.8.1   Differential Diagnosis of Polymyalgia

	Polymyalgia rheumatica (2)	Fibromyalgia (3)	Inflammatory conditions (1) (e.g., polymyositis/ dermatomyositis)
Epidemiology (4)	More common in the elderly, rarely <50 y	Middle age (usually <50 y)	40–60 y
	Affects women more than men 700/100,000 >50 y	Affects women more than men 2%–8% adults (where studied)	2:1 women:men 1/100,000
Pathophysiology	Large vessel vasculitis	Unclear	Inflammation of striated muscle
		Sensitization of central nervous system	If it involves the skin it is "dermatomyositis"
History	Sudden onset	Systemic: fatigue, sleep disturbance, headaches, frequently multiple symptoms	Insidious
	Systemic: fever, malaise, anorexia, weight loss, depression	Widespread pain	Systemic: fever, malaise, weight loss in acute phase
	Specific: proximal symmetrical shoulder ± hip girdle pain and **stiffness**, worse in the morning or after rest		Specific: proximal pain (50%) and weakness (worse after use)
			Dysphagia (50%)
			Respiratory muscles

(continued)

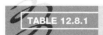

TABLE 12.8.1	Differential Diagnosis of Polymyalgia *(Continued)*		

	Polymyalgia rheumatica (2)	Fibromyalgia (3)	Inflammatory conditions (1) (e.g., polymyositis/ dermatomyositis)
Physical	Proximal tenderness	**Tender "trigger" points**	Proximal tenderness
	NO weakness	No weakness	**Proximal weakness**
			Muscle atrophy
			Rash (dermatomyositis), Gottron's papules, heliotrophic rash on eyelids
Laboratory tests	Elevated ESR >50 mm/h (rarely normal)	No specific test	ESR, creatine phosphokinase
	Normochromic normocytic anemia	Normal ESR	Electromyography
			Muscle biopsy
Treatment	Rapid response to oral prednisone (60–80 mg/d)	No response to steroids	Admission, steroids, cytotoxics
		Multifaceted individualized programme	Splinting of joints and gradual rehabilitation
Associations	Temporal arteritis (15% patients)	Irritable bowel syndrome	Systemic lupus erythematosus, rheumatoid arthritis, systemic sclerosis
		Myofascial pain syndrome	Malignancy (lung, ovary, breast, stomach)
		Chronic fatigue syndrome	

ESR, erythrocyte sedimentation rate.

A. History

1. Ask about onset (acute or insidious) and the muscles affected (diffuse, proximal muscles of shoulder/hip girdle). To assess proximal muscle weakness, ask about difficulty going up stairs, getting up from chairs, and raising hands above the head.
2. Enquire about the presence of systemic symptoms (fever, weight loss, fatigue). Is there joint involvement (and which ones)?
3. Is there a significant past medical history? Ask about medication and family history. In the social history, it is important to enquire about occupation and sources of stress.

B. Physical examination.
Pay particular attention to the musculoskeletal system. Inspect for muscle atrophy and palpate for muscle tenderness (including the scalp and temporal artery). The presence or absence of muscle weakness is the key clinical finding. Distinguish between soft tissue pain (myalgia) and joint pain (arthralgia). In the latter, synovitis is a frequent finding. Is a rash present?

C. Testing.
Frequently, laboratory tests fail to elucidate the cause. Baseline investigations may include a complete blood count, erythrocyte sedimentation rate, C-reactive protein, glucose, liver function tests, creatine phosphokinase, thyroid function tests, and a chest radiograph. If muscle weakness is present, consider an electromyogram and/or muscle biopsy. Consideration may be given to obtaining serologies for infectious diseases, depending on risk factors.

IV. DIAGNOSIS. The differential diagnosis is wide ranging (Table 12.8.1). Apart from the aforementioned, the following should be considered. Major rheumatologic disorders (rheumatoid arthritis, systemic lupus erythematosus) can be distinguished by the presence of joint pain. Other possibilities include underlying malignancy, serious infections, endocrine disorders (e.g., hyperthyroidism), and depression.

References
1. Nirmalananthan N, Holton JL, Hanna MG. Is it really myositis? A consideration of the differential diagnosis *Curr Opin Rheumatol* 2004;16(6):684–691.
2. Salvarani C, Cantini F, Boiardi L, et al. Polymyalgia rheumatica. *Best Pract Res Clin Rheumatol* 2004;18(5):705–722.
3. Mease P. Fibromyalgia syndrome: review of clinical presentation, pathogenesis, outcome measures, and treatment. *J Rheumatol Suppl* 2005;75:6–21.
4. Lawrence RC, Helmick CG, Arnett FC, et al. Estimates of the prevalence of arthritis and selected musculoskeletal disorders in the United States. *Arthritis Rheum* 1998;41:778.

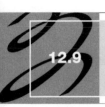

12.9 SHOULDER PAIN
Kalyanakrishnan Ramakrishnan and Andrew D. Jones

I. BACKGROUND. Six to twenty-five percent of the general population report shoulder pain (1). Significant disability including inability to carry out day-to-day household activities may result (1). Most patients (85%) with shoulder pain have a disorder intrinsic to the shoulder.

II. PATHOPHYSIOLOGY
  A. The shoulder joint's principal articulation, the glenohumeral joint, is small and provides only a limited degree of bony stability. Therefore, many causes of shoulder pain are related to stress on its soft tissue support structures, principally the rotator cuff. This musculotendinous cuff helps stabilize the shoulder joint. The subacromial bursa protects these tendons from compression between the acromion and humeral head. Repetitive overhead activities, acute trauma, or instability may result in impingement of the rotator cuff tendon and subacromial bursa between humerus and acromion, resulting in pain and inflammation.
  B. In younger patients, especially in those involved in sports requiring overhead motions (baseball, tennis, football, or swimming), pain and instability are often due to repetitive microtrauma involving the labrocapsular structures (2). Psychosocial factors may contribute to persistence of pain long after the injury or inflammation has resolved. With advancing age, focal degeneration and ischemia of the rotator cuff may occur.
  C. Other sites of significant shoulder pain due to trauma or overuse include the biceps tendon, acromioclavicular (AC) joint, brachial plexus. Pain may also be referred to sources in the neck, thorax, and abdomen (*vide infra*).

III. EVALUATION
  A. History. History should include pain onset, type, location, severity, effect on activities or work, any therapy, history of injury, and associated symptoms. Anatomic localization of the pain is important. Inspection should focus on the cranium, cervical spine, and the entire upper limb, including the designated painful site.
  B. Physical examination. The shoulder is examined for atrophy, loss of muscle tone, fasciculations, reflex, and sensory changes. The upper limb is then inspected for swelling, skin changes, and abnormal posture. Active range of motion (flexion, extension, adduction, abduction, medial and lateral rotation) is observed, as is the

| **TABLE 12.9.1** | **Special Tests to Confirm Shoulder Pathology** |

Test	Maneuver	Pathology
Neer test (impingement sign)	Examiner stabilizes patients acromion with one hand, performs maximum passive shoulder abduction and internal rotation with the other.	Subacromial inflammation, impingement
Hawkin's impingement sign	Forced internal rotation with the shoulder flexed forward to 90°	Impingement
Jobe's test (empty can test)	Deltoid assessed with arm at 90° abduction and neutral rotation. Shoulder then internally rotated and angled forward 30°; thumbs pointing toward the floor. Downward pressure of examiner's hand resisted.	Supraspinatus weakness due to injury, pain due to rotator cuff pathology
Cross-body adduction test	Shoulder flexed to 90° and adducted across the patient's body	Rotator cuff/acromioclavicular pathology
Lift-off test	Patient's arm behind back, with volar surface of the hand resting on the sacrum. Weakness in lifting the hand away from the spine	Subscapularis muscle weakness/injury
Yergason test	Supination of the pronated forearm against resistance with the elbow flexed at 90°	Biceps tendonitis/tear
Speed's test	Extension and supination of the elbow as the examiner resists flexion of the humerus	Biceps tendonitis/tear
Apprehension test	Abduction to 90° and external rotation of the shoulder with the examiner's hand applying forward pressure to the scapula. The patient resists further shoulder extension	Positive anterior instability
Drop arm test	The arm is passively abducted to 90°, and the support is suddenly discontinued. A positive test is reported if the arm drops abruptly	Rotator cuff tear or axillary nerve injury

scapular motion from the rear. Glenohumeral motion is assessed by stabilizing the scapula with the examiner's hand. The sternoclavicular and AC joints, coracoid process, spine of scapula and clavicle, acromion, rotator cuff, and other shoulder joint muscles are all palpated. Special tests performed to detect clinical entities specific to the shoulder are described in Table 12.9.1. The Neer impingement sign is most reliable in diagnosing impingement (3).

1. Pathology involving the greater tuberosity or subacromial structures often results in pain on abduction. A painful arc (pain between 30° and 90° of abduction) suggests impingement of the greater tuberosity under the acromion or supraspinatus tendonitis.

2. In rotator cuff tears, active abduction is often limited, and there is weakness with abduction against resistance.

3. AC joint pathology is indicated by pain on top of the shoulder, which may refer to the neck and jaw, and local joint tenderness exaggerated by adduction of the arm.
4. Crepitus over the shoulder while rotating the humerus may indicate severe rotator cuff disease with secondary glenohumeral osteoarthritis.

C. Testing

1. **Laboratory tests.** A complete blood count and analysis of synovial or bursal aspirate for cell count, Gram stain, and culture are obtained in suspected septic arthritis or bursitis. In suspected inflammatory arthritis, an erythrocyte sedimentation rate or C-reactive protein, rheumatoid factor, and antinuclear antibody tests may be helpful, and the joint aspirate may be examined for crystals.

2. **Imaging studies.** Standard anteroposterior (AP) and lateral x-rays of the shoulder detect most bone and joint pathology. Axillary or special Y views are needed in suspected posterior dislocation; AP views with the arm in internal and external rotation are useful following trauma (4). Views with and without weights better assess AC joint separation. Arthrography may be useful in planning surgery for rotator cuff tears. Ultrasound is a noninvasive, relatively inexpensive modality; it diagnoses most full-thickness rotator cuff tears (sensitivity 87%, specificity 96%) (2,5). Magnetic resonance imaging also has high sensitivity (80%–100%) and specificity (88%–94%) in rotator cuff injuries (2,5). Magnetic resonance arthrography (sensitivity 95%, specificity 93% in complete rotator cuff tears) may also be used.

IV. EVALUATION

A. Differential diagnosis.
The differential diagnosis includes musculoskeletal injury, trauma, infection, and inflammatory conditions. Referred sources should also be considered and include cervical disc disease, myocardial ischemia, reflex sympathetic dystrophy, diaphragmatic irritation and intrathoracic tumors, thoracic outlet syndrome, and gallbladder disease.

B. Clinical manifestations

1. **Impingement/subacromial bursitis/rotator cuff tendonitis/tear.** Pain is typically severe at night and worse with overhead activities. Rotator cuff tears should be distinguished from impingement/bursitis, because subsequent evaluation and treatment may be different. Pain elicited by the Neer test confirms impingement; it resolves on subacromial injection of 10 mL of lidocaine. Rotator cuff tendonitis is seen more often in middle-aged or older patients and often causes loss of active range of motion most pronounced in abduction, forward flexion, and internal rotation (3). The Neer impingement and Jobe's tests are positive, and there may be weakness to resisted abduction due to pain. Pain and weakness are reversed with subacromial lidocaine injection. Rotator cuff tears may present with severe pain worse at night, weakness, and decreased active shoulder motion; passive range of motion may be normal. The Neer test is usually positive; subacromial lidocaine injection may result in pain relief, but weakness to resisted abduction persists.

2. Shoulder stiffness (frozen shoulder, adhesive capsulitis) is often seen in older patients and in patients with diabetes (3) following upper limb immobilization, causing aching pain and reductions in both active and passive ranges of motion.

3. **Shoulder dislocation, instability.** Most dislocations are anterior (subcoracoid) and follow a fall on the outstretched hand or forced abduction/rotation injuries. Labral and rotator cuff tears may coexist. The arm is fixed in abduction/external rotation, the shoulder is flattened, and there is a subcoracoid bulge. Radiographs are confirmatory and may reveal associated fractures. Posterior dislocations follow forced adduction internal rotation, as occurring during a seizure. Inferior dislocations follow muscle atrophy associated with neurologic disorders. Shoulder instability follows lesser grades of injury associated with sporting activities. A positive apprehension sign is confirmatory. Recurrent instability is seen more often in younger patients (3).

4. Glenohumeral arthritis also produces shoulder pain that worsens at night, joint crepitus, and decreased active and passive ranges of motion. X-rays may show features of arthritis such as subchondral sclerosis, bone cysts, and osteophytes.

5. AC separation results from a fall onto the acromion, separating it from its distal clavicular articulation. The AC and coracoclavicular (conoid and trapezoid) ligaments are stretched or torn. In type I separation, there is ligament sprain, joint tenderness, and normal x-rays. In type II, there is AC ligament tear and prominence of the distal clavicle, which is higher than the acromion on x-ray. In type III separation, complete ligament disruption occurs and the distal clavicle is prominent and tender and is seen above its acromial articulation on x-ray (6).

6. AC osteoarthritis follows an AC separation or excessive weight training and is indicated by pain localized at the top of the shoulder, worsens with activity and is exacerbated by adduction. AC joint palpation causes pain. Radiographs show osteoarthritis of the joint.

7. Biceps tendonitis or tendon rupture typically follows repetitive motion or trauma. Rupture presents with pain and an abnormal bulge in the anterior arm and tendonitis with shoulder pain and tenderness to palpation of the bicipital groove.

8. Polymyalgia rheumatica is seen in older patients, who may also have pain and stiffness in the contralateral shoulder or other joints. Temporal arteritis may also present with shoulder pain in association with headache and visual changes.

References

1. Van der wint DAWM, Thomas E, Pope DP, et al. Occupational risk factors for shoulder pain: a systematic review. *Occup Environ Med* 2000;57:433–442.
2. Oxner KG. Magnetic resonance imaging of the musculoskeletal system: Part 6. The shoulder. *Clin Orthop* 1997;334:354–373.
3. McMahon PJ, Sallis RE. The painful shoulder. Zeroing in on the most common causes. *Postgrad Med* 1999;106:36–49.
4. Stevenson HJ, Trojian T. Evaluation of shoulder pain. *J Fam Pract* 2002;51:605–611.
5. Dinnes J, Loveman E, McIntyre L, Waugh N. The effectiveness of diagnostic tests for the assessment of shoulder pain due to soft tissue disorders: a systematic review. *Health Technol Assess* 2003;7(29), http://www.cinahl.com/cexpress/hta/summ/summ729.pdf.
6. Steinfeld R, Valente RM, Stuart MJ. A commonsense approach to shoulder problems. *Mayo Clin Proc* 1999;74:785–794.

Dermatologic Problems

Michael L. O'Dell

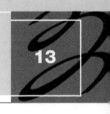

13

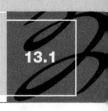

I. **BACKGROUND.** Alopecia, or hair loss, is a common problem. It should be considered a sign of illness and not a diagnosis. Hair loss can be divided into two patterns: generalized and localized.

II. **PATHOPHYSIOLOGY**

   A. **Etiology.** Hair follicles have three phases of growth: anagen, catagen, and telogen. Normally, hairs are shed at the end of telogen phase and the cycle restarts. Alopecia disorders can be divided into two categories on the basis of whether cyclic hair growth is abnormal or the hair follicle is damaged (1). Generalized hair loss has normal hair follicles. Localized hair loss can have either normal or abnormal hair follicles. **Generalized alopecia** includes telogen effluvium, loose anagen syndrome, female pattern androgenic alopecia, and postpartum alopecia. It can be induced by chemotherapy, radiation therapy, analgesics, anticoagulants, antiepileptics, psychotropics, selective serotonin reuptake inhibitors, oral contraceptives and estrogens, proton-pump inhibitors, cardiovascular drugs, immunosuppressants, as well as physical and/or mental stressors (1). **Localized alopecia with normal hair follicles** includes androgenic alopecia, alopecia areata, and traction alopecia. **Localized alopecia with abnormal hair follicles** includes aplasia cutis congenital, infections (e.g., kerion), autoimmune (e.g., discoid lupus), trauma (e.g., thermal burns), skin carcinomas, metastatic adenocarcinoma, lymphoma, and cicatricial pemphigus.

   B. **Epidemiology.** Alopecia is a common problem affecting both genders, all races, and all ages. A variety of illnesses result in alopecia, each with its own distinct age, sex, and race characteristics and patterns of morbidity and mortality.

III. **EVALUATION**

   A. **History.** The important questions to ask are as follows: Is the hair loss generalized or local? Was the loss gradual over time or sudden? Were any new medications, prescription, or over-the-counter drugs taken? Were any new hair grooming products, procedures, or treatments used? Were any family members known to have had similar patterns of hair loss? Were any preceding psychosocial or physical stressors present? **Generalized hair loss** can be seen in these conditions. Acute telogen effluvium is usually described as finding "handfuls" of lost hairs in the shower, in the hair brush, on the pillow or bathroom floor, which causes considerable emotional distress. Telogen effluvium can unmask localized alopecia that has been hidden by the previously thicker hair growth (1). Both male and female **androgenic alopecia** are insidious at onset. Most other etiologies are more sudden at onset. History or presence of known iron deficiency, thyroid problems, sprue, or malnutrition may lead to the etiology. *Stressors* leading to telogen effluvium include a severe acute or chronic illness, major surgery, anorexia (malnutrition), crash dieting, excessive exercising leading to amenorrhea, and severe psychologic stress. Any new medications or hair treatments that are temporally related to the hair loss need to be considered as possible causes. Use of chemical or thermal hair treatments such as hair straightening, curling, or permanent waving can lead to cumulative damage. Hair weaving or braiding that is too tight can lead to traction alopecia.

   B. **Physical examination.** The texture, length, and thickness of individual hairs may suggest the cause of hair loss. Shorter, fine hairs may be found in areas of thinning in androgenic alopecia. "Exclamation point hairs" which have a distal broken shaft and a proximal club-shaped hair root, are seen at the periphery of hair loss in alopecia areata (2). Short broken hairs in the area of loss occur with trichotillomania and tinea capitis. Long eyelashes and straightening of scalp hair can be seen in human immunodeficiency virus (HIV) infection. All areas of the body must be carefully examined for hair growth patterns and changes. Trichotillomania can be seen in the scalp, eyebrow areas, and even eyelashes. Patterns of hair loss in male pattern androgenic alopecia typically range from bitemporal recession, to frontal and vertex thinning, and to loss of all hair except for occipital and temporal fringes. Female pattern alopecia is seen as diffuse thinning that is more prominent in the frontal or parietal areas, with sparing of the frontal fringe (2). In women, watch for signs of virilization that can be associated with androgenic alopecia. Virilization can also cause acne, hypertrichosis in other areas, deepening of the voice, and clitoromegaly. Rashes or other changes in the skin either at the area of hair loss or elsewhere may suggest various causes. Scaling and flaking suggest tinea, psoriasis, or drying of the skin as a result of heat or chemicals. Scarring of the areas of hair loss suggest trauma, infection, or discoid lupus. A "moth eaten" pattern of hair loss on either scalp or face should suggest syphilis, sarcoid, or discoid lupus. Telogen effluvium can be detected by the "pull test", which is performed by grasping approximately 60 hairs between thumb and fingers and pulling gently but firmly. Normal shedding should yield six or fewer hairs. Hair should not have been shampooed within 24 hours of this test (1).

C. Testing

1. Laboratory tests should be ordered on the basis of clinical findings. A typical androgenic alopecia pattern of hair loss with normal skin in men and women without evidence of virilization requires no further testing. Women who show evidence of virilization should have a free testosterone, total testosterone, prolactin, and dehydroepiandrosterone sulfate (DHEA-S) levels drawn first. If these are abnormal, then workup should continue. Patients with nonandrogenic patterns of alopecia should have thyroid function tests, a complete blood count, ferritin level, and an antinuclear antibody done. The need for syphilis serology should also be considered on the basis of history and examination. If these tests are all normal, other nutritional deficiencies such as zinc deficiency should be considered (1). Bacterial and fungal cultures of any drainage should be obtained. Potassium hydroxide microscopic evaluation of skin scrapings for fungal elements and/or fungal cultures of scaling areas can confirm the diagnosis of fungal infection.

2. Scalp biopsy is often helpful especially where scarring is associated with hair loss; biopsy can distinguish between sarcoid, discoid lupus, and lichen planopilaris. The biopsy should be taken with a 4 to 5 mm punch of the active area of a lesion. Areas of infiltration may be scleroderma or a local or metastatic carcinoma. Follicular structure and number as well as the stages of hair growth can be evaluated.

D. Genetics. The hair follicle is the most complex organ of the epidermal structures. There are more than 300 genetic abnormalities that affect hair (3).

IV. DIAGNOSIS

A. Differential diagnosis. The key consideration in diagnosis is whether the hair loss is localized or generalized. Subsequent examinations as noted earlier allow a definitive diagnosis.

B. Clinical manifestations. Most cases of alopecia are caused by either androgenic alopecia or telogen effluvium. These etiologies do not require treatment. Early diagnosis and intervention can be critical in the remaining cases if caused by thyroid disorder, carcinoma, metastatic adenocarcinoma, melanoma, syphilis, or HIV. Permanent hair loss may be prevented or limited by early institution of therapy when alopecia is caused by excessive traction, infection, or other infiltrative or scarring processes. If the alopecia is caused by a drug, hair loss can be reversible if the drug is stopped early in the process. Treatment, if desired, for androgenic alopecia works best if started early on in hair loss. Resolution of the stressful event that precipitates acute telogen effluvium is often difficult and, in some cases, can only be managed by time. Reassurance and support are the best therapy.

References
1. Thiedke C. Alopecia in women. *Am Fam Physician* 2003;67(5):1017–1018.
2. Bertolino A. Alopecia areata. *Postgrad Med* 2000;107(7):81–90.
3. Irvine A, Christiano A. Hair on a gene string: recent advances in understanding the molecular genetics of hair loss. *Clin Exp Dermatol* 2001;26:59–71.

ERYTHEMA MULTIFORME
Ray T. Perrine

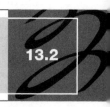

13.2

I. BACKGROUND. Erythema multiforme (EM) describes a syndrome of symptoms. It is a hypersensitivity reaction triggered by various stimuli or by reactivation of a latent infection. EM minor is an eruption that is confined to the skin as typical acral target lesions with or without mucosal involvement. EM major is a much more serious illness and includes the syndromes of erythema multiforme majus (EMM), Stevens-Johnson syndrome (SJS), and toxic epidermal necrolysis (TEN). Many now believe that SJS and TEN are a single entity distinguished only by the severity of the illness. Although EMM is a severe form, it is considered to be a separate entity from SJS/TEN in that it differs in demographics and causes (1).

II. PATHOPHYSIOLOGY
  A. Etiology. EM minor, EMM, SJS, and TEN are believed to be hypersensitivity reactions triggered by various stimuli or by reactivation of a latent infection. Recent herpetic infections are the most common triggers; recent work implicates transport of viral particles to the skin by CD34 cells (2). Oxicam nonsteroidal anti-inflammatory drugs, allopurinol, phenobarbital, phenytoin, and sulfonamides are drugs that are highly suspect in leading to more severe diseases (1). Drug-related EM appears to invoke a tumor necrosis factor mechanism, whereas herpes simplex virus (HSV)–related illness does not (3).
  B. Epidemiology. EM Minor, EMM, SJS, and TEN occur worldwide, in individuals of any age, although most patients are younger than 40 years of age. Drug-related illness tends to be more severe and more often associated with TEN (1). SJS/TEN are accompanied by higher morbidity and mortality rates.

III. EVALUATION
  A. History. The primary focus of the history is on whether there were any prodromal symptoms. EM minor is often asymptomatic. Some patients may experience itching or tenderness. The condition is of sudden onset and generally does not cause systemic symptoms. In EMM/SJS/TEN, two-thirds of patients present without experiencing a prodrome. In the one-third of cases in which prodromal symptoms occur, these usually appear in the form of an upper respiratory illness with fever, malaise, and myalgias. Another focus is on recent exposures. Has the patient been exposed to any drugs 1 to 3 weeks prior to onset? These most often include sulfonamides, penicillin, anticonvulsants, and nonsteroidal anti-inflammatory drugs. Has the patient been ill recently? Most cases of EM minor, particularly those with recurrence, are associated with HSV infection. *Mycoplasma* pneumonia, tuberculosis (TB), β-hemolytic streptococcus, staphylococcal infections, radiation therapy, collagen vascular diseases, pregnancy, carcinomas, and the bacillus Calmette-Guérin vaccine have also been implicated.

B. **Physical examination.** Characteristics of the rash are important to determine the disease. The classic appearance of EM, the target lesion, is a dusky, reddish, central papule surrounded by a red ring. The lesions blanch partially with pressure. No scaling is seen. EM minor manifests as target or iris lesions that often appear at the extremities (e.g., palms, soles) and sometimes on the face or trunk. The distribution is symmetric. The lesions develop over 10 days or more and resolve on their own, usually in 1 to 6 weeks. Recurrences are common and may continue for years. Lesions that are irregular, or occur in large erythematous patches, blister, or bullae with sloughing in large sheets are highly suggestive of SJS and the more severe TEN. SJS/TEN lesions are erythematous or purpuric macules with irregular shape and size. Blisters often occur on all or part of the macule. Lesions are widespread. In TEN, confluent blisters result in the detachment of the epidermis and erosions on 10% to more than 30% of the body surface area. Large erythematous areas without discrete lesions can be present. Systemic signs of high fever, involvement of the eyes with corneal ulceration, pulmonary findings, widespread cutaneous involvement, or pneumonia are present in EM major.

C. **Testing.** Punch biopsy may be useful in the case of atypical lesions. Typical findings include vacuolization of the basal cell layer, with lymphocytes along the dermal–epidermal junction (4). Necrosis of individual keratinocytes is seen in the epidermis, whereas perivascular lymphocytic infiltrates may be present in the dermis. If underlying infection is suspected, other laboratory tests may be indicated, including a complete blood count, throat culture, antistreptolysin-O titer, and a slide test for infectious mononucleosis, and hepatitis screen may be indicated. A chest x-ray may be needed if *Mycoplasma pneumoniae,* histoplasmosis, coccidiomycosis, or TB is suspected. Skin tests or serum complement fixation titers for infectious agents may be needed.

D. **Genetics.** There is no well-defined genetic basis to EM minor, SJS, or TEN. The triggering agent in most cases appears to be infectious or drug-related exposure.

IV. **DIAGNOSIS**

A. **Differential diagnosis.** A systemic, fixed, discrete, round, erythematous rash, which lasts 1 to 6 weeks from onset to healing and is self-limited, acute, or episodic, satisfies the clinical criteria for EM minor. Biopsy may be needed for confirmation. A systemic, erythematous rash, with irregular and target lesions, blisters, sloughing when the patient is systemically ill is much more indicative of SJS/TEN.

B. **Clinical manifestations.** Determining which subtype of EM is present helps dictate treatment and anticipate prognosis. EM minor is a limited illness with little morbidity and mortality, although recurrences are common. SJS/TEN are often life-threatening illnesses with considerable morbidity.

References

1. Auquier-Dunant A, Mockenhaupt M, Nalda L, et al. Correlations between clinical patterns and causes of erythema multiforme majus, Stevens-Johnson syndrome, and toxic epidermal necrolysis: results of an international prospective study. *Arch Dermatol* 2002;138:1019–1024.

2. Ono F, Sharma B, Smith C, et al. CD34+ Cells in the peripheral blood transport herpes simplex virus DNA fragments to the skin of patients with erythema multiforme (HAEM). *J Invest Dermatol* 2005;124(6):1215–1224.

3. Kokuba H, Aurelian L, Burnett J. Herpes simplex virus associated erythema multiforme (HAEM) is mechanistically distinct from drug-induced erythema multiforme: interferon- is expressed in HAEM lesions and tumor necrosis factor- in drug-induced erythema multiforme lesions. *J Invest Dermatol* 1999;113(5):808–815.

4. Katta R. Taking aim at erythema multiforme. *Postgrad Med* 2000;107(1):87.

MACULOPAPULAR RASH
James R. Lundy

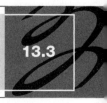

13.3

I. **BACKGROUND.** Maculopapular describes a rash that contains both macules and papules. A maculopapular reaction is usually a large area that is red and has small, confluent bumps.

II. **PATHOPHYSIOLOGY**

   A. **Etiology.** When fever is present, the rash is usually due to infection. Rashes not accompanied by fever regularly result from allergic reactions. Rarely, a maculopapular rash is a systemic sign of an underlying malignancy. Serious infectious illnesses, such as meningococcemia, disseminated gonorrhea, and Rocky Mountain spotted fever (RMSF) can initially present with acute onset of maculopapular rash and fever. Anaphylaxis occasionally presents early in the course with a maculopapular rash, with palmar or pharyngeal itching.

   B. **Epidemiology.** Maculopapular rash is the result of varied diseases. The prevalence, morbidity, and mortality in various ages, sexes, and race populations reflect the underlying disease.

III. **EVALUATION**

   A. **History.** Pertinent history of present illness includes where the rash started; how far it has spread; what associated symptoms, such as fever, itching, burning or pain, accompany the lesions; and its previous occurrence. If it has appeared before, it helps determine what treatment was used and the patient's response as well as the existence of any sick contacts. Other questions of importance include the following: does the patient have any chronic medical conditions; what are the patient's current medications, including over-the-counter and herbal therapies and have any of these drugs been started recently; and does the patient have any known allergies. The social history including occupation, hobbies, new sexual partners, and travel may also be significant.

   B. **Physical examination.** A general physical examination should be conducted. Examination should focus on the distribution of the rash. Consider centrally and peripherally distributed eruptions separately (1). A central rash (face and the trunk) is characteristic of viral illnesses including measles and rubella. A peripheral rash starts on the extremities. The rash of meningococcemia often starts peripherally, presenting as a macule with central petechiae, which then progresses to a nodule as the rash then appears and spreads widely. A maculopapular rash occurring on the palms should prompt concern about syphilis, RMSF, or disseminated gonorrhea. The lesions of gonorrhea are usually acral (affecting limbs and digits) and quickly become pustular.

      1. **Head, eyes, ears, nose, and throat (HEENT) examination.** The scalp is a common location for ticks, which lends support to the diagnosis of RMSF. Mucous membrane swelling may indicate early anaphylaxis. Koplik's spots in the oropharynx are pathognomonic for measles.

      2. **Lung examination.** Wheezing on examination can indicate anaphylaxis.

      3. **Genitourinary examination.** Purulent discharge or evidence of pelvic inflammatory disease indicates gonorrhea. A chancre indicates primary syphilis, although palmar lesions (secondary syphilis) often occur well after the healing of the initial chancre.

      4. **Extremities examination.** Evidence of joint swelling indicates meningococcemia, gonococcemia, or rheumatologic conditions.

      5. **Neurologic examination.** Evidence of meningitis indicates meningococcemia or RMSF.

C. **Testing.** The complete blood count (CBC) is valuable. An elevated white blood cell count with a left shift may indicate a bacterial infection; lymphocytosis may indicate a viral infection; eosinophils are sometimes increased with allergic reactions; and rarely, myelogenous leukemias can present with rash and abnormalities on CBC. Other testing should be performed on the basis of the most likely causes of the rash. Consider the rapid plasma reagin test and gonococcemia in sexually active patients. Consider a smear and culture of any pustules, especially if meningococcemia or gonococcemia is suspected. Cerebrospinal fluid examination is useful if meningococcemia is suspected; it is usually negative in RMSF. Consider an erythrocyte sedimentation rate if there is joint involvement.

D. **Genetics.** Maculopapular rash is the result of varied diseases. Any genetic basis is reflective of the underlying disease. Most underlying causes are infectious and lack a genetic basis.

IV. DIAGNOSIS

A. **Differential diagnosis.** Maculopapular eruptions are most frequently seen in viral illnesses and immune-mediated syndromes. However, the differential diagnosis includes bacteria, spirochetes, rickettsia, and rheumatologic diseases.

1. **Viral exanthems.** These viral etiologies of rashes include rubeola, rubella, Fifth disease, and roseola among others (2). The rash of rubeola (measles) begins around the fourth febrile day, with discrete lesions that become confluent as they spread from the hairline downward, sparing the palms and soles. The exanthem typically lasts 4 to 6 days, with lesions fading gradually in the order of appearance, leaving a residual yellow-tan coloration or faint desquamation, accompanied by the presence of Koplik's spots in the oral mucosa. Rubella (German measles) is similar to rubeola but is less severe and of shorter duration. However, rubella can cause severe birth defects if an expectant mother becomes infected. Roseola has a prodrome of asymptomatic fever lasting 3 to 4 days. Within 2 to 3 days following defervescence, a diffuse rash, sparing the face and hands, appears which resolves spontaneously. Human herpes virus 6 is the causative agent.

2. **Allergic eruptions.** A dull rash that is often accompanied by central vesicles or bullae; this appears commonly on the hands, including palms, as well as soles, arms, knees, and genitals in a symmetric distribution. The rash, which is intensely pruritic, usually appears within the first week after the offending drug is started and typically resolves within days after the drug is discontinued.

3. **Bacterial infection.** This diagnosis is usually serious, with meningococcus and gonococcus being the most common in the United States. Consider this diagnosis in acutely ill patients with high fever, tachypnea, tachycardia, hypotension, leukocytosis, and meningeal signs. Secondary syphilis can be diffuse, with localized eruptions occurring on the head, neck, palms, and soles. The lesions are typically brownish-red or pink macules and papules, but they may be papulosquamous, pustular, or acneiform. The eruption usually occurs 2 to 6 months after the primary infection and 2 to 10 weeks after the primary chancre (3). Additional signs and symptoms include fever, lymphadenopathy, and splenomegaly. Recurrent episodes with symptom-free periods in between may occur.

4. **Rocky Mountain spotted fever.** The rash begins as pinkish-red maculopapules on the wrists and ankles but spreads toward the trunk and progresses to petechiae. Involvement of the palms and soles occurs late in disease. The onset is typically abrupt with fever, severe headache, myalgias, bradycardia, and leukopenia. The rash appears around the fourth day of illness. *Rickettsia rickettsii* is the causative agent.

5. **Kawasaki's disease.** Kawasaki's disease manifests as a maculopapular to scarlatiniform rash with mucous membrane involvement. It is accompanied by high fever lasting 5 days or more, conjunctivitis, lymphadenopathy, desquamation of the hands, and/or strawberry tongue. It usually occurs in younger children. The etiology is unknown.

B. **Clinical manifestations.** These vary according to the underlying disease process.

References
1. Bolognia J, Braverman I. Skin manifestations of internal disease. In: Braunwald E, ed. *Harrison's principles of internal medicine*. 15th ed. New York, NY: McGraw-Hill, 2001.
2. McKinnon H, Howard T. Evaluating the febrile patient with a rash. *Am Fam Physician* 2000;62(4):804–816.
3. Pickering L, ed. AAP-Committee-on-Infectious-Disease. *Red book: report of the committee on infectious disease*. 25th ed. Elk Grove, IL: American Academy of Pediatrics, 2000.

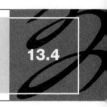

PIGMENTATION DISORDERS
Karen Hughes

13.4

I. BACKGROUND. Patients often present complaining of patches of skin that are lighter or darker.

II. PATHOPHYSIOLOGY

A. Etiology. Disorders of hyperpigmentation include pityriasis versicolor, *café au lait* macules, melasma, *acanthosis nigricans*, solar lentigines, drug eruptions, phytophotodermatitis, and postinflammatory hyperpigmentation. Disorders of hypopigmentation include vitiligo, pityriasis alba, ash leaf macules, halo nevus, idiopathic guttate hypomelanosis, and postinflammatory hypopigmentation.

B. Epidemiology. Prevalence as well as morbidity and mortality rates vary with the specific disease. Pigmentation disorders affect all races, all ages, and both genders.

III. EVALUATION

A. History. The first step in diagnosing a pigmentation disorder is to classify the complaint as hyperpigmentation or hypopigmentation (1). Table 13.4.1 provides other necessary history, including onset, exacerbating factors, relieving factors, and associated symptoms.

B. Physical examination

1. **Hyperpigmented disorders.** *Café au lait* macules are 0.2 to 10 cm, uniform, well-demarcated brown areas found on sun-protected sites of the trunk and extremities. Melasma appears on the malar eminence and other sun-exposed areas. *Acanthosis nigricans* appears as dirty or unwashed skin and as thickened plaques in a symmetric pattern in the axillae, neck, and folds of the breast and groin. Pityriasis versicolor begins as a reddish macule, generally on the upper back, appearing darker than the surrounding skin during winter and lighter than tanned skin during summer. Minocycline-induced hyperpigmentation occurs in old scars, on the lower extremities and forearms, or diffusely in sun-exposed areas. Fixed-drug eruptions occur in the same place with each exposure: they are often vesicobullous, resolving as a hyperpigmented patch (1). Phytophotodermatitis initially resembles sunburn, followed by prolonged hyperpigmentation. Postinflammatory hyperpigmentation is generally light brown to black discoloration.

2. **Hypopigmented disorders.** Vitiligo appears as depigmented macules with scalloped edges, initially on the face, hands, wrists, axillae, umbilicus, and genitalia. The macules then coalesce with time into larger depigmented areas. Pityriasis alba appears as small macules that do not tan, are pale pink to light brown with irregular borders and a powdery scale located on the face, and are seen more often in darkly pigmented skin types. Ash leaf macules are hypopigmented lesions appearing with one end rounded and the other pointed (lance ovate) resembling an ash tree leaf; its size and shape remain stable with age (1). They can occur in normal children but if accompanied by acnelike lesions, they are suspects for

TABLE 13.4.1	**Factors Used to Differentiate between Hyperpigmentation and Hypopigmentation**			
	Onset	**Exacerbating factors**	**Relieving factors**	**Associated symptoms**
Hyperpigmented disorders				
Café au lait spots	Birth or early childhood	None	Regress over time	None
Melasma	Onset of liver dysfunction, pregnancy, phenytoin use, oral contraceptive use	Worsening liver disease or ongoing exposure	May improve with removal of offending agents, but rarely disappears entirely	Usually none
Acanthosis nigricans	Increased weight, insulin use	Weight gain or the use of insulin, nicotinic acid, glucocorti-coids, or estrogens	Improves with weight loss and removal of offending agents	Diabetes-related symptoms
Halo nevus	Severe sun exposure in a youth, especially in Turner's syndrome	Ongoing sun exposure	Tends to disappear with time	Usually none
Solar lentigines	Older age with earlier age sun exposure	Ongoing sun exposure	None	Usually none
Pityriasis versicolor	Exposure to humidity and heat	Ongoing exposure to humidity and heat	Lower humidity, treatment	Occasionally mild pruritus
Drug-induced hyperpigmentation	Drug exposure, especially to minocycline or zidovudine	Reexposure to causative agent	Occasionally fades with removal of offending agents. Minocycline-induced changes are often permanent	Usually none
Fixed-drug eruption	Drug exposure, (phenolphthalein, salicylates, tetracyclines, and sulfonamides)	Reexposure to causative agent	May fade with removal of offending agents, but often remains	Sometimes painful
Phytophotodermatitis	Exposure to topical agents containing furocoumarins (oil of bergamot, psoralens, limes)	Ongoing exposure to topical agents containing furocoumarins (oil of bergamot, psoralens, limes)	Topical or oral steroids, antihistamines.	Sometimes painful
Inflammation	With inflammation	Ongoing inflammation	Relief of inflammation	Pain from inflammation

(continued)

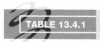

TABLE 13.4.1		Factors Used to Differentiate between Hyperpigmentation and Hypopigmentation *(Continued)*		
	Onset	Exacerbating factors	Relieving factors	Associated symptoms
Hypopigmented disorders				
Pityriasis alba	Young children (especially those with eczema)	Drying agents, sunlight	May fade with moisturizers, tends to disappear at puberty	Occasionally itchy or burning
Ash leaf macule	Childhood	None	None	If underlying tuberous sclerosis: mental retardation, seizures, and adenoma sebaceum
Vitiligo	10–30 years of age	Stress, illness, personal crises, skin trauma	Progressive illness	
Guttate hypomelanosis	Middle age and older	None (idiopathic lesions)	None (idiopathic lesions)	None

tuberous sclerosis. A halo nevus is an area of depigmentation surrounding a typical pigmented nevus. Guttate hypomelanosis is seen as small 5-mm or less porcelain-white macules (2).

3. Ophthalmologic examination is important for patients with vitiligo, because pigmentation abnormalities of the choroid and retina can lead to poor visual acuity or blindness. Lung examination of children with pityriasis alba is useful, because atopy and asthma often coexist.

4. Neurologic examination is necessary in individuals with *café au lait* macules or ash leaf spots. A complete physical examination, searching for underlying malignancy, is necessary in patients with rapid onset of *acanthosis nigricans*, especially if it occurs without weight loss or in the absence of diabetes.

C. Testing

1. Hyperpigmented disorders. Skin scraping of pityriasis versicolor may reveal the characteristic "spaghetti and meatballs" appearance *of Malassezia furfur*; Wood's light illumination often reveals a yellow-gold luminescence (1). More than six *café au lait* macules larger than 0.5 cm in length should prompt an evaluation for neurofibromatosis (1). Evaluate the patient with unexplained *acanthosis nigricans*, diabetes, for underlying tumor, especially gastrointestinal adenocarcinomas.

2. Hypopigmented disorders. Vitiligo can be associated with hyperthyroidism or hypothyroidism, diabetes, pernicious anemia, and other endocrine disorders (2). Have patients with ash leaf macules screened for tuberous sclerosis.

D. Genetics. Examples of the many known genetic defects causing hypomelanosis include piebaldism, vitiligo, tuberous sclerosis complex, pigmentary mosaicism (hypomelanosis of Ito). Some defects resulting in hypermelanosis include *café au lait* macules and neurofibromatosis. Pigmentary defects associated with lentigines include Peutz-Touraine-Jeghers syndrome and freckles (3).

IV. DIAGNOSIS

A. Differential diagnosis. Patients with pigmentary disorders are initially best classified into disorders of excessive pigmentation or hypopigmentation. History is useful in eliciting inciting factors, especially drug- or inflammation-induced changes. Characteristic appearances of the lesions further define the illness. Biopsy of lesions is generally not necessary, although selected lesions may require further testing for underlying diseases.

B. Clinical manifestations. These vary according to the illness.

References
1. Kim N, Pandya A. Pigmentary diseases. *Med Clin North Am* 1998;82(5):1185–1207.
2. Hacker S. Common disorders of pigmentation: when are more than cosmetic cover-ups required? *Postgrad Med* 1996;99(6):177–186.
3. Passeron T, Mantoux F, Ortonne H-P. Genetic disorders of pigmentation. *Clin Dermatol* 2005;23(1):56–67.

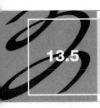

13.5 PRURITUS
James R. Lundy

I. BACKGROUND. Pruritus, a sense of the need to scratch, is an unpleasant cutaneous sensation that has numerous causes. The itch can be either local or generalized and mild or sufficiently annoying to impair sleep.

II. PATHOPHYSIOLOGY

    A. Etiology. Pruritus can be classified into one of four categories on the basis of the origin of the itch: pruritoceptive, neuropathic, neurogenic, or psychogenic (1).

        1. Pruritoceptive itch originates in the skin and is caused by inflammation, dryness, or other skin damage. Examples include aquagenic pruritus, bullous pemphigoid, contact dermatitis, dermatitis herpetiformis, fiberglass dermatitis, insect bites, miliaria (prickly heat), pediculosis (lice), scabies, urticaria (hives), xerosis (dry skin), drug reactions, folliculitis, fungal infections, lichen planus, lichen simplex chronicus, mycosis fungoides, pemphigus foliaceus, pityriasis rosea, pruritic urticarial papules, and plaques of pregnancy, psoriasis, and sunburn.

        2. Neuropathic itch originates in the afferent pathway through a specific disease mechanism. Examples include postherpetic neuralgia, multiple sclerosis, and some brain tumors.

        3. Neurogenic itch originates centrally without any indication of a specific neural lesion. Examples include biliary disease caused by drugs, pregnancy, or cirrhosis; chronic renal failure; hyperthyroid disease; lymphoreticular disorders (Hodgkin's and non-Hodgkin's lymphoma); and visceral malignancy (2).

        4. Psychogenic itch has no origin. This can range from mild cases like the itchiness we all seem to have while discussing a patient with scabies to part of a psychiatric disorder where the patient's arms are scarred by constant clawing at the skin (3).

    B. Epidemiology. Pruritus is a rather common complaint, and it seems unlikely that any individual with intact cognition will not have at least one brief episode of a sensation of needing to scratch an itch during any given year.

III. EVALUATION

    A. History

        1. History of the present illness. Determine the location and duration of the pruritus. For example, scabies involves the interdigital webs, volar wrists, and genitalia, whereas atopic dermatitis occurs in the antecubital or popliteal fossae. Pityriasis rosea typically has a "herald patch" on the trunk. Fungal infections tend to occur in warm, dark, moist body surfaces (e.g., genitalia, feet, and inguinal folds).

2. **Exacerbating and alleviating factors.** Symptoms during or immediately following bathing are distinctive of aquatic pruritus.
3. **Time of year.** Onset or worsening of the itching in winter would suggest xerosis. Are there other individuals or pets with similar symptoms?
4. **Other history.** Are there chronic medical problems such as diabetes mellitus, chronic renal failure, or hepatic disorders? Is the patient taking current medications as well as over-the-counter drugs and herbals?
5. **Social history.** What are the patient's occupation, travel, and bathing habits? Has there been exposure to chemicals, new soaps, or detergents that can cause allergic or irritant dermatitis?
6. **Family history.** Is there a family history of atopy (allergic rhinitis, asthma, and/or atopic dermatitis) or cancer?
7. **Menstrual history.** Remember to ask about potential pregnancy.

B. **Physical examination**
1. **Head, eyes, ears, nose, and throat (HEENT) examination.** Look for scleral icterus as a sign of hepatic disease. Evaluate mucous membranes for signs of allergies.
2. **Lung examination.** Listen for stridor in acute presentations, which is an ominous sign of anaphylaxis.
3. **Gastrointestinal examination.** Palpate for organomegaly and particularly hepatomegaly.
4. **Lymph nodes.** Check for lymphadenopathy of the cervical, axillary, and inguinal regions. The differential diagnosis of lymphadenopathy includes mycosis fungoides, lymphoma, and chronic irritation.
5. **Mental status/psychiatric examination.** Is there any indication of anxiety, drug withdrawal, or psychosis?
6. **Skin examination.** Perform a thorough assessment of the undressed patient with good lighting. Notice skin areas not easily observed or reached by the patient. Pay attention to new, unscratched lesions, because chronically excoriated skin owing to any cause has comparable secondary changes. Are there dermatographism and wheals that characteristically indicate urticaria (hives)? Flat-topped polygonal papules with subtle white lines (Wickham's striae) are distinctive of lichen planus. Silver plaques on an erythematous base with a positive Auspitz sign (punctate bleeding of the scale after blunt scraping) are typical of psoriasis. The application of tangential pressure on superficial, crusting lesions resulting in dislodging the epidermis (Nikolsky's sign) indicates pemphigus foliaceus. Pustular lesions above hair follicles are a sign of folliculitis.

C. **Testing.** If the history and physical examination do not reveal the diagnosis, it may be sensible to try an empiric course of therapy before proceeding with tests.
1. **Skin scraping.** Using a scalpel, cells are scraped away from a recent lesion onto a slide. The slide can then be treated with potassium hydroxide for cellular disruption so that hyphae and budding yeasts may emerge in cases of fungal infection.
2. Skin punch biopsies often yield useful information.
3. **Blood studies.** If a systemic disorder is suspected, include the following in the evaluation: a complete blood count with differential; complete metabolic panel; thyroid-stimulating hormone; human immunodeficiency screen; and serologic test for syphilis.
4. **Other studies may be warranted.** If the history and physical examination imply other systemic diagnoses, additional recommended tests to consider include chest x-ray, fecal occult blood test, urinalysis, serum iron studies, stool for ova and parasites, serum glucose, and serum electrophoresis. Additional diagnostic tests for systemic disorders can be considered to rule out the more obscure diagnoses listed in the preceding text.

D. **Genetics.** A family history of atopy is useful for diagnosis, especially in children. The spectrum of diseases that can cause pruritus is broad, and genetic testing should be pursued only once an illness with a strong genetic basis is strongly suspected.

IV. DIAGNOSIS

   A. Differential diagnosis. The potential causes of pruritus are numerous. The listing included in the section on etiology represents the more frequent and common causes. Unfortunately, sometimes no cause can be found. Often, a trial of treatment is needed on the basis of the most likely cause and diagnosis is honed on the response to treatment.

   B. Clinical manifestations. In addition to itching, secondary changes of the skin are often induced by the patient's scratching. Scarring is common in severe cases.

References

1. VonderPool V. Pruritus. In: Taylor R, ed. *The 10-minute diagnosis manual.* Philadelphia, PA: Lippincott Williams & Wilkins, 2000.
2. Charlesworth E, Beltrani V. Pruritic dermatoses: overview of etiology and therapy. *Am J Med* 2002;113(9A):25s–33s.
3. Yosipovitch G, Greaves M, Schmelz M. Itch. *Lancet* 2003;361:690–694.

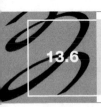

13.6   RASH ACCOMPANIED BY FEVER
Michael L. O'Dell

I. BACKGROUND. Fever with an accompanying rash represents a diagnostic challenge for even the most experienced clinician because this combination of signs may represent either a trivial or a life-threatening illness.

II. PATHOPHYSIOLOGY. A useful way of approaching the differential diagnosis is to distinguish among the various entities that cause fever and illness by the types of rash they commonly cause. Although various febrile diseases may present by more than one type of rash, this grouping allows the clinician to look at fewer causes rather than the entire spectrum of possible causes (1).

   A. Petechial rashes are commonly associated with the following:

     1. Treatable infections, including endocarditis, meningococcemia, gonococcemia, septicemia from any bacteria, rickettsiosis (especially Rocky Mountain spotted fever [RMSF]) (2)

     2. Infectious causes not subject to acute treatment, including enterovirus, dengue fever, hepatitis B virus, rubella, and Epstein-Barr virus (EBV)

     3. Noninfectious causes, including urticaria, thrombocytopenia, scurvy, Henoch-Schönlein disease, hypersensitivity vasculitis, acute rheumatic fever, and systemic lupus erythematosus (SLE)

   B. Maculopapular rashes are commonly associated with the following:

     1. Treatable infections, including typhoid, secondary syphilis, meningococcemia, gonococcemia, mycoplasma, Lyme disease, psittacosis, rickettsiosis (especially RMSF)

     2. Infectious causes not subject to acute treatment, including enterovirus, parvovirus B-19, human herpesvirus 6, rubeola, rubella, adenovirus, EBV, primary human immunodeficiency virus (HIV)–1

     3. Noninfectious causes, including allergy, erythema multiforme, SLE, dermatomyositis, serum sickness, and juvenile rheumatoid arthritis

   C. Vesicobullous rashes are commonly associated with the following:

     1. Treatable infections, including staphylococcal large vesicle impetigo and toxic shock syndrome, gonococcemia, rickettsialpox, varicella-zoster, herpes simplex virus, *Vibrio vulnificus* sepsis, and folliculitis

  2. Infectious causes not subject to acute treatment, including enterovirus, parvovirus B-19, and HIV (although none of these three commonly present in this manner)

  3. Noninfectious causes, including eczema vaccinatum and erythema multiforme bullosum

  D. Diffuse erythematous rashes are commonly associated with the following:

  1. Treatable infections, including streptococcal scarlet fever, toxic shock syndrome, ehrlichiosis (3), *Streptococcus viridans* (chemotherapy patients), *Corynebacterium haemolyticum* pharyngitis, and Kawasaki's disease

  2. Infectious causes not subject to acute treatment, including enteroviral infections

  3. Noninfectious causes of erythema are only rarely associated with fever

  E. Urticaria rashes are commonly associated with the following:

  1. Treatable infections, including mycoplasma and Lyme disease

  2. Infectious causes not subject to acute treatment, including enteroviral infections, adenoviral infections, EBV, HIV, and hepatitis

  3. Noninfectious causes of urticaria only rarely associated with fever

III. EVALUATION

  A. History. History is quite important and should include standard items, such as onset, duration, aggravating factors, relieving factors, and associated symptoms. Additionally, other factors should be considered, such as the following:

  1. Exposure history. Are any other family members or close contacts ill? Is there a history of exposure to brackish water, mosquitoes, or foreign travel?

  2. Are there any underlying illnesses or is there a significant chance of immunologic compromise, such as undiagnosed HIV infection?

  B. Physical examination. The lesions and their distribution should be carefully examined. The rash should be classified as petechial, maculopapular, vesicobullous, erythematous, or urticarial. The distribution of the rash should be noted. For instance, rubella and rubeola generally begin on the face and spread to the trunk, whereas RMSF petechiae tend to occur on the ankles and wrists first.

  1. A general physical examination should be conducted. Areas of particular concern are as follows:

  a. Head, eyes, ears, nose, and throat (HEENT) examination. Koplik's spots are pathognomonic for rubeola. The discovery of a tick lends support to the diagnosis of RMSF. Sinusitis may represent a source for meningococcemia. Pharyngitis in a young adult with diffuse erythema may be due to *C. haemolyticum.* The presence of mucous membrane swelling may indicate early anaphylaxis.

  b. Lung examination. Wheezing on examination, especially in a patient who has recently received medications or contrast dye, can indicate anaphylaxis. Evidence of pneumonia is consistent with psittacosis and mycoplasma.

  c. Cardiac examination. Cardiovascular collapse is associated with meningococcemia and other sepsis. A new murmur may indicate subacute bacterial endocarditis in a patient with subungual or scleral petechiae.

  d. Genital examination. Purulent urethral drainage or evidence of pelvic inflammatory disease supports the consideration of gonorrhea. A chancre supports a diagnosis of syphilis, although palmar lesions often occur well after the healing of the initial chancre.

  e. Joint examination and extremities. A petechial rash near the ankles and wrist is suggestive of RMSF. Evidence of joint swelling supports a diagnosis of meningococcemia or gonococcemia. A maculopapular rash may be seen in juvenile rheumatoid arthritis and other rheumatological conditions as well.

  f. Neurologic examination. Evidence of meningitis supports a diagnosis of meningococcemia. Patients with RMSF may also have meningeal signs.

  C. Testing. Testing should be directed by the suspected illnesses, with life-threatening illnesses being tested for upon reasonable suspicion. A complete blood count is generally useful, although life-threatening sepsis often presents without significant elevation of the white blood cell count. In general, a blood culture should be obtained in all patients with petechial rashes and in those with signs of cardiovascular collapse.

IV. DIAGNOSIS. On the basis of the history and physical examination, the likelihood of various illnesses can be assessed. Patients who appear toxic should be treated as septic until initial laboratory tests and culture results can be evaluated (4).

References
1. Schlossberg D. Fever and rash. *Infect Dis Clin North Am* 1996;10(1):101–110.
2. Drolet BA, Baselga E, Esterly NB. Painful, purpuric plaques in a child with fever. *Arch Dermatol* 1997;133(12):1500–1501.
3. *Am J Med.* Fever, nausea, and rash in a 37-year-old man [clinical conference]. *Am J Med* 1998;104(6):596–601.
4. Dellinger RP. Current therapy for sepsis. *Infect Dis Clin North Am* 1999;13(2):495–509.

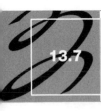

URTICARIA

13.7 *Ray T. Perrine*

I. BACKGROUND. Urticaria is defined by the appearance of wheal, a lesion that is generally circular, made up of reddish lesions, usually surrounded by redness (flare), spongy to the touch, and often changes in appearance rapidly. Lesions are often completely gone within minutes to hours, but other lesions appear in other locations over that same time frame. These are generally intensely pruritic.

II. PATHOPHYSIOLOGY

A. Etiology. Urticaria can be classified as immunologic, nonimmunologic, or idiopathic. *Immunologic urticaria* includes immunoglobulin E (IgE)- and complement-mediated hypersensitivity and physical and contact urticaria. *Nonimmunologic urticaria* includes mast cell release, physical agents, and contact urticaria. A major advance in the understanding of chronic urticaria has been the demonstration of circulating IgG autoantibodies directed against the α-subunit of the high-affinity IgE receptor or anti-IgE autoantibodies in a subset of patients. Approximately 40% to 50% of patients with chronic urticaria are now considered to have chronic autoimmune urticaria, with the remaining having idiopathic chronic urticaria (1).

B. Epidemiology. Urticaria is a common illness, and 15% to 20% of the population is estimated to have one episode of hives during their lifetime. Urticaria occurs most frequently between 20 and 40 years of age, and it is more common in women than men. There are two primary forms of urticaria: acute and chronic. Acute urticaria lesions last <6 weeks. Chronic urticaria lasts >6 weeks. Only 50% of the cases of chronic urticaria are likely to remit within 1 year, and up to 40% of the cases that last >6 months are likely to persist for 10 years or more.

III. EVALUATION

A. History

1. Food or drug exposures are common causes of urticaria. Certain systemic diseases can cause urticaria, including but not limited to connective tissue diseases, endocrine disorders, and neoplastic diseases. Insect stings and bites are another common cause of urticaria. Does anything specific trigger the rash? Is it localized or systemic? Does it respond to any treatment?

2. Symptom chronology is also important. When does urticaria occur? How long does it last? Is it in association with physical trauma? Has the patient been on any medication that has helped relieve symptoms (e.g., antihistamines)?

B. Physical examination. A complete physical examination is required to rule out infection or other systemic diseases. The cardinal features of urticaria that distinguish it from any other type of inflammatory eruption are the repeated occurrence of short-lived cutaneous wheals and the accompanying redness and itching. Wheals are lesions ranging from a few millimeters to several centimeters in diameter, although if they run together and become confluent, much larger plaques may occur. If angioedema is present, it can last for several days. The skin returns to normal once the wheal has disappeared.

C. **Testing**

1. Blood studies are generally not helpful in confirming the diagnosis. Studies should be performed when there is concern about the diagnosis or atypical features. Measurement of complete blood count, erythrocyte sedimentation rate, serum chemistry values, complement C3 and C4, and thyrotropin level should be considered to exclude systemic disease. In some cases, tests for antinuclear antibodies and hepatitis are also necessary (2).

2. Specific allergy or provocative tests (e.g., additive challenge, exercise, pressure, cold) may be required to further clarify the diagnosis. Skin tests for food and latex sensitivities are often indicated, especially in chronic urticaria.

3. Punch biopsy of an urticarial lesion often provides useful information.

4. Diagnostic imaging studies, such as chest x-ray, computed tomography, sinus, and dental films may help rule out underlying cancer and infection.

D. **Genetics.** It is useful to ask whether there are any members of the family who suffer from a connective tissue disorder? There is a marked increase in the incidence of chronic urticaria in first-degree relatives (3). Do any complement disorders occur in the family, such as hereditary angioedema? Is there a family history of atopy?

IV. **DIAGNOSIS**

A. **Differential diagnosis.** The lesions of urticaria are generally distinctive. The differential diagnosis usually focuses on underlying causes. These include cancer, endocrine disorders, connective tissue diseases, and infections. The most significant factors in diagnosing acute urticaria are the history and physical examination. Facts must be obtained regarding food or drug ingestion, insect stings, current infections, or physical triggers such as cold, heat, or exercise. At present, demonstration of circulating IgG autoantibodies is directed against the α-subunit of the high-affinity IgE receptor or anti-IgE autoantibodies in a subset of patients; the testing lacks applicability clinically. Approximately 30% to 40% of patients with chronic urticaria have the anti-FceRIa autoantibodies and 10% have anti-IgE autoantibodies (4).

B. **Clinical manifestations.** Although the lesions of urticaria are distinctive, the various underlying conditions that trigger the skin's response are numerous and varied in their clinical manifestations. Virtually all patients with urticaria complain of pruritus in addition to the rash.

References

1. Kaplan AP. Chronic urticaria: pathogenesis and treatment. *J Allergy Clin Immunol* 2004;114(3):465–474.
2. Kaplan AP. Chronic urticaria and angioedema. *N Engl J Med* 2002;346(3):175–179.
3. Riboldi P, Asero R, Tedeschi A, et al. Chronic urticaria: new immunologic aspects. *Isr Med Assoc J* 2002;4(11suppl):872–873.
4. Greaves M. Chronic urticaria. *J Allergy Clin Immunol* 2000;105(4):664–672.

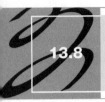

VESICULAR AND BULLOUS ERUPTIONS
Michael L. O'Dell

13.8

I. **BACKGROUND.** Vesicular and bullous eruptions (VBLs) are blistering illnesses.

II. **PATHOPHYSIOLOGY**

A. **Etiology.** VBLs occur as a result of bacteria, viruses, systemic illnesses (e.g., allergic vasculitis), or injury (especially sun or heat exposure). Special precipitators can lead to VBL. Sunlight can precipitate recurrent herpes simplex (HS) (as can wind, menses, dry skin, smoking, drinking alcohol, lack of sleep, and fever). Many drugs or alcohol can trigger porphyria cutanea tarda (PCT) (1). Drug ingestion can also precipitate allergic vasculitis, Stevens-Johnson syndrome (SJS)/toxic epidermal necrolysis (TEN), and PCT. Contact with skin precipitates dermatitis due to *Rhus*, nickel, and perfume.

B. **Epidemiology**

1. In patients of certain ages, particular diagnoses should be considered:
   a. **Newborns.** Epidermolysis bullosa, pemphigus neonatorum, and syphilitic pemphigus
   b. **Children.** Varicella (if unimmunized), primary HS, hand, foot, and mouth (HFM) disease, and bullous impetigo (BI)
   c. **Adults.** Recurrent HS, PCT, pemphigus vulgaris (PV), dyshidrotic eczema (DE), dermatitis herpetiformis (DH), linear immunoglobulin A (LIgA) disease
   d. **Elderly.** Bullous pemphigoid (BP) and herpes zoster (HZ)
2. In patients of any age, allergic contact dermatitis, allergic vasculitis, SJS/TEN, insect bites, and second-degree burns should be considered.
3. There is seasonal variation as well.
   a. **Fall and winter.** Varicella, HFM, and primary HS are often seen in epidemics after gatherings of children, such as return to school.
   b. **Spring and summer.** BI (due to staphylococcal infection) and DE (increased sweating of hands and feet). Contact dermatitis due to *Rhus* species parallels yard work.

III. **EVALUATION**

A. **History**

1. **Pain or pruritus.** Itching is common, especially in contact dermatitis. Pain is common before, during, and after the eruption of HZ.
2. **Onset and duration.** Many VBLs occur acutely without preceding episodes: SJS/TEN, varicella, BI, HZ, allergic vasculitis, HFM, and PV. Some diseases are chronic with exacerbations, such as DH, DE, BP, epidermolysis bullosa, and PCT. Acute contact dermatitis and HS often recur in episodes. DH is more common in patients with gluten-sensitive enteropathy (2).

B. **Physical examination**

1. **Appearance.** In patients who look sick, toxic, or ill, consider possible diagnoses of SJS/TEN, PV, or primary HS (particularly in toddlers).
2. **Presence of fever.** Patients with varicella and HFM may have low-grade fever. Patients with SJS/TEN or primary HS may have preceding and/or concurrent fever.
3. **Presence of oral lesions.** Oral lesions tend to signify more serious consequences and more significant illness, such as SJS/TEN, PV, TEN, varicella, and HFM. The skin lesions of PV may appear months after the onset of oral lesions (2).
4. **Characteristics of the lesions.** Vesicles are <1 cm; bullae are >1 cm. The fluid in the lesion may be clear, purulent, or hemorrhagic. Rupture of VBLs may lead to erosions, ulcers, and/or crusts. Vesicular diseases may represent HS,

varicella, HZ, contact dermatitis, DE, hemorrhagic vasculitis, HFM, Kaposi's varocelliform eruption (KVE), and DH. Bullous diseases are generally PV, BP, BI, PCT, SJS/TEN, TEN, and epidermolysis bullosa. There is considerable overlap in lesion size in some diseases, but the finding of larger bullae tends to be confined to the group listed as bullous diseases. Some lesions are distinctive. The bullae of BI are thin, fragile, short lived, and easily ruptured, leaving a thin, varnishlike often honey-colored crust with occasionally a delicate remnant of the blister roof at its rim. Contact dermatitis lesions are often excoriated by the time the patient presents because of intense pruritus. Varicella is characterized by lesions in various stages—the newest ones vesicular ("dew drop on a rose petal"), the older ones becoming purulent, then crusting over. The bullae of BP are large and tense. Bullae of PV are flaccid and easily ruptured, leaving large denuded, bleeding, and weeping erosions. The lesions of PCT, DH, and allergic vasculitis may be hemorrhagic and secondarily crusted. Umbilication is generally characteristic of a viral etiology—HS, HZ, varicella, and KVE. Chronic urticarial lesions progressing to bullae often signal BP. In TEN, light pressure on normal appearing skin may cause it to wrinkle, slide laterally, and separate from the dermis (Nikolsky's sign).

5. **Location and distribution of the lesions**
   a. **Localized.** Lesions in sun-exposed areas are often due to contact dermatitis, insect bites, or PCT. Contact dermatitis is localized to the area of contact. Allergic vasculitis lesions are dependent. HFM has hand, foot, and mouth lesions. DH occurs primarily on the shoulders, buttocks, elbows, and posterior upper back. HZ follows a sensory (cutaneous) dermatome which does not cross the midline. DE involves the lateral aspects of the fingers, palms, and soles. KVE occurs at sites of preexisting dermatitis, especially areas of atopic dermatitis. LIgA disease commonly occurs in the genital area, with up to 50% of cases also having oral lesions (2).
   b. **Generalized** (some diseases begin in one area and then become generalized). Varicella begins on the trunk or head, and successive crops erupt more distally. SJS/TEN often begins in the oral cavity, groin, or axilla. PV may also begin in the oral cavity. BP occurs mostly in the flexor surfaces, axilla, and groin but can be generalized.

C. **Testing**
   1. **The Tzanck smear** may be used to diagnose viral dermatoses. The smear may be obtained by the following procedure: unroof an early intact vesicle, one without infection or trauma. Scrape the base of the lesions lightly with a scalpel. Smear the material on the scalpel blade onto a clean glass slide. Air-dry the smear and fix and follow by stain with Wright or Giemsa. The test is positive if multinucleated giant cells are noted (3).
   2. **Biopsy** of the edge of the blister and subsequent immunofluorescent staining is helpful for diagnosing PV, BP, and SJS/TEN (4).

D. **Genetics.** Some bullous or vesicular illnesses have a genetic basis, especially PCT (autosomal dominant illness, generally with incomplete penetrance).

IV. **DIAGNOSIS**
   A. **Differential diagnosis.** Diagnosis is reached considering the age of the patient, the location of the lesions, whether the lesions are bullous or vesicular, and whether the patient appears toxic.
   B. **Clinical manifestations.** These vary widely according to the underlying disease or agent.

References

1. Robson KJ, Piette WW. Cutaneous manifestations of systemic diseases. *Med Clin North Am* 1998;82(6):1359–1379, vi–vii.
2. Bickle KM, Roark TR, Hsu SH. Autoimmune bullous dermatoses: a review. *Am Fam Physician* 2002;65(9):1861–1870.
3. Brodell RT, Helms SE, Devine M. Office dermatologic testing: the Tzanck preparation. *Am Fam Physician* 1991;44(3):857–860.
4. Gellis SE. Bullous diseases of childhood. *Dermatol Clin* 1986;4(1):89–98.

Endocrine and Metabolic Problems

Richard D. Blondell

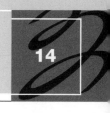

14

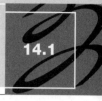

DIABETES MELLITUS

J. Steven Cramer and Andrea Manyon

14.1

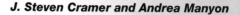

I. BACKGROUND. Diabetes mellitus (DM) is a group of metabolic diseases (type 1, type 2, gestational, and "others"). It is characterized by hyperglycemia resulting from defects in insulin secretion (type 1), insulin action (type 2), or both (1).

II. PATHOPHYSIOLOGY

  A. Etiology

    1. Type 1 diabetes (immune-mediated insulin deficiency). Type 1 DM is thought to be caused by a gradual autoimmune destruction of pancreatic β cells, leading to deficiency in the production of insulin. Autoantibodies to islet cells, insulin, glutamic acid decarboxylase, and tyrosine phosphatases are seen in 85% to 90% of these patients.

    2. Type 2 diabetes (insulin resistance). The hallmark of type 2 DM is insulin resistance with a relative, rather than absolute, insulin deficiency. Risk factors for type 2 DM include obesity (especially with a central distribution), lack of physical activity, increasing age, a family history of type 2 DM, and prior gestational diabetes.

  B. Epidemiology. Approximately 18.2 million people in the United States have DM and of these, 5.2 million are undiagnosed (2). The lifetime risk of developing diabetes for those born in 2000 is estimated to be 32.8% for men and 38.5% for women (3). Type 1 DM accounts for 5% to 10% of patients with diabetes and its prevalence in people younger than 20 years of age is approximately 1 in 400. Type 1 DM has no seasonal variation and gender differences are not clinically significant. Type 2 DM accounts for 90% to 95% of all those with diabetes. Its prevalence varies among different racial and ethnic groups (African-American: 11.4%, Latino: 8.2%, and Native American: 14.9%) (2). The incidence of type 2 DM in children and adolescents appears to be increasing. In one study of adolescents, the incidence rose from 0.7/100,000 per year in 1982 to 7.2/100,000 per year in 1994 (4).

III. EVALUATION

  A. History. The initial presentation of DM can vary. Both type 1 and type 2 can present with the classic symptoms of polyuria, polydipsia, and unexplained weight loss.

    1. Type 1 diabetes. Patients with type 1 DM usually present as children or young adults, but the disease can occur at any age. The emergence of symptoms varies, depending on the rate of β cell destruction. Serum ketoacidosis is often the first manifestation of the disease in younger patients in whom β cell destruction is more rapid and may present with life-threatening ketoacidosis as the first manifestation of the disease. Modest elevations in fasting hyperglycemia can rapidly change to severe hyperglycemia or ketoacidosis in the face of infection or other stress. Enuresis may be a clue for polyuria in a child who was previously toilet trained. Lethargy, weakness, and weight loss are other common features.

    2. Type 2 diabetes. Patients with type 2 DM traditionally present after 40 years of age. The diagnosis is often made in an asymptomatic patient as a result of routine blood tests that reveal an elevation of plasma glucose. Other patients may present with symptoms of hyperglycemia such as extreme hunger, fatigue, and irritability. The patient may have a history of recurrent skin infections or persistent monilial vulvovaginitis. Minor skin infections are often slow to heal. Other common symptoms include altered sensation in the extremities, nocturia, erectile dysfunction, and visual disturbances

319

(Chapters 4.6, 5.1, 10.3, and 10.5). The use of glucocorticoids, β-adrenergic agonists, or thiazide diuretics can precipitate symptoms and unmask latent type 2 DM.

B. Physical examination. Patients often present with similar physical findings in both type 1 and type 2 DM, owing to hyperglycemia. In type 1 DM, the young child may fail to grow or gain weight. Others may appear ill and lethargic with signs of dehydration (tachycardia, hypotension, and dry mucous membranes with reduced skin turgor). In ketosis, an acetone or fruity odor may be noted on the patient's breath. The patient with type 2 DM tends to be obese (especially central obesity) and may appear fatigued and flushed with muscle weakness or blurry vision. Monilial infections may be found in the vagina and intertriginous regions. The neurologic examination in previously undiagnosed advanced cases may reveal extremities with altered sensation or frank diabetic foot ulcers.

C. Testing. A "casual" plasma blood glucose level is obtained at any time of the day without regard to the time of the last meal and a "fasting" level is obtained after a fast of at least 8 hours. The American Diabetes Association (ADA) diagnostic criteria for diabetes are either symptoms of diabetes and a casual plasma glucose ≥200 mg/dL (11.1 mmol/L) or a fasting plasma glucose ≥126 mg/dL (7.0 mmol/L), or a plasma glucose ≥200 mg/dL (11.1 mmol/L) 2 hours after an oral glucose load (75 g) as described by the World Health Organization (5). If the only criterion is hyperglycemia, confirmation should be made by repeat testing on a different day. The ADA also recommends screening individuals older than 45 years of age with a body mass index ≥25 kg/m^2 or those with risk factors such as inactivity, a family history, a personal history of gestational diabetes, or hypertension (1).

D. Genetics. Type 1 DM has strong human leukocyte antigen (HLA) associations and linkages to the *DQA* and *DQB* genes and is influenced by the *DRB* genes (1). Type 2 DM is associated with a family history of the disease and is associated with a high risk for gestational diabetes in women. These predispositions have not yet been linked with any specific genetic pattern.

IV. DIAGNOSIS

A. Clinical manifestations. The presence of polyuria, polydipsia, weight loss, and hyperglycemia with ketosis is sufficient to establish the diagnosis of type 1 DM. If the diagnosis of type 1 DM is not clear, a low or absent C-peptide level may help confirm the diagnosis. The key to the diagnosis of type 2 DM is the detection of hyperglycemia in the face of the classic risk factors.

B. Differential diagnosis. Assigning a type of diabetes to an individual begins with a clear understanding of the epidemiology and an awareness of the patient's circumstances. Clinicians must first account for the age of the patient, body habitus, risks associated with past medical history (as with gestational diabetes), and family history.

 1. Type 1 diabetes. Not all children with hyperglycemia have diabetes. Some children with a severe illness (e.g., severe dehydration from diarrhea or asthma treated with corticosteroids) may have elevated serum glucose and ketosis. An elevated HbA$_{IC}$ can provide a strong circumstantial case for the diagnosis of DM but is not recommended as a screening test because of the associated costs.

 2. Type 2 diabetes. The diagnosis can be made according to the ADA criteria. "Prediabetic" patients have impaired glucose tolerance with a fasting plasma glucose of 100 to 125 mg/dL (5.6–6.9 mmol/L) (1). Lifestyle modification for this group is paramount and includes exercise and a suggested weight loss of 5% to 10%.

References

1. American Diabetes Association Position Statement. Diagnosis and classification of diabetes mellitus. *Diabetes Care* 2005;28(Suppl 1):S37–S42.
2. Centers for Disease Control and Prevention. *National diabetes fact sheet: general information and national estimates on diabetes in the United States, 2000.* CDC [Internet]. Available at: www.cdc.gov/diabetes/pubs/ndfs.pdf, accessed on October 12, 2003.

3. Venkat Narayan KM. Lifetime risk for diabetes mellitus in the United States. *JAMA* 2003;290:1884–1890.
4. Pinhas-Hamiel O, Dolan LM, Daniels SR, et al. Increased incidence of non-insulin-dependent diabetes mellitus among adolescents. *J Pediatr* 1996;128:608–615.
5. World Health Organization. *Laboratory diagnosis and monitoring of diabetes.* World Health Organization. Available at: http://whqlibdoc.who.int/hq/2002/9241590483.pdf, accessed on June 1, 2005

GYNECOMASTIA
Charles M. Kodner

14.2

I. **BACKGROUND.** Gynecomastia is the palpable enlargement of the breast tissue in men. There are three peak age-groups for presentation, corresponding to the common physiologic causes of breast enlargement. After the neonatal period, the most common causes of gynecomastia are idiopathic (25%), pubertal factors (25%), medications (10%–20%), cirrhosis or malnutrition (8%), or primary hypogonadism (8%) (1).

II. **PATHOPHYSIOLOGY.** Gynecomastia is caused by a relative increase of estrogen over androgen, usually from the aromatization of testosterone and androstenedione to estradiol.

  A. **Etiology.** Most cases of gynecomastia represent a transient, physiologic imbalance between circulating estrogens and androgens.

   1. Normal physiologic conditions are associated with transient gynecomastia. In the neonatal period, transplacental estrogen causes transient breast tissue enlargement in most newborns; this may be associated with nipple discharge and typically resolves over 3 to 4 weeks. No additional evaluation is necessary. During puberty, hormonal changes and breast tissue proliferation cause transient gynecomastia in adolescent boys; this may be asymmetric and tender. The condition usually resolves within 1 year, but may persist for up to 2 years. Older men (50–80 years of age) may have palpable breast tissue enlargement that is often physiologic due to a relative increase in body fat and increased aromatization of estrogen precursors, but medication effects or medical disorders should be considered (2).

   2. Medications may cause gynecomastia. Examples include alcohol, marijuana, estrogens, digitoxin, cimetidine, spironolactone, anabolic steroids, finasteride, ketoconazole, and antiandrogens (1). Prostate cancer may be associated with gynecomastia, because the treatment with orchiectomy, estrogens, or antiandrogens may cause gynecomastia as a side effect.

   3. Medical disorders (renal failure, liver disease, or starvation/malnutrition) may be associated with gynecomastia. Some cancers (lung, liver, and kidney) may produce ectopic human chorionic gonadotropin (HCG), which stimulates aromatase activity, causing gynecomastia.

   4. Endocrine disorders (hyperthyroidism and primary testicular failure) may also be associated with gynecomastia.

  B. **Epidemiology.** The overall prevalence of palpable gynecomastia is approximately 36% and may be up to 48% in boys 10 to 15 years of age or 57% in men older than 44 years of age (3). Obesity is a risk factor for gynecomastia, with up to 80% of those with a body mass index over 25 kg/m^2 affected.

III. **EVALUATION.** Gynecomastia that is persistent or symptomatic or presents outside the expected age ranges may represent a pathologic process requiring diagnostic evaluation.

  A. **History.** The history should be directed toward identifying symptoms suggestive of breast cancer or an underlying endocrine disorder and any specific causative factors (as described in the preceding text). Persistent or rapid breast tissue enlargement may necessitate further evaluation if no diagnosis is apparent. Mild pain or tenderness by itself does not indicate a concerning underlying cause.

B. Physical examination. A focused physical examination should exclude cancer of the breast or testes, as well as some endocrine disorders. The physical examination should also differentiate true gynecomastia from pseudogynecomastia. The breast is grasped between thumb and forefinger and the digits are moved toward the nipple; a firm, rubbery, mobile, disk-shaped mass of tissue beneath the nipple indicates true breast tissue enlargement, rather than softer, less-defined breast enlargement due to adipose tissue deposition (1). The testicles should be examined carefully. Congenital anorchia is a rare cause of gynecomastia. Small bilateral testes suggest gonadal failure. Testicular atrophy may be due to mumps, leprosy, or other granulomatous disorders (2). Asymmetry or a palpable mass suggests testicular cancer.

C. Testing. If pathology is suspected, additional testing may be needed. Tests of liver, kidney, and thyroid function should be assessed if clinically indicated. If an underlying endocrine disorder is suspected, serum HCG, testosterone, estradiol, and luteinizing hormone (LH) should be checked (1). A high LH and a normal-to-low testosterone indicate testicular insufficiency. Elevated estradiol, with small firm testes, behavioral abnormalities or mental retardation, and an arm span greater than the height should prompt a diagnostic chromosome analysis for possible Klinefelter's syndrome. A high LH and high testosterone suggest an androgen resistance syndrome. A high HCG level may indicate an HCG-secreting tumor of the lung, stomach, liver, or kidney, or a testicular or extragonadal germ cell tumor (2). An elevated HCG should prompt a search for one of these cancers, by chest x-ray, abdominal computed tomography, and detailed physical examination. Mammography has recently been found to be accurate in distinguishing between malignant and benign male breast disease and may be useful in limiting the need for biopsy if physical examination and mammography suggest benign disease (4). Fine needle aspiration of a mass may be considered to diagnose breast cancer.

D. Genetics. Klinefelter's syndrome increases the risk of breast cancer, but other causes of gynecomastia are not associated with an increased risk of breast cancer (1).

IV. DIAGNOSIS

A. Differential diagnosis. If true gynecomastia appears in the expected age ranges, it is likely to be physiologic, and only reassurance and observation over 1 to 2 years are necessary before specific treatment is initiated. The medical history at the time of presentation should screen for medical or endocrine disorders that suggest a diagnosis and identify medications that may be the cause of gynecomastia. The physical examination focuses on ruling out breast cancer and testicular examination, and screening for endocrine disorders. If these steps are unrevealing, no related diagnosis is suggested, and the patient is otherwise asymptomatic, reassure and observe for 1 to 2 years, expecting that the condition will resolve spontaneously.

Pseudogynecomastia can be detected by the typical findings on physical examination or the presence of obesity, which is usually adequate to identify true breast tissue enlargement against enlargement of the male breasts due to adipose tissue in obese men.

Breast cancer presents as a unilateral, eccentric mass that is hard or firm, fixed to underlying tissue, or associated with overlying skin dimpling, nipple discharge or retraction, or axillary lymphadenopathy. A biopsy is indicated.

B. Clinical manifestations. Gynecomastia is bilateral in more than 50% of affected men, but it may be unilateral or symmetric. It presents as a firm, mobile, or rubbery mass that may be slightly tender and forms a symmetrical mound around the nipple. Most patients with normal physiologic gynecomastia can be readily identified, and no further evaluation is required. If the condition does not resolve with observation, if it is progressive or of rapid onset, or if history and examination suggest a general medical disorder, then an underlying pathologic process should be sought.

References

1. Braunstein GD. Gynecomastia. *N Engl J Med* 1993;328:490–495.
2. Frantz AG, Wilson JD. Disorders of breasts in men. In: Wilson JD, Foster DW, eds. *Williams textbook of endocrinology*, 9th ed. Philadelphia, PA: WB Saunders Company, 1998:885–900.
3. Wise GJ. Male breast disease. *J Am Coll Surg* 2005;200:255–269.
4. Evans GFF. The diagnostic accuracy of mammography in the evaluation of male breast disease. *Am J Surg* 2001;181:96–100.

HIRSUTISM

Richard D. Blondell and Vinod R. Patel

14.3

I. **BACKGROUND.** Hirsutism is excessive male-pattern hair growth in women of reproductive age. Pathologic causes of hirsutism may be associated with *virilization* (the development of other secondary male sex characteristics) or *defeminization* (the loss of secondary female sex characteristics).

II. **PATHOPHYSIOLOGY**
   A. **Etiology.** Hirsutism may be idiopathic or due to exogenous androgens, increased production of androgens by the ovaries or adrenal glands, or increased hair follicle sensitivity to androgens. Common causes are summarized in Table 14.3.1.
   1. **Common causes.** The most common causes of hirsutism are polycystic ovary syndrome (PCOS) and idiopathic forms (1). Less common causes include hyperandrogenic insulin-resistant acanthosis nigricans (HAIRAN) and various forms of 21-hydroxylase deficient adrenal hyperplasia.
   2. **Other causes.** Androgen-secreting tumors of the ovaries (Sertoli-Leydig cell tumors, granulosa-theca cell tumors, and hilus-cell tumors), adrenal glands, or lungs are not common, even among referral populations (1). Hirsutism may be observed among patients who have hypothyroidism, hyperprolactinemia, or Cushing's syndrome. Mild hirsutism may be constitutional (as a variant of normal menopause, pregnancy, or obesity).
   B. **Epidemiology.** The prevalence of hirsutism depends on the methods used to define it and the population studied, but it is estimated to affect between 4% and 8% of women in their childbearing years (2, 3). Approximately 50% of women with minimal unwanted hair growth have an androgen excess disorder (2).

III. **EVALUATION**
   A. **History.** The history of hirsutism (age at onset, rate of progression) and the menstrual history (age at menarche, regularity of menstrual cycles) may provide important diagnostic clues. Infertility and weight gain suggest PCOS. Certain medications such as danazol and oral contraceptives that contain androgenic progestins (e.g., levonorgestrel) can cause hirsutism. Highly competitive women athletes may abuse anabolic steroids. Some forms of hirsutism are familial.
   B. **Physical examination.** During examination, the height and weight should be documented and the body mass index calculated. The distribution of hair growth on nine areas of the body (upper lip, chin, chest, abdomen, superior pubic triangle, upper arms, thighs, upper back, and buttocks) are used to quantify hirsutism (3). Androgen excess may cause acne. Signs of virilization (male-pattern balding, deepening of the voice, increased muscle mass, and clitoromegaly) or defeminization (loss of breast tissue, vaginal atrophy) should be noted. Some diagnoses may be suggested by other physical findings: Cushing's syndrome (truncal obesity, buffalo

TABLE 14.3.1   The Common Causes of Hirsutism

Diagnosis	Frequency[a] (%)	Clinical manifestations	Laboratory tests
Polycystic ovarian syndrome	82	Abnormal menses, infertility, obesity, diabetes	Elevated androgens, ultrasound showing multiple ovarian cysts
Idiopathic hirsutism	12	Normal menses and normal examination	Normal serum progesterone in luteal phase (20–24 d)
Normal androgen levels	6.8		
Elevated androgen levels	4.7		
Hyperandrogenic insulin-resistant acanthosis nigricans	3	Family history of diabetes, obesity, brown velvety skin patches	Elevated insulin levels
Late-onset 21-hydroxylase deficient nonclassic adrenal hyperplasia	2	Family history, virilization, defeminization	Elevated 17 α-hydroxyprogesterone
Congenital 21-hydroxylase deficient adrenal hyperplasia	1	Congenital virilization	Elevated 17 α-hydroxyprogesterone
Androgen-secreting tumor	<1	Rapid-onset hirsutism, virilization	Diagnostic images demonstrating a tumor
All other causes	<2	See text	See text

[a]Frequency data from Azziz R, Sanchez ES, Knochenhauer C, et al. Androgen excess in women: experience with over 1,000 consecutive patients. *J Clin Endocrinol Metab* 2004;89:453–462.

hump), hyperprolactinemia (galactorrhea), HAIRAN (velvety hyperpigmentation of the axilla, groin, neck, or umbilicus), and ovarian tumor (pelvic mass).

C. Testing. If the patient's history and physical examination are unremarkable, serum levels of total testosterone and dehydroepiandrosterone sulfate (DHEA-S) can be obtained to exclude an androgen-producing tumor. Elevated levels of androgens over twice the normal values should prompt an evaluation for an ovarian or adrenal tumor. High-resolution pelvic ultrasonography with a transvaginal probe can identify ovarian follicles and cysts as small as 3 to 5 mm in diameter. Basal body temperature charts and serum progesterone levels in the luteal phase (20–24 days) of the menstrual cycle can be used to document the normal ovarian function of women who are thought to have idiopathic hirsutism. A clinical suspicion of hypothyroidism, hyperprolactinemia, or Cushing's disease requires confirmatory testing. Referral and further diagnostic testing may be warranted for patients with early onset, severe, or rapidly progressive hirsutism.

D. Genetics. A familial pattern can be associated with idiopathic hirsutism, PCOS, HAIRAN, and late-onset nonclassic congenital adrenal hyperplasia, which is a disorder particularly associated with Ashkenazi Jewish women.

IV. DIAGNOSIS

A. Differential diagnosis. Most hirsute women have either PCOS or idiopathic hirsutism. The challenge is to identify the small number of women who have some other cause.

1. Hirsutism. PCOS and idiopathic hirsutism are diagnoses of exclusion. PCOS can be diagnosed if two of the following are present: oligo-ovulation or anovulation (usually manifested as oligomenorrhea or amenorrhea), elevated levels of androgens or signs of androgen excess (hyperandrogenism), and polycystic ovaries as defined by ultrasonography (4). Therefore, polycystic ovaries are not always present in PCOS and their presence alone does not establish the diagnosis.

2. Hypertrichosis. This condition, which may be familial, is described as excessive growth of androgen-independent hair (5). It is usually vellus and prominent in nonsexual areas. Causes include hypothyroidism, anorexia nervosa, malnutrition, porphyria, dermatomyositis, and medications (phenytoin, penicillamine, diazoxide, minoxidil, or cyclosporine).

B. Clinical manifestations. Several clinical findings suggest one of the rare and more serious causes of hirsutism: (1) abrupt onset, short duration (typically <1 year), or progressive worsening of hirsutism; (2) onset in the third decade of life or later, rather than near puberty; (3) symptoms or signs of virilization or defeminization; (4) more severe hirsutism (ovarian hyperthecosis); (5) symptoms and signs of cortisol excess, such as obesity, hypertension, striae, that suggest the presence of Cushing's syndrome; and (6) moderately elevated (or higher) serum androgen concentrations. Serum testosterone values above 150 ng/dL (5.2 nmol/L), serum-free testosterone values above 2 ng/dL (0.07 nmol/L), or DHEA-S values greater than 700 µg/dL (13.6 µmol/L) in young women raise the possibility of an androgen-secreting tumor.

References

1. Azziz R, Sanchez LA, Knochenhauer ES, et al. Androgen excess in women: experience with over 1000 consecutive patients. *J Clin Endocrinol Metab* 2004;89:453–462.
2. Souter I, Sanchez LA, Perez M, et al. The prevalence of androgen excess among patients with minimal unwanted hair growth. *Am J Obstet Gynecol* 2004;191:1914–1920.
3. Azziz R. The evaluation and management of hirsutism. *Obstet Gynecol* 2003;101: 995–1007.
4. Ehrmann DA. Polycystic ovary syndrome. *N Engl J Med* 2005;352:1223–1236.
5. Wendelin DS, Pope DN, Mallory SB. Hypertrichosis. *J Am Acad Dermatol* 2003;48: 161–179.

HYPOTHYROIDISM

14.4

Richard W. Pretorius and Stephen F. Wheeler

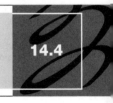

I. BACKGROUND.
Hypothyroidism is the clinical syndrome resulting from thyroid hormone deficiency.

II. PATHOPHYSIOLOGY.
Thyrotropin-releasing hormone, secreted by the hypothalamus, stimulates the anterior pituitary to produce the thyroid-stimulating hormone (TSH), which mediates the production of thyroxine (T_4).

A. Etiology. *Primary hypothyroidism* is the result of thyroid gland failure (1). The most common cause is autoimmune thyroiditis, or Hashimoto's disease, which results from the gradual destruction of the thyroid by abnormal T cells. Iatrogenic hypothyroidism from either radioactive iodine or surgery is the next most common cause. Goitrous hypothyroidism from iodine deficiency is rare in the United States since the introduction of iodized salt. *Secondary* or *tertiary hypothyroidism* is caused by pituitary or hypothalamic disease, respectively. The most common cause of secondary hypothyroidism is a pituitary tumor; other common causes include pituitary surgery, cranial radiation therapy, postpartum hemorrhage (Sheehan's syndrome), head trauma, granulomatous diseases, metastatic disease (breast, lung, colon, and prostate), and infectious diseases (tuberculosis and others). Multiple endocrine end-organ failure caused by the autoimmune destruction of endocrine glands (Schmidt's syndrome) is a rare cause of primary hypothyroidism that mimics secondary disease.

B. Epidemiology. Overt hypothyroidism is found in 0.5% of middle-aged women between 40 and 60 years of age, increasing to 2% in women older than 70 years of age (2). It is slightly less common among men, Hispanics, and blacks.

III. EVALUATION

A. History. Symptoms generally correspond directly to the duration and severity of disease.

   1. The probability of thyroid disease is directly related to the number of typical symptoms manifested by the patient, including weakness, lethargy, fatigue, skin changes (dry, coarse, cold, yellow), coarseness or loss of hair, cold intolerance, weight gain, constipation, memory or concentration impairment, depression, hoarseness, goiter, menstrual abnormalities (most commonly menorrhagia), and fluid infiltration of tissues (eyelids, face, periphery). Secondary or tertiary hypothyroidism is suggested by loss of axillary or pubic hair, headaches, visual field defects, amenorrhea, galactorrhea, and symptoms of postural hypotension.

   2. Patients with an increased risk include women 4 to 8 weeks postpartum, women older than 50 years of age, patients with immunologically mediated diseases (diabetes mellitus type 1, pernicious anemia, vitiligo, Addison's disease, and rheumatoid arthritis), and persons with a family history of thyroid disease.

B. Physical examination

   1. Observation. A welcoming handshake may reveal cold skin and further observations uncover altered affect, hoarseness, facial or eyelid edema, hair loss (scalp and eyebrows), and physical or mental slowing.

   2. General examination. Vital sign abnormalities commonly include weight gain, diastolic hypertension, and bradycardia. A systematic head-to-toe examination is helpful, because all major organ systems are affected by thyroid hormone deficiency. The heart may be enlarged owing to either dilation or pericardial effusion, which may be indicated by a cardiac rub or distant heart sounds. Adynamic ileus can cause constipation and abdominal distention and, rarely, can result in megacolon or intestinal obstruction. Even carpal tunnel syndrome can occur from the generalized edema owing to tissue glycosaminoglycan accumulation and reduced lymphatic clearance of interstitial proteins. Hyporeflexia may be present in addition to a prolonged relaxation phase of the deep tendon reflexes, creating the characteristic "hung-up reflex." Secondary or tertiary disease is suggested by orthostatic hypotension, visual field defects, and galactorrhea.

   3. Thyroid examination. The thyroid is palpated by using the fingers or thumbs while standing in front of or behind the patient. If felt between the cricoid cartilage and the suprasternal notch, the thyroid isthmus can be used to help locate the gland. The location, size, consistency, mobility, and tenderness of any nodules should be noted. Having the patient swallow during both inspection and palpation causes the thyroid to move and aids in developing a three-dimensional impression of gland's shape and size.

C. Testing. The most useful test for the diagnosis of thyroid disease is an elevated TSH of >10 mIU/L, which has a high sensitivity (98%) and specificity (92%) in a referral office. Its positive predictive value, however, is low when used for screening primary care populations. A free T_4, or occasionally the much more expensive free T_3, does not need to be ordered routinely but can confirm the presence of hypothyroidism when the TSH is elevated or in the rare situation when hypothyroidism is suspected in the presence of a normal TSH. Although antibodies to thyroid peroxidase are elevated in 95% of patients with Hashimoto's thyroiditis, determining their presence is usually not necessary in the evaluation of patients with hypothyroidism, because management is unchanged (3). Similarly, because radioactive iodine uptake is typically low in hypothyroidism of any cause, radionuclide scans are also not normally helpful. Although the TSH is characteristically elevated in primary hypothyroidism, pitfalls can occur. Starvation, corticosteroid administration, and use of dopamine can lower TSH, even in patients with hypothyroidism. In some hospitalized patients with severe nonthyroidal illness, low peripheral thyroid hormone levels may suggest hypothyroidism, although the TSH is usually normal in this setting. The U.S. Preventive Services Task Force finds the evidence for either benefit or harm insufficient to recommend for or against routine screening for thyroid disease in asymptomatic adults (4).

   D. **Genetics.** The molecular defects have been identified in only a few cases of human hypothyroidism (5). Hypothyroidism remains primarily an acquired disease associated with aging.

IV. DIAGNOSIS

   A. **Differential diagnosis.** Because the symptoms of hypothyroidism are nonspecific, its differential diagnosis is large and includes depression, emotional or physical stress, chronic infections, autoimmune disorders, anemia, cardiovascular disease, occult malignancies, adverse reactions to medication, and other endocrine disorders such as diabetes. Because of the multisystem involvement of hypothyroidism, the clinician might focus attention on changes, such as constipation, in one organ system, the gastrointestinal system, which can divert attention to the presence of signs and symptoms of hypothyroidism in other organ systems.

   B. **Clinical manifestations.** Most patients have only mild or moderate disease at the time of diagnosis. *Subclinical hypothyroidism* occurs when the TSH is mildly elevated (4.5–10.0 mIU/L) and there are no associated signs or symptoms. If not treated to prevent progression, these patients can be monitored every 2 to 5 years to detect the cases that will progress to overt hypothyroidism at a rate of up to 5% per year (2). *Primary hypothyroidism* can be diagnosed by the typical findings on history and physical examination, coupled with an elevated TSH and a low free T$_4$. *Secondary hypothyroidism* should be suspected when both the TSH and the free T$_4$ are low. *Myxedema coma* is a life-threatening complication of long-standing hypothyroidism, which is rare in warm climates and uncommon in cold climates. These patients may present with stupor, areflexia, respiratory depression, hypercapnia, and profound hypothermia that may go undetected with standard medical thermometers. Prompt diagnosis, hospitalization, and rapid treatment are required to prevent death. Factors that predispose to myxedema coma include infection, trauma, cold exposure, and central nervous system depressants.

References
1. Hollowell JG, Stachling NW, Flanders WD, et al. Serum TSH, T4, and thyroid antibodies in the United States population (1988 to 1994): National Health and Nutrition Examination Survey (HHANES III). *J Clin Endocrinol Metab* 2002;87:489–499.
2. Helfand M, Redfern CC. Screening for thyroid disease. *Ann Intern Med* 1998;129: 144–158.
3. LeGrys VA, Hartmann K, Walsh JF. The clinical consequences and diagnosis of hypothyroidism. *Clin Lab Sci* 2004;17(4):203–208.
4. Agency for Healthcare Research and Quality. U.S. Preventive Services Task Force. *Recommendation statement: screening for thyroid disease (January 2004).* Available at: http://www.ahrq.gov/clinic/3rduspstf/thyroid/thyrrs.htm, accessed on July 7, 2005.
5. Moreno JC, de Vijlder JJ, Vulsma T, et al. Genetic basis of hypothyroidism: recent advances, gaps and strategies for future research. *Trends Endocrinol Metab* 2003; 14(7):318–326.

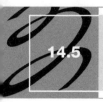

POLYDIPSIA
14.5
Soraya P. Nasraty

I. **BACKGROUND.** Polydipsia is excessive drinking of water owing to abnormal thirst that can be attributed to medical or psychogenic causes.

II. **PATHOPHYSIOLOGY**

A. **Epidemiology.** Polydipsia is a common symptom among patients with diabetes mellitus (DM) and prominent in patients with diabetes insipidus (DI). Polydipsia has a prevalence of 3% to 39% among chronic psychiatric inpatients (1).

B. **Etiology.** Initially, the physician should try to classify and identify the etiology of polydipsia, which is usually accompanied by polyuria.

1. **Poorly resorbed solutes.** Glucose, mannitol, or sorbitol can cause an osmotic diuresis. DM should be suspected in any patient with polydipsia and polyuria of recent onset.

2. **Primary polydipsia.** This may be caused by psychotic delusions, a hyperactivity of hypothalamic thirst centers, or a dry month due to the anticholinergic effects of medications.

3. **Diabetes insipidus (DI).** This may be due to either a central (neurogenic DI) or renal (nephrogenic DI) cause. Central (complete or partial) DI is caused by a defect in the secretion of antidiuretic hormone (ADH) by the pituitary gland. Neurogenic DI can be idiopathic, genetic, or secondary to intracranial pathology such as a brain tumor, head trauma, toxic brain injury, metastatic cancer, granulomatous disease (tuberculosis, sarcoidosis), or from a complication of a neurosurgical procedure. Vasopressinase-induced DI occurs in the last trimester of pregnancy and is often associated with pre-eclampsia.

   Nephrogenic DI can be caused by the nephrons not responding to ADH from an inherited defect, can result from an acquired problem secondary to medications (lithium, methoxyflurane, demeclocycline), or can result from systemic disease (hypokalemia, hypercalcemia).

4. **Iatrogenic polydipsia.** This can occur because of patients misinterpreting physician's instructions to "drink plenty of water" (2).

III. **EVALUATION**

A. **History.** In eliciting the history, the clinician should take note of neurologic symptoms (problems with visual fields, headaches, numbness); a prior history of cancer, particularly metastatic brain cancer; a history of trauma; neurosurgery; and infections such as encephalitis. The patient's psychiatric history may also be relevant. Polydipsia usually starts abruptly in central DI, and patients often have a preference for ice cold water (3).

B. **Physical examination.** A good general physical examination, including vital signs, is helpful in making the diagnosis, but the emphasis is on the neurologic examination (i.e., visual fields, cranial nerve deficits, oculomotor palsies, and reflexes). Signs of recent weight loss or the presence of peripheral neuropathy suggest the diagnosis of DM.

C. **Testing**

1. **Laboratory tests.** A urinalysis needs to be performed to check for glucosuria of DM or the low specific gravity associated with DI. A chemistry panel is helpful in checking for elevated serum glucose levels of DM or an elevated creatinine seen with renal disease and nephrogenic DI. A calcium level could be useful if hypercalcemia is suspected. Serum and urine osmolality are useful in differentiating between DI, which presents with increased serum osmolality and an in appropriately low urine osmolality (specific gravity <1.005), and

excessive water intake, which presents with low or normal serum osmolality and an appropriately low urine osmolality. Normal serum values are between 285 and 295 mOsm/L.

2. **Imaging.** Magnetic resonance imaging (MRI) of the head may be indicated to exclude pituitary or hypothalamic tumors. In DI associated with pituitary disease, MRI is quite specific, because the normal bright spot of a functioning pituitary gland is absent (3).

3. **Water deprivation test.** This test may be useful in the diagnosis of DI and to differentiate between neurogenic and nephrogenic DI by determining the effects of water deprivation (mild dehydration) on ADH secretion by measuring serum, urine osmolality, urine specific gravity, and serum sodium in a controlled environment (3). This test needs to be carefully supervised by someone able to treat severe hypertonic dehydration, if necessary. Patients with mild polydipsia are placed on fluid restriction starting at midnight prior to testing but in those with severe polydipsia fluids are restricted only during the day. Baseline body weight, plasma osmolarity, serum sodium, and urine osmolarity are determined. Urine osmolarity and weight are assessed on an hourly basis. Adequate dehydration is noted by a decrease in body weight by 5% and serum osmolarity >275 mOsm/L. A normal response would show normal plasma osmolarity and sodium concentration with decreased urine output and increasing urine osmolarity to >800 mOsm/L (i.e., two to four times greater than the plasma). In contrast to healthy patients, patients with DI cannot concentrate their urine in response to dehydration. Patients with central DI respond to desmopressin (a synthetic analog of vasopressin) administered intranasally, whereas patients with nephrogenic DI do not (4). Patients do not fall into definite categories sometimes (e.g., partial central DI). The direct form of testing where ADH levels are measured after infusing hypertonic saline is rarely performed.

D. **Genetics.** An inherited autosomally dominant form of neurogenic DI is caused by mutations in the *AVP neurophysin II* gene (*AVP-NPII* gene), and hereditary nephrogenic DI can be caused by V2 receptor problems (X-linked mode of inheritance or a defect in the ADH-sensitive aquaporin-2 water channels) (3).

IV. DIAGNOSIS

A. **Differential diagnosis.** Often, important clues about the cause of polydipsia can be obtained with a directed clinical history with particular attention to the onset of symptoms, the presence of nocturia, and the medication history. The value of the physical examination is limited unless there are signs of defects due to a pituitary tumor (e.g., progressive headaches, visual field defects) or endocrinologic symptoms (e.g., amenorrhea, galactorrhea, acromegaly, Cushing's syndrome). The diagnosis is often made with routine laboratory tests. Sometimes, a water deprivation test needs to be performed to make the diagnosis, but this test should be performed in a hospital setting with the patient monitored closely for dehydration.

B. **Clinical manifestations.** Thirst associated with polyuria is the chief complaint in patients with DM, DI, and psychogenic polydipsia. Nocturia occurs more frequently with DM and DI than with psychogenic polydipsia. Patients with psychogenic polydipsia may have delusions leading to increased fluid intake of up to 20 L/day (1).

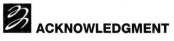 **ACKNOWLEDGMENT**

The author thanks Lara O. Fakunle, MD, for her help in reviewing this chapter.

References

1. Greendyke RM, Bernhardt AJ, Tasbas HE, et al. Polydipsia in chronic psychiatric patients: therapeutic trials of clonidine and enalapril. *Neuropsychopharmacology* 1998;18:272–281.

2. Olapade-Olaopa EO, Morley RN, Ahiaku EK, et al. Iatrogenic polydipsia: a rare cause of water intoxication in urology. *Br J Urol* 1997;79:488.
3. Robertson GL. Disorders of the neurohypophysis. In: Kasper DL, Fauci AS, Longo DL, eds. *Harrison's principles of internal medicine*, 16th ed. New York: McGraw-Hill, 1998:2098–2103.
4. Adam P. Evaluation and management of diabetes insipidus. *Am Fam Physician* 1997;55:2146–2153.

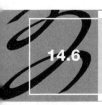

THYROID ENLARGEMENT/GOITER

Jeri R. Reid and Stephen F. Wheeler

14.6

I. BACKGROUND. Goiter, an enlarged thyroid gland, is the most common thyroid abnormality. Goiter is termed *endemic* if it occurs in more than 10% of a population. Endemic goiter most commonly results from dietary iodine deficiency and is extremely rare in the United States. *Sporadic* goiter arises in nonendemic areas and from various causes (1). *Simple* goiter describes a diffusely enlarged thyroid gland. *Multinodular* goiter is an enlarged gland with multiple areas of nodularity. The functional status of a goiter is usually normal (*nontoxic*) but can be hypothyroid or hyperthyroid (*toxic*). The mean weight of the thyroid gland in iodine-sufficient populations is 10 g, with the upper limit of the normal being 20 g (2).

II. PATHOPHYSIOLOGY

A. Etiology. Any process that impedes thyroid hormone synthesis or release can cause goiter. By far the most important risk factor for the development of goiter is iodine deficiency. Goitrogens, substances that interfere with thyroid hormone production and action, can cause sporadic goiter. This category includes certain drugs (thioamide derivatives, lithium, iodides, amiodarone, and others) and foods (rutabagas, cabbage, turnips, soybeans, kelp, and others) (1). Cigarette smoking has been linked to the development of goiter in iodine-deficient areas and is believed to interfere with iodine uptake of the thyroid gland. Pregnancy-induced goiter is related to the exacerbation of the existing iodine deficiency and proliferative effect of estrogen on the thyroid gland. However, the use of oral contraceptives has been found to be associated with reduced incidence of goiter (3).

B. Epidemiology. The prevalence of goiter in the United States is estimated at 4% to 7% but varies widely, depending on the regional iodine intake. One autopsy study of thyroid glands that were thought to contain no pathology demonstrated a 38% incidence of multinodular goiter (2). Goiter prevalence increases with age and is 5 to 10 times more common in women than men (1).

III. EVALUATION

A. History. Although simple goiters are usually euthyroid, typical symptoms of hypothyroidism or thyrotoxicosis should be sought. Generalized thyroid pain suggests subacute thyroiditis, whereas sudden localized pain and swelling are consistent with hemorrhage into a nodule (4). A family history of goiter and a personal history of residing in an endemic goiter area or ingesting goitrogens may be significant.

B. Physical examination. Physical signs consistent with hypothyroidism or thyrotoxicosis may be present. Pemberton's sign can be induced by having the patient raise both arms above the head for one minute. The patient develops facial and neck plethora if venous outflow is obstructed by the thyroid gland. Inspect the neck below the thyroid cartilage from the front, using cross lighting to accentuate shadows and masses. Full extension of the neck enhances the visibility of the gland. Inspection from the side with measurement of any prominence of the normally smooth and straight contour between the cricoid cartilage and the suprasternal notch is useful. Palpitation is performed using the technique with which the examiner is most experienced and skilled. The thyroid is palpated by using the fingers or thumbs while standing in front of or behind the patient. If felt between the cricoid cartilage and the suprasternal notch, the thyroid isthmus can be used to help locate the gland. Palpation of the lobes can be improved by relaxation of the sternocleidomastoid; for example, the left lobe can be defined better by having the patient slightly flex and rotate the neck to the left. Other useful maneuvers include measuring the circumference of the neck or the dimensions of each lobe. The location, size, consistency, mobility, and tenderness of any nodules should be noted. Having the patient swallow during both inspection and palpation causes the thyroid to move and aids in developing a three-dimensional impression of the gland's shape and size. This maneuver can also make a low-placed gland accessible. The patient should be placed in the supine position to determine the inferior extent of the gland (2, 5).

- **C. Testing**
    - **1. Laboratory tests.** The highly sensitive thyroid-stimulating hormone (TSH) assay is the single best test to evaluate the thyroid status. An elevated TSH is highly suggestive of hypothyroidism. If TSH is suppressed, an elevated free thyroxine index (FTI) or free thyroxine (fT_4) measured directly, confirms thyrotoxicosis. In a patient with a suppressed TSH and a normal FTI or fT_4, serum triiodothyronine (T_3) should be measured to assess for possible T_3 thyrotoxicosis. Antithyroid antibodies are usually low or absent but the presence of elevated levels can help predict those patients at a higher risk of developing thyroiditis, hypothyroidism, or Graves' disease.
    - **2. Imaging.** Nuclear scans and ultrasound studies are not warranted in the routine evaluation of simple or multinodular goiter. Ultrasonography may be helpful in patients with equivocal findings on palpation. Symptoms suggestive of substernal mechanical pressure require evaluation, usually by computed tomography or magnetic resonance imaging (4).
    - **3. Other tests.** Fine needle biopsy should be performed in cases of a solitary or dominant nodule found by palpation. Pulmonary function tests are warranted with evidence of inspiratory impairment. Barium swallow is indicated to evaluate goiter-associated dysphagia (4).
- **D. Genetics.** Currently, no genetic markers are used in evaluating goiter. Family and twin studies have demonstrated that genetic factors play a role in the development of goiter, but at present, the results cannot be extrapolated to the general population (5).

IV. DIAGNOSIS

- **A. Differential diagnosis.** A cystic hygroma or a thyroglossal duct cyst, which may transilluminate, and lymphadenopathy can be confused with a goiter. Primary thyroid cancers, lymphomas, or metastatic cancers may present as a firm mass in the neck. Patients with thyroiditis (Hashimoto's, subacute, or silent) can present with an enlarged thyroid gland. An asymptomatic patient with a simple or multinodular goiter associated with a normal metabolic state does not necessarily require further diagnostic studies or treatment. Periodic assessment, at least annually, to evaluate growth, function, and symptoms is warranted. In two studies, it was shown that 10% of patients with nodular goiter developed thyrotoxicosis during a 7- to 10-year follow-up period (1).
- **B. Clinical manifestations.** In simple goiter, patients are asymptomatic or, if the gland is sufficiently enlarged, present with symptoms caused by mechanical pressure. Substernal goiters are frequently responsible for tracheal pressure symptoms, including dyspnea and inspiratory stridor. They can also obstruct the large cervical veins at the thoracic inlet, causing suffusion of the face, giddiness, and syncope (Pemberton's sign). Esophageal compression can lead to dysphagia. Hoarseness caused by compression of or traction on the recurrent laryngeal nerve is rare in simple goiter and suggests a malignancy. Goiter with compressive or cosmetic symptoms usually requires surgical consultation but referral for radioiodine therapy could be considered especially in older patients. The natural history of simple goiter may

include spontaneous resolution or no clinical change but may also involve gradual thyroid growth, nodule formation, and the development of functional autonomy. The use of thyroid hormone suppression in goiter is controversial. Nodules within a multinodular goiter may become toxic in the presence of a supplemental thyroid hormone (4, 5).

References

1. Hermus AR, Huymans DA. Pathogenesis of nontoxic diffuse and nodular goiter. In: Braverman LE, Utiger RD, eds. *Werner and Inbar's the thyroid*, 9th ed. Philadelphia. PA: Lippincott Williams & Wilkins, 2005:873–878.
2. Day TA, Chu A, Hoang KG. Multinodular goiter. *Otolaryngol Clin North Am* 2003; 36:35–54.
3. Knudsen N, Laurberg P, Perrild H, et al. Risk factors for goiter and thyroid nodules. *Thyroid* 2002;12:879–888.
4. Hermus AR, Huymans DA. Clinical manifestations and treatment of nontoxic diffuse and nodular goiter. In: Braverman LE, Utiger RD, eds. *Werner and Inbar's The Thyroid*, 9th ed. Philadelphia, PA: Lippincott Williams & Wilkins, 2005:879–885.
5. Hegedus L, Bonnema SJ, Bennedbaek FN. Management of simple nodular goiter: current status and future perspectives. *Endocr Rev* 2003;24:102–132.

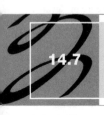

THYROID NODULE
14.7
Jeri R. Reid and Stephen F. Wheeler

I. **BACKGROUND.** A thyroid nodule is a palpable swelling in an otherwise normal thyroid gland. The types of thyroid nodules are summarized in Table 14.7.1. The most common nodule is the colloid nodule, which is not associated with an increased risk of cancer.

II. **PATHOPHYSIOLOGY**

    A. **Etiology.** Exposure to ionizing radiation or external beam radiation therapy (especially before 20 years of age) increases the incidence of both benign and malignant

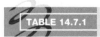

TABLE 14.7.1   Types of Thyroid Nodules

Adenoma	Carcinoma	Colloid nodule
Macrofollicular adenoma (simple colloid)	Papillary (75%)	Dominant nodule in a multinodular goiter
Microfollicular adenoma (fetal)	Follicular (10%)	**Other**
Embryonal adenoma (trabecular)	Medullary (5%–10%)	Inflammatory disorders
Hürthle cell adenoma (oxyphilic, oncocytic)	Anaplastic (5%)	Subacute thyroiditis
Atypical adenoma	Thyroid lymphoma (5%)	Chronic lymphocytic thyroiditis
Adenoma with papillae	**Cyst**	Granulomatous disease
Signet-ring adenoma	Simple cyst	Developmental abnormalities
	Cystic/solid tumors (hemorrhagic, necrotic)	Dermoid
		Rare unilateral lobe agenesis

Reproduced with permission from Welker MJ, Orlov D. Thyroid nodules. *Am Fam Physician* 2003;67:559–66.

thyroid nodules at a rate of 2% annually and peaks 15 to 20 years after exposure (1). Nodules are observed in 25% of patients with Graves' disease, and approximately 15% of these are malignant (2). Iodine deficiency results in increased thyroid-stimulating hormone (TSH) levels, increased thyroid cell replication, and an increased incidence of nodules (2).

B. Epidemiology. Palpable nodules are present in 4% to 7% of adults. Nodules found incidentally on diagnostic imaging are estimated to occur as often as 19% to 67%. Approximately 5% of all nodules are carcinomas, regardless of how they are discovered (1). Benign thyroid nodules are present four to five times more often in women but are more likely to be cancerous in men (3). Age younger than 20 years or older than 65 years, male gender, exposure to radiation, and previous history of thyroid cancer are risk factors for thyroid cancer.

III. EVALUATION. The evaluation of nodular thyroid disease focuses on the functional status of the gland and detection of thyroid cancer. Hypothyroidism or hyperthyroidism may be suggested by the history and physical examination.

A. History. Rapid growth of a nodule or symptoms of local invasion (hoarseness, neck pain, dysphagia, stridor, or dyspnea) increases the suspicion of cancer. Sudden onset of localized swelling, pain, or tenderness suggests hemorrhage into a preexisting nodule or cyst.

B. Physical examination. The neck is inspected below the thyroid cartilage from the front and side, using cross lighting to accentuate shadows and masses. Full extension of the neck enhances the visibility of the gland. The patient is approached from either the front or behind during palpation which is accomplished using the fingers or thumbs. Having the patient swallow during both inspection and palpation causes the thyroid to move and aids in developing a three-dimensional impression of the gland. The location, size, consistency, mobility, and tenderness of all nodules should be documented. A nodule that is hard, irregular, nontender, >4 cm, fixed to surrounding structures or that is associated with local lymphadenopathy suggests malignancy (1).

C. Testing

1. **Laboratory tests.** Serum TSH, performed by a sensitive method, should be assessed in every patient. It is the best screening test for both hypothyroidism (elevated TSH; Chapter 14.4) and thyrotoxicosis (suppressed TSH; Chapter 14.8). A family history of medullary thyroid cancer or multiple endocrine neoplasia type II warrants a basal serum calcitonin (4).

2. **Fine needle biopsy.** In euthyroid patients with a nodule, a fine needle biopsy (FNB) should be performed. FNB has demonstrated a sensitivity of 68% to 98% and specificity of 72% to 100% (1). The use of FNB has decreased the number of surgical procedures for thyroid nodules by 50% and increased the rate of detecting carcinoma after surgery by 50% (4,5).

3. **Imaging.** Diagnostic imaging cannot reliably differentiate benign from malignant nodules; however, incidentally discovered nodules smaller than 1 cm are usually not biopsied if there are no major risk factors for cancer. Ultrasonography can be useful when findings on palpation are inconclusive regarding the presence of a single nodule or a dominant one in a multinodular gland. It can distinguish between solid and cystic lesions with accuracy, evaluate nodule size, and facilitate FNB. Ultrasound-guided FNB decreases the incidence of indeterminate specimens from 15% to 4% (1). Some authors have suggested ultrasound to be performed by an operator and that could proceed with a biopsy if indicated (2). An ^{123}I radionuclide scan should only be performed in the initial evaluation of thyroid nodules if the TSH level indicates hyperthyroidism. A hyperfunctioning nodule with suppressed uptake in the rest of the gland suggests a toxic nodule and reduces the risk of cancer to <1% (5). However, such lesions constitute <10% of all nodules (4).

D. Genetics. Most autonomously functioning nodules are caused by a mutation in the TSH receptor. Other mutations that may explain the causes of papillary and follicular carcinomas have been identified (2). Approximately 4% to 8% of cases of papillary cancer are familial, and a high incidence has been reported in patients with adenomatous polyposis coli (Gardner's syndrome) and multiple hamartoma syndrome (Cowden disease). Medullary cancer, usually as part of multiple endocrine neoplasia type II, often occurs in a hereditary pattern (3).

IV. DIAGNOSIS

A. Differential diagnosis. Even in experienced hands, up to 15% of biopsies are unsatisfactory and need to be repeated, preferably using ultrasound guidance (5). If the results of FNB demonstrate a malignancy or are suspicious, indeterminate, or repeatedly unsatisfactory, then an immediate surgical referral is warranted (3). Sometimes, radionuclide scanning is used to evaluate a suspicious biopsy result, and hyperfunctioning nodules are observed rather than removed (5). If the biopsy is clearly benign, an examination of the neck, an ultrasound, and a TSH measurement should be performed every 6 to 12 months (4).

B. Clinical manifestations. Subacute thyroiditis is suggested by fever, a preceding viral illness, or a gradual onset of swelling, pain, and tenderness. Typical symptoms of hypothyroidism suggest Hashimoto's thyroiditis, whereas thyrotoxicosis suggests toxic adenoma or toxic multinodular goiter (3). The presence of hyperthyroidism or hypothyroidism lowers the suspicion of cancer but does not exclude it. Any nodule that enlarges or becomes clinically suspicious should be rebiopsied.

References
1. Welker MJ, Orlov D. Thyroid nodules. *Am Fam Physician* 2003;67:559–566.
2. Weiss RE, Lado-Abeal J. Thyroid nodules: diagnosis and therapy. *Curr Opin Oncol* 2002;14:46–52.
3. Kaplan MM. Clinical evaluation and management of solitary thyroid nodules. In: Braverman LE, Utiger RD, eds. *Werner and Inbar's The Thyroid*, 9th ed. Philadelphia, PA: Lippincott Williams & Wilkins, 2005:996–1010.
4. Hegedus L. The thyroid nodule. *N Engl J Med* 2004;351:1764–1771.
5. Walsh RM, Watkinson JC, Franklyn J. The management of the solitary thyroid nodule: a review. *Clin Otolaryngol* 1999;24:388–397.

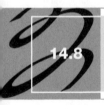

14.8 HYPERTHYROIDISM/THYROTOXICOSIS
Barbara A. Majeroni and Stephen F. Wheeler

I. BACKGROUND. Hyperthyroidism is excessive thyroid hormone secretion. Thyrotoxicosis is the clinical syndrome of increased metabolism caused by excess thyroid hormone activity, regardless of the source.

II. PATHOPHYSIOLOGY. Causes of thyrotoxicosis are summarized in Table 14.8.1.

A. Etiology

1. **Graves' disease,** an autoimmune disorder and the most common cause of hyperthyroidism, results when thyrotropin receptor antibodies stimulate thyroid growth, leading to the synthesis and release of the thyroid hormone.

2. **Toxic adenoma and toxic multinodular goiter** are characterized by the development of areas of focal or diffuse hyperplasia of thyroid follicular cells, which function without regulation by thyroid-stimulating hormone (TSH). In trophoblastic tumors, TSH receptors may be stimulated by the overproduction of the human chorionic gonadotropin (HCG) or other placental proteins.

3. **Thyroiditis** results in the release of preformed thyroid hormone from the thyroid gland. It is of viral or postviral origin (subacute granulomatous thyroiditis) or from an autoimmune process (subacute lymphocytic thyroiditis). Subacute

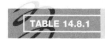

TABLE 14.8.1	Causes of Thyrotoxicosis and Associated Radioactive Iodine Uptake Findings
Cause	**Radioactive iodine uptake**
Graves' disease (most common)	Homogeneous increase
Toxic multinodular goiter	Increased heterogeneous pattern
Toxic adenoma	One area increased, rest of the gland suppressed
Exogenous	Low or absent uptake
Iatrogenic (overtreatment)	
Factitious (patient taking excess)	
Thyroiditis	
Acute suppurative (rare)	Normal
Subacute (de Quervain's)[a]	Low (transient)
Silent thyroiditis[a]	Low (transient)
Excess iodine	Low or absent
Thyroid carcinoma	Variable
Functioning bone metastases	Absent
TSH-secreting pituitary tumor	Increased
Struma ovarii	Reduced in thyroid (increased over pelvis)
Activating mutation of TSH receptor	Increased
Thyroid hormone resistance syndrome	Increased

[a]Transient, followed by hypothyroidism, then return to normal.
TSH, thyroid-stimulating hormone.

thyroiditis can also be caused by chemical toxicity from drugs such as amiodarone, by radiation, or by drugs that interfere with the immune system, such as interferon alfa.

B. Epidemiology. Hyperthyroidism affects up to 2% of women and 0.2% of men. The prevalence increases with age and is highest in patients older than 80 years of age (1). Graves' disease accounts for 60% to 80% of cases of thyrotoxicosis, occurs typically in patients between 20 and 50 years of age, and is less prevalent in areas of low iodine intake (2). Toxic nodular goiter is the next most common cause of thyrotoxicosis (10%–40%) and is the most common cause of thyrotoxicosis in patients older than 40 years of age. Thyroiditis accounts for 5% to 20% of the cases. The other causes of thyrotoxicosis are much less common.

III. EVALUATION

A. History. Symptoms vary and are nonspecific. Elderly patients may present with fewer typical symptoms than younger patients. More than 50% of patients exhibit some of the common symptoms, which include nervousness, increased sweating, heat intolerance, palpitations, dyspnea, fatigue, weight loss, diarrhea, polyuria, oligomenorrhea, loss of libido, and eye complaints.

B. Physical examination. Vital signs may reveal weight loss, tachycardia, and systolic hypertension with a widened pulse pressure. Patients may appear nervous or restless. Sinus tachycardia is the most frequent arrhythmia. Atrial fibrillation occurs in 5% to 15% and may be the presenting problem. The risk of atrial fibrillation or flutter is higher in men than women (1.8–1) and increases with age (3). Despite complaints of exertional dyspnea, the lung examination is usually normal unless there is concomitant congestive heart failure. The skin may be warm and moist with palmar erythema. Pretibial myxedema, painless raised swelling of subcutaneous tissues, most often found on the anterior lower leg or dorsal foot of patients with Graves' disease, causes a *peau d'orange* texture, which can be pruritic and hyperpigmented. A fine tremor is most evident in the fingertips when the hands are extended. Hypokalemic periodic paralysis is most commonly seen in Asian men. The neck is inspected below the thyroid cartilage from the front and side. During palpation, the patient is approached from behind using the fingers. Making the patient swallow during the examination causes the thyroid to move and aids in distinguishing it from excess fatty tissue or neck muscle. Auscultation of a bruit over the gland correlates with increased vascularity.

C. Testing. Measuring serum thyrotropin (TSH) is the most sensitive test for screening for hyperthyroidism. A normal result virtually excludes hyperthyroidism except in the rare instances where it is due to thyrotropin hypersecretion. An undetectable level of TSH is the hallmark of hyperthyroidism, which is confirmed by an elevated free thyroxine (T_4). If the free T_4 is normal and suspicion is high, a serum free triiodothyronine (T_3) should also be measured to rule out T_3 toxicosis. Drugs such as glucocorticoids, levodopa, and dopamine can cause a low TSH in patients who are euthyroid. A low TSH with a normal free T_4 and T_3 may indicate subclinical hyperthyroidism. A thyroid scan with radioactive iodine uptake can help differentiate the causes of thyrotoxicosis as indicated in Table 14.8.1 (4). Ultrasonic examination of the thyroid is useful to detect the presence of nodules or cysts.

D. Genetics. A combination of genetic factors, including HLA-DR and CTLA-4 polymorphisms, and environmental factors contribute to Graves' disease. Activating mutations of Gs-α proteins have been identified in many toxic adenomas. Activating somatic mutations of the genes for TSH receptor have been identified in both toxic adenomas and toxic multinodular goiters.

IV. DIAGNOSIS

A. Differential diagnosis. Thyrotoxicosis must be differentiated from other causes of unexplained weight loss, including malignancies, psychiatric disorders, alcohol or drug abuse, diabetes, occult infections, gastrointestinal disorders, and chronic renal, hepatic, cardiac, or pulmonary disease.

B. Clinical manifestations. The signs and symptoms are extremely variable.

   1. Graves' disease is suggested by a characteristic stare with widened palpebral fissures, lid lag, and visualization of the sclera on all sides of the iris. Typically, the thyroid is increased in size and is smooth and nontender. A bruit is present in 50% of patients.

   2. Toxic nodular goiter presents with a gland that is typically enlarged and non-tender with multiple nodules. A single toxic nodule is more common in younger people.

   3. Thyroiditis, which usually refers to subacute granulomatous thyroiditis (de Quervain's thyroiditis), presents with an enlarged, tender thyroid. In subacute lymphocytic thyroiditis (painless or silent thyroiditis), the gland is enlarged but nontender.

References

1. Flynn RWV, MacDonald TM, Morris AD, et al. The thyroid epidemiology, audit, and research study: thyroid dysfunction in the general population. *J Clin Endocrinol Metab* 2004;89:3879–3884.
2. Cooper DS. Hyperthyroidism. *Lancet* 2003;362:459–468.
3. Frost L, Vestergaard P, Mosekilde L. Hyperthyroidism and the risk of atrial fibrillation or flutter: a population based study. *Arch Intern Med* 2004;164:1675–1678.
4. Intenzo CM, dePapp AE, Jabbour S, et al. Scintigraphic manifestations of thyrotoxicosis. *Radiographics* 2003;23:857–869.

Vascular and Lymphatic System Problems

Gregory J. Babbe

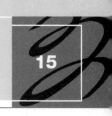

15

LYMPHADENOPATHY, GENERALIZED
Kristy D. Edwards

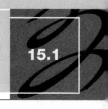

I. **BACKGROUND.** Lymphadenopathy, enlarged, tender, or inflamed lymph nodes, is a common presenting complaint. In primary care, patients presenting with nonspecific lymphadenopathy are mainly younger than 40 years of age, and one-fourth of the patients have generalized lymphadenopathy. Generalized lymphadenopathy is diagnosed when abnormal lymph nodes are identified in two or more noncontiguous areas (e.g., neck and groin). Generalized lymphadenopathy should prompt further investigation of systemic disease by the physician.

II. **PATHOPHYSIOLOGY.** Infectious, autoimmune, granulomatous, malignant diseases, or medication reactions can cause generalized lymphadenopathy. The overall risk of cancer in patients with generalized lymphadenopathy is low; however, the risk of malignancy increases with age. There is a 4% cancer risk in those patients older than 40 years of age with generalized lymphadenopathy (1). A good complete history and physical examination can often lead to a diagnosis of the cause of lymphadenopathy.

III. **EVALUATION**

A. **History.** The history should focus on the common causes of generalized lymphadenopathy.

1. **History of present illness** should focus on the duration, location, quality, and context of the lymphadenopathy. Enlarged, tender lymph nodes present for <2 weeks are often due to infectious causes. Lymphadenopathy present for more than a year is usually from nonspecific causes. Associated signs and symptoms such as rash, fever, night sweats, weight loss, sore throat, and arthralgias may help identify a specific cause of the generalized lymphadenopathy (2).

2. **Past medical history** should focus on known illness and medication usage. Common chronic illnesses (e.g., lupus erythematosus, rheumatoid arthritis, and human immunodeficiency virus [HIV]) can also cause generalized lymphadenopathy. Drug reactions resulting in lymphadenopathy can occur with certain antibiotics and seizure and hypertension medications (1).

3. **Social history** may identify risk factors for hepatitis B, secondary syphilis, and early HIV. All of these diseases can present with generalized lymphadenopathy.

4. **Family history** is important to identify illness with a genetic predisposition such as lipid storage diseases and immunologic diseases (e.g., Niemann-Pick disease, rheumatoid arthritis). Any known exposures to family members with infectious diseases (e.g., tuberculosis, infectious mononucleosis, or hepatitis B) can also yield important information when trying to identify a causative etiology of lymphadenopathy.

5. **Review of systems** should focus on constitutional symptoms such as weight loss, fatigue, night sweats, malaise, arthralgias, nausea, and vomiting.

B. **Physical examination**

1. **General.** A comprehensive physical examination should be performed on all patients with generalized lymphadenopathy. It should focus on identifying systemic diseases. Vital signs are important, because fever may suggest infectious etiology and weight loss may suggest systemic disease. Skin rashes or lesions, mucous membrane ulcers, and inflammatory arthritis are important physical findings in establishing a differential diagnosis for the adenopathy. An abdominal examination for splenomegaly can yield useful information. Patients with generalized lymphadenopathy and splenomegaly implies systemic illness (e.g., infectious mononucleosis, lymphoma, leukemia, lupus, sarcoidosis,

toxoplasmosis, or cat-scratch disease) and virtually excludes nonhematologic metastatic disease (1, 2).

2. **Nodal examination.** In generalized lymphadenopathy, lymph node size, location, and consistency can help in establishing a diagnosis.

   a. **Size.** Lymph nodes >1.5 cm in diameter have a 38% risk of cancer involvement and require further workup (2). Lymph nodes 1 cm in diameter and smaller can be normal and can usually be observed.

   b. **Location.** The anatomic location of lymphadenopathy is sometimes helpful in establishing a diagnosis. However, with generalized lymphadenopathy, the anatomic location is less helpful. Anterior cervical, submandibular, and inguinal nodes may normally be palpable. However, lymph nodes palpated in certain areas are always alarming. For example, supraclavicular lymphadenopathy has a 90% risk of cancer in patients older than 40 years of age.

   c. **Consistency.** Rock hard nodes particularly in older patients are worrying for metastatic disease (2). Firm rubbery nodes are found with lymphomas. Soft tender nodes tend to occur with infectious causes; however, this should not be considered diagnostic. Pain is not a reliable indicator of the cause of lymphadenopathy.

C. Testing

1. **Laboratory tests.** Laboratory testing in patients with generalized lymphadenopathy should be purposeful and specific. Tests should be directed by the patient's signs and symptoms of an underlying disease process (3). A complete blood count (CBC) with peripheral smear is almost always indicated (4). Elevated neutrophils suggest pyogenic etiologies, lymphocytosis suggests viral infection, and pancytopenia suggests leukemia or HIV infection. An erythrocyte sedimentation rate is nonspecific, but if it is persistently elevated, further investigation is indicated. Disease-specific serologic tests, including antibody testing for Epstein - Barr virus, cytomegalovirus, HIV, rubella virus, syphilis (FTA-ABS), and others, are useful. Antibody testing can be diagnostic and can differentiate between acute and chronic illness. Chest x-rays are rarely positive but should be ordered to look for mediastinal lymph node involvement in sarcoid disease, metastatic disease, lymphomas, or granulomatous disease. Purified protein derivative (PPD) testing is used to identify tuberculin disease (2).

2. **Lymph node biopsy.** If the laboratory testing is nondiagnostic, then lymph node biopsy may be indicated. The largest and most pathologic node should be removed. Axillary and inguinal nodes should be avoided, because they often reveal only reactive hyperplasia. Biopsy should be avoided in cases of suspected infectious mononucleosis and drug reaction because the histologic picture is easily confused with malignant lymphoma (2). Experienced hematologists or hematopathologists should handle all specimens. The value of fine needle aspiration is controversial, with reasonable arguments both for and against this procedure (5).

IV. DIAGNOSIS. The thorough history and examination should establish a differential diagnosis including infectious, autoimmune, granulomatous, and malignant etiologies. Investigation should be limited to specific diseases because generalized lymphadenopathy is often a sign of a specific systemic illness. In the event that the cause is unclear, infectious etiologies must be considered and a CBC and mononucleosis spot ordered. If these are negative, then immunologic and granulomatous etiologies are considered with serologic testing, a chest x-ray, and PPD. A lymph node biopsy must be considered in those cases where the node is rock hard or larger than 1.5 cm × 1.5 cm in size (1). Biopsy should be avoided in those cases in which viral causes are clinically suggested.

References
1. Ferrer R. Lymphadenopathy: differential diagnosis and evaluation. *Am Fam Physician* 1998;58:1313–1320.
2. Pangalis GA, Vassilalopoulos TP, Boussiotis VA, et al. Clinical approach to lymphadenopathy. *Semin Oncol* 1993;20:570–582.

3. Williamson HA. Lymphadenopathy in a family practice. *J Fam Pract* 1985;20:449–452.
4. Simon HB. Evaluation of lymphadenopathy. In: Goroll AH, May LA, Mulley AG, eds. *Primary care medicine: office evaluation and management of the adult patient*, 3rd ed. Philadelphia, PA: JB Lippincott, 1995:54–58.
5. Henry P, Longo D. *Enlargement of lymph nodes and spleen. Harrison's on line* 1999;61. www.harrisonsonline.com/

LYMPHADENOPATHY, LOCALIZED
Kristy D. Edwards

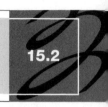

15.2

I. **BACKGROUND.** Lymph nodes are normally palpated in children and may be normally felt in the neck, axilla, and inguinal regions of adults. Three-fourths of primary care patients presenting with unexplained lymph node enlargement have regional lymphadenopathy. Localized or regional lymphadenopathy occurs when enlarged lymph nodes are identified in one anatomic location. The most common anatomic locations for localized lymphadenopathy are the head and neck (55%) and inguinal (14%) regions. Once lymphadenopathy is identified, a complete lymph node examination should be performed to rule out generalized lymphadenopathy. A thorough history and physical examination including regions drained by the lymph nodes should be performed (1).

II. **PATHOPHYSIOLOGY.** The cause of localized lymphadenopathy can be separated by the age of the patient and its location. Reactive hyperplasia and benign etiologies make up 80% of the causes of lymphadenopathy in children and adults younger than 30 years of age. Older patients, especially those older than 40 years of age, are at increased risk of malignancy (2). In localized lymphadenopathy, the location can aid in determining a causative etiology. Knowledge of the patterns of lymphatic drainage and region-specific conditions are essential in the investigation of localized lymphadenopathy (3). The context in which lymphadenopathy occurs is very important in establishing a differential diagnosis. A detailed history including present illness, review of systems, past medical history, social history, and thorough physical examination of the region should be performed.

III. **EVALUATION**

A. **History.** It is important to elicit a detailed history. Lymphadenopathy that is present for months to years suggests underlying malignancy or systemic disease, whereas lymphadenopathy that is present for a few weeks is usually due to infectious etiologies. History of exposure to a cat scratch or sexually transmitted disease can explain lymphadenopathy in the axilla or inguinal regions. History of recent cold symptoms or local signs of redness, swelling, or discharge may suggest infection, whereas nonspecific signs of fever, chills, or night sweats may suggest systemic illness.

B. **Physical examination.** The examination of lymph nodes should include size, location, pain, consistency, and whether matting is present (1).

1. **Size.** As with generalized lymphadenopathy, lymph nodes >1 cm in diameter should arouse suspicion.

2. **Location.** The location of the abnormal lymph node helps focus the examination. A thorough examination of the anatomic region drained by the affected lymph node is of the highest yield for diagnosis. Cervical lymph nodes drain the oropharynx, tongue, and ears. Cervical lymphadenopathy without a known source should be treated with antibiotic coverage for *Staphylococcus aureus* and group A β hemolytic streptococci. However, bilateral cervical lymphadenopathy is often caused by viral or streptococcal pharyngitis (4). Lymphadenopathy in the neck posterior to the sternocleidomastoid muscle is a more ominous finding and

warrants further evaluation (3). Palpated supraclavicular lymph nodes (SCLNs) are also worrisome. Left SCLNs drain intra-abdominal regions and right SCLNs drain the lungs, mediastinum, and the esophagus. Inguinal lymph nodes heighten the concern for venereal disease or lower extremity infection. Axillary lymph nodes suggest breast pathology or upper extremity infection. Other areas of lymphadenopathy, such as abdominal or mediastinal lymph nodes, may not be palpable but may be identified with radiologic studies.

3. Pain. Pain is often associated with lymphadenitis, tender, warm, soft, enlarged lymph nodes. This is usually a result of pyogenic infection (2).

4. Consistency. Consistency of lymph nodes is difficult to assess. Traditionally, firm and hard nodes are associated with malignancy and rubbery nodes suggest lymphoma. Matted or fixed nodes are particularly worrisome for metastatic disease (5).

C. Testing. Laboratory testing is often performed to uncover pathology involving the region of the body drained by the affected lymph nodes. For example, a monospot for Epstein-Barr virus or throat culture for streptococcal pharyngitis may be obtained in a patient with cervical lymphadenopathy. A mammogram may be ordered in older females with axillary lymphadenopathy. Screening for sexually transmitted diseases should be performed in patients with persistent inguinal lymphadenopathy. If the initial evaluation for localized lymphadenopathy does not reveal a diagnosis, it is usually acceptable to observe the patient for 2 to 4 weeks rather than perform unnecessary tests (6). Any testing performed should be specific to identify regional pathology. The test of choice is an excisional biopsy of the node or nodes involved when the diagnosis is unknown and a serious condition is suspected. Usually, the biopsy site is determined by location and size. Large nodes that have recently enlarged are preferred for biopsy (5).

IV. DIAGNOSIS. Localized lymphadenopathy is a common presenting complaint in clinical practice. Usually, a thorough history and physical examination lead to a diagnosis. If the diagnosis is not readily identifiable, then disease-specific tests may be helpful. Biopsy is a last resort if serious disease is suspected. Watchful waiting is acceptable and preferred as long as a serious condition is not suspected.

References

1. Ferrer R. Lymphadenopathy: differential diagnosis and evaluation. *Am Fam Physician* 1998;58:1313–1320.
2. Simon HB. Evaluation of lymphadenopathy. In: Goroll AH, May LA, Mulley AG, eds. *Primary care medicine: office evaluation and management of the adult patient*, 3rd ed. Philadelphia, PA: JB Lippincott, 1995:54–58.
3. Sills R, Jorgensen S. *Lymphadenopathy*. eMedicine from WebMD. Available at: http://www.emedicine.com/ped/topic1333.htm. Last updated April 11, 2005.
4. Leung AK, Robson WL. Childhood cervical lymphadenopathy. *J Pediatr Health Care* 2004;18(1):3–7.
5. Pangalis GA, Vassilalopoulos TP, Boussiotis VA, et al. Clinical approach to lymphadenopathy. *Semin Oncol* 1993;20:570–582.
6. Williamson HA. Lymphadenopathy in a family practice. *J Fam Pract* 1985;20:449–452.

PETECHIAE AND PURPURA
John L. Smith

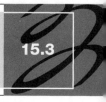

15.3

I. BACKGROUND. Purpura are discolorations in the skin as a consequence of red blood cells extravasating into the skin or the mucous membranes. A petechiae is a purpura that is <2 mm in diameter, and an ecchymosis is a purpura that is >1 cm in diameter.

II. PATHOPHYSIOLOGY. Petechiae most often result from a platelet disorder–either too few (usually <50,000/μL) or abnormally functioning platelets. Localized increases in intravascular pressure or capillaritis may also be responsible. Ecchymoses are usually due to a disorder in the coagulation cascade. Disorders of the vascular system as well as connective tissue disease can also occasionally result in purpura (1).

III. EVALUATION

A. History

1. A time sequence and past history of purpura as well as any indications of abnormal bleeding are important, because the cause of purpura can be either congenital or acquired. A recent viral or bacterial infection may affect platelets or the vessel integrity. Establish a history of easy or prolonged bleeding or bruising, or menorrhagia in women. von Willebrand's disease is the most common inherited disorder of hemostasis and occurs in up to 1% of the population. The disease is symptomatic in up to 10% of these (2). Ten to 20% of early-onset menorrhagia may be associated with an inherited bleeding disorder.

2. Medications may decrease the platelet production or increase their destruction. Associated medications are many, but acetylsalicylic acid, nonsteroidal antiinflammatory drugs, sulfa, heparin, and, classically, quinidine and quinine are frequently noted. A family history of inherited bleeding tendencies or indicators of liver disease may be clues to a coagulation disorder.

B. Physical examination. Initially, determining that the patient is stable and checking vital signs is imperative, because life-threatening causes of purpura such as disseminated intravascular coagulation (DIC), Rocky Mountain spotted fever, meningococcemia, sepsis from *Staphylococcus aureus*, and thrombotic thrombocytopenic purpura (TTP) may be present. Attention should then be directed at the purpuric lesions themselves and also at the location of the lesions. Palpable petechiae are seen with various forms of vasculitis. Purpura do not blanch like intravascular blood seen in angiomas, telangiectasias, and hyperemia. Purpura isolated to eyelids may be secondary to coughing, vomiting, or straining as in childbirth or weight lifting. Purpura limited to forearms are most likely secondary to poor stromal support as is frequently seen in senile purpura in the older population or those with much previous sun exposure. Facial or periorbital purpura may be secondary to a cryoglobulinemia, or amyloidosis.

C. Testing

1. Initial laboratory tests should include a complete blood count, platelet count, peripheral smear, prothrombin time (PT), activated partial thromboplastin time (APTT), and possibly a bleeding time or other evaluation of platelet function such as a PFA 100 analysis.

2. If the lesions are palpable, and vasculitis is a consideration, a sedimentation rate or C-reactive protein determination should be obtained.

3. In vasculitis, a skin biopsy may need to be obtained because the laboratory findings are often nonspecific.

4. Urinalysis and serum creatinine screen must be performed for any renal involvement and liver function tests for liver abnormalities.

D. Genetics. The multitude of disorders causing purpura may be acquired or congenital. Antibodies to factors in the coagulation cascade, as well as infectious diseases, and medications are examples of acquired abnormalities. Hereditary disorders are present with von Willebrand's disease and hemophilia.

IV. DIAGNOSIS

A. Differential diagnosis. The causes of purpuric lesions are numerous and have clinical implications, which may potentially be lethal. A thorough history and physical examination along with some basic laboratory studies and occasional skin biopsy are all that are frequently needed to establish a likely diagnosis.

1. In patients with isolated thrombocytopenia and prolonged bleeding time, idiopathic thrombocytopenic purpura is the probable diagnosis after ruling out drug-induced thrombocytopenia, human immunodeficiency virus infection, and pregnancy-induced thrombocytopenia.

2. An isolated increased APTT is seen in deficiencies or inhibitors of factors VIII, IX, and XI. von Willebrand's disease may have an increased bleeding time with an increased APTT (3). Heparin administration is included in the differential diagnosis.

3. An isolated PT elevation is seen in liver disease, vitamin K deficiency, warfarin (Coumadin) administration, and a factor VII deficiency or inhibitor.

4. When the PT and APTT are both elevated, consider DIC and liver failure along with the various deficiencies in the coagulation cascade.

5. In newborns with purpura, evaluation for sepsis, serologies for the TORCH (toxoplasmosis, other infections, rubella, cytomegalovirus infection, and herpes simplex syndrome), and coagulation factors are recommended. Purpura fulminans and leukemia are also included in the differential diagnosis (4).

B. Clinical Manifestations

1. In addition to those manifestations noted above, certain constellations of clinical and laboratory findings should be mentioned. TTP and hemolytic uremic syndrome (HUS) are seen in many clinical situations, including pregnancy, cancer, infections, and chemotherapy. The signs include the pentad of fever, thrombocytopenia, microangiopathic hemolytic anemia, hemorrhage (including purpura), and neurologic abnormalities. Because of serious consequences, diagnosis should be considered if thrombocytopenia and fragmented red blood cells are seen on the peripheral smear. TTP-HUS has a normal PT, APTT, and d-dimer as opposed to DIC.

2. With regard to coagulation factor abnormalities, hemophilia A and B can cause increased bruising and ecchymoses but not nearly as frequently as von Willebrand's disease. Patients with mild cases of von Willebrand's disease may have a normal bleeding time. Because this disease is caused by a glycoprotein that helps protect factor VIII from breakdown and interferes with platelet aggregation, the APTT is sometimes elevated. With the sudden onset of large ecchymoses and hematomas in an adult with normal platelets, an acquired factor VIII deficiency (autoantibody) should be investigated in cases of a prolonged PT and APTT.

3. Vasculitis causing palpable purpura in children is most common with Henoch-Schönlein purpura.

References

1. Burns T, Breathnach S, Cox N, et al., eds. *Rook's textbook of dermatology*, 7th ed. Chapter 48. Oxford: Blackwell Publishing, 2004.
2. Ewenstein B. von Willebrand's disease. *Annu Rev Med* 1997;48:525–542.
3. Loserh JM. Screening and diagnosis of coagulation disorders. *Am J Obstet Gynecol* 1996;175:778–783.
4. Baselga E, Drolet BA, Esterly NB. Purpura in infants and children. *J Am Acad Dermatol* 1997;37:673–705.

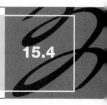

SPLENOMEGALY
Kimberly J. Jarzynka

15.4

I. BACKGROUND

A. Definition. Splenomegaly refers to the enlargement of the spleen to a craniocaudal measurement of 13 cm or more, or to a weight of >400 to 500 g. When the spleen reaches >20 cm in length or 1,000 g, it is termed *massive splenomegaly* (1–4).

B. Anatomy and physiology. Normally, the spleen is a reticuloendothelial organ located in the left upper quadrant of the abdomen at the level of the 8th to 11th ribs. It lies adjacent to the diaphragm, stomach, splenic flexure of the colon, left kidney, and tail of the pancreas. It weighs an average of 150 g, measures approximately 11 cm in greatest diameter, and is palpable in only 2% to 5% of the population (1–4). Essential functions of the spleen include the clearance of senescent red blood cells, micro-organisms, and other particulate matter from circulation (red pulp); generation of a cellular and humoral immune response (white pulp); extramedullary hematopoiesis; and platelet sequestration (1–4).

II. PATHOPHYSIOLOGY

A. Etiology. The many diverse causes of splenomegaly can be grouped into the following categories: structural, inflammatory, hyperplastic, congestive, infiltrative, and infectious. *Structural abnormalities* causing splenomegaly include hemangiomas, hamartomas, cysts, and hematomas. *Inflammatory splenomegaly* is caused by reticuloendothelial cell proliferation and lymphoid hyperplasia from an increase in the antigen clearance and antibody production. *Hyperplastic splenomegaly*, otherwise known as *work hypertrophy*, results from the normal sequestration of increased amounts of abnormal blood cells or extramedullary hematopoiesis. Increased venous pressure results in *congestive splenomegaly*. Macrophages can become engorged with indigestible material or tumor, causing *infiltrative splenomegaly*. Abscess formation within the spleen, most often due to filtered encapsulated organisms, causes *infectious splenomegaly* (3,4).

B. Epidemiology. There is no race, age, or sex predilection for splenomegaly. Epidemiologic data is dependent on the primary etiology (4).

III. EVALUATION

A. History. A thorough past medical, family, and social history including a history of recent travel can often reveal a possible cause of splenomegaly. Splenomegaly itself is often asymptomatic. However, symptoms of vague, colicky left upper quadrant abdominal pain and fullness, early satiety, and pain while lying on the side may be present (3,4). Acute pleuritic left upper quadrant pain can suggest perisplenitis, splenic abscess, or infarction (4). Other symptoms related to the primary illness causing splenomegaly may be present. For example, a febrile illness can suggest an infectious cause, whereas weight loss and constitutional symptoms may be related to a neoplastic etiology. A history of chronic liver disease, alcoholism, congestive heart failure, or pancreatitis can be associated with congestive splenomegaly. Hyperplastic splenomegaly is often associated with symptoms of cytopenia including pallor, dyspnea, easy bruising, or petechial rash (4).

B. Physical examination

1. Examination of the spleen is performed with the patient supine, lying at a slight incline, and/or in the right lateral decubitus position with the knees, hips, and neck flexed and the arms down at the sides. From the patient's right side, lightly palpate under the left costal margin with the right hand while lifting the left costovertebral angle with the left hand. During deep inspiration, palpate gently inward toward the descending spleen. It is often necessary to also palpate from

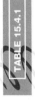

TABLE 15.4.1 Differential Diagnosis of Splenomegaly

Structural and infectious	Inflammatory	Hyperplastic	Congestive	Infiltrative
Hemangiomas, hamartomas, cysts, hematomas abscesses	Viral hepatitis, infectious mononucleosis, cytomegalovirus, AIDS, tuberculosis, subacute bacterial endocarditis, bacterial septicemia, congenital syphilis, malaria, histoplasmosis, leishmaniasis, trypanosomiasis, ehrlichiosis. Rheumatoid arthritis (Felty's syndrome), lupus, other collagen vascular diseases, autoimmune hemolytic anemias, thrombocytopenias, and neutropenias, serum sickness, drug reactions, sarcoidosis, angioimmunoblastic lymphadenopathy, thyrotoxicosis, and interleukin-2 therapy.	Sickle cell anemia, thalassemia major, ovalocytosis, spherocytosis, other hemoglobinopathies, paroxysmal nocturnal hemoglobinuria, and nutritional anemias. Extramedullary hematopoiesis can be seen in leukemias, myelofibrosis, Gaucher's disease, marrow infiltration by tumors, and marrow damage	Hepatic, portal, and splenic vein obstruction; congestive heart failure, cirrhosis, splenic artery aneurysm, hepatic schistosomiasis, portal hypertension of any etiology	Hodgkin's disease, lymphomas, leukemias, myeloproliferative syndromes, angiosarcomas, metastatic tumors, hyperlipidemias, amyloidosis, Gaucher's disease, Niemann-Pick disease, Tangier disease, histiocytosis X, mucopolysaccharidoses, eosinophilic granulomas. Berylliosis

AIDS, acquired immunodeficiency syndrome.

the left lower quadrant up toward the costal margin, as well as in the midline, to identify the lower pole and medial border of a severely enlarged spleen (1,2,5,6).
   2. The ability to palpate the spleen usually suggests splenomegaly, although 2% to 5% of normal spleens are palpable (1–4).
   3. Dullness to percussion in the lowest intercostal space in the anterior axillary line on full inspiration also suggests splenomegaly (Castell's method) (1). Findings of splenomegaly on physical examination are recorded in centimeters below the left costal margin at a point specified by the examiner (i.e. in the midclavicular line).
C. **Testing (1,2,4)**
   1. Complete blood count with differential and platelet count
   2. Peripheral smear
   3. Liver function tests
   4. Urinalysis
   5. Human immunodeficiency virus testing (should be considered)
   6. Appropriate tests for primary disease
   7. Tissue pathology
D. **Imaging studies (1,2,4)**
   1. Ultrasound for initial evaluation
   2. Computed tomography (CT) for preoperative evaluation. CT is better for detecting lesions, masses, or inflammation
   3. Nuclear scans for determining size and function. These scans are used to detect a space-occupying lesion and accessory spleen
   4. Splenoportography for determining portal vein patency and collateral circulation
   5. Angiography for detecting splenic tumors and circulation abnormalities
E. **Genetics.** Splenomegaly itself has no genetic link. However, many of the primary diseases that cause splenomegaly do (e.g., hereditary spherocytosis) (1,2,4).

IV. DIAGNOSIS
A. **Differential diagnosis.** The differential diagnosis of splenomegaly is presented in Table 15.4.1.
B. **Clinical manifestations.** Hypersplenism is an increase in normal splenic function associated with splenomegaly. It results in varying degrees of anemia, leucopenia, and/or thrombocytopenia owing to the increased destruction and sequestration of cells. The bone marrow is either normal or hyperplastic, and improvement in cell counts is seen postsplenectomy (1–4). Other clinical manifestations depend on the primary etiology.

References
1. Kasper DL, Braunwald E, Fauci AS, et al., eds. *Harrison's principles of internal medicine*, 16th ed. Available at: http://www.accessmedicine.com/resourceTOC.aspx?resourceID=4. McGraw-Hill's AccessMedicine, 2004–2005.
2. Landaw SA. Approach to the patient with splenomegaly. UpToDate Online 13.2. May 2, 2005. Available at: http://www.utdol.com/utd/content/topic.do?topicKey=red_cell/30042&type=A&selectedTitle=1~116.
3. Way LW, Doherty GM. *Current surgical diagnosis and treatment online*, 11th ed. San Francisco: California Medical Association, 2004–2005.
4. Kaplan LJ, Coffman D. *Splenomegaly*. eMedicine from WebMD. Available at: http://www.emedicine.com/med/topic2156.htm. Last updated: October 5, 2004.
5. Brottmiller WG, et al., eds. *Mosby's guide to physical examination*, 2nd ed. St Louis, MO: Mosby Year Book, Inc, 1991.
6. Yang JC, Rickman LS, Bosser SK. The clinical diagnosis of splenomegaly. *West J Med* 1991;155:47–52.

Laboratory Abnormalities: Hematology and Urine Determinations

Carol A. LaCroix

16

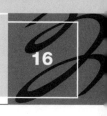

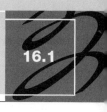

I. **BACKGROUND.** Anemia, simply put, is too few red blood cells (RBCs). In men, it is usually defined as hemoglobin of <13.5 g/dL or a hematocrit of <41.0%, and in women, as hemoglobin <12.0 g/dL or a hematocrit of <36.0%. It is important to remember that anemia is only a symptom of a disease, not the disease itself. Whenever anemia is found, the cause must be sought.

II. **PATHOPHYSIOLOGY.** The causes for anemia can be broken down into three main categories:

   A. **Decreased production.** Anemia results when the rate of RBC production is less than the rate of RBC destruction. Decreased production may be due to many causes, including lack of nutrients. Decreased intake or malabsorption of nutrients such as iron, vitamin B_{12}, or folate may cause decreased RBC production. A bone marrow disorder such as aplastic anemia, myelodysplasia, or tumor infiltration may decrease RBC production as well. Patients who are undergoing chemotherapy or radiation may have bone marrow suppression.

   B. **Increased RBC destruction.** The normal RBC life span is 120 days; certain situations may decrease the survival of RBCs. Hemolytic anemia is the result of increased RBC destruction. There are hereditary causes of hemolytic anemia, including hereditary spherocytosis, sickle-cell anemia, and thalassemia. Acquired hemolytic anemias include autoimmune, thrombotic thrombocytopenic purpura and hemolytic uremic syndrome.

   C. **Blood loss.** Blood loss is by far the most common cause of anemia. Sometimes the source of bleeding may be obvious, such as in a trauma, or it may be occult such as in a gastrointestinal bleed. In women, menstrual bleeding should always be considered.

III. **EVALUATION**

   A. **History.** A thorough history should include questions regarding symptoms such as fatigue, light-headedness, fever, weight loss, and night sweats. A gynecologic history should be taken in women. Patients should be asked whether they have ever been anemic before or have a family history of anemia or bleeding disorders. A nutritional history should also be obtained to evaluate for possible malnutrition; this is especially important in elderly and alcoholic patients. Concomitant conditions that may also contribute to the development of anemia include renal failure, cancer treatment, and immunosuppression. A thorough medication history should also be taken; any herbal supplements taken by the patient should be noted.

   B. **Physical examination.** Pertinent findings include pallor of the skin and conjunctivae. Examination of the patient in natural light may reveal jaundice. Petechiae may indicate a platelet abnormality as well. Cardiovascular examination may reveal a systolic flow murmur, tachycardia, or strong peripheral pulses. An abdominal examination may be significant for splenomegaly, which may suggest a lymphoproliferative disorder.

   C. **Testing.** Finding the etiology of anemia requires a few basic laboratory values. First, a complete blood count (CBC) is essential. This not only gives the value of hemoglobin and hematocrit but also gives the white blood cell count and platelet count. These are important in the evaluation of pancytopenia. The CBC should also include the mean corpuscular volume (MCV), which indicates the average size of the RBCs and helps with diagnosis. A reticulocyte count is also helpful in determining whether the bone marrow is responding appropriately to the level of anemia. Additional testing may include iron studies: ferritin, total iron-binding

351

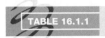

TABLE 16.1.1	Etiology of Anemia Based on Mean Corpuscular Volume		
Mean Corpuscular Volume (fL)	**<80**	**80–100**	**>100**
Possible etiology	Iron deficiency Thalassemia Myelodysplastic syndrome Sideroblastic anemia Chronic disease	Acute hemorrhage Chronic renal insufficiency Chronic disease Iron deficiency (early)	Vitamin B_{12} deficiency Folate deficiency Sickle-cell disease Reticulocytosis Liver disease Endocrine dysfunction Alcohol abuse

capacity (TIBC), and percent iron saturation. Vitamin deficiencies may be evaluated by vitamin B_{12} and folate levels. If a hereditary disorder is suspected, hemoglobin electrophoresis may be required. A peripheral blood smear is also helpful in many cases.

IV. DIAGNOSIS

   A. The simplest way to determine the diagnosis in anemia is to follow a three-step approach.

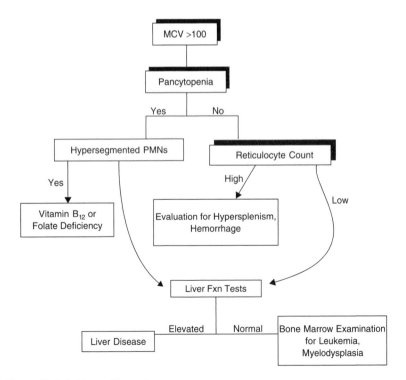

Figure 16.1.1. Macrocytic anemia.

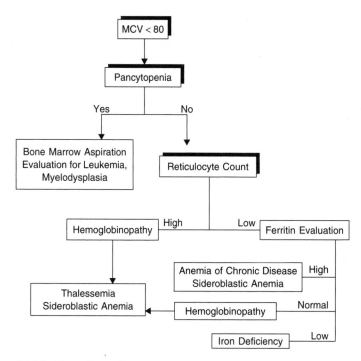

Figure 16.1.2. Microcytic anemia.

1. **Step one.** Categorize the anemia as microcytic, normocytic, or macrocytic on the basis of the MCV. See Table 16.1.1.
2. **Step two.** Determine whether pancytopenia is present. If there is also a decrease in the number of white blood cells and platelets, this indicates a depression of all cell lines produced by bone marrow. If pancytopenia is found, a bone marrow examination is almost always necessary.
3. **Step three.** Determine a cause for the anemia by evaluating the reticulocyte count. This value helps determine whether the bone marrow response to the anemia is appropriate.

B. Cause of anemia

1. **Microcytic anemias** (Figure 16.1.2)
   a. **Anemia of chronic disease.** Decreased iron and decreased TIBC; increased ferritin
   b. **Sideroblastic anemia.** Increased iron and normal TIBC; increased ferritin. Peripheral smear shows basophilic stippling and ringed sideroblasts.
   c. **Iron deficiency anemia.** Decreased iron and increased TIBC. Ferritin <12 μg/L is very suggestive of iron deficiency.
   d. **Thalassemia.** Very low MCV (usually <70 fL); normal iron studies. The peripheral smear may reveal basophilic stippling. Hemoglobin electrophoresis is needed for diagnosis.

2. **Normocytic anemias**
   a. **Hemorrhage.** Look for source of blood loss, perform a Hemoccult's stool
   b. Glucose-6-phosphate deficiency
   c. **Autoimmune hemolytic anemia.** Positive Coombs
   d. **Membranopathies.** Hereditary spherocytosis with splenomegaly on physical examination

3. **Macrocytic anemias** (Figure 16.1.1)
   a. **Vitamin B$_{12}$ or folate deficiency.** Low serum vitamin B$_{12}$ and folate levels. The peripheral smear reveals hypersegmented neutrophils. Vitamin B$_{12}$ deficiency may also have neurologic findings.
   b. **Liver disease.** Elevated liver function tests, aspartate aminotransferase, and alanine aminotransferase. The peripheral smear may reveal target and spur cells.

Suggested Readings

Farley P. Iron deficiency anemia: how to diagnose and correct. *Anemia* 1990;87:89–101.

Schrier SL. Approach to the adult patient with anemia Up to Date Patient Information. Available at: http://patients.update.com/topic.asp?file=red_cell/2950&title=Anemia. Last updated June 2006.

Braunwald E, Harrison TR, Armitage JO, et al. *Principles of internal medicine*, 15th ed.349–352.

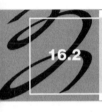

16.2 EOSINOPHILIA

Tina M. Flores

I. **BACKGROUND.** Eosinophilia, an accumulation of eosinophils in the peripheral blood at levels greater than the normal range, can occur in a multitude of diseases. Eosinophilia can be classified as mild (351–1,500 cells/mm^3), moderate (1,501–5,000 cells/mm^3), or severe (greater than 5,000 cells/mm^3) (1). There is little concern about mild eosinophilia if an identifiable cause is found and the eosinophilia resolves with treatment. Moderate to severe eosinophilia should be evaluated carefully, because it can lead to eosinophilic infiltration of the eyes, heart, liver, lungs, gastrointestinal tract, or central nervous system, resulting in permanent end-organ damage (2).

II. **PATHOPHYSIOLOGY**
A. **Etiology.** The causes of eosinophilia can be broken down into two categories: primary and secondary. Primary causes include clonal disorders (myeloid cancers) and the idiopathic hypereosinophilic syndrome. Secondary causes include parasitic infections, allergic diseases, drug reactions, autoimmune disorders, nonmyeloid cancers, and adrenal insufficiency (3).
B. **Epidemiology.** In the Unites States, allergic diseases contribute to most cases of eosinophilia. In developing countries, the most common cause is still parasitosis (1).

III. **EVALUATION**
A. **History.** Any patient with eosinophilia warrants a thorough travel, medication, and family histories, and a review of systems.
B. **Physical examination.** A complete physical examination should also be performed.
C. **Testing.** A complete blood count with differential should be performed to determine the degree of eosinophilia. All further testing should be guided by clues given in the history and physical examination; it may include the following:
   1. **Stool studies for ova and parasites (three samples).** If these are negative, but parasitic infection is strongly suspected, consider small bowel biopsy or muscle biopsy in cases of trichinosis.
   2. Urinalysis with examination for schistosome eggs
   3. Serology for parasites
   4. Sputum evaluation for eosinophils
   5. Blood cultures to evaluate for bacterial infection
   6. Chest x-ray with or without chest computed tomography scan to evaluate for pulmonary involvement

    7. 12-lead electrocardiogram and echocardiogram to evaluate for cardiac involvement

    8. Liver function panel and renal profile to evaluate for end-organ damage

    9. Bone marrow biopsy to evaluate for clonal disorders

  D. Genetics. Allergic diseases such as asthma and some malignancies appear to have a strong hereditary component as well as an environmental cause. Ten percent of solid tumors are inherited. Studies have shown the heritability component of asthma to be between 36% and 72% (4). Research in this area continues to attempt at determining the exact mechanism of transmission of asthma.

IV. DIAGNOSIS. It is important to consider the differential diagnosis of eosinophilia, because the prognosis and treatment vary greatly, depending on the cause. If the diagnosis of eosinophilia still remains elusive after an extensive workup, consider referral to infectious disease or hematology.

  A. Primary eosinophilia

    1. Clonal disease. This includes eosinophilic leukemias and myeloid disorders. Clinical manifestations of leukemia include weight loss, fever, lymphadenopathy, night sweats, recurrent infections, and easy bruising.

    2. Hypereosinophilic syndrome. Patients typically present with a moderate to severe eosinophilia. Symptoms must be present for more than 6 months with end-organ damage and no identifiable cause of the eosinophilia. Men are more than two times more likely than women to be diagnosed with this disease (2).

  B. Secondary eosinophilia

    1. Allergic diseases. These include asthma, atopic dermatitis, and allergic rhinitis. Patients with asthma may complain of dyspnea, wheezing, or cough. Sneezing, rhinorrhea, and nasal itching are the hallmark of allergic rhinitis. Patients with atopic dermatitis may complain of rash, dry skin, and itching.

    2. Drug reaction. Certain medications such as sulfonamides, phenytoin, gold compounds, aspirin, allopurinol, and some toxins may lead to eosinophilia.

    3. Tissue-invasive parasitic infections. These include schistosomiasis, visceral toxocariasis, strongyloidiasis, filariasis, ancylostomiasis, fascioliasis, trichinellosis, and paragonimiasis (5). Symptoms vary depending on the invasion site and may include abdominal pain, diarrhea or constipation, fever, rash, muscle aches, dysuria, and lymphadenopathy.

    4. Bacterial/viral infections. This is a less common cause of eosinophilia, although *Borrelia* infections and human immunodeficiency virus (HIV) have been implicated. HIV can manifest with weight loss, fever, night sweats, and recurrent infections.

    5. Autoimmune disorders. This includes Wegener's granulomatosis, Kimura's disease, Churg-Strauss syndrome, scleroderma, sarcoidosis, polyarteritis nodosum, and inflammatory bowel disease. The symptoms are dependent on the organ involved in the disease process.

    6. Cancer. This includes Hodgkin's lymphoma and metastatic cancers (lung, cervical, breast, liver, pancreas, and kidney). The patient may exhibit fever, weight loss, and night sweats.

    7. Adrenal insufficiency. This can lead to hyperpigmentation of the skin, fatigue, weight loss, weakness, and abdominal pain.

References

1. Rothenberg ME. Eosinophilia. *N Engl J Med* 1998;38:1592–1599.
2. Sutton S, Assa'ad A, Rothenberg M. Anti-IL-5 and hypereosinophilic syndromes. *Clin Immunol* 2005;115:51–60.
3. Tefferi A. Blood eosinophilia: a new paradigm in disease classification, diagnosis, and treatment. *Mayo Clin Proc* 2005;80:75–83.
4. Blumenthal M. The immunopathology and genetics of asthma. *Minn Med* 2004;87: 53–56.
5. Grathwol K, LeBrun C, Tenglin R. Eosinophilia of the blood. *Postgrad Med* 1995;97: 169–172.

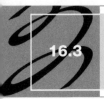

NEUTROPENIA
16.3
Sara Graybill

I. BACKGROUND. Neutropenia is defined as an absolute neutrophil count (ANC) of <1,500/μL. The ANC is calculated using the total white blood cell count and the fraction of polymorphonuclear (PMN) cells and band forms from the differential. The formula follows (1):

$$ANC = WBC \ (cells/\mu L) \times percent \ (PMNs + bands) \div 100$$

II. PATHOPHYSIOLOGY

  A. Etiology. The three basic processes leading to neutropenia include (a) decreased production, (b) enhanced peripheral destruction, and (c) pooling of neutrophils in the vascular endothelium or tissue (2).

  B. Epidemiology. Blacks and people from the Middle East may normally have ANCs as low as 1,500/μL yet have no problems with recurrent infections.

III. EVALUATION

  A. History. Recent, recurrent, or frequent infections point to immune dysfunction. History of current and prior medications should be taken. Several illnesses also

---

TABLE 16.3.1   **Differential Diagnosis of Neutropenia (1)**

Acquired

  Infection

  Collagen vascular diseases (e.g., Felty's syndrome, systemic lupus erythematosus)

  Complement activation (e.g., hemodialysis, acute respiratory distress syndrome)

  Drug-induced (e.g., sulfonamides, chlorpromazine, clozapine, diuretics, gold)

  Toxins (e.g., benzene)

  Autoimmune

  Transfusion reaction

  Pure white cell aplasia

  Hypersplenism

  Nutritional deficiency (e.g., alcoholism, vitamin B_{12}/folate deficiency)

  Diseases affecting bone marrow (e.g., leukemia, chemotherapy, aplastic anemia, tumor replacement)

Congenital

  Cyclic neutropenia

  Chédiak-Higashi syndrome

  Severe congenital neutropenia (Kostmann's syndrome)

  Severe infantile agranulocytosis

Revised from Baehner R. *Overview of neutropenia.* In: Rose B, ed. UpToDate. Wellesley, MA: UpToDate, 2005.

have neutropenia as a related feature or as a consequence of their treatment. A history of heavy alcohol use and possible exposure to occupational toxins should be elicited. Finally, family history may point to rare hereditary conditions.

B. Physical examination. Splenomegaly may be present. The oral cavity should also be explored as gingivitis, stomatitis, and abscesses are often the first presenting sequelae of mild neutropenia.

C. Testing. A manual differential and peripheral blood smear can confirm the diagnosis of neutropenia. If pancytopenia exists, a bone marrow biopsy is required. If the neutropenia is mild (ANC >1,000/μL), and the patient has no infections, ANC measurements three times per week may be done to see whether the condition resolves. If counts normalize, surveillance for the next year should include a complete blood count at the first sign of infection to look for recurrence. If neutropenia fails to resolve after 8 weeks, recurrent infections develop, or lower ANC (<1,000/μL) counts are noted, further workup is needed. Additional laboratory tests may include bone marrow biopsy (even if not pancytopenic), antinuclear antibodies, complement levels, rheumatoid factor, antineutrophil antibodies, immunoglobulins, human immunodeficiency virus serology, vitamin B_{12} and folate levels, and bone marrow culture (1).

D. Genetics. Hereditary neutropenia is rare. Two main forms include cyclic neutropenia and severe congenital neutropenia (Kostmann's syndrome). *ELA2* gene mutations have been linked to both disorders (3).

IV. DIAGNOSIS

A. Differential diagnosis. A practical approach to the differential diagnosis of neutropenia is listed in Table 16.3.1.

B. Clinical manifestations. The hallmark of neutropenia is recurrentneutropenia! infections. However, on examination of the patient with severe neutropenia, the classic signs of infection may be absent. The inflammatory response is blunted, which may cause diminished fever, peritoneal signs, and radiologic findings. As a result, the patient's infection may go undetected until late in the course. Infections in patients also progress more rapidly and a patient with neutropenia must be treated more aggressively than a patient without it.

References

1. Baehner R. *Overview of neutropenia*, UpToDate Patient Information 14.2. Available at: http://patients.update.com/topic.asp.?file=whitecel/5073&title=Neutropenia. Last updated June 2006.
2. Holland SM, Gallin JI. Disorders of granulocytes and monocytes. In: Kasper D, Harrison TR, Armitage JO, et al., eds. *Harrison's principles of internal medicine*, 16th ed. New York, NY: McGraw-Hill, 2005.
3. Berliner N, Horwitz M, Loughran TP, *Congenital and acquired neutropenia*. American Society of Hematology Education Program, 2004:63–79. Available at: http://www.asheducationbook.org/cgi/content/full/2004/1/63.

POLYCYTHEMIA
Katrina Carter

16.4

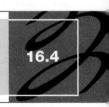

I. BACKGROUND. Polycythemia occurs when the serum hematocrit is very high. This is generally greater than 48% in women and 52% in men. A hemoglobin >16.5 g/dL in women and 18.5 g/dL in men is also considered polycythemic. This elevation in hemoglobin or hematocrit may be relative or absolute. Relative polycythemia occurs when there is no true increase in the red blood cell (RBC) mass but rather a contraction of the plasma volume. Absolute polycythemia occurs when there is a true increase in the RBC mass due to either primary or secondary causes (1).

II. PATHOPHYSIOLOGY

A. Primary polycythemia results from an acquired or inherited abnormality of RBC precursors. Simply put, the RBCs undergo clonal expansion. Although the RBC is the most prominent feature, the white blood cells and platelets multiply as well. The increase in cell mass results in hyperviscosity of the blood. This causes most of the symptoms experienced by the patient such as headache, dizziness, pruritus, and stroke (2).

B. Secondary polycythemia occurs in response to increased erythropoietin (EPO). EPO is produced in the kidneys in response to hypoxia. This is a mechanism to increase the oxygen-carrying capacity of the circulation. In response to a hypoxic insult, EPO is released, but it may be released for other reasons as well. Inappropriate release of EPO may occur with renal tumors or hepatomas.

III. EVALUATION

A. History. The most common cause of polycythemia is related to hypoxia, therefore a thorough evaluation of the respiratory status should be sought. Patients should be asked if they have a history of asthma or chronic obstructive pulmonary disease (COPD). Additional symptoms such as shortness of breath, dyspnea on exertion, or cyanosis should be ascertained. A thorough smoking history should be elicited, including how many cigarettes patients smoke daily and how many years they have smoked, and if they are no longer smoking, how many years ago did they stop. Many jobs predispose patients to environmental exposures. Patients should be asked about their occupation and if they are exposed to substances such as carbon monoxide at work. Particular persons who are at high risk are industrial

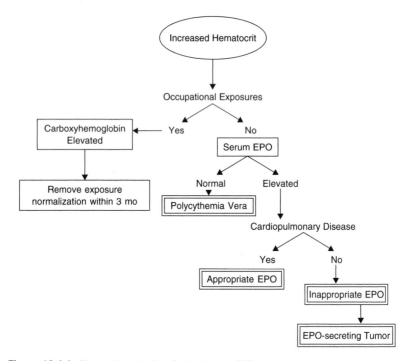

Figure 16.4.1. Diagnostic evaluation of polycythemia. EPO, erythropoietin.

workers and individuals who work in poorly ventilated areas. Patients may also report increased itching all over their body, particularly after showering (2, 3).

B. Physical examination. The physical examination in patients with polycythemia may be notable for cyanosis of lips, earlobes, and extremities. Clubbing may also be evident. A thorough abdominal examination for hepatosplenomegaly and a heart examination evaluating for murmurs or bruits should be performed.

C. Testing. The most important laboratory tests are hemoglobin, hematocrit, and RBC count. These values should be adjusted for the sex and age of the patient. One should also obtain a white blood cell count and platelet count. A urinalysis should be obtained, looking for hematuria. Liver function tests should also be obtained. If cardiopulmonary disease is suspected, a chest x-ray may be helpful to assess the patient for COPD or congestive heart failure. If the patient has significant exposures, a serum carboxyhemoglobin should be obtained.

IV. DIAGNOSIS. Whenever a laboratory value comes back grossly elevated, it should be repeated. Once an increase in hemoglobin and hematocrit is confirmed, an evaluation of possible causes must begin (see Figure 16.4.1).

A. If the patient has occupational exposures and the carboxyhemoglobin is elevated, a trial of stopping the exposures should be done. Resolution of abnormal blood values should occur within 3 months.

B. If the patient has no exposure, and the carboxyhemoglobin is within normal limits, a serum EPO level should be obtained. If it is low, the diagnosis is polycythemia vera, or primary polycythemia. If EPO levels are high, it is indicative of either a hypoxic response (appropriate response) or overproduction by a tumor (inappropriate). Depending on the circumstances, further evaluation may not be necessary. For example, if the EPO level is mildly elevated, and the patient has COPD, then there is a low suspicion of a tumor. If, on the other hand, the patient has no risk factors for cardiopulmonary disease and a highly elevated EPO, evaluation for a tumor should be done. Abdominal ultrasound or abdominal computed tomography scan is recommended in patients with a high suspicion for an EPO-secreting tumor. EPO-secreting tumors are usually hepatocellular carcinoma, pheochromocytoma, hemangioblastoma, uterine myomata, and, most commonly, renal cell carcinoma (1, 2).

References
1. Rakel R. *Textbook of family practice*, 6th ed. Philadelphia, PA: WB Saunders. 2002:1262–1266.
2. Harrison TR, et al. *Principles of internal medicine*. 15th ed. McGraw-Hill Professional. 2001:353–354.
3. Tefferi A. *Diagnostic approach to the patient with polycythemia*. Up to Date 2006.

THROMBOCYTOPENIA
Teresa Stump

16.5

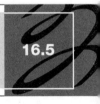

I. BACKGROUND. Thrombocytopenia occurs when there is an abnormal decrease in the number of platelets. This condition is encountered when the platelet count is <100,000 μL. A unique relation exists between platelet count and bleeding tendencies. For example, patients with platelet counts of >50,000 μL are generally asymptomatic and are diagnosed incidentally, whereas patients whose platelet counts are <10,000 μL are at risk of spontaneous bleeding (1–3).

II. PATHOPHYSIOLOGY

A. Etiology. Thrombocytopenia occurs through one of the following mechanisms (1–3): inadequate number of platelets produced by the bone marrow, increased destruction of platelets, entrapment in the spleen, or a dilution effect.

1. Autoimmune thrombocytopenic conditions arise through explicit autoantibodies, resulting in either increased destruction of platelets or impairment of specific proteins. This leads to platelet aggregation and thrombus formation (4).
2. Drug-induced thrombocytopenia may be caused by a plethora of medications. The most frequent culprit, especially in hospitalized patients, is heparin. Although drug-induced thrombocytopenia is also an antibody-mediated syndrome, it is transient, typically resolving when the offending agent is discontinued (1,2,4).

B. **Epidemiology.** Immune thrombocytopenic purpura (ITP) is a relatively common autoimmune thrombocytopenic disease that occurs in the acute and chronic setting with a prevalence of one in ten thousand persons. Acute ITP is seen solely in children 2 to 9 years of age with a peak incidence at 3 to 5 years of age. It affects men and women equally. Acute ITP typically follows an acute viral syndrome and has a self-limiting course. In contrast, chronic ITP has a female predominance of 3:1, affects adults 20 to 50 years of age, and rarely results in spontaneous remission (1,2,4).

III. EVALUATION

A. **History.** A meticulous history must be obtained with particular focus on the following:
   1. A thorough review of all medications currently being taken and the date prescribed
   2. Menstrual and pregnancy history
   3. The presence of the following: epistaxis and bleeding gums; reddish or purplish discoloration of the skin; excessive bruising; and hematuria, melena, hematochezia, and bright red blood from the rectum
   4. Alcohol use

B. **Physical examination.** A thorough physical examination is warranted with special emphasis on the following:
   1. Skin examination looking for petechiae, purpura, and ecchymoses
   2. Abdominal examination to assess for splenomegaly and hepatomegaly
   3. Neurologic examination to ascertain if hemorrhage has occurred, although rare

C. **Testing.** A complete blood count with differential and peripheral smear is essential for evaluating thrombocytopenia. Imaging studies are rarely indicated. Bone marrow biopsy is beneficial in patients with splenomegaly and in those who follow an uncharacteristic course.

IV. DIAGNOSIS (1–5).

Determining the etiology of thrombocytopenia may seem daunting initially. A comprehensive history and physical examination along with a few laboratory tests often leads to the correct diagnosis.

A. Inadequate number of platelets produced by the bone marrow. Diagnoses include the following:
   1. Leukemia
   2. Lymphoma
   3. Aplastic and megaloblastic anemia
   4. Heavy alcohol use

B. Increased destruction of platelets. Diagnoses include the following:
   1. Immune thrombocytopenia purpura (diagnosis of exclusion)
   2. Human immunodeficiency virus/acquired immunodeficiency syndrome
   3. Medications (e.g., heparin, quinine, rifampin, gold salts)
   4. Disseminated intravascular coagulation, HELLP (hemolysis, elevated liver enzymes, low platelet count) syndrome
   5. Thrombotic thrombocytopenic purpura
   6. Hemolytic-uremic syndrome

C. Entrapment in the spleen. Diagnoses include the following:
   1. Cirrhosis
   2. Myelofibrosis
   3. Gaucher's disease

D. Dilution effect: large blood replacement with too few platelets

E. Laboratory error: clotted specimen, wrong patient, or technical/equipment errors

References

1. George JN. *Evaluation and management of thrombocytopenia by primary care physicians.* www.uptodate.com, 2004.
2. Thiagarajan P. *Platelet disorders.* www.emedicine.com/med/topic987.htm. Last updated September 2004.
3. *Thrombocytopenia: bleeding and clotting disorders.* The Merck Manual of Medical Information. Available at: http://www.merck.com/mmhe/sec14/ch173/ch173d.html. Last updated February 2003.
4. Kravitz MS, Shoenfeld Y. Thrombocytopenic conditions-autoimmunity and hypercoagulability: commonalities and differences in ITP, TTP, HIT, and APS. *Am J Hematol* 2005;80:232–242.
5. Vesely SK, Perdue JJ, Rizvi MA, et al. Management of adult patients with persistent idiopathic thrombocytopenic purpura following splenectomy: a systematic review. *Ann Intern Med* 2004;140:112–121.

ERYTHROCYTE SEDIMENTATION RATE AND C-REACTIVE PROTEIN

16.6

Elisabeth L. Backer

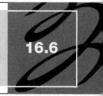

I. BACKGROUND. The erythrocyte sedimentation rate (ESR) and C-reactive protein (CRP) are currently the most widely used indicators of the acute phase protein response, used to detect illnesses associated with acute and chronic infection, inflammation, tissue destruction, and advanced neoplasm. The CRP is a more sensitive and rapidly responding indicator than the ESR, often showing an earlier and more intense increase than the ESR in an acute inflammatory process. With recovery, the disappearance of the CRP precedes the normalization of the ESR (1).

II. PATHOPHYSIOLOGY. The acute phase response is a major pathophysiologic phenomenon that accompanies inflammation and other disorders (2). Focus on this phenomenon first occurred with the discovery of elevated serum concentrations of CRP during the acute phase of pneumococcal pneumonia (3). The initial concept of an ESR dates back to 1918. The Westergren method is still considered the gold standard for measuring the ESR (4).

III. EVALUATION

A. Physical examination. Acute phase reactant measurements are useful in conjunction with a thorough physical examination. Because the ESR and CRP levels are influenced by multiple factors, the results should be interpreted in the light of the clinical findings.

B. Testing

1. The ESR, which measures the distance in millimeters that erythrocytes fall during 1 hour, is a simple but nonspecific laboratory test ordered frequently in clinical practice. The CRP is a nonspecific (3) acute phase reactant protein used to diagnose infectious and inflammatory disorders; it also serves as a cardiovascular disease (CVD) marker (5). The ESR has the advantages of familiarity, simplicity, and extensive literature compiled over many decades (3). The CRP is standardized, inexpensive, and widely available.

2. Although elevations in multiple components of the acute phase response commonly occur together, not all happen uniformly in all patients, and discrepancies between ESR and CRP are found fairly frequently (2) (e.g., an elevated ESR together with a normal CRP may reflect a false-positive value for the ESR). Currently, the optimal use of the acute phase reactants may be to obtain several measurements and interpret the results in the light of the clinical context (3,5).

3. CRP levels can be affected by lifestyle choices, concurrent disease, pharmacotherapy, age, gender (female), and possibly ethnicity (e.g., African Americans).

   a. Factors known to increase CRP values include smoking, elevated body mass index, elevated blood pressure, dyslipidemia, metabolic syndrome, type 2 diabetes, hormone use, chronic infections (bronchitis), and chronic inflammation (rheumatoid arthritis) (5).

   b. Factors known to decrease CRP values include moderate alcohol consumption, physical exercise, weight loss, and medications (statins, fibrates, thiazolidinediones, anti-inflammatory agents, salicylates, and steroids) (5).

4. ESR levels can be affected by menstruation and pregnancy, hematologic disorders, medications, gender, age, ethnicity, and obesity (1, 3). Conditions with an ESR of >100 mm/hour include abscess formation, subacute bacterial endocarditis, osteomyelitis, temporal arteritis, collagen vascular disease, multiple myeloma, leukemia/lymphoma, neoplasms, and drug hypersensitivity reactions.

   a. Factors known to increase ESR values include chronic renal failure (nephritis, nephrosis), macroglobulinemia, hyperfibrinogenemia, iron/vitamin B_{12} deficiency anemias, medications (dextran, heparin, methyldopa, oral contraceptives, penicillamine, procainamide, theophylline, vitamin A), female gender, advanced age, African-American ethnicity, and hyperlipidemia (1).

   b. Factors known to decrease ESR levels include sickle-cell anemia, spherocytosis, hypofibrinogenemia, polycythemia vera, medications (aspirin, cortisone, quinine), and chronic heart failure (1).

IV. DIAGNOSIS

A. Despite the lack of diagnostic specificity, measuring acute phase protein levels is useful in differentiating between inflammatory and noninflammatory conditions and in evaluating the response to and the need for therapeutic interventions. In general, the ESR increases as the disease worsens and decreases as it improves. The CRP may be useful when the ESR is equivocal or inconsistent with the clinical impressions (1). Results should be expressed as the average of two tests performed 2 weeks apart. Patients with levels >10 mg/L should be examined for sources of inflammation before repeating the test (5). Acute phase reactants should not be ordered for screening purposes in asymptomatic patients (1).

1. Normal ESR rates for men between 20 and 65 years of age can be empirically calculated as age/2; for women it would be (age plus 10)/2 (1). Most healthy subjects have a CRP level of <3 mg/L. Levels of 3 to 10 mg/L may indicate minor degrees of inflammation or other influences. Levels >10 mg/L suggest significant inflammation (3).

2. CRP testing is also recommended as an adjunct to traditional risk factor assessment in CVD. It has been found to be the strongest marker of future CVD, *de novo* atherosclerosis, and plaque rupture. Additionally, it has independent prognostic value for future strokes and peripheral vascular disease (5). The relative risk category based on CRP levels is shown in Table 16.6.1.

TABLE 16.6.1	Risk of cardiovascular disease based on C-reactive protein level

Risk	C-reactive protein (mg/L)
Low	<1
Average	1.0–3.0
High	>3.0

B. Specific applications of acute phase reactant measurements include disease processes such as Crohn's disease, rheumatoid arthritis (CRP superior to ESR), polymyalgia rheumatica, and giant cell arteritis (ESR often >100 mm/hour, but CRP may be more sensitive for disease detection), and the noninvasive prognostic assessment in patients with malignancy (3). Systemic lupus erythematosus represents an exception in that CRP levels are often not elevated, except during bacterial infections (3).

References

1. Pagana KD, Pagana TJ. *Mosby's manual of diagnostic and laboratory tests.* St. Louis, MO: Mosby, 1998.
2. Kushner I. The phenomenon of the acute phase response. *Ann N Y Acad Sci* 1982; 389:39–48.
3. www.UpToDate.com, accessed on June 30, 2005.
4. Bedell SE, Bush BT. Erythrocyte sedimentation rate. From folklore to facts. *Am J Med* 1985;78(6 Pt 1):1001–1009.
5. Brunton S. The value of C-reactive protein in the clinical assessment of cardiovascular disease risk. *Female Patient* 2005;30:11–16.

PROTEINURIA
Carol A. LaCroix

16.7

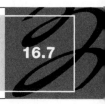

I. BACKGROUND. It is normal for an adult to excrete 80 to 150 mg of protein in the urine per day. Usually, the excreted protein consists of 40% albumin, 40% uromodulin (also known as *Tamm-Horsfall mucoprotein* from the loop of Henle), and 20% small-molecular-weight globulins (1, 2). Microalbuminuria refers to an excretion rate of 30 to 300 mg of albumin per day, whereas the nephrotic range is more than 3,000 mg per day (3).

II. PATHOPHYSIOLOGY. Proteinuria may be transient or persistent. Transient proteinuria can occur with exercise, cold exposure, fever, and congestive heart failure. Persistent proteinuria is diagnosed when a value of >300 mg/dL has been documented in three urine specimens. There are three types of proteinuria: glomerular, tubular, and overflow. Glomerular proteinuria involves increased permeability to plasma proteins in the glomeruli and may range from the minimal to the nephrotic range. Tubular proteinuria occurs when the proximal tubule is unable to reabsorb proteins. Overflow proteinuria results from an overproduction of immunoglobulins, particularly in multiple myeloma (1).

III. EVALUATION

    A. History. Proteinuria is usually identified on a urinalysis obtained for a routine physical examination. Sometimes the patient reports foamy urine, which is due to an alteration of the surface tension by the proteins.

    B. Physical examination. Check vital signs, especially blood pressure. Perform a funduscopic examination, checking for diabetic retinopathy or vascular changes from hypertension. Edema of the legs or face may be due to hypoalbuminemia. Check the abdomen for masses (such as polycystic kidneys) and renal artery bruits. Look for evidence of rheumatologic joint changes.

    C. Testing

        1. A dipstick test of the urine preferentially identifies albumin. It can be falsely negative when the urine is dilute (specific gravity <1.015) and when the proteins are of low molecular weight. The dipstick can be falsely positive with alkaline urine, gross hematuria, pus, semen, vaginal secretions, and the presence of penicillin and sulfonamides. The proteinuria is graded as 30 mg/dL (1+), 100 mg/dL (2+), 300 mg/dL (3+), and 1,000 mg/dL (4+).

2. After persistent proteinuria has been confirmed, a quantitative measurement should be obtained. The gold standard has been the 24-hour urine collection. Another option is the urine protein-to-creatinine ratio (UPr/Cr), which can be determined on a random urine specimen. A ratio <0.2 is normal, whereas a ratio more than 3.0 is in the nephrotic range. The flag for microalbuminuria has been set at 30 mg/24 hours (4).

3. The next step is to look for an underlying cause that can be treated. The differential diagnosis includes diabetes mellitus, glomerulonephritides with low complement levels, streptococcal glomerulonephritis, systemic lupus, multiple myeloma, and sarcoidosis. Hematuria may indicate infection, stones, or nephritis (4, 5).

4. Any adult or child with proteinuria or hematuria without a clear diagnosis should have a nephrology consult. This is especially true if the proteinuria is >2 g/day, because the person most likely has some type of glomerular disease. Most of these patients will need a renal biopsy. One exception is patients with postinfectious glomerulonephritis, which is usually self-limiting (4).

IV. DIAGNOSIS

A. Transient proteinuria does not require further evaluation or monitoring. Orthostatic proteinuria accounts for up to 60% of asymptomatic proteinuria in individuals 6 to 30 years of age. This condition appears to be benign, although yearly follow-up is recommended.

B. Dehydration, fever, intense physical activity, emotional stress, and seizures can cause benign proteinuria. Secondary glomerulonephropathy occurs with diabetes mellitus, lupus, amyloidosis, preeclampsia, recent streptococcal infections, endocarditis, human immunodeficiency virus, and hepatitis B and C. Tubular nephropathy may be due to hypertension, sickle-cell disease, or urate stones.

C. Gold, penicillamine, lithium, and heroin can cause glomerulonephropathy. Nonsteroidal anti-inflammatory drugs and heavy metals can damage both the glomeruli and the tubules. Patients with glomerulonephropathy should be closely monitored with regard to proteinuria and hyperlipidemia.

D. A history of polycystic kidney disease, hypertension, diabetes, or autoimmune disease such as lupus may point to the diagnosis (5).

References

1. Devuyust O, Dahan K, Pirson Y. Tamm-Horsfall protein or uromodulin. *Nephrol Dial Transplant* 2005;20(7):1290–1294.
2. Loghman-Adham M. Evaluating proteinuria in children. *Am Fam Physician* 1998;58(5): 1145–1158.
3. Molitch MR, DeFrazo RA, Franz MJ, et al. Nephropathy in diabetes. *Diabetes Care* 2004;27(suppl 1):S79–83. Available at: http://care.diabetesjounals.org/cgi/content/full/27/suppl_1/s79#BIBL.
4. Hassan A. Proteinuria. *Postgrad Med* 1997;101(4):173–180.
5. Carroll MF, Temte JL. Proteinuria in adults. *Am Fam Physician* 2000;62(2):1333–1342.

Laboratory Abnormalities: Blood Chemistry and Immunology

17

Judith A. Fisher

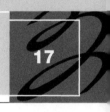

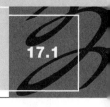

ALKALINE PHOSPHATASE, ELEVATED
Joseph B. Straton and Peter F. Cronholm

17.1

I. **BACKGROUND.** Serum alkaline phosphatase (ALP) arises primarily from the liver and bone although small amounts are derived from the intestines and the vascular endothelium. The normal range of serum ALP varies by age and clinical history. The normal ranges for adolescents, adults older than 60 years, and pregnant women, are higher than for nonpregnant women younger than 60 years. Normal ranges are—infant: 50–165 U/L, child: 20–150 U/L, adult: 20–70 U/L, adult older than 60 years: 30–75 U/L.

Serum ALP should be ordered only if bone or liver disease is suspected. ALP results should be compared with appropriate normal ranges on the basis of the age and clinical history. Abnormal results should be repeated, because spurious elevations can be caused by a recent albumin infusion, the use of an anticoagulant tube for the blood collection, or by serum samples left standing at room temperature for prolonged periods.

II. **PATHOPHYSIOLOGY**
   A. To identify the source of ALP elevations, one can use ALP isoenzyme testing. Alternatively, one can use the results of γ-glutamyltransferase (GGT) or 5'-nucleotidase testing to identify the source. In liver disorders, GGT or 5'-nucleotidase are usually elevated with ALP. ALP elevation in the setting of normal GGT or 5'-nucleotidase suggests a bone source of ALP.
   B. Uncommon causes of ALP elevation include hyperthyroidism, vitamin D deficiency, hepatic infiltration (due to lymphoproliferative disorders, granulomatous disease, or primary and secondary malignancies of the liver), intestinal conditions such as bowel obstruction, and infarction. Additionally, infarction of any solid organ may cause ALP elevation owing to the presence of ALP in the vascular endothelium.

III. **EVALUATION.** Further testing should be performed on the basis of the results of a careful history and physical examination and should be targeted to specific clinical suspicions (Table 17.1.1).

IV. **DIAGNOSIS.** See Table 17.1.1.

 **TABLE 17.1.1**   Evaluation of the Patient with Elevated Alkaline Phosphatase

History	Physical examination	Testing	Diagnosis
A. Bone disorders (1)			
■ Asymptomatic or bone pain ■ Male ■ Hearing/vision problems ■ Headaches ■ Pain increased with walking (tibia involved)	■ Frontal bossing ■ Dilated superficial vessels ■ Saber tibia ■ Deafness ■ Congestive heart failure	■ 24-h urine hydroxyproline ■ Serum phosphate ■ Serum calcium (normal) ■ X-ray involved bone(s) ■ Bone scan	Paget's disease

(continued)

TABLE 17.1.1 Evaluation of the Patient with Elevated Alkaline Phosphatase *(Continued)*

History	Physical examination	Testing	Diagnosis
▪ Female ▪ >60 y ▪ Diffuse aches and pains ▪ Vague abdominal pain ▪ Depressive symptoms ▪ Renal calculi	▪ Neck mass (rare) ▪ Muscle weakness ▪ No clinical evidence of malignancy	▪ Parathyroid hormone ▪ Serum calcium ▪ Urinary calcium/blood ▪ Serum phosphate ▪ Serum chloride	Hyperparathyroidism
▪ >50 y ▪ Unexplained weight loss ▪ Smoker ▪ Cough ▪ Hemoptysis ▪ Shortness of breath	▪ Decreased air entry (wheeze) ▪ Pleural effusion ▪ Dull to percussion ▪ Horner's syndrome	▪ Chest x-ray ▪ Chest CT scan ▪ Bone scan ▪ Serum calcium	▪ Lung cancer
▪ Female ▪ >50 y ▪ Family history ▪ Breast mass	▪ Breast mass ▪ Axillary/supraclavicular nodes ▪ Liver enlargement	▪ Mammogram ▪ Bone scan ▪ Serum calcium	▪ Breast cancer
▪ Female ▪ >45 y ▪ Family history ▪ Abdominal bloating ▪ Unexplained weight loss	▪ Ovarian mass ▪ Ascites	▪ Pelvic ultrasound ▪ Pelvic CT scan ▪ CA-125 ▪ CT scan ▪ Serum calcium	▪ Ovarian cancer
▪ Male ▪ >50 y ▪ Hematuria ▪ Flank/abdominal pain	▪ Unilateral flank mass ▪ Conjunctival pallor	▪ Urinalysis ▪ Abdominal CT scan ▪ Serum calcium	▪ Renal cell carcinoma
▪ Male ▪ >50 y ▪ Urinary complaints ▪ Family history	▪ Prostate mass on rectal examination or diffusely enlarged hard prostate	▪ Serum calcium ▪ Prostate-specific antigen ▪ Ultrasound-guided prostate biopsy ▪ Bone scan	▪ Prostate cancer
▪ 10–30 y ▪ Male ▪ Pain near joint ▪ Very high ALP	▪ Mass near joint ▪ Tender over mass	▪ X-ray area (mixed sclerotic/lytic lesion of bone) ▪ Magnetic resonance imaging of affected region ▪ Bone scan ▪ Biopsy	▪ Osteosarcoma

(continued)

TABLE 17.1.1	Evaluation of the Patient with Elevated Alkaline Phosphatase *(Continued)*		
History	**Physical examination**	**Testing**	**Diagnosis**
■ Recent trauma	■ Bone pain in area	■ X-ray (callous formation)	■ Healing fracture
B. Biliary/liver disease (2)			
■ ALP 2 times normal ■ Alcohol use/abuse (chronic) ■ Family history of liver disease ■ Risky sexual practices ■ Blood transfusions ■ Intravenous drug use ■ Obesity ■ Fatigue ■ Weight loss	■ Spider nevi ■ Leukonychia ■ Dupuytren's contracture ■ Tender RUQ ■ Liver may be enlarged ■ Jaundice	■ Serum AST/ALT levels ↑ in early disease ↓↔ late disease ■ Bilirubin (elevated) ■ Hepatitis screen (A, B, C) ■ Coagulation screen ■ Liver biopsy	■ Cirrhosis ■ Hepatitis ■ Fatty liver
■ Female ■ >40 y ■ Obese ■ Family history of gallstones ■ Pain after meals/episodic ■ Bloating/gas	■ RUQ abdominal tenderness + Murphy's sign (only in acute cholecystitis) ■ Jaundice	■ AST/ALT may be elevated ■ Bilirubin elevated ■ Ultrasound of gallbladder	■ Gallstones ■ Biliary colic ■ Acute cholecystitis
■ ALP 5 times normal ■ 10–25 y old ■ Fever ■ Sore throat/fatigue ■ History of contact with infected friend/relative	■ Fever ■ Tender RUQ ■ Splenomegaly ■ Lymphadenopathy (mainly cervical)	■ Monospot test ■ AST/ALT ■ Complete blood count ■ Toxoplasma titers	■ Infectious mononucleosis ■ Toxoplasmosis ■ Cytomegaloviral infection
■ ALP 10 times normal ■ Weight loss ■ Anorexia ■ Back or RUQ pain ■ Jaundice	■ Palpable gallbladder ■ Cachectic ■ Epigastric mass ■ Jaundice	■ Abdominal CT scan ■ Elevated bilirubin ■ CT scan or ultrasound-guided biopsy	■ Pancreatic carcinoma ■ Gallbladder carcinoma

(continued)

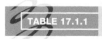

| TABLE 17.1.1 | Evaluation of the Patient with Elevated Alkaline Phosphatase *(Continued)* |

History	Physical examination	Testing	Diagnosis
■ ALP 10–20 times normal ■ Chlorpropamide use ■ Antineoplastic agents ■ Immune modulators	■ Frequently normal ■ RUQ tenderness	■ AST/ALT ■ Liver biopsy if problem persists (3)	■ Drug-induced elevation of ALP
■ ALP 5–20 times normal ■ Female ■ 35–60 years of age (90%) ■ Frequently asymptomatic ■ Itching (palms/soles first) ■ Fatigue ■ Bone pain ■ Steatorrhea ■ Jaundice	■ Excoriations ■ Jaundice ■ Skin pigmentation ■ RUQ tenderness ■ Xanthelasma ■ Liver/spleen enlarged	■ Antimitochondrial antibodies ■ Liver biopsy ■ Elevated bilirubin (late) ■ Elevated liver enzymes (late) ■ Cholesterol elevated	■ Primary biliary cirrhosis
■ ALP >5–20 normal ■ Male ■ 30–60 y of age ■ RUQ pain ■ Jaundice ■ Pruritus ■ Inflammatory bowel disease ■ Fatigue	■ RUQ tenderness ■ Jaundice	■ Endoscopic retrograde cholangiopancreatography	■ Sclerosing cholangitis (primary or secondary)

CT, computed tomography; ALP, alkaline phosphatase; AST, aspartate aminotransferase; ALT, alanine aminotransferase; RUQ, right upper quadrant.

References
1. Taylor AK, Lueken SA, Libanati C, et al. Biochemical markers of bone turnover for the clinical assessment of bone metabolism. *Clin Rheum Dis* 1994;20:589–607.
2. Pratt DS, Kaplan MM. Evaluation of abnormal liver-enzyme results in asymptomatic patients. *N Engl J Med* 2000;342:1266.
3. Sorbi D, McGill DB, Thistle JL, et al. An assessment of the role of liver biopsies in asymptomatic patients with chronic liver test abnormalities. *Am J Gastroenterol* 2000;95:3206.

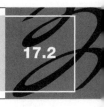

AMINOTRANSFERASE LEVELS, ELEVATED
Peter F. Cronholm and Joseph B. Straton

17.2

I. **BACKGROUND.** Liver function tests (LFTs) are a misnomer in that hepatocellular injury and cholestasis are actually the conditions being measured rather than its function. These tests include aspartate aminotransferase (AST) (or serum glutamic-oxaloacetic transaminase [SGOT]), alanine aminotransferase (ALT) (or serum glutamic-pyrunic transaminase [SGPT]), alkaline phosphatase, and serum bilirubin.

II. **PATHOPHYSIOLOGY.** Evaluation of abnormalities should include an assessment of medication use (including over-the-counter and herbal medications), travel, alcohol consumption and recreational drug use, sexual behavior, signs and symptoms of hepatic injury, and a thorough physical examination. ALT and AST may also be elevated in myocardial infarctions, hemolytic anemia, after trauma, and intramuscular injections.

III. **EVALUATION.** A thorough clinical history and examination are essential in guiding the testing and interpreting the results, because patterns of abnormalities in liver testing are better predictors of clinical disease than any single component. For further details, see Table 17.2.1.

IV. **DIAGNOSIS.** See Table 17.2.1.

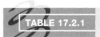 **TABLE 17.2.1** **Evaluation of the Patient with Elevated Aminotransferase**

History	Physical examination	Testing	Diagnosis
■ ALT and AST can be markedly elevated with ratio usually less than one ■ Alkaline phosphatase and serum bilirubin may be elevated or normal ■ Patient often asymptomatic or experiences transient flulike illness ■ Antecedent illness of several days to weeks with nausea, vomiting, anorexia, malaise, diarrhea, arthralgias, or low-grade fever ■ Recent shellfish ingestion ■ Risky sexual practices ■ Past or present intravenous drug use ■ History of blood transfusions or tattoos	■ Jaundice ■ Clay-colored stools ■ Dark urine ■ Left upper quadrant tenderness ■ Hepatomegaly ■ Urticaria ■ Maculopapular skin eruptions ■ Isolated joint swelling, redness, or tenderness	■ Serial testing of amino-transferases ■ CBC ■ Hepatitis A IgM ■ Hepatitis B surface antigen, IgM anti–hepatitis B surface antigen antibody, and IgM anti–hepatitis B core antibody ■ IgG anti–hepatitis C antibody ■ Epstein-Barr virus or cytomegalovirus titers ■ Liver biopsy if diagnosis cannot be determined or to guide treatment for hepatitis C	■ Acute viral hepatitis

(continued)

| | **Evaluation of the Patient with Elevated Aminotransferase** **(Continued)** | | |

History	Physical examination	Testing	Diagnosis
■ ALT and AST can (1) be markedly elevated with ratio usually less than one ■ Excessive somnolence ■ Obtundation ■ History of rectal or upper GI bleeding ■ Rapidly progressive course in 65%–95% of patients ■ Symptoms of sepsis with or without multiorgan failure ■ Prior hepatitis ■ History of aspirin ingestion in children younger than 17 y with influenza or chickenpox ■ Toxic doses of acetaminophen	■ Liver may be reduced in size ■ Ascites ■ Refractory hypotension ■ Petechia ■ Bleeding from mucous membranes ■ Edema	■ Prothrombin time (profoundly prolonged) ■ Low blood glucose ■ Low total serum protein and serum albumin ■ CBC ■ Serum ammonia (may be severely elevated)	■ Fulminant hepatitis ■ Acute hepatic failure associated with Reye's syndrome ■ 1% of the elderly or immunocompromised patients with hepatitis
■ AST:ALT >2:1 (2) ■ Chronic or acute alcohol ingestion ■ Younger age drinker ■ History of pancreatitis or erosive gastritis ■ Cirrhotic liver disease ■ Anorexia ■ Nausea ■ Vomiting ■ Abdominal pain	■ Jaundice ■ ± Fever ■ Weight loss ■ Hepatomegaly with mild tenderness ■ Advanced disease can be characterized by spider angiomas, ascites, palmar erythema, caput medusae, gynecomastia, parotid enlargement, and testicular atrophy	■ γ-Glutamyl transferase ■ CBC (possible anemia)	Alcoholic hepatitis
■ ALT and AST are variably elevated ■ Often asymptomatic ■ Previous episode of acute hepatitis ■ Coagulopathy	■ May be no findings (3) ■ Thin ■ Jaundiced ■ Small, nodular liver	■ Hepatitis B surface antigen, IgM anti–hepatitis B surface antigen antibody, and IgM/G anti–hepatitis B core and envelope antibody ■ IgG anti–hepatitis C antibody ■ Albumin (often low) ■ Prothrombin time (may be elevated) ■ Liver biopsy (4)	Chronic hepatitis

(continued)

TABLE 17.2.1	**Evaluation of the Patient with Elevated Aminotransferase (Continued)**		

History	Physical examination	Testing	Diagnosis
■ Alkaline phosphatase elevated more than the ALT or AST ■ Elevated serum bilirubin ■ RUQ pain ■ Gallstones ■ Middle aged ■ Overweight ■ Female	■ Jaundice ■ Intermittent fever ■ Rigors ■ RUQ tenderness ± rebound	■ CBC ■ RUQ ultrasound ■ Endoscopic retrograde cholangiopancreatography or imaging equivalent ■ HIDA scan can demonstrate biliary function in the setting of an obstructive presentation but an indeterminate ultrasound	Biliary tract obstruction with or without an infection (cholestasis vs. cholangitis)
■ Can present as hepatocellular injury, obstructive or a combination profile ■ Known or unknown malignancy ■ Abdominal pain ■ Weakness ■ Anorexia ■ History of hepatitis B or C infection	■ Weight loss ■ Ascites ■ GI malignancies can be left supraclavicular (Virchow's) or periumbilical (Sister Mary Joseph) lymph node enlargement ■ Other findings specific to the primary site malignancy site	■ MRI ■ Serum α-fetoprotein ■ Determination of primary source of malignancy with testing specific to primary in question	Malignancy (primary or metastatic)
Use of: ■ HMG-CoA Reductase inhibitor ■ Isoniazid ■ Phenothiazine ■ Erythromycin ■ Progesterone ■ Halothane ■ Opiates ■ Indomethacin ■ Corticosteroids	■ Often none	■ Repeat ALT and AST after discontinuation of the medication ■ Other testing specific to medication effects (e.g., creatinine kinase levels with toxicity of HMG-CoA reductase inhibitors)	Medication effect
■ Fatigue, malaise, and vague right upper abdominal discomfort ■ AST:ALT ratio <1 ■ Hepatitis with no clear etiology	■ Obesity ■ Hepatomegaly ■ Splenomegaly	■ Ultrasound, CT scan, or MRI ■ Liver biopsy is necessary to determine inflammation	Hepatic steatosis and nonalcoholic steatohepatitis
■ Polyuria, polyphagia, and polydipsia ■ Weakness and lethargy ■ Arthralgia ■ Impotence in men	■ Weakness ■ Skin hyperpigmentation ■ Diabetes mellitus ■ Electrocardiographic abnormalities	■ Serum iron ■ TIBC ■ Iron saturation (ratio of serum iron to TIBC) >45% ■ Ferritin ■ Liver biopsy for determination of hepatic iron index ■ Hb A_{1c}	Hemochromatosis

(continued)

TABLE 17.2.1	Evaluation of the Patient with Elevated Aminotransferase (Continued)		
History	**Physical examination**	**Testing**	**Diagnosis**
■ May describe muscle pain or weakness	■ Muscle pain or weakness on examination	■ Creatine kinase ■ Aldolase ■ Muscle biopsy	Muscle disorders
■ Unintentional weight loss or gain ■ Skin and hair changes ■ Heat or cold intolerance	■ Goiter and/or thyroid nodule(s) in certain conditions ■ Hair loss ■ Abnormal reflexes	■ TSH ■ Thyroid function testing if TSH is abnormal	Thyroid disorders (5)
■ Hepatitis or liver failure ■ Emphysema when young or out of proportion with smoking history	■ Physical examination ranging from acute hepatitis to end-stage liver disease ■ Pulmonary examination suggestive of end-stage pulmonary disease	■ α-1-antitrypsin phenotype ■ Serum protein electrophoresis	α-1-antitrypsin deficiency
■ Child or young adult (5–25 y) ■ Hepatitis ■ Dysarthria ■ Dysphagia	■ Kayser-Fleischer rings in cornea ■ Tremors	■ Liver function tests often nonspecific ■ Ceruloplasmin (reduced in 85% of patients) ■ 24-h urine for quantitative copper excretion (>100 µg/d is suggestive)	Wilson's disease

ALT, alanine aminotransferase; AST, aspartate aminotransferase; CBC, complete blood count; IgM, immunoglobulin M; GI, gastrointestinal; RUQ, right upper quadrant; MRI, magnetic resonance imaging; HMG-CoA, 3-hydroxy-3-methylglutaryl coenzyme A; TIBC, total iron binding capacity; TSH, thyroid-stimulating hormone.

References

1. Kaplan MM. Alanine aminotransferase levels: what's normal? (editorial). *Ann Intern Med* 2002;137:50.
2. Cohen JA, Kaplan MM. The SGOT/SGPT ratio an indicator of alcoholic liver disease. *Dig Dis Sci* 1979;24:835.
3. Pratt DS, Kaplan MM. Evaluation of abnormal liver-enzyme results in asymptomatic patients. *N Engl J Med* 2000;342:1266.
4. Sorbi D, McGill DB, Thistle JL, et al. An assessment of the role of liver biopsies in asymptomatic patients with chronic liver test abnormalities. *Am J Gastroenterol* 2000;95:3206.
5. Huang MJ, Liaw YF. Clinical associations between thyroid and liver diseases. *J Gastroenterol Hepatol* 1995;10:344.

ANTINUCLEAR ANTIBODY TITER, ELEVATED
Peter F. Cronholm and Joseph B. Straton

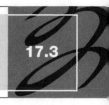

17.3

I. **BACKGROUND.** Antinuclear antibodies (ANAs) include antibodies to double-stranded DNA, histones, chromatin, along with other nuclear proteins and RNA–protein complexes. The presence of significant ANA titers is a necessary component in diagnosing systemic autoimmune diseases, but they can also be found in otherwise normal individuals. Because of the low specificity of a positive ANA titer, an ANA titer should only be ordered when there is clinical suspicion of a disease process in which the ANA value plays a significant role (1).

II. **PATHOPHYSIOLOGY.** ANA-staining patterns are not as useful as was once believed in correlating patterns with clinical disease, but are often reported with titers. It is important to remember that the specificity of a positive ANA titer for all rheumatic diseases is only 50%. Five percent of young adults and 18% of individuals older than 65 years have a mildly elevated ANA and no disease process (a falsely positive ANA) (2).

III. **EVALUATION.** A careful history and physical examination along with an understanding of the prevalence of systemic autoimmune diseases should guide the ordering and interpretation of ANA titers. For further details, see Table 17.3.1.

IV. **DIAGNOSIS.** See Table 17.3.1.

TABLE 17.3.1 | **Evaluation of the Patient with an Elevated Antinuclear Antibody Titer**

History	Physical examination	Further testing	Diagnosis
A. Connective tissue disorders			
▪ Fatigue ▪ Fever ▪ Weight loss ▪ Pain, redness, or heat in two or more joints ▪ Photosensitivity reaction ▪ Rash ▪ Oral ulcers ▪ Chest pain ▪ Shortness of breath ▪ Seizures or psychosis without history of offending medications or drug use ▪ Abdominal pain ▪ More common in women and African-Americans	▪ Malar rash (presents in 1/3–1/2 of patients) ▪ Discoid rash ▪ Joint effusion or derangement in chronic disease (present in 2/3 of patients) ▪ Focal neurologic deficits (15% of patients) ▪ Pleural effusions ▪ Cardiac or pleural rubs	▪ Anti-ds-DNA (high specificity for SLE) ▪ Urinalysis with 24-h collection (look for persistent proteinuria or casts) ▪ CBC (look for evidence of anemia) ▪ Specialized nuclear antigen tests: ribonucleoprotein, antibodies to anti-Smith, anti-SS-A/Ro, anti-SS-B/La (patients with SLE may produce different autoantibodies) ▪ Creatinine (look for occult renal disease) ▪ X-rays of involved joints	SLE

(continued)

TABLE 17.3.1 Evaluation of the Patient with an Elevated Antinuclear Antibody Titer *(Continued)*

History	Physical examination	Further testing	Diagnosis
■ Systemic symptoms: fever, weight loss, and fatigue ■ Morning stiffness ■ Chronic, symmetric joint complaints (three or more for 6 or more wk) ■ Joint symptoms are often intermittent and migratory	■ ± Red, hot, swollen joint(s) (most common are the wrist, metacarpophalangeal, or proximal interphalangeal joints) ■ Subcutaneous nodules (usually on the extensor or pressure surfaces)	■ Rheumatoid factor (20% of patients with RA are negative) ■ CBC (look for an anemia of chronic disease) ■ X-rays of involved joints (typically demonstrates erosions or bone loss) ■ Joint aspiration (inflammatory profile to synovial fluid)	RA
■ Excessive dryness of eyes and/or mouth ■ Recurrent oral ulcers ■ Sensation disturbance over the hands and/or feet ■ Vaginal dryness and dyspareunia ■ Dysphagia	■ Enlarged salivary glands ■ Dry mucous membranes ■ Decreased salivation ■ Decreased tearing ■ Purpura ■ Peripheral neuropathy	■ Anti-SS-A/Ro ■ Anti-SS-B/La ■ Biopsy of salivary glands or lip to assess lymphocytic infiltration ■ CBC (looking for anemia of chronic disease) ■ Cryoglobulins (if positive, should screen for hepatitis C) ■ Immunoglobulin electrophoresis (to demonstrate a monoclonal spike) ■ Objective testing of tear and saliva production (Schirmer test and salivary scintigram) ■ Chest x-ray to differentiate from possible sarcoidosis	Sjögren's syndrome
■ Fever and malaise ■ Weight loss ■ Muscle tenderness ■ Muscle weakness is usually symmetric, gradual in onset, greater loss in lower limbs ■ Skin rash ■ Arthralgia ■ Chest pain or shortness of breath with pulmonary involvement	■ Muscle strength may be diminished ■ Tenderness to palpation over affected areas ■ Skin rashes: heliotrope rash on eyelids or erythematous papules over extensor surfaces of joints (proximal interphalangeal, elbow, or knee)	■ Presence of anti-U1-RNP in MCTD ■ ANA likely to have a high titer and a speckled pattern in MCTD in contrast to DM or PM where high titers are suggestive of a separate overlapping inflammatory condition ■ Muscle biopsy can be definitive for a diagnosis. ■ Specific patterns on electromyelogram in DM	■ Idiopathic inflammatory myopathy (e.g., DM, PM) ■ MCTD

(continued)

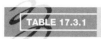

TABLE 17.3.1	**Evaluation of the Patient with an Elevated Antinuclear Antibody Titer** *(Continued)*		
History	**Physical examination**	**Further testing**	**Diagnosis**
B. Drugs Patient is more likely to be older and men Patient likely to be taking: ■ Procainamide (10% develop lupus, 50% have elevated ANAs) ■ Chlorpromazine ■ Quinidine ■ Hydralazine Symptoms consistent with SLE described above	Physical examination as per SLE	■ Anti–histone antibodies (present in 95% of cases) ■ Erythrocyte sedimentation rate is often elevated ■ Anti-ds-DNA testing is usually negative and can be used to differentiate this condition from SLE ■ Antibodies to neutrophil cytoplasmic antigens may be positive	Drug-induced lupus
C. Systemic illness ■ Fever (in 50%–80%) ■ Malaise ■ Weight loss ■ Night sweats ■ Cough (nonproductive in early stages, may eventually be productive of sputum and/or blood tinged) ■ Pleuritic pain ■ Dyspnea ■ Extrapulmonary involvement (15% of cases)	■ Pleural effusion ■ ± Adventitial lung sounds ■ Lymph node enlargement with or without tenderness ■ Organ-specific findings	■ Tuberculin skin test ■ Chest x-ray if positive skin test ■ Acid-fast staining and culture of induced sputum for mycobacteria ■ Possibly bronchoscopy ■ CBC looking for anemia ■ Electrolytes may demonstrate hyponatremia in patients complicated by the syndrome of inappropriate adrenocortical hormone secretion	Tuberculosis
■ Fatigue ■ Fever ■ Chills ■ Nonspecific sore throat ■ Headache ■ Sleep disturbances	■ Often normal ■ May have lymphadenopathy ■ Right upper quadrant tenderness or liver enlargement	■ CBC (may demonstrate lymphocytosis) ■ Viral titers (Epstein-Barr or cytomegalovirus) ■ Other laboratory abnormalities are unusual but may be specific to the particular viral agent suspected	Chronic viral infections (e.g., Epstein-Barr virus, cytomegalovirus)

(continued)

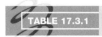

TABLE 17.3.1	Evaluation of the Patient with an Elevated Antinuclear Antibody Titer *(Continued)*

History	Physical examination	Further testing	Diagnosis
■ Women (95% for PBC and common for AH) and young (AH) ■ Abdominal pain ■ Fever ■ Amenorrhea ■ Diarrhea ■ Pleuritic pain and/or polyarthritis	■ Jaundice ■ Hepatomegaly ■ Splenomegaly ■ Advanced disease can be characterized by spider angiomas, ascites, palmar erythema, caput medusae, gynecomastia, parotid enlargement, and testicular atrophy	■ Liver function testing (AST, ALT, gamma-glutamyl transferase, alkaline phosphatase) ■ Serial testing of aminotransferases if elevated ■ CBC ■ Hepatitis testing (A, B and C) ■ Anti-ss-DNA and anti–smooth muscle antibody testing ■ Anti–mitochondrial antibodies hallmark of PBC ■ Liver biopsy	Liver disease (PBC, AH, and primary autoimmune cholangitis)
■ Weight loss ■ Fatigue ■ Malaise ■ Cigarette smoking ■ Family history of cancer	Physical findings are dependent on the type of malignancy suspected	Laboratory testing is dependent on the type of malignancy suspected	Malignancy (positive ANA is a rare finding) (3)

AH, autoimmune hepatitis; ALT, alanine aminotransferase; AST, aspartate aminotransferase; CBC, complete blood count; RNP, antiribonucleoprotein; DM, dermatomyositis; MCTD, mixed connective tissue disorder; PBC, primary biliary cirrhosis; PM, polymyositis; RA, rheumatoid arthritis; SLE, systemic lupus erythematosus; ANA, antinuclear antibodies.

References
1. Phan TG, Wong RC, Adelstein S. Autoantibodies to extractable nuclear antigens: making detection and interpretation more meaningful. *Clin Diagn Lab Immunol* 2002;9:1.
2. Solomon DH, Kavanaugh AJ, Schur PH. Evidence-based guidelines for the use of immunologic tests: antinuclear antibody testing. *Arthritis Rheum* 2002;47:434.
3. Lane SK, Gravel JW Jr, Clinical utility of common serum rheumatologic tests. *Am Fam Physician* 2002;65(6):1073–1080.

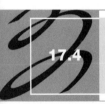

17.4 BRAIN NATRIURETIC PEPTIDE
Nicole Otto and Perry W. Sexton

I. **BACKGROUND.** Brain natriuretic peptide (BNP) was first discovered in the brains of pigs. In humans, BNP is produced in the ventricles of the heart and released as cardiac myofibrils which are stretched during volume or pressure overload. There are three other known human natriuretic peptides (atrial, C-type, and dendroaspis).

II. **PATHOPHYSIOLOGY.** Physiologic levels of BNP cause sodium and water excretion through the kidneys although its primary effect is through venous dilation, subsequently decreasing cardiac preload. BNP is secreted in increasing amounts as healthy individuals age. Women secrete more BNP than men. The role of BNP in medicine is evolving; although it was initially used solely in the diagnosis of congestive heart failure (CHF), other uses continue to be established. BNP is also useful in diagnosing, predicting prognosis, and managing left ventricular dysfunction (LVD) and coronary ischemia. Some experts suggest that BNP could be used to monitor symptomatic and asymptomatic patients with cardiovascular risk factors and predict their overall risk of death from cardiovascular events. Recent evidence suggests that BNP may even have a role in diagnosing and treating children with CHF in renal disease (1).

III. **EVALUATION.** Current BNP tests are rapid immunofluorescence, which cost about $26.00 per kit. Within 30 minutes, the anti-BNP antibodies bind quantitatively to the BNP in the serum and fluoresce proportionally to the amount of BNP present (see Table 17.4.1). In the patient with CHF and coronary ischemia, rapid bedside BNP measurement in the emergency department setting has been found to decrease morbidity and mortality. The half-life of BNP is only 22 minutes; therefore, serial testing can be informative (2).

IV. **DIAGNOSIS**

　　A. **Congestive heart failure.** BNP is currently used for diagnosis, guide treatment, and predict prognosis in CHF. An elevated BNP is 86% sensitive and 98% specific for CHF. A normal BNP has 96% negative predictive value and can be used to rule out CHF in the patient with dyspnea.

　　　　1. CHF is most often diagnosed through history and physical examination and then confirmed by chest x-ray. In patients who present with symptoms of cough or dyspnea, an elevated BNP can help distinguish a cardiac cause from other differential diagnoses (such as pulmonary embolus, a history of chronic obstructive lung disease, asthma, or pneumonia). Adding BNP to clinical judgment increases the diagnostic accuracy from 74% to 81%. A BNP value of <100 pg/nL may be normal, whereas most patients with dyspnea with CHF achieve values of >400 pg/nL (see Table 17.4.1) (3).

　　　　2. BNP levels fall after effective therapeutic intervention. Morbidity, mortality, and hospital admission and readmission are dependent on aggressive treatment of CHF, and a decline in BNP levels often correlate with clinical improvements. A suggested goal at hospital discharge is a BNP <500 pg/nL.

　　　　3. BNP measured at initial clinical presentation provides useful prognostic information on patients with chronic heart failure. Persistently elevated BNP, despite optimal medical intervention carries a poorer prognosis. Note that patients with chronic heart failure may have persistently elevated BNP but may be clinically

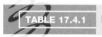

| **TABLE 17.4.1** | **Helpful Values for Brain Natriuretic Peptide** |

BNP level (pg/nL)	Interpretation	Other
<100	May be normal	96% negative predictive value for CHF
>100	Possible CHF	84.3% positive predictive value for CHF
		See text for discussion of confounding factors
>400	Most patients with dyspnea due to heart failure	These patients should be under intense monitoring and treatment in either the outpatient or inpatient setting (see Chapter 7.5)
<500	Goal at hospital discharge	—
>700	Severely decompensated CHF	—

BNP, brain natriuretic peptide; CHF, congestive heart failure.

stable. A series of BNP levels is often more helpful in understanding the relative trend in a particular patient.

B. Left ventricular dysfunction.

1. Elevated BNP levels can help predict the existence of LVD in both symptomatic and asymptomatic patients. Some authors suggest that measurement of BNP can be used as a screening test for LVD in patients with cardiovascular risk factors. The evidence and parameters to support this claim are currently emerging and are controversial.

2. BNP levels correlate strongly with left ventricular mass (including left ventricular hypertrophy) and left ventricular distension. Therefore, many other conditions (primary pulmonary hypertension, primary hyperaldosteronism, Cushing's syndrome, or athletic heart) might precipitate and increase the BNP. BNP increases as LVD worsens in severe sepsis despite the frequent preservation of ejection fraction (4).

C. Acute coronary syndromes and known coronary ischemia. In the patient presenting with chest pain and questionable coronary ischemia, BNP may be elevated. Elevated levels denote ongoing or recent ischemia when measured 6 hours to 10 days after an event. This can be especially helpful in patients who have nonspecific ST-T wave changes, a non–q wave myocardial infarction, or symptoms of atypical chest pain. Patients with any condition causing cardiac ischemia may have an elevated BNP value. Some experts even believe that BNP may be more useful than the measurement of troponin in cardiac ischemia. It is not yet known whether the level of BNP predicts the severity and ultimate the prognosis of the cardiac ischemia in these populations (5).

D. Special considerations.

1. Older individuals and women have normally higher BNP levels. BNP is elevated in primary and secondary pulmonary hypertension, renal disease, and cirrhosis. Patients with renal failure (on dialysis or awaiting transplantation) may have unreliable BNP levels, likely resulting from chronic volume expansion. However, patients with nondialysis-dependent renal dysfunction have BNP levels that reliably correlate with echocardiographic evidence of heart failure. Patients with cirrhosis have BNP levels three times that of healthy subjects in some studies.

2. Cardiac inflammation of any type of myocarditis, including cardiac transplant rejection, Kawasaki disease, or an arrhythmogenic right ventricle with decreased ejection fraction, may lead to increased BNP.

3. Obese patients (body mass index >30) with heart failure tend to have lower levels of BNP when compared with nonobese patients with failure.

4. Other potential uses of BNP are being studied and developed, including the use of pharmacologic doses of BNP (known as *nesiritide*) to treat CHF (6).

References

1. Wieczorek SJ, Wu AH, Christenson R, et al. A rapid B-type natriuretic peptide assay accurately diagnoses left ventricular dysfunction and heart failure: a multicenter evaluation. *Am Heart J* 2002;144:834.
2. McCullough PA, Nowak RM, McCord J, et al. B-type natriuretic peptide and clinical judgment in emergency diagnosis of heart failure: analysis from Breathing Not Properly (BNP) multinational study. *Circulation* 2002;106:416–422.
3. Hobbs RE. Using BNP to diagnose, manage, and treat heart failure. *Cleve Clin J Med* 2003;70(4):333–336.
4. Koglin J, Pehlivani S, Schwaiblmair M, et al. Role of brain natriuretic peptide in risk stratification of patients with congestive heart failure. *J Am Coll Cardiol* 2001;38:1934.
5. De Lemos JA, Morrow DA, Bentley JH, et al. The prognostic value of B-type natriuretic peptide in patients with acute coronary syndromes. *N Engl J Med* 2001;345:1014.
6. Topol EJ. Nesiritide—not verified. *N Engl J Med* 2005;353(2):113–116.

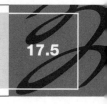

D-DIMER
Perry W. Sexton and Nicole Otto

17.5

I. BACKGROUND. A D-dimer is a degradation product of cross-linked fibrin that has undergone fibrinolysis in the final stages of the clotting cascade. Although the D-dimer test is useful in the diagnosis of venous thromboembolism (VTE) (deep vein thrombosis and/or pulmonary embolism), venogram, Doppler ultrasound, impedance plethysmography, arteriogram, and/or high-resolution chest computed tomography (CT) scan are the definitive diagnostic tests for these conditions. The challenge of some of these diagnostic tests is that the results are operator dependent and can sometimes be "indeterminate." The D-dimer test was developed to potentially eliminate the need for further diagnostic testing in those who present with an unsure diagnosis of suspect VTE.

II. EVALUATION
  A. The first step in approaching a patient with VTE is to establish the pretest probability on the basis of clinical criteria such as the Wells Criteria (see Table 17.5.1). In patients with a low clinical pretest probability of VTE, a D-dimer level can be obtained to guide the diagnosis. A result of <500 ng/mL by rapid enzyme-linked immunosorbent assay (ELISA) has a negative predictive value of 95% (see Table 17.5.2) and eliminates the need for further testing. Patients with a low pretest probability and a D-dimer of ≥500 ng/mL should go on to the appropriate imaging study (venogram, Doppler ultrasound, impedance plethysmography, arteriogram, and/or high-resolution chest CT scan). Patients with a high pretest probability of VTE should be evaluated first by an imaging study; D-dimer is used only when the imaging results are "indeterminate."
  B. Two types of D-dimer assays exist. The latex agglutination assay utilizes antibodies specific for D-dimer. The alternate method of D-dimer testing is the ELISA. Second-generation latex agglutination tests for D-dimer are as sensitive (95%) as the current ELISA, and the costs are comparable.

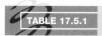

TABLE 17.5.1	Wells Criteria for Predicting Pulmonary Embolus in the Symptomatic Patient

Criteria	Number of points
Clinical signs and symptoms of deep venous thrombosis	3.0
An alternative diagnosis that is less likely than pulmonary embolism	3.0
Pulse rate >100 beats/min	1.5
Immobilization or surgery in the previous 4 wk	1.5
Previous deep venous thrombosis/pulmonary embolism	1.5
Hemoptysis	1.0
Malignancy	1.0

≤4 points, pulmonary embolism unlikely (pretest probability with prevalence for pulmonary embolism of 5% to 8%).
>4 points, pulmonary embolism likely (pretest probability with prevalence for pulmonary embolism of 39% to 41%).

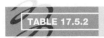

D-dimer value[a]	Pretest probability for VTE, deep venous thrombosis, or pulmonary embolism	Interpretation	Diagnostic decision
<500 ng/mL	Low pretest probability	Normal	Can safely exclude the diagnosis of VTE
(Any value)	Malignancy or <3 mo postsurgery	VTE cannot be excluded	Need further imaging
>500 ng/mL	Any clinical probability	VTE cannot be excluded	Need further imaging

[a]By enzyme-linked immunosorbent assay (ELISA) testing.
VTE, venous thromboembolism.

C. It is important to note that a low D-dimer test is able to rule out VTE. By contrast, an elevated D-dimer level is not able to establish a diagnosis of VTE (this test is not sufficiently specific). There are many other systemic causes of an elevated D-dimer (see Table 17.5.3).

III. DIAGNOSIS. The D-dimer test is a quick, noninvasive, and non–operator-dependent laboratory test that can exclude the diagnosis of VTE when negative in patients with low pretest probability but does not have sufficient specificity to rule in VTE with certainty when positive.

Increase false-positive results	Increase risk of false-negative results	Shown not to increase false-positive or false-negative results
Inflammatory states	Patient at high risk for deep venous thrombosis (known hypercoagulable state, malignancy, recent surgery, pregnancy)	Chronic renal failure
Pregnancy	Presence of small subsegmental emboli (vs. large pulmonary emboli)	Intravenous placement
Infection	—	Osteoarthritis
Sepsis		
Superficial thrombophlebitis	—	—
Trauma	—	—
Wounds (postoperative patient's normal range is 200–500 ng/mL)		
Hospitalization	—	—

Many conditions affect the predictive value of a positive D-dimer test. These conditions and their effect are shown in Table 17.5.3.

Suggested Readings

American Thoracic Society. The diagnostic approach to acute venous thromboembolism. Clinical practice guideline. *Am J Respir Crit Care Med* 1999;160(3): 1043–1066.

Kruip MJ, Leclercq MG, van der Heul C, et al. Diagnostic strategies for excluding pulmonary embolism in clinical outcomes studies. *Ann Intern Med* 2003;138:941.

Ginsberg JS, Brill-Edwards PA, Demers C, et al. D-dimer in patients with clinically suspected pulmonary embolism. *Chest* 1993;104:1679.

Schutgens RE, Esseboom EU, Haas FJ, et al. Usefulness of a semiquantitative D-dimer test for the exclusion of deep venous thrombosis in outpatients. *Am J Med* 2002;112:617.

Brotman DJ, Segal JB, Jani JT, et al. Limitations of D-dimer testing in unselected inpatients with suspected venous thromboembolism. *Am J Med* 2003;114:276.

Fedullo PF, Tapsen VF. Evaluation of suspected pulmonary embolism. *N Engl J Med* 2003;349(13):1247–1256.

Charles LA, Edwards T, Macik BG, et al. Evaluation of sensitivity and specificity of six D-dimer latex assays. *Arch Pathol Lab Med* 1994;118(11):1102–1105.

Wildberger JE, Vorwerk D, Kilbinger M, et al. Bedside testing (SimpliRED) in the diagnosis of DVT. Evaluation of 250 patients. *Invest Radiol* 1998;33(4):232–235.

Janssen MC, Wollersheim H, Verbruggen B, et al. Rapid D-dimer assays to exclude deep vein thrombosis and pulmonary embolism: current status and new developments. *Semin Thromb Hemost* 1998;24(4):393–400.

Wells PS, Anderson DR, Rodger M, et al. Evaluation of D-dimer in the diagnosis of suspected deep vein thrombosis. *N Engl J Med* 2003;349(13):1227–1235.

Wolf, SJ. Prospective validation of Wells criteria in the evaluation of patients with suspected pulmonary embolism. *Ann Emer Med* 2004;44(5):503–510.

HYPERCALCEMIA
Joseph B. Straton and Peter F. Cronholm

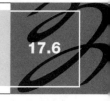

17.6

I. **BACKGROUND.** The normal range of serum calcium is 8.5–10.5 mg/dL. Hypercalcemia, defined as serum calcium concentrations above 10.5 mg/dL, occurs when the calcium enters the circulatory system more rapidly than it is excreted in urine or deposited in bones. An initial elevated calcium level should be repeated to confirm the abnormality (1).

II. **PATHOPHYSIOLOGY.** Nine out of ten cases of hypercalcemia in adults are caused by either hyperparathyroidism or malignancy. Hyperparathyroidism causes most of the hypercalcemia in the outpatient setting. Malignancy causes most of the hypercalcemia found in hospitalized patients. Less common causes of hypercalcemia are chronic renal failure, hyperthyroidism, hypervitaminosis A, hypervitaminosis D, immobilization, Paget's disease, and granulomatous diseases. Pseudohypercalcemia occurs when patients have increased serum calcium-binding proteins. For example, dehydration severe enough to cause hyperalbuminemia may result in high serum calcium levels. Such pseudohypercalcemia should resolve after the hemoconcentration is corrected.

III. EVALUATION

A. History. Patients are often asymptomatic until the calcium level rises above 12 mg/dL, and the symptoms are often nonspecific: generalized muscle weakness, muscle aches, decreased coordination, decreased level of consciousness, headache, loss of appetite, nausea, vomiting, constipation, increased salivation, dysphagia, and abdominal pain or distension. A review of systems may turn up a history of a renal calculus or a history of a malignancy (2).

B. Physical examination. Depending on the severity of hypercalcemia, physical examination may reveal mental confusion, poor memory, slurred speech, acute psychotic behavior, lethargy or coma, ataxia, poor overall muscle strength, hypotonia, hyperextensible joints, increased deep tendon reflexes, positive Babinski's reflexes, incoordination, decreased pain or vibration sense, calcium deposits on the conjunctiva near the palpebral fissure or on the cornea around the iris, or an acute abdomen or an ileus.

C. Testing. See Table 17.6.1.

IV. DIAGNOSIS.

See Table 17.6.1. Calcium levels above 12.5 mg/dL can be life threatening. In such situations, one should perform an electrocardiogram and begin treatment immediately, because cardiac arrest, convulsions, or coma can occur. Further testing can be performed while the serum calcium is lowered.

TABLE 17.6.1	Evaluation of the Patient with Hypercalcemia		
History	**Physical examination**	**Testing**	**Diagnosis**
A. Spurious			
■ Excessive thirst ■ Vomiting or diarrhea with poor oral intake	■ Dry mucous membranes ■ Decreased skin turgor ■ Confusion/lethargy	■ Repeat calcium after rehydration	■ Pseudohypercalcemia due to dehydration
B. Endocrine disorders			
■ Female ■ >60 y ■ Aches and pains ■ Vague abdominal pain ■ Depressive symptoms ■ Renal calculi	■ Neck mass (unlikely) ■ No clinical evidence of malignancy	■ Serum calcium <14.5 mg/dL ■ Parathyroid hormone (elevated) ■ Serum chloride >102 mg/dL ■ Alkaline phosphatase (normal) ■ Serum phosphate ■ Bicarbonate ■ X-ray hands and clavicles	■ Hyperparathyroidism (3) (primary or secondary)
■ Anxiety/tremor ■ Weight loss ■ Family history ■ Heat intolerance ■ Vision problems	■ Exophthalmos ■ Eyelid tremor ■ Tachycardia ■ Perspiration ■ Hyperreflexia	■ Thyroid-stimulating hormone, free T_4	■ Thyrotoxicosis

(continued)

TABLE 17.6.1 Evaluation of the Patient with Hypercalcemia *(Continued)*

History	Physical examination	Testing	Diagnosis
■ Fatigue ■ Weight loss ■ Family history ■ Nausea/vomiting	■ Hypotension ■ Lethargy ■ Increased mucosal or skin pigmentation	■ Elevated potassium ■ Decreased sodium ■ Decreased blood glucose ■ Abnormal adrenal cortical hormone stimulation test	■ Addison's disease
C. Malignancy (4)			
■ >50 y ■ Weight loss ■ Smoker ■ Family history ■ Other symptoms specific to particular tumor site	■ Weight loss ■ Signs specific to particular tumor site	■ Serum calcium >14 mg/dL ■ Serum chloride <100 mg/dL ■ Alkaline phosphatase >2 times normal ■ Parathyroid hormone <2 times normal ■ CBC (anemia frequent) ■ Further workup according to the suspected site of primary tumor ■ Bone scan	Malignancy with or without metastasis ■ Lung cancer ■ Renal cell carcinoma ■ Squamous cell carcinoma
■ >50 y ■ Female	■ Weight loss ■ Signs specific to particular tumor site	■ Further workup according to the suspected primary tumor site ■ Alkaline phosphatase ■ Bone scan	■ Breast cancer ■ Ovarian cancer ■ Metastatic disease
■ >50 y ■ Male ■ Urinary complaints	■ Prostate mass on rectal examination or a diffusely enlarged hard prostate	■ Prostate-specific antigen ■ Alkaline phosphatase ■ Bone scan ■ Ultrasound-guided prostate biopsy	■ Prostate cancer
■ >60 y ■ Bone pain ■ Weight loss ■ Fatigue	■ Pallor ■ Hepatomegaly ■ Splenomegaly ■ Tenderness over bones	■ CBC (anemia) ■ Serum and urine protein electrophoresis ■ Creatinine ■ Erythrocyte sedimentation rate	■ Multiple myeloma (5)
D. Medications/ vitamins			
■ Lithium ■ Furosemide ■ Thiazide diuretics ■ Aminophylline	■ Physical examination normal or shows signs of hypercalcemia	■ Repeat serum calcium (elevated) ■ Other serum electrolyte values may be abnormal	■ Medication use
■ Calcium-based antacids	■ Normal or shows signs of hypercalcemia	■ Phosphate ■ BUN ■ Creatinine ■ Bicarbonate	■ Milk-alkali syndrome

(continued)

TABLE 17.6.1 Evaluation of the Patient with Hypercalcemia *(Continued)*

History	Physical examination	Testing	Diagnosis
■ Vitamin pill use ■ Bone pain ■ Headaches	Normal physical examination or ■ Tenderness over bones ■ papilledema	■ Repeat serum calcium ■ Serum phosphate and chloride levels ■ For vitamin A overuse, CT scan of the head	■ Vitamin D overdose ■ Vitamin A overdose
E. Other			
■ Prolonged bed rest or chair rest	■ Physical examination normal or shows signs of hypercalcemia	■ Consider DEXA scan for osteoporosis	■ Immobilization
■ History of acute renal failure	■ Physical examination normal or shows signs of hypercalcemia	■ BUN ■ Creatinine ■ Urinalysis	■ Chronic or diuretic phase of acute renal failure
■ Fever ■ Fatigue ■ Malaise ■ Anorexia ■ Cough ■ Dyspnea ■ Retrosternal chest discomfort ■ Polyarthritis	■ Findings dependent on sites involved ■ Erythema nodosum ■ Uveitis ■ Lymphadenopathy	■ CBC (lymphocytopenia) ■ Chest x-ray ■ Pulmonary function testing ■ Transbronchial biopsy	■ Sarcoidosis or other granulomatous disease
■ Family history of hypercalcemia	■ May be normal or show signs of hypercalcemia	■ Low 24-h urine calcium level	■ Familial hypocalciuric hypercalcemia

CBC, complete blood count; BUN, blood urea nitrogen; CT, computed tomography; DEXA, dual energy x-ray absorptiometry.

References

1. Bushinsky DA, Monk RD. Calcium. *Lancet* 1998;352:306–311.
2. Shane E. Hypercalcemia: pathogenesis, clinical manifestations, differential diagnosis, and management. In: Favus MJ, ed. *Primer on the metabolic bone diseases and disorders of mineral metabolism*, 4th ed. Philadelphia, PA: Lippincott Williams & Wilkins, 1999:183–187.
3. Al Zahrani A, Levine MA. Primary hyperparathyroidism. *Lancet* 1997;349:1233–1238.
4. Stewart AF, Clinical practice. Hypercalcemia associated with cancer. *N Engl J Med* 2005;352:373–379.
5. Mundy GR, Guise TA. Hypercalcemia of malignancy. *Am J Med* 1997;103:134–145.

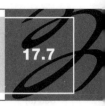

HYPERKALEMIA
David Webner

17.7

I. BACKGROUND. Hyperkalemia is defined as a serum potassium (K^+) >5.0 mEq/L. Hyperkalemia can be life threatening when K^+ is >6.5 mEq/L (1).

II. PATHOPHYSIOLOGY. Hyperkalemia can be divided into four etiologic groups: spurious causes, redistribution abnormalities, renal disorders, and hormone deficiencies. Spurious hyperkalemia is hyperkalemia in a healthy patient; it is manifested as thrombocytosis, leukocytosis (also may cause hypokalemia), hemolysis, and repeated fist clenching in blood drawing. The most common redistribution abnormality is acidosis. The most frequently occurring renal disorders are renal insufficiency or failure with a concomitant potassium load. The primary cause of endocrinologic hyperkalemia is uncontrolled diabetes.

III. EVALUATION. Hyperkalemia is usually not sustained unless there is a disorder of the potassium regulatory system. In an otherwise healthy individual, routine screening of potassium is not indicated. Potassium should be monitored in patients on certain medications (see Table 17.7.1), with acid–base disorders, abnormalities in renal function, and disorders of aldosterone secretion. These patients are at risk of potentially fatal hyperkalemia (5).

 TABLE 17.7.1   **Evaluation of the Patient with Hyperkalemia**

History	Physical examination	Testing	Diagnosis
A. Spurious (2)			
Laboratory reading is "hemolysis" on electrolyte panel	Healthy patient	Repeat serum K^+ testing; normalized in redrawn sample	Hemolysis in collection tube
Platelet count >1 million	Healthy patient, except for disorder causing thrombocytosis	Repeat platelet count with heparinized specimen	Thrombocytosis (platelets release K^+ during clotting)
WBC count >200,000	Healthy patient, except for underlying disorder causing leukocytosis	Repeat WBC count with rapid processing/spinning down specimen	Leukocytosis
K^+ normalized in repeat draw with careful draw technique	Healthy patient	Repeat serum K^+	Tight or prolonged tourniquet or fist clenching during blood draws

(continued)

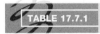

	TABLE 17.7.1	Evaluation of the Patient with Hyperkalemia *(Continued)*

History	Physical examination	Testing	Diagnosis
B. Redistribution (3)			
Acidosis	Often no signs specific to acidosis in an otherwise ill patient	■ Immediate ECG ■ Monitor cardiac rhythm ■ ABG ■ Sequential testing	pH < 7.35
■ β-Blockers ■ Angiotensin-converting enzyme inhibitors ■ Angiotensin-receptor blockers ■ Cardiac glycosides ■ Neuromuscular blocking agents ■ Salt substitutes ■ Trimethoprim ■ Pentamidine	No signs of hyperkalemia Physical examination may reveal underlying illness leading to medication use	■ Immediate ECG ■ Cardiac rhythm should be monitored	Medication/diet effect
■ Crush injury ■ Tissue breakdown	Bruising, other signs of trauma, or a necrotic wound	■ Immediate ECG ■ Monitor cardiac rhythm	Cell breakdown
Rhabdomyolysis	Signs cell injury, heat stroke, crush injury	■ Urinalysis for myoglobin ■ BUN/creatinine ■ Immediate ECG ■ Monitor cardiac rhythm	Cell breakdown and kidney dysfunction
Large bruise or hematoma	Hematoma	■ Immediate ECG ■ Monitor cardiac rhythm	Hematoma breakdown
Muscle contraction in marathon runners	Endurance athlete		Cell breakdown and muscle release of K^+
■ Cachexia ■ Symptoms related to the etiology of the cachexia	■ Cachetic ■ Signs related to reason for cachexia	■ Immediate ECG ■ Monitor cardiac rhythm	Tissue catabolism
Hemolytic anemia	■ Pallor ■ Petechiae ■ Orthostatic hypotension ■ Bleeding from any orifice	■ Immediate ECG ■ Monitor cardiac rhythm ■ CBC	Hemolysis

(continued)

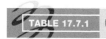

TABLE 17.7.1	Evaluation of the Patient with Hyperkalemia *(Continued)*

History	Physical examination	Testing	Diagnosis
	■ Other signs as related to the etiology of hemolytic anemia		
Hyperkalemic periodic paralysis (4)	Quadriplegia with sparing of the cranial nerves		Transient hyper K^+
C. Renal disorders			
Use of potassium-sparing diuretics (e.g., triamterene, spironolactone)		■ BUN ■ Creatinine ■ Creatinine clearance may be low ■ FE_{K+}	Diuretic use
History of treatment for a *Pneumocystis carinii* infection		■ BUN ■ Creatinine ■ Normal creatinine clearance	Trimethoprim or pentamidine effect
Known creatinine clearance <50		■ Creatinine clearance ■ Immediate ECG, monitor cardiac rhythm	Renal insufficiency or failure with a potassium load
Systemic lupus erythematosus	■ Malar rash ■ Discoid rash ■ Recurrent oral ulcers ■ Focal neurologic deficits	■ ABG ■ Creatinine clearance ■ FE_{K+} ■ Evaluation of underlying disease	Decreased GFR
Sickle-cell disease or trait		■ BUN ■ Creatinine ■ Creatinine clearance may be low ■ Low FE_{K+} ■ Evaluation of underlying disease	Decreased GFR
Amyloidosis	Signs due to amyloidosis	■ BUN ■ Creatinine ■ Creatinine clearance may be low ■ Low FE_{K+} ■ Evaluation of underlying disease	Decreased GFR

(continued)

TABLE 17.7.1   Evaluation of the Patient with Hyperkalemia *(Continued)*

History	Physical examination	Testing	Diagnosis
D. Hormone deficiency			
Diabetes	Signs of DKA	▪ Evaluate for DKA ▪ Check ECG/cardiac rhythm ▪ Sequential testing	Acidosis causing redistribution with K^+/H^+ exchange
Pseudo and actual aldosterone deficiency	▪ Hyperpigmentation ▪ Hypotension ▪ Weight loss ▪ Vomiting	▪ Aldosterone levels ▪ Renin levels ▪ Check ECG/cardiac rhythm ▪ Cosyntropin stimulation test	Addison's disease
Heparin use		▪ Aldosterone levels ▪ Check ECG/cardiac rhythm	Aldosterone excretion low second to heparin

WBC, white blood cell; ECG, electrocardiogram; CBC, complete blood count; ABG, arterial blood gases; BUN, blood urea nitrogen; FE_{K+}, low fractional excretion of potassium; GFR, glomerular filtration rate; DKA, diabetic ketoacidosis.

IV. DIAGNOSIS. Hyperkalemia is usually asymptomatic. Lower levels of K^+ elevation may change normal cardiac function, producing electrocardiographic (ECG) changes that become progressively more life threatening. Patients with a $K^+ \geq 6.5$ mEq/L require immediate cardiac evaluation. The earliest ECG changes are elevation of T waves, followed by a widening of the QRS complex, atrioventricular conduction delays; this slower rhythm may lead to lethal ventricular fibrillation and asystole. Arrhythmias occur at high levels of K^+ and if K^+ rises very rapidly in its concentration. As in hypokalemia, severe cases of hyperkalemia can also occur with an ascending paralysis.

References

1. Halperin ML, Kamel KS. Potassium. *Lancet* 1998;352(9122):135–140.
2. Wallach J, ed. *Interpretation of diagnostic tests*, 6th ed. New York: Little, Brown and Company, 1996.
3. Gennari F. Disorders of potassium homeostasis: hypokalemia and hyperkalemia. *Crit Care Clin* 2002;18:273–288.
4. Evers S, Engelien A, Karsch V, et al. Secondary hyperkalemic paralysis. *J Neurol Neurosurg Psychiatry* 1998;64(2):249–252.
5. Martinez-Maldonado M. Approach to the patient with hyperkalemia. In: Kelley WN, ed.*Textbook of internal medicine*. Philadelphia PA: Lippincott-Raven, 1997.

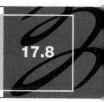

HYPOKALEMIA
David Webner

17.8

I. BACKGROUND. Hypokalemia is one of the most common electrolyte abnormalities found in basic laboratory electrolyte panels. Although the definition varies, hypokalemia is generally said to occur when serum potassium (K^+) concentration falls below 3.6 mEq/L.

II. PATHOPHYSIOLOGY. With the exception of factitious causes (leukemic patients with extreme leukocytosis, where K^+ is taken up by the abnormal white blood cells), true hypokalemia results from increased potassium excretion, transcellular shift, or decreased dietary intake of potassium. Most commonly, hypokalemia is caused by abnormal losses of potassium through the gastrointestinal tract or kidney (see Table 17.8.1). The most common of these causes is diuretic use leading to K^+ depletion. Both the loop (blocked resorption in the loop of Henle) and thiazide diuretics (block resorption in early distal tubule) contribute to the development of hypokalemia. Sodium and chloride delivery are increased by the diuretics, resulting in the secretion of K^+. Further K^+ loss is fostered by increased magnesium excretion, which is also linked to the loop and thiazide diuretics. Other medications, metabolic alkalosis, renal tubular acidosis, and aldosteronism due to systemic diseases and genetic disorders are implicated in the development of hypokalemia (1).

III. EVALUATION. See Table 17.8.1.

IV. DIAGNOSIS. See Table 17.8.1.

TABLE 17.8.1   **Evaluation of the Patient with Hypokalemia**

History	Physical examination	Testing	Diagnosis
A. Gastrointestinal losses (2)			
■ Emesis ■ Nasogastric drainage ■ Pyloric/duodenal obstruction ■ Pancreatic fistulas ■ Diarrhea ■ Laxative abuse ■ Colonic neoplasms	■ Often no signs on physical examination ■ Generalized muscle weakness ■ Constipation ■ Cachexia ■ Abdominal examination for signs of peritonitis or localized pain	■ Serum electrolytes ■ Spot urine electrolytes if needed ■ Urine and serum osmolality as needed ■ Stool electrolytes as appropriate ■ Electrocardiogram (look for "U" waves, or, if rapidly replacing potassium by the intravenous route, look for arrhythmias)	Gastrointestinal potassium losses

(continued)

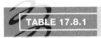

TABLE 17.8.1 Evaluation of the Patient with Hypokalemia *(Continued)*

History	Physical examination	Testing	Diagnosis
B. Renal losses ■ Diuretics (loop or thiazide) ■ Osmotic diuresis (uncontrolled diabetes) ■ Metabolic alkalosis (vomiting/diarrhea) ■ Primary hyperaldosteronism ■ Cortisol responsive aldosteronism ■ Congenital adrenal hyperplasia ■ Liddle's syndrome ■ 11 β-hydroxysteroid dehydrogenase deficiency ■ Bartter syndrome ■ Gitelman's syndrome ■ Inappropriate secretion of antidiuretic hormone ■ Hypomagnesemia ■ Licorice use ■ Corticosteroids ■ Renal tubular acidosis ■ Renal artery stenosis	■ As above ■ May also ask about history of diabetes or use of loop or thiazide diuretics	■ As above ■ May also check for ketones, blood sugar, serum pH	Renal potassium losses and congenital syndromes
C. Transcellular shift (3) ■ Bronchodilators ■ Antihistamines ■ Tocolytics ■ Theophylline ■ Caffeine ■ Insulin ■ Delirium tremens ■ Hyperthyroidism ■ Familial hypokalemic periodic paralysis ■ Barium toxicity ■ Pancreatitis ■ Congestive heart failure ■ Toxic shock ■ Pleural effusion	■ As above ■ May also ask about alcohol abuse and careful medication history	■ As above ■ May also check for serum alcohol level, drug screen as appropriate	Drug therapy and systemic diseases

(continued)

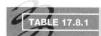

TABLE 17.8.1	Evaluation of the Patient with Hypokalemia *(Continued)*		

History	Physical examination	Testing	Diagnosis
▪ Ascites ▪ Anasarca ▪ Burns (second/third degree) **D. Inadequate intake** ▪ Anorexia/bulimia ▪ Forced vomiting or diarrhea for any reason ▪ Neurotic spitting ▪ Poor diet	▪ As above ▪ May also check for evidence to support the history such as weight loss, staining, or pitting of the teeth	▪ As above	Patient excesses

References

1. Gennari F. Current concepts: hypokalemia. *N Engl J Med* 1998;339(7):451–458.
2. Gennari F. Disorders of potassium homeostasis: hypokalemia and hyperkalemia. *Crit Care Clin* 2002;18:273–288.
3. Rastergar A, Soleimani M. Hypokalemia and hyperkalemia. *Postgrad Med J* 2001;77:759–764.

Diagnostic Imaging Abnormalities

Enrique S. Fernandez

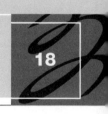

18

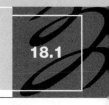
I. BACKGROUND. Bone cysts present either as incidental lesions on x-rays obtained for other diagnostic purposes or as the underlying cause of a pathologic fracture. When confronted with a bone cyst, the physician has to decide if further diagnostic testing is required to confirm the diagnosis, whether treatment is required, and what type of follow-up plan is needed (1).

II. PATHOPHYSIOLOGY

A. Etiology. The cause of simple bone cysts is unknown. Typically, a bone cyst expands the cortex of the bone, with the periosteum covering the thin cortical shell of the cyst. A membrane lines the cyst, and if traumatized, may leak blood or fluid into the cyst or develop septations within the cyst that may give the cyst a more complex appearance on x-ray or computed tomography (CT) scan (2).

B. Epidemiology. Most cysts occur during the first or second decades, most commonly in children younger than 10 years of age. The most common location is the humerus, followed by the femur, and rarely the tibia, fibula, radius, and ulna. Older patients more commonly present with bone cysts in the ileum and calcaneus. Multiple cysts may occur in the same patient. Within the long bones, the most common locations are the proximal metaphysis, but involvement of the epiphysis can occur.

III. EVALUATION

A. History. Bone cysts are typically asymptomatic unless a spontaneous fracture has occurred through the cyst. Pain associated with a bone lesion may simply be due to rapid growth of a benign lesion but may be a more ominous sign of a malignant bone tumor.

B. Physical examination. Examination of the affected extremity should include an inspection of the overlying soft tissue for evidence of associated soft tissue mass. Presence of an associated mass should alert the physician to the possibility of a more significant pathology, because bone cysts are confined to the bone itself. Similarly, associated inflammatory reactions, including tenderness, induration, or erythema, may be warning signs of more serious conditions. Limb lengths should be measured and documented so that serial monitoring for limb length discrepancy can be accomplished, particularly with lesions adjacent to or involving the epiphysis.

C. Testing. Plain x-ray is usually the only diagnostic test required to establish the diagnosis of bone cyst. The x-ray shows a well-defined, well-circumscribed lesion with a thin sclerotic margin without reaction or disruption of the periosteum. Suspected cysts in the spine or pelvis may require magnetic resonance imaging (MRI) to elicit the anatomic detail necessary for the diagnosis. If an associated soft tissue lesion is suspected in a long bone, an MRI can be helpful in determining the presence or absence of associated mass. An MRI is indicated if the cyst appears adjacent to or involves the epiphysis, because such cysts that involve the growth plate need referral for intervention or, at the least, more careful monitoring for growth impairment. If any additional imaging is required, MRI is superior to CT scan for this indication. Nuclear medicine studies, including positron-emission tomography, are not usually helpful (3).

IV. DIAGNOSIS

A. Differential diagnosis. The diagnosis of bone cysts is confirmed by plain x-ray. The differential diagnosis includes malignant bone tumor or metastases. The diagnostic dilemma when bone cysts are identified incidentally is to distinguish a benign condition from a malignancy. The therapeutic dilemmas when bone cysts are identified are to determine which cysts require intervention to prevent pathologic fracture, how to treat pathologic fractures through bone cysts when they occur, and how to monitor for and prevent a growth discrepancy (4).

1. Refer pathologic fractures through bone cysts for the treatment by orthopaedic surgeon.
2. Order an MRI of the affected extremity if the bone lesion detected on x-ray is painful, tender to palpation, or has an associated soft tissue mass. Any atypical characteristics detected on MRI warrant referral.
3. Refer large bone cysts that have expanded and thinned the overlying cortex for treatment in order to prevent pathologic fracture.
4. Carefully document limb lengths when the bone cyst is adjacent to or involves the epiphysis and arrange for serial follow-up.
5. Refer for treatment if limb length or growth discrepancy occurs.

B. Clinical manifestations. Bone cysts that present with pathologic fractures may have to be treated by curettage of the cyst and packing with bone graft in addition to standard fracture immobilization. Large cysts with thinning of the cortex need prophylactic treatment with curettage and bone grafting, cryotherapy, and injection of bone marrow or steroids in order to resolve the cyst and prevent pathologic fracture.

References
1. Teo, ELH, Peh WCG. *Simple Bone Cyst.* eMedicine from WebMD. Available at: http://www.emedicine.com/radio/topic642.htm. Last updated: January 5, 2005.
2. Capanna R, Campanacci DA, Manfrini M. Unicameral and aneurysmal bone cysts. *Orthop Clin North Am* 1996;27:605–614.
3. Mettler F. *Primary care radiology.* Philadelphia, PA: WB Saunders, 2000.
4. Novelline RA. *Squire's fundamentals of radiology.* Cambridge: Harvard University Press, 1997.

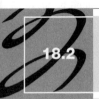

18.2   MEDIASTINAL MASS
Ronnie Coutinho and Enrique S. Fernandez

I. BACKGROUND. Most mediastinal masses are discovered incidentally during routine radiographic studies. Because these are frequently malignant, it is imperative to initiate a timely investigation of any symptoms that may be associated with a mediastinal process. When a mediastinal mass is suspected or detected, knowledge of the boundaries of individual mediastinal compartments and their contents facilitates the formulation of a differential diagnosis. Causes of a mediastinal mass are numerous, ranging from infectious etiologies to benign cystic lesions to malignancies.

The *mediastinum* is the space in the thorax between the pleural cavities. It extends from the sternum anteriorly to the vertebral column posteriorly and contains all the thoracic viscera except the lungs. Traditionally, the mediastinum has been divided into the *anterior mediastinum* (the space in front of the pericardium), the *middle mediastinum* (the portion that contains the pericardium and its contents), and the *posterior mediastinum* (the portion behind the pericardium). It is vital to establish the location of the mass in a particular compartment, as masses in the anterior compartment are more likely to be malignant than those found in other compartments (1).

II. PATHOPHYSIOLOGY. The pathophysiology of mediastinal masses is determined by both the age of the patient and location of the mass itself. On the chest x-ray, a line drawn through the anterior aspect of the trachea and the posterior aspect of the heart may be considered to be in the middle mediastinum. A line drawn through the anterior margins of the vertebral bodies is in the posterior mediastinum. It is often difficult to tell if an abnormality is in the middle or the posterior mediastinum. Therefore, these two compartments may at times be considered together when formulating a differential diagnosis.

A. Anterior mediastinum. The anterior mediastinum contents include the thymus gland, a quantity of loose areolar tissue, lymphatic vessels, a few anterior mediastinal lymph glands, branches of the internal mammary artery, and the sternopericardial ligaments. Lesions seen in this region include thymic lesions (including thymic cysts), lymphoid proliferations, thyroid lesions, parathyroid lesions, and germ cell tumors. Additional tumors that may be seen in the anterior mediastinum include lymphangiomas, hemangiomas, and lipomas. One should consider infectious etiologies, such as tuberculous lymphadenitis, as well as noninfectious etiologies, such as sarcoidosis. Common anterior mediastinal lesions include thymomas, teratomas (also called *teratoid* lesions), lymphomas, and thyroid lesions (2).

   1. Thymoma. This is the most common neoplasm of the mediastinum, and often it is discovered incidentally. Besides thymomas, other tumors of the thymus include thymic carcinomas, thymic lymphomas, thymic cysts, and thymolipomas. Approximately 25% of all mediastinal masses are thymomas and around half of the anterior mediastinal masses are thymomas. Thymomas generally present in the fifth decade, equally in men and women; they are rare in children. Most thymomas are benign lesions.

   2. Teratoma. Frequently, anterior mediastinal masses are teratomas (also referred to as *teratoid lesions*). Teratomas are germ cell tumors that usually arise in young adults from abnormally derived embryonic layers. They are often asymptomatic, but if large, they may have a mass effect with compression of adjacent structures. Histologically, most teratomas contain ectodermal components (e.g., sebum, hair, teeth). Computed tomography (CT) scan shows the cystic component as well as regions of calcification. The treatment of teratoma is surgical excision, and the prognosis is excellent.

   3. Lymphomas. These constitute approximately 10% to 20% of all anterior mediastinal masses. In children, lymphomas account for approximately 25% of mediastinal masses. In adolescents, acute lymphoblastic lymphoma usually presents as an anterior mediastinal mass, often with thymic involvement. In adults, most mediastinal lymphomatous masses are seen in patients between 30 and 40 years of age. One of the most common lymphomatous lesions in relatively young adults, especially women, that most often presents in the anterior mediastinum, is Hodgkin's lymphoma.

   4. Thyroid lesions. Presenting as mediastinal masses, these are usually substernal goiters extending into the anterior mediastinum. A thyroid mass here may be asymptomatic, or if large enough, may present with pain or dysphagia. Most patients are women, usually older than 40 years of age at presentation. Besides the common types of lesions mentioned, various other types of cystic neck masses may be present. These vary in their histology and embryogenesis. CT scan and radionucleotide studies are helpful in making a determination (3).

B. Middle mediastinum. Approximately 20% of all mediastinal masses are located in the middle mediastinum. These include the heart; the great vessels to and from the heart; the bifurcation of the trachea into the bronchi; the pericardium; the phrenic nerve around the pericardium; portions of the vagus nerve; the esophagus; and the lymph nodes in this region, which include the paratracheal and the tracheobronchial lymph nodes. The lesions that may arise from the middle mediastinum include aortic aneurysms, dilation of the superior vena cava, dilation of the pulmonary artery, or dilation/enlargement of the azygos and the hemiazygos veins. Lymphomas, tumors of the heart, pericardial cysts, and metastatic lesions are other diagnostic considerations in this compartment.

C. Posterior mediastinum. Approximately 20% to 25% of all mediastinal masses present in the posterior mediastinum. Contents of the posterior mediastinum include the esophagus, the descending portion of the thoracic aorta, the thoracic duct, a portion of the vagus nerves, and lymph nodes. Neurogenic tumors predominate in the posterior mediastinum. These include neuroblastomas, ganglioneuromas, ganglioneuroblastomas, neurofibromas, schwannomas, and pheochromocytomas (4). Less frequently occurring lesions include paragangliomas, chemodectomas, and giant lymph node hyperplasia (Castleman disease). Benign mesenchymal lesions such as lipomas, fibromas, myxomas, and leiomyomas may also be seen. Malignant versions include liposarcomas, fibrosarcomas, and leiomyosarcomas.

D. Mediastinal widening. Aortic dissection is an important cause of mediastinal widening. Other causes of mediastinal widening include aortic rupture, sternal fracture, pulmonary contusions, mediastinal masses, tumors of the lung, idiopathic mediastinal fibrosis, cardiac tamponade, and leaking aortic aneurysms. Also, lymphomas and metastatic lesions can cause mediastinal widening. Sarcoidosis is an important autoimmune consideration. Infectious etiologies of hilar lymphadenopathy and/or mediastinal widening include mycobacterium tuberculosis, tularemia, pertussis, viral diseases (including human immunodeficiency virus [HIV] and Epstein-Barr virus), rickettsial infections, varicella pneumonia, and fungal infections (including histoplasmosis, coccidioidomycosis), and tropical eosinophilia. Anthrax and plague are important infectious considerations in the age of bioterrorism. Other miscellaneous entities causing mediastinal widening include Goodpasture's syndrome, histiocytosis X, cystic fibrosis, and idiopathic pulmonary hemosiderosis. Finally, occupational lung diseases such as silicosis and berylliosis should be considered.

III. EVALUATION. A carefully directed history and physical examination is essential before investigative studies are performed to determine the likely causes of a mediastinal mass.

A. History. A history of constitutional symptoms, including a documentation of fever, sweat, and weight loss is important.

B. Physical examination. Check vital signs at the time of examination. Check for skin lesions and evaluate for signs of skin pallor or conjunctival pallor. Examine the neck for thyromegaly, masses, or adenopathy. Auscultate the lungs for wheezes, rales, rhonchi, or pleural friction rubs. Listen for pericardial rubs. On abdominal examination, evaluate for liver or spleen enlargement. On genitourinary and pelvic examinations, evaluate for testicular and/or scrotal masses or ovarian masses. Significance should be attached to the presence of localized as well as generalized lymphadenopathy (due to metastatic disease, HIV or other viral infections, or when considering a diagnosis of lymphoma). One should recognize the significance of a pathologic lymph node (1 cm or larger, persisting for at least 4 weeks).

C. Testing

1. Laboratory tests. Routine laboratory tests should include a complete blood count with differential, and an erythrocyte sedimentation rate, as well as specific tests to be performed, depending on the type of lesion suspected. These may include lactate dehydrogenase, α fetoprotein, β fraction human growth hormone, serum calcium, parathormone, γ globulins, serum antiacetylcholine receptor antibody, purified protein derivative skin test, and HIV antibody screening. Suspicious or pathologic peripheral lymph nodes should be biopsied.

2. Diagnostic imaging. CT scan is a very useful and precise tool for localizing and characterizing mediastinal masses and for providing helpful clues as to their nature (5). CT scan is better than plain films at demonstrating the calcification of lymph nodes that commonly follows tuberculosis and fungal infections (6). Magnetic resonance imaging is less often used to evaluate mediastinal masses but may help in the evaluation of patients with superior vena caval obstruction, aortic aneurysms, and larger intrathoracic blood vessels. Transthoracic ultrasound is useful in evaluating the thymus in adults and children and can help distinguish cystic from solid mediastinal masses; it can also aid in distinguishing cardiac from paracardiac masses. Barium swallow and endoscopic ultrasound studies are useful adjuncts for evaluating masses within the middle mediastinum as well as for evaluating esophageal masses and lymph nodes adjacent to the esophagus (6).

3. Biopsy. Suspicious or pathologic peripheral lymph nodes should be biopsied.

IV. DIAGNOSIS

A. Widening of the mediastinum can be due to numerous conditions. When evaluating a suspicious lesion, look for clues that help differentiate a mediastinal origin from a lung, pleural, or chest wall origin. Masses with irregular, nodular, or spiculated borders tend to arise in the lung, whereas broad-based masses with smooth edges are more likely to arise in the mediastinum or mediastinal pleura.

B. To make a definitive diagnosis, a biopsy of the mediastinal mass may be necessary. Histologic diagnosis guides more specific laboratory and imaging studies. A tissue diagnosis is also important for disease staging and to inform treatment options for the specific condition.

ACKNOWLEDGMENT

The authors appreciate the input and assistance from Pepi Granat, MD

References
1. Davis RD Jr, Oldham HN Jr, Sabiston DC Jr. Primary cysts and neoplasms of mediastinum; recent change in clinical presentation, methods of diagnosis, management and results. *Ann Thorac Surg* 1987;44(3):229–237.
2. Suto Y, Araya S, Sakuma K, et al. Myasthenia gravis with thymic hyperplasia and pure red cell aplasia. *J Neurol Sci* 2004;224(1–2):93–95.
3. Lev S, Lev MH. Imaging of cystic lesions. Department of Radiology, Nassau County Medical Center, East Meadow, New York, USA. *Radiol Clin North Am* 2000;38(5): 1013–1027.
4. Topcu S, Alper A, Gulhan E, et al. Neurogenic tumors of the mediastinum: a report of 60 cases. *Can Respir J* 2000;7(3):261–265.
5. Hoerbelt R, Keunecke L. The value of a noninvasive diagnostic approach to mediastinal masses. *Ann Thorac Surg* 2003;75(4):1086–1090.
6. Armstrong P, Padley S. *Grainger & Allison's diagnostic radiology: a textbook of medical imaging*, 4th ed. New York: Churchill Livingstone, 2001.

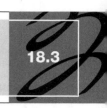

OSTEOPENIA
Scott Ippolito

18.3

I. BACKGROUND. Fifteen million patients have osteoporosis and another 34 million patients have low bone mass, or osteopenia (1). Osteoporosis is considered to be a chronic progressive condition: when left untreated, it results in decreased bone mass and skeletal fragility. It is preceded by osteopenia, a low bone density condition. Osteopenia occurs when resorption occurs at a faster rate than formation. It has been thought of as low bone mass or decreased calcification of bone without the clinically increased risk of fracture (1). If this imbalance in the bone remodeling cycle continues, osteopenia progresses to osteoporosis (2). If left unchecked, osteoporosis can lead to fracture, deformity, and disability (3).

II. PATHOPHYSIOLOGY

A. Etiology. The process of bone thinning is a natural part of aging: however, it can be delayed medically or minimized by lifestyle changes (3). The development of osteoporosis results from defective bone remodeling. Osteoblasts are responsible for the formation of osteoid, or bone matrix. Mineralization of this osteoid matrix produces bone, and the osteoblasts that remain following mineralization are termed *osteocytes*. Osteoblasts respond to a variety of humoral factors such as estrogen, vitamin D, cytokines, and various growth factors that stimulate bone growth (1).

Osteoclasts act in direct opposition to osteoblasts and respond to many signals, most importantly osteoprotegerin ligand, granulocyte colony-stimulating factor, and interleukins that are necessary for cell development. Osteoclasts attach to endosteal bone and secrete acid to dissolve calcium crystals. Enzymes such as metalloproteineases then act to break down the protein matrix, and the osteoclast undergoes apoptosis. The breakdown materials from this protein degradation can be measured as possible markers of bone resorption (1).

The imbalance of osteoclastic and osteoblastic activity can be caused by several age- and disease-related conditions. These causes are often classified into three main categories: **primary osteoporosis** (normal aging processes decrease gonadal function, resulting in decreased bone formation without declining osteoclastic action), **postmenopausal osteoporosis** (declining estrogen causes an increase in osteoclastic activity and a resulting imbalance between formation and resorption), and **secondary osteoporosis** (due to secondary causes, often from diseases, [see differential diagnosis], nutritional deficiencies or medications that have effects on calcium, and other factors related to bone formation or resorption) (1,4).

B. Epidemiology. Osteoporosis mainly affects postmenopausal women, although younger women and men can also be affected. The prevalence of osteoporosis based on bone density at the femoral neck is 18% to 28% in women and 6% to 22% in men older than 50 years of age and increases with increasing age. Fractures are the most serious consequence of osteoporosis. Currently, it has been estimated that more than 50% of women and 20% of men at the age of 50 will experience at least one osteoporotic fracture in their lifetimes (5). The disease currently results in more than 350,000 hip fractures and 700,000 vertebral fractures each year in the United States (4). Because men and women older than 65 years of age are the fastest growing segment of the population worldwide, the annual number of fractures is expected to double by 2025 (6). With respect to race, white women are the most often affected and African-American women have the lowest prevalence of osteoporosis (1).

Numerous risk factors predict low bone mineral density (BMD) and the development of osteoporosis and resulting fracture. Risk factors include age, white race, tobacco use, female gender, low body weight, physical inactivity, family history of osteoporosis, medications (i.e., glucocorticoids, anticonvulsants, excess thyroid hormone), previous fracture, estrogen deficiency, excessive alcohol intake, and low calcium, phosphorus, or vitamin D intake (1,3,4). Consuming large quantities of soft drinks has been linked to causing low bone density, because they contain high levels of phosphoric acid, which interferes with calcium absorption. Vitamin A, taken in excess of 1,200 µg a day, accelerates bone loss. Finally, testosterone protects men; nevertheless, bone loss may occur when hormone levels decline (3).

III. EVALUATION

A. History. Ask female patients about their menstrual history, age of menarche and menopause, periods of amenorrhea, pregnancy, lactation, and oral contraceptive. Ask all patients about illnesses, medications, falls, anorexia and other eating disorders, steroid use, calcium and vitamin D intake, alcohol and tobacco use, exercise, and family history of osteoporosis. Ask male patients about symptoms suggestive of low testosterone levels.

B. Physical examination. Observe for abnormal gait, posture, and balance. Look for kyphosis, abnormal spinal curvature, and asymmetry of the paravertebral musculature. Focal tenderness on palpation over the vertebral processes may suggest vertebral fracture. Observe other bones for deformities. Note signs of poor nutrition. Examine for any physical manifestations of low testosterone in male patients.

C. Testing

1. **Diagnostic imaging.** Bone densitometry is a noninvasive technique that is used to measure the bone mineral content in order to predict fracture risks and the need for medical therapy. BMD is typically expressed as the T score (e.g., the number of standard deviations (SDs) below the mean for nonosteopenic, healthy young women) (7). Similarly, a Z score is the number of SDs from the mean bone density for age-matched, sex-matched, and ethnic-matched patients (1). The World Health Organization defines osteopenia as a T score of between −1.0 and −2.5 SD, and osteoporosis as a score of −2.5 SD or more (7). Recently, several diagnostic techniques have come to the market, most notably the dual-energy

x-ray absorptiometry (DEXA). However, ultrasound, computed tomography (CT) scan, magnetic resonance imaging (MRI), radiographic absorptiometry, dual-photon absorptiometry, and dual x-ray and laser have also been suggested as methods of bone measurement (1).

a. DEXA is the most commonly used "gold standard" technique to measure BMD. DEXA uses two x-ray beams of different energy levels to scan the region of interest and measure the amount of x-ray absorbed by the bone as the beam passes through the body (7). DEXA measures the sum of cortical and trabecular bone and can detect as little as 2% bone loss (1). The current practice is to perform DEXA of the lumbar vertebrae (L1-4); the hip, including the femoral neck, Ward's triangle, the greater trochanter, and the total hip (which includes all these measures); or both. The results are presented visually, including both T scores and Z scores (8).

b. CT scan depends on the differential absorption of radiation by calcified bone and is used for central measurements only. Compared to DEXA, CT scan is less readily available and is associated with relatively high radiation exposure (7).

c. MRI in diagnosing osteoporosis is still evolving. More research must be done to improve the sensitivity and specificity of MRI as well as to calculate appropriate T and Z scores (1).

d. Ultrasound measures the bone mass and strength and assesses the bone microarchitecture by detecting the transmission of high-frequency sound waves through bone (7). The calcaneus is the primary site of measurement (1). However, this technique has not been shown to be useful in monitoring skeletal response to the different therapies used to treat osteoporosis (7).

e. Radiographic absorptiometry provides radiologic assessment of the metacarpals and phalanges on the basis of plain film. However, radiographs are an insensitive measure of bone loss and may demonstrate abnormalities only after 30% of bone loss has occurred. Generally, it is not recommended as a screening test for osteoporosis or osteopenia (1).

f. Dual-photon absorptiometry measures bone mineral content at the spine and hip using photons emitted at low energy levels. It is also used to measure the total body calcium and provides a measurement of the mineral density in both long bones and bones such as the heel by measuring the total mineral content in the path of the beam (7).

g. Dual x-ray and laser is a new technique that is presently being researched. It uses two x-ray beams in combination with a laser. Researchers have suggested that this technique has the advantage of filtering out any influence that adipose tissue may have on the accuracy of DEXA measurements (7).

2. Laboratory tests. Laboratory assessment is not routinely used to screen for the presence of osteoporosis but it may be useful in patients with low bone density with the goal of identifying secondary causes (such as elevated serum calcium levels, suggesting hyperparathyroidism) or factors that can aggravate bone fragility (such as a low level of 25-hydroxyvitamin D). Biochemical markers of increased bone resorption (i.e., collagen cross-links, calcium, and hydroxy-proline) or increased bone formation (i.e., bone-specific alkaline phosphatase and osteoclastin) are associated with an increased fracture risk. However, these markers show substantial variability, and there are insufficient data to support their use in deciding for or against bone densitometry or pharmacotherapy (8).

IV. DIAGNOSIS. The radiographic finding of generalized loss of bone density (osteopenia) is not specific and can be seen in various conditions. Disorders associated with generalized loss of bone density include disorders of multiple or uncertain cause (senile osteoporosis, juvenile osteoporosis, osteogenesis imperfecta), adrenal cortex disorders (Cushing's disease, Addison's disease), gonadal disorders (postmenopausal osteoporosis, hypogonadism), pituitary disorders (acromegaly, hypopituitarism), diabetes mellitus, thyroid disorders (hyperthyroidism, hypothyroidism), hypoparathyroidism, marrow replacement and expansion (myeloma, leukemia, lymphoma, metastatic disease, Gaucher's disease), anemias (sickle cell, thalassemia, hemophilia), drugs and other substances (steroids, heparin, anticonvulsants, immuno-suppressants, alcohol), and chronic diseases (chronic renal disease, hepatic insufficiency, gastrointestinal malabsorption syndromes, chronic inflammatory polyarthropathies, amyloidosis, sarcoidosis, chronic debility or immobilization) (4, 9).

References

1. Osteoporosis: diagnosis and treatment. *Contin Med Educ Resour* 2004;118(10):27–41, www.NetCE.com.
2. *Bone density/osteoporosis*. From the Diagnostic Imaging Associates' website. Available at: http://www.diaxray.com/bone-density.html.
3. Lamontanaro DM. Imaging osteoporosis. *RT Imaging* 2005;18(27), www.rt-image.com.
4. Keller M. Treating osteoporosis in post-menopausal women: a case approach. *Cleve Clin J Med* 2004;71(10):829–835.
5. Osteoporosis: assessment for diagnosis, evaluation and treatment. WPMH GmbH. 2004;1(2–3):204–214.
6. Rosen C. *Osteoporosis. Rakel: conn's current therapy*, 57th ed. Philadelphia, PA: Elsevier; 2005.
7. *Unicare:medical policy: bone mineral density measurement and screening for vertebral fractures using dual energy X-Ray absorptiometry*; Policy # RAD.00004, 07/14/2005, www.medpolicy.unicare.com.
8. Raisz L. Screening for osteoporosis. *N Engl J Med* 2005;353:164–171.
9. Generalized Decrease in Bone Density. *Grainger & Allison's diagnostic radiology: a textbook of medical imaging*, 4th ed. St. Louis, MO: Churchill Livingstone, Inc., 1929–1930.

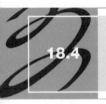

18.4 SOLITARY PULMONARY NODULE
Mark R. Needham

I. **BACKGROUND.** Pulmonary nodules, generally considered to be isolated and circum-scribed lesions <3 cm in diameter in the lungs, are a common and somewhat vexing clinical finding. Also called "coin" lesions, they are typically found incidentally on chest x-rays obtained for other purposes. They are also very commonly detected; computed tomography (CT) scan is used for purposes of screening for lung cancer. The entire purpose of any evaluation is to resect potentially curable lesions while avoiding unnecessary and risky interventions. Toward that end, the physician needs to determine which of the following three approaches to use: observation with serial monitoring, biopsy, or immediate excision. The primary medical–legal pitfall is to ig-nore a potentially respectable and curable early-stage lung cancer. However, an overly aggressive approach may lead to unnecessary procedures and complications such as pneumothorax or pulmonary hemorrhage.

II. **PATHOPHYSIOLOGY.** Pulmonary nodules may be of either benign or malignant etiology. All types of lung cancer may present initially as a solitary nodule, including carcinoid tumor and metastasis to the lung. Benign causes include infection, particularly fungal and granulomatous disease, hamartomas or benign tumors of the lung, lipomas, vascular lesions, rheumatoid arthritis, sarcoidosis, and bronchogenic cyst (1).

III. **EVALUATION**

   A. **History.** History is not definitive but can assist in moving the odds toward benign or malignant. Age younger than 40 years probably carries <3% chance of malig-nancy. Age older than 60 years carries >50% chance of malignancy. Past smoking history is strongly associated with malignancy. Asbestos or occupational carcinogen exposure increases the probability of malignancy. A previously diagnosed malignancy increases the odds that the nodule is a metastasis. A lesion larger than 3 cm is highly likely to be malignant. Doubling time is a significant historical observation that may contribute to the decision-making process, thereby making the review of any available prior chest x-rays essential. Benign lesions have either a very rapid growth rate, with doubling times <20 days seen in infectious conditions, or extremely long doubling times. Malignant nodules generally have doubling times between 20 days and 2 years. A nodule that has been present and is unchanged for 2 years is almost certain to be benign. Note that because plain x-rays project an image of a sphere onto a two-dimensional plane, an increase of 26% in diameter, for example, from 1 cm to 1.3 cm, is equivalent to one doubling in volume of the nodule. Well-circumscribed borders favor benign lesions, whereas irregular or spiculated borders favor malignancy (2).

B. Physical examination. The presence of fever suggests a possible infectious etiology. Extrapulmonary manifestations of certain diseases such as tuberculosis, sarcoidosis, or rheumatoid arthritis may give some additional clues to the diagnosis. However, the contribution of physical diagnosis is limited.

C. Testing. If the nodule is detected on plain x-ray, then subsequent additional studies can include CT scan, fiberoptic bronchoscopy, percutaneous fine needle aspiration, magnetic resonance imaging (MRI), ultrasound, single photon emission computed tomography (SPECT), positron emission tomography (PET), and video-assisted thoracic surgery (VATS) for excision.

1. A CT scan can be useful in that small nodules not seen on plain x-ray may be detected by it. The presence of multiple nodules favors a benign cause, except with the history of prior neoplasm, in which case metastatic disease is more likely. A CT scan may also demonstrate certain patterns of calcification within the nodule that cannot be visualized on plain x-ray. A stippled or eccentric pattern of calcification favors malignancy, whereas other characteristic patterns may favor a benign etiology. Benign lesions tend to have higher Hounsfield units on CT scan, a measure of density, but there is no distinct cutoff point between benign and malignant lesions.

2. Fiberoptic bronchoscopy generally has low yield, particularly with peripheral nodules.

3. Fine needle aspiration has a reasonable yield with peripheral nodules >2 cm but carries a significant risk of pneumothorax.

4. MRI and ultrasound do not play much of a role in the diagnostic evaluation.

5. SPECT and PET, with fluorodeoxyglucose used as a biological marker, are promising techniques for noninvasive diagnosis but are limited by false-positive results in metabolically active nodules such as infectious granulomas and inflammatory conditions. False-negative results can occur because of the limited special resolution of PET, which can form an image only down to approximately 8 mm, thereby possibly not detecting malignancies smaller than about 1 cm. In addition, some tumors, such as carcinoid and bronchoalveolar carcinoma, have very low metabolic rates and can be missed (3).

6. The advantage of VATS is that the procedure is both diagnostic and therapeutic. However, it is more costly and more invasive with inherent complications of pneumothorax and hemorrhage (4).

IV. DIAGNOSIS. The diagnosis of solitary pulmonary nodule is usually made through plain x-ray. The differential diagnosis includes primary or metastatic lung malignancy. Further evaluation or monitoring depends on the clinical setting. Whenever possible, obtain old chest x-rays for comparison. A nodule unchanged over a period of 2 years is almost certain to be benign. Other recommendations include the following:

A. For nodules detected in patients younger than 40 years of age, with no prior smoking history, no occupational exposure risks, no known prior malignancies, and smooth well-circumscribed borders, consider serial monitoring. However, the patient must be stable in the practice such that serial chest x-rays at 3-, 6-, 12-, and 24-month intervals may be obtained. Elect VATS for resection for nodules increasing in size over prior x-ray.

B. For nodules detected in patients older than 40 years of age, with prior smoking history, any occupational cancer risks, known prior malignancies, and speculated borders or suspicious calcification patterns, proceed to VATS for resection. If the patient is at a high surgery risk because of impaired pulmonary reserve or other complication, consider biopsy to verify diagnosis prior to resection for nodules >2 cm in size located in the periphery.

C. For patients who have nodules that do not fit into the first two categories, the options are not as clear, and patient preference can play a role in establishing the work-up. Choices include CT scan; the presence of multiple nodules, density >160 HU, or characteristic calcification pattern may favor benign etiology. Absence of these findings may suggest malignancy. For nodules larger than 1 cm in an otherwise indeterminate situation, consider PET, recognizing that false-negative and false-positive results may occur.

D. In situations in which the choice is made to not proceed with VATS and resection, immediately follow the patient with serial chest x-rays at 3, 6, 12, and 24 months and proceed to resection for any change in nodule size (5).

References

1. Weinberger MD, Steven E. Differential diagnosis and evaluation of the solitary pulmonary nodule. *Up to Date Online Reference*, 2005.
2. Manocha Sanjay. Solitary Pulmonary Nodule. E Medicine Online Reference, 2005.
3. Gould MK, Maclean CC, Kuschner WG, et al. Accuracy of positron emission tomography in the diagnosis of pulmonary nodules and mass lesions: a meta analysis. *JAMA* 2001;21:914–924.
4. Bernard A. Resection of pulmonary nodules using video assisted thoracic surgery. *Ann Thorac Surg* 1996;61:202.
5. Hartman TE. Evaluation of the solitary pulmonary nodule. *Radiol Clin North Am* 2005; 43(3):459–465.

Note: Page numbers followed by *f* indicate figures; those followed by *t* indicate tables.